NURSING RESEARCH
Principles and Methods

NURSING RESEARCH
Principles and Methods

FOURTH EDITION

Denise F. Polit, Ph.D.
President
Humanalysis, Inc.
Saratoga Springs, New York

Bernadette P. Hungler, R.N., Ph.D.
Boston College School of Nursing
Chestnut Hill, Massachusetts

 J.B. LIPPINCOTT COMPANY Philadelphia
New York   London   Hagerstown

Acquisitions Editor: David P. Carroll
Coordinating Editorial Assistant: Amy Stonehouse
Project Editor: Dina Kamilatos
Indexer: Lillian R. Rodberg
Design Coordinator: Kathy Kelley-Luedtke
Cover and Interior Designer: Terri J. Siegel
Production Manager: Caren Erlichman
Production Coordinator: Sharon McCarthy
Compositor: Circle Graphics
Printer/Binder: R.R. Donnelley & Sons Company

4th Edition

3   5   6   4

Library of Congress Cataloging-in-Publication Data

Polit-O'Hara, Denise.
    Nursing research : principles and methods / Denise F. Polit,
Bernadette P. Hungler.—4th ed.
        p.   cm.
    Includes bibliographical references and index.
    ISBN 0-397-54820-6
    1. Nursing—Research—Methodology.   I. Hungler, Bernadette P.
II. Title.
    [DNLM: 1. Nursing Research.   WY 20.5 p769n]
RT81.5.P64   1991
610.73'072—dc20
DNLM/DLC
for Library of Congress   90-13624
                                                        CIP

Any procedure or practice described in this book should be applied by the health-care practitioner under appropriate supervision in accordance with professional standards of care used with regard to the unique circumstances that apply in each practice situation. Care has been taken to confirm the accuracy of information presented and to describe generally accepted practices. However, the authors, editors, and publisher cannot accept any responsibility for errors or omissions or for any consequences from application of the information in this book and make no warranty, express or implied, with respect to the contents of the book.

Every effort has been made to ensure drug selections and dosages are in accordance with current recommendations and practice. Because of ongoing research, changes in government regulations and the constant flow of information on drug therapy, reactions and interactions, the reader is cautioned to check the package insert for each drug for indications, dosages, warnings and precautions, particularly if the drug is new or infrequently used.

To the nurse researchers
leading us into the 21st century

Preface

This fourth edition of *Nursing Research: Principles and Methods* introduces numerous changes that make this book, we believe, a state-of-the-art textbook on research methods for nurses in the 1990s. This edition retains all of the features that have made this textbook popular in the past, while including several improvements and innovations.

In keeping with the direction of nursing research, we have continued to expand the discussion of qualitative research. Perhaps the single greatest addition to this edition is a new chapter, which we believe is pathbreaking, on the integration of qualitative and quantitative research. We are persuaded that nurse researchers of the future will increasingly need to adopt research designs and data collection strategies that combine the strengths of these two basic approaches to knowledge discovery.

Two other chapters have been added to this edition. The first is a chapter specifically devoted to ethical considerations in research with human subjects. This chapter discusses key ethical principles, and also raises the important issue of ethical dilemmas that confront scientists, who are sometimes faced with balancing the rights of subjects with the need for scientific rigor. The second is a chapter on research utilization. This chapter discusses some of the barriers to utilization, strategies for overcoming those barriers, and criteria for undertaking a utilization project.

In addition to these three new chapters, new materials have been integrated into virtually every chapter of this edition. Of particular note are

state-of-the-art discussions on powerful new designs, data collection approaches, and analytic techniques.

Despite the many improvements, this edition reflects many of the same basic convictions that shaped earlier editions. First, we have an unshaken belief that, more than ever before, the development of research skills is critical to the nursing profession. Second, we are convinced that research is an intellectually and professionally rewarding enterprise. We try to reflect our enthusiasm for the research process throughout this book. And third, we believe that learning about research methods need be neither intimidating nor dull.

As in the previous three editions, we have tried to present the fundamentals of research methods in a way that both facilitates understanding and stimulates interest and curiosity. We know of no better way to accomplish both aims than to incorporate actual and hypothetical research studies that illustrate concepts under discussion. In fact, this edition features such illustrations to an even greater degree than earlier editions. We have also maintained other aspects of our basic teaching style: concepts are introduced carefully and systematically; difficult ideas are presented with some redundancy, but from several vantage points; and the readers are assumed to have no prior exposure to technical terms.

We have tried to keep in mind the needs of both consumers and producers of nursing research. The uses to which the first three editions have been put suggest that we have reached both audiences. We have paid attention to the problems frequently encountered by students in reading, understanding, and evaluating research reports, and have included in this edition an early discussion on how to "translate" difficult-to-read research reports into a more manageable form. However, as before, the organization of the book is intended as a guide to those nursing students who are learning to conduct their own research projects.

This edition is organized into six main sections that lead the reader sequentially through the steps in the research process. Part I introduces the reader to the rationale underlying the scientific approach in general and to the basic aims of nursing research in particular. The purpose of these chapters is to help students understand and appreciate the manner in which the scientific approach can be applied to the solution of problems and to develop an enthusiasm for the kinds of knowledge and discoveries that research can produce. Part I also provides a general overview of research terminology and of the phases of the research process. In Part II, the preliminary steps of a research project—those that are primarily conceptual in nature—are discussed. This includes the selection of a problem, the development of hypotheses, the conduct of a literature review, and the development of a theoretical or conceptual framework. Part III focuses on research design issues, and also introduces students to various types of research, including survey research, field studies, evaluations, and secondary analyses. Part IV covers the major techniques in the collection of data for nursing research studies, as well as principles of measurement. Part V is devoted to the analysis of research data. It includes chapters on quantitative and qualitative analysis, as well as the new chapter on the integration of the two. Part V also includes a thoroughly revised chapter on preparing data for analysis; the chapter covers such issues as data transformations, dealing with missing data, and evaluating data quality and biases. The final section of the book focuses on communication in research: writing about research, critiquing written reports, preparing research proposals, and using the results of published studies.

We hope that the content and organization of this book will continue to meet the needs of a broad spectrum of nursing students and nurse researchers.

DENISE F. POLIT, Ph.D.
BERNADETTE P. HUNGLER, R.N., Ph.D.

Acknowledgments

This fourth edition, like the first three, depended on the contribution of many individuals. We are deeply appreciative of those who made all four editions possible. In addition to all those who assisted us with the earlier editions, the following individuals deserve special mention.

Many faculty and students who used the text during the past decade have made invaluable suggestions for its improvement, and to all of you we are very grateful. In particular, we would like to acknowledge the continuing feedback from the nursing students and faculty at Boston College. Anne Lippman, Marilyn Grant, and the late Mary Pekarski made important contributions to Chapter 6. Several of the examples used in the text and in the accompanying study guide were developed from ideas provided by Sarah Cimino, Susan Kelly, and Mary Jane Daly. Thomas Knapp pointed out some needed changes in the chapters on statistical analysis. We again wish to note our deep

appreciation for the mentorship of Peter W. Airasian, without whose fine teaching and clear writing this book would not be possible.

We also extend our warmest thanks to those who helped to turn the manuscript into a finished product. Rob Sherman and Jean Cummings served as able assistants in the preparation of this edition. The staff at J. B. Lippincott has been outstanding in the support they have given to us over the years. We would like to express our deepest gratitude in particular to David Carroll. We are also indebted to Amy Stonehouse, Dina Kamilatos, and all the others behind the scenes for their fine contributions.

Finally, we thank our friends and family, who provided support and encouragement throughout this enterprise. A special word of thanks to the clan at Phila Street—Joe, Nate, Molly, Brigitte, Sasha, Scarlet, Max, and Maxine.

Contents

Part VI
Communication in the Research

NURSING RESEARCH
Principles and Methods

Part I

The Scientific Research Process

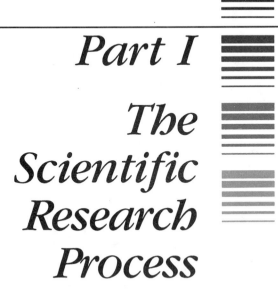

1
Nursing and the Role of Research

Nursing research has experienced remarkable growth in the past two decades. During this time, the focus of nursing research has been directed toward problems relating to nursing practice. Nurses today are being schooled in the scientific method to a greater degree than ever before. Today, there appears to be a more orderly progression of research functions demanded of graduates from associate, baccalaureate, master's, and doctoral programs in nursing.

To produce scientific research, it is necessary to develop skills in the scientific method. But it is not only nursing researchers who need to understand the scientific approach and methods of research. Nurses engaged in the practice of nursing, nursing administrators, and nursing educators all have a responsibility to identify problems that warrant scientific investigation. Professional accountability demands that nurses utilize the findings of research to perform their roles. In addition, as consumers of research, nurses are called upon to evaluate the methods used to carry out research projects to estimate the confidence that can be placed in the results. The purpose of this book is to acquaint potential consumers and producers of nursing research with the fundamentals of scientific research methods.

In this introductory chapter, we discuss the important role that research plays in establishing a scientific base for the practice of nursing, the historical development of nursing research, the current status of nursing research, and possible future directions of nursing research as suggested by nursing leaders.

≡ IMPORTANCE OF RESEARCH IN NURSING

The ultimate goal of any profession is to improve the practice of its members so that the services

3

provided to its clientele will have the greatest impact. Any profession seeking to enhance its professional image undertakes the continual development of a scientific body of knowledge fundamental to its practice. The emergence of such a body of scientific knowledge can be instrumental in fostering a commitment and accountability to the profession's clientele.

Professionalism

Nursing, like other occupations seeking to establish themselves as professions, is concerned about the development of a service orientation, the continual growth of a scientific base from which members practice, and the evolution of a fairly distinct body of knowledge that separates nursing from other professions. The increasing awareness of nurses of research as an integral part of professional nursing behavior is accelerating rapidly in several areas. Nurses recognize the need to extend the base of nursing knowledge as part of professional responsibility and are endorsing scientific investigations as a way to broaden the body of knowledge.

Accountability

Gortner (1974) pointed out that the quality of nursing care cannot be improved until scientific accountability becomes as much a part of nursing's tradition as humanitarianism. She noted that scientific accountability is essential for the teacher in dealing with students; for the nurse practitioner in dealing with clients or patients; and for the nurse administrator in dealing with clients, patients, or professionals in the health-care delivery system.

Social Relevance of Nursing

Nurses today are being asked more than ever before to document their role in the delivery of health services. Consumers of health care, in recent years, are recognizing health care as a right rather than a privilege and, with the spiral-ing costs of health care, are asking various groups of health professionals how their services contribute to the total delivery of health care. This increased interest in examining health-care practices makes it essential for nurses to evaluate the efficacy of their practices and to modify or abandon those practices shown to have no effect on the health status of individuals.

Research and Decision Making in Nursing Practice

Many nurses use the Standards of Nursing Practice established by the American Nurses' Association (ANA) Congress for Practice (1973) both as their method of clinical practice and to evaluate the quality of their nursing care. The process requires nurses to engage in many decision-making activities. What will be assessed? What nursing diagnoses result from the assessment? What plan of care is most likely to produce the desired outcomes? What nursing interventions are necessary? How will the results be evaluated in terms of their effectiveness? Research can play an important role at each phase of the nursing process. The findings from research aid nurses in making more informed decisions in the delivery of nursing care and help document the unique role of nursing in the health-care system.

ASSESSMENT PHASE

The assessment phase of the nursing process dictates the systematic collection of information. The information may come from a variety of sources, such as clients, families, records, or nurses' observations. Currently, many different forms and methods exist for collecting assessment information. For example, Gordon (1982) suggested using a functional pattern assessment. Bates (1983) focused on a body systems approach. Nursing research can help nurses select alternative methods or forms for particular types of clients, settings, and situations. Research can help to determine the extent to which the forms produce comparable and useful information.

DIAGNOSIS PHASE

Based on an analysis of the information collected at the assessment phase of the nursing process, nurses are expected to develop nursing diagnoses.

Research can play an important role in helping nurses make more accurate nursing diagnoses by validating the etiology of each diagnosis against the recorded assessment information. In addition, nursing research can help determine the frequency of occurrence for each defining characteristic or cue associated with each diagnosis. The documentation will be helpful to the profession of nursing, which has only recently begun the task of building up its taxonomy of diagnoses.

PLANNING PHASE

The planning phase of the nursing process involves decisions concerning *what* nursing actions or interventions are needed and *when* the nursing actions are most appropriately instituted for each nursing diagnosis. The last step of this phase generally involves the delineation of behavioral outcomes for the client. Nursing research can help nurses evaluate the holism of the nursing-care plan and make more informed decisions about whether the goals set are realistic for the type of facility and the characteristics of the client involved.

INTERVENTION PHASE

Professionally accountable nurses base as many of their nursing interventions as possible on research findings. Consider, for example, the many decisions made by night nurses working in a nursing home. At what point do they decide that the nursing interventions are no longer producing the desired results for a resident in the process of dying? When is it time to notify the family or physician? What alterations in nursing interventions are available that facilitate, with as much ease as is possible, the transition from a state of life to a state of death? What approach might be used with families? What response might be expected from other residents of the home and how might their stresses be appropriately helped? The systematic documentation of nursing interventions that have been found to be effective may benefit other nurses facing the same kind of situation.

EVALUATION PHASE

The last stage of the nursing process evaluates the degree to which the behavioral outcomes or goals developed at the planning stage have been met. Research can help document success or failure in meeting the various outcomes. When success occurs with relative frequency, it offers other nurses the opportunity to implement the plan in other comparable situations with a fair degree of confidence. When the plan has been unsuccessful, then nurses are redirected to examine the accuracy of the assessment, the nursing diagnoses, the goals, the plan, and the nursing interventions. Such information, collected systematically, may aid other nurses in avoiding the same dilemmas and should lead to improvements in nursing care.

In summary, research conducted by nurses can play a critical role in improving both the quality of care delivered and the process of delivering that care. Although most nursing studies of the 1980s and 1990s have involved inquiries into the nursing process, this focus is relatively recent. The next section provides an overview of the history of nursing research.

≡ *HISTORICAL EVOLUTION OF NURSING RESEARCH*

Most people would agree that research in nursing began with Florence Nightingale, who maintained detailed recorded observations about the effects of nursing actions during the Crimean War and, on the basis of her observations, was able to effect some changes in nursing care. During several years following her work, however, little was added to the nursing literature concerning nursing research.

The pattern that nursing research followed, subsequent to Nightingale, was closely aligned to the problems confronting nursing. For example, as more nurses received university-based education and advanced academic preparation, studies concerning students—their differential characteristics, problems, and satisfactions—became more numerous. Most of the early nursing leaders received their advanced nursing preparation in the field of education and, thus, it is not surprising that the studies they conducted focused on the nurse or nursing student rather than on the practice of nursing. Also, tests and other tools from education were already available for use by these early nursing researchers. It has been only recently that research on the practice of nursing has become a high priority.

Early Years

Most of the studies conducted between 1900 and 1940 concerned nursing education. During these years, much of the nursing students' preparation was service oriented rather than education oriented, and nurse educators did not hold advanced educational preparation. One group, the Committee for the Study of Nursing Education (1923), at the request of the National Organization for Public Health Nursing and with financing from the Rockefeller Foundation, studied on the national level the educational preparation of nurse teachers, administrators, and public health nurses and the clinical experiences of nursing students. The committee, which identified many inadequacies in the educational backgrounds of the groups studied, concluded that advanced educational preparation was essential. Their report is referred to as the Goldmark Report. Simmons and Henderson (1964) pointed out that the school of nursing at Yale University came into being as a result of that investigation. Partly as a result of that study, hospitals began employing registered nurses to give nursing care that freed student nurses from heavy service demands.

The 1940s

During the 1940s, studies concerning nursing education continued. However, World War II and the increase in the number of hospital admissions created an unprecedented demand for nursing personnel, and researchers began to investigate the supply and demand of nurses, the hospital environment, and the status of staff nurses in various regions of the country.

For example, Brown (1948), a social anthropologist, reassessed nursing education in her study initiated at the request of the National Nursing Council for War Service and funded by the Carnegie Foundation. The findings from the study, like those of the Goldmark Report, revealed that inadequacies existed in nursing education. Brown recommended that the education of nurses occur in collegiate settings. Many subsequent research investigations concerning the functions performed by nurses, nurses' roles and attitudes, hospital environments, and nurse–patient interactions stemmed from the Brown report (Abdellah & Levine, 1978).

Simmons and Henderson (1964) reported that nearly every state nurses' association conducted its own fact-finding study concerning nursing needs and resources during this period. Comparisons of the findings from these studies revealed that wide variations in the quantity and quality of nursing care existed; that personnel policies varied greatly for staff nurses; and that the functions of nurses were often ill defined. These studies initiated further research by bringing together nurses and other groups to promote more uniform and systematic research on the national level, by pointing out areas and issues in nursing that needed further research, and by establishing a beginning point for periodic state checks on the changing needs and resources in nursing.

The 1950s

A number of forces combined during the 1950s to put nursing research on a rapidly accelerating upswing that is still being experienced today. An increase in the number of nurses with advanced educational degrees, the establishment of a nursing research center by the government, an increase in the availability of funds from the government and private foundations, the inception of the American Nurses' Foundation, and the appearance of the journal *Nursing Research* occurred during this period and provided impetus to the research movement in nursing.

Not only were more nurses enrolling in undergraduate nursing programs during the 1950s but more master's programs in nursing were being developed with courses in research methods included in the curriculum. Funding from the federal government during the late 1950s enabled more nurses to pursue master's-level preparation, and most of the programs required a thesis or research project as part of the program. A growing awareness of the need for nursing research was being introduced to an ever increasing number of nurses.

The first nursing unit (established at the Walter Reed Army Institute of Research) to focus its efforts on research in nursing practice hoped to parallel the research conducted by other professionals, such as physicians and dentists, at the institution. Werley (1972) noted that, despite the unique opportunity, nursing research did not flourish to the same extent as research in other professions. She attributed the lack of growth of nursing research, in part, to lack of experienced nurse researchers able to cope with the issues and problems and able to develop research projects. Nonetheless, research in nursing practice was becoming established as an important area.

ANA undertook a 5-year research project in which it studied the activities and functions performed by nurses. The report resulting from this lengthy study served as the basis for the functions, standards, and qualifications statements for nurses prepared by ANA (Hughes, 1958). Individual nurses provided the financial support for the study, demonstrating the conviction that nursing had something to gain from a systematic scrutiny of its activities.

ANA created the American Nurses' Foundation, which is devoted exclusively to the promotion of nursing research. The increasing number of research studies being conducted during the 1950s created the need for a vehicle in which the findings from these studies could be published; thus, *Nursing Research* came into being in 1952.

In education, Montag (1954) developed and evaluated the effectiveness of establishing 2-year programs leading to an associate degree in nursing. Funding from the federal government provided universities the opportunity to develop curricula (Sands & Belcher, 1958) and to increase the research competencies in faculty.

Nursing research took a twist in the 1950s not experienced by research in other professions, at least not to the same extent as in nursing. Nurses studied themselves: Who is the nurse? What does the nurse do? Why do individuals choose to enter nursing? What are the characteristics of the ideal nurse? How do other groups perceive the nurse?

The 1960s

The 1960s was the period during which terms such as "conceptual framework," "conceptual model," "nursing process," and "theoretical base of nursing practice" began to appear in nursing literature. Nurse researchers collaborated more than in the past with members of other professions on nursing research projects. Funding continued to be available both for the educational preparation of nurses and for nursing research projects. Nursing leaders expressed concern about the lack of research in nursing practice, and the professional nursing organizations established priorities for research investigations.

A nurse and a team of social scientists collaborated in an important research project that studied dying patients and hospital personnel. The findings from the study revealed that interaction between a dying patient and hospital personnel changes according to the dying person's level of awareness of his or her condition (Glaser & Strauss, 1966). The findings from the study served as the basis for further investigations into the area of death and dying.

The 5-year study undertaken by Hall (1963)

focused on an alternative to acute-care hospitalization for a carefully selected group of chronically ill elderly people. Only professional nurses gave nursing care, and the nurses and patients decided when the services of a physician were needed. At a time when staff nurse shortages were acute, the Loeb Center in New York, where the study was conducted, had no difficulty in recruiting nurses.

During the 1960s, nurse educators continued to study nursing students' characteristics. Councils of nurse educators received funds to conduct workshops for faculties and to examine the characteristics of graduate nursing education. Nurse investigators compared students enrolled in the various types of nursing programs and compared nursing students with other students, such as education students, in terms of personality and attitudinal characteristics. The Western Interstate Council for Higher Education in Nursing (WICHEN) developed content for graduate education in the clinical areas of community health, maternal–child, medical–surgical, and psychiatric nursing, and conducted workshops for faculty on the application of scientific knowledge.

The Mugar Library at Boston University established a nursing archive in the late 1960s; one purpose of the archive is to foster nursing research. This is the first archive for nursing history and was initially supported through a grant from the federal government.

The 1970s

The 1970s witnessed a series of accomplishments in a number of areas germane to nursing research. ANA and the National League for Nursing (NLN) had established a national commission for the study of nursing and nursing education in the late 1960s. The commission's report, completed in 1970, recommended that increased research should be undertaken in both the areas of nursing practice and nursing education. The commission urged that funding be sought for nursing research (Lysaught, 1970).

Various groups discussed what direction nursing research should take. Lindeman (1975),

for example, conducted a study to ascertain the views of nursing leaders concerning the focus of scientific nursing studies. Clinical problems were identified as the highest priorities for nursing research. Similar themes emerged in the resolution passed by the delegates to the 1974 ANA convention (ANA, 1974). Actual research appeared to be consistent with these views: Carnegie (1978) reported a steady increase in the number of clinical investigations published in *Nursing Research*.

The research preparation of nurses received attention from a number of sources. Both ANA and NLN addressed the importance of research in the education of nurses. The ANA Commission on Nursing Research (1976) recommended preparation for research in undergraduate, graduate, and continuing education programs. NLN began reviewing the research component of curricula as part of the accreditation process. The cadre of nurses with earned doctorates steadily increased, especially during the later part of the 1970s. The availability of both predoctoral and postdoctoral research fellowships facilitated advanced preparation in research skills.

The rapidly accelerating pace of nursing research was also evident in the number and types of activities undertaken by regional groups of nurses. Regional meetings and workshops provided nurses who shared mutual interests with both support and an opportunity to exchange ideas. For example, WICHEN began a 7-year project that focused on increasing the quality and quantity of clinical nursing research. Other activities of the western regional group included the compilation of a two-volume work that contained data collection tools for measuring various aspects of health care and a similar compendium of data collection instruments for measuring nursing education-related concepts (Elliot, Krueger, & Kearns, 1980).

The growing number of nurses conducting research studies and the discussions of theoretical and contextual issues surrounding nursing research created the need for additional sources of communication. Examples of nursing journals that focus on nursing research established during the 1970s are *Advances in Nursing Science, Research in Nursing and Health,* and the *Western Journal of Nursing Research.*

In the 1970s, the change in emphasis from such areas as teaching, administration, curriculum, recruitment, and nurses themselves to the improvement of client or patient care may be attributed to the growing awareness by nurses of the need for a scientific base from which to practice. Many questions might be raised about the role that research currently plays in nursing: If the knowledge of a discipline is best investigated by members of the discipline, are nurses studying nursing? Have nurse researchers produced any knowledge that is applicable to the practice of nursing? We can say with increasing confidence that the answers to these questions are "yes."

The 1980s

The 1980s were an exciting time in the history of nursing research. A major event was the establishment in 1986 of the National Center for Nursing Research (NCNR) at the National Institutes of Health (NIH) by congressional mandate. The purpose of NCNR is to promote and support research training and research relating to patient care. NCNR is organized into four branches. One branch is devoted to the continued research development of nurse scientists by its National Research Service Awards in the form of predoctoral and postdoctoral fellowships. The other three branches are devoted to the conduct of basic or clinical nursing research in the broad classifications of health promotion and disease prevention, acute and chronic illness, and nursing systems and special projects. Such a center helps put nursing research more into the mainstream of research activities enjoyed by other health disciplines. Its creation acknowledges the integral role that nursing and nursing research play in health care.

Several nursing groups developed priorities for nursing research during the 1980s. The ANA Commission on Nursing Research (1980) identified priorities that helped focus research more precisely on aspects of nursing practice. The

group recommended that the generation of knowledge for the practice of nursing should be in the areas of health promotion, prevention of illness, development of cost-effective health-care delivery systems, and the development of strategies that provide effective nursing care to high-risk groups.

The same group, known as the ANA Cabinet on Nursing Research (1985), expanded the priorities for nursing research. The 11 priorities include not only areas related to nursing practice but also research concerned with alternative ways to educate nurses for broad-based practice as well as specialist practice, and for involvement in developing health-care policy. The 11 priorities identified by this group are presented in Box 1-1.

Several nursing specialty groups also developed research priorities within their domain of practice. For example, the Nurses' Association of the American College of Obstetrics and Gynecologists recommended that priority for research be in the areas of obstetric nursing, women's health nursing, and neonatal nursing (Raff & Paul, 1985). Other research priorities have been identified for the areas of childbirth research (Thomas, 1984), critical-care nursing (Lewandowski & Kositsky, 1983), the long-term care of the elderly (Brower & Crist, 1985), and nursing administration (Henry et al., 1987).

Nurses at all levels are increasingly being called upon to develop research skills. The ANA Commission on Nursing Research (1981) issued several guidelines relating to the ability of nurses to integrate research into clinical practice. For example, the commission suggested that baccalaureate nurses, as consumers of research, be able to evaluate research in terms of its applicability to nursing practice, to identify problems for future investigation, to incorporate research findings into their practice, and to share research findings with their colleagues. The group also suggested that nurses with master's degrees conduct scientific investigations, assist others in their research endeavors, help others apply research findings in their practice, and work toward developing a climate that is conducive to the conduct of research.

BOX 1-1 THE 11 PRIORITIES FOR RESEARCH

1. Promote the health, well-being, and ability to care for oneself among all age, social, and cultural groups.
2. Minimize or prevent behaviorally and environmentally induced health problems that compromise the quality of life and reduce productivity.
3. Minimize the negative effects of new health technologies on the adaptive abilities of individuals and families experiencing acute or chronic health problems.
4. Ensure that the care needs of particularly vulnerable groups, such as the elderly, children with congenital health problems, individuals from diverse cultures, mentally ill people, and the poor, are met in effective and acceptable ways.
5. Classify nursing practice phenomena.
6. Ensure that principles of ethics guide nursing research.
7. Develop instruments to measure nursing outcomes.
8. Develop integrative methodologies for the holistic study of human beings as they relate to their families and life styles.
9. Design and evaluate alternative models for delivering health care and for administering health-care systems so that nurses will be able to balance high quality and cost-effectiveness in meeting the nursing needs of identified populations.
10. Evaluate the effectiveness of alternative approaches to nursing education for the kind of practice that requires broad knowledge and a wide repertoire of skills and for the kind of practice that requires specialized knowledge and a focused set of skills.
11. Identify and analyze historical and contemporary factors that influence the shaping of nursing professionals' involvement in national health policy development.

From American Nurses' Association Cabinet on Nursing Research. (1985). *Directions for nursing research: Toward the twenty-first century.* Kansas City, MO: Author, with permission.

Several other trends were discernible among nursing studies of the 1980s. The conceptual models of nursing that were developed in the 1960s and 1970s began to receive increasing attention by researchers. In particular, the conceptual models of such nursing theorists as Dorothea Orem, Dorothy Johnson, Martha Rogers, Sister Callista Roy, Betty Neuman, and Rosemary Parse have been subjected to validation efforts by nurse researchers (see Chapter 7).

There also emerged in the 1980s a growing interest in intensive, process-oriented studies that try to gain an in-depth understanding of a given problem or situation through naturalistic observation of people in their environments. This research approach often has its roots in such disciplines as anthropology or ethnography. This emerging interest has given rise to a debate about whether the "appropriate" research approach for nurse researchers lies in these descriptive, qualitative methods or in more controlled, quantitative procedures. Nursing leaders are suggesting that both major types of research approaches are needed to develop a scientific base for nursing practice.

The establishment of journals beneficial to nurse researchers continued in the 1980s. Examples are *Nursing Scan in Research, Nursing Science Quarterly, Applied Nursing Research,* and *Research Review: Studies for Nursing Practice.*

≡ FUTURE DIRECTIONS OF NURSING RESEARCH

The trend toward clinical research is destined to continue. The ANA Standards of Nursing Practice will continue to be evaluated in terms of their application to nursing. Studies will compare various assessment tools in terms of their ability to collect comparable information and their suitability for different types of clients and clinical situations. Jones, Lepley, and Baker (1984) suggested that nursing diagnoses could be used as a framework for clinical research. The validation of the diagnoses could help identify nursing actions that are within the realm of nursing practice and help delineate nursing's unique role in health care.

Studies concerning the effect of nursing interventions on client or patient outcomes will undoubtedly continue. There is also a growing interest in building a firmer knowledge base by repeating studies, using the identical procedures of previous research but with different clients, in various types of clinical settings and at different times. When findings from several studies are similar, nurses will be able to develop greater confidence that their nursing actions will have an effect on client outcomes.

It is likely that research will be increasingly directed toward the continuing development of nursing theories that are grounded in practice. The nursing profession is likely to encourage efforts to develop theories capable of guiding nursing practice. An increasing number of studies will focus on testing the applicability of current frameworks for practice proposed by nursing leaders to various types of clinical situations.

The development of measuring tools that adequately and accurately assess client or patient outcomes is also likely to be a high priority of the future. Tool construction will be directed toward the measurement of both short- and long-term outcomes. Valid and effective instruments are sorely needed to collect information about the effectiveness of nursing interventions.

The establishment of NCNR holds promise for an increased number of nurses prepared to undertake scientific investigations and to plan a career that includes a program of research in a patient care area. The result should improve the scientific base for nursing practice.

The involvement of nurses in health-care policy research seems destined to increase in the future. The creation of the Agency for Health Care Policy and Research in 1989 at the federal level offers nurses greater opportunities to examine health-care policies related to nursing-care delivery.

In essence, the future of nursing research looks bright and challenging. Nursing research is more likely to be directed toward the practice of nursing than it was in the past. Perhaps such direction will not only improve the quality of nursing practice but also will alter existing curricula of nursing schools. Future nursing students may learn the art and science of nursing practice from perspectives that are completely different from those of today.

☰ SUMMARY

Research has an important role to play in helping nursing establish a scientific base for its practice. The ANA Standards of Nursing Practice provide nurses with a method of clinical practice, a means to evaluate the quality of nursing care, and a rich variety of clinical research problems.

Nursing research began slowly. Most people trace its roots to the work of Florence Nightingale during the Crimean War. The early focus of nursing research closely paralleled the problems faced by the nursing profession. The majority of early research studies were conducted in the areas of nursing education and nursing administration. Only in recent years has the major focus of nursing research shifted toward nursing practice.

Nursing research came to be accepted as part of professional nursing behavior during the 1950s, and such acceptance has continued at a rapidly accelerating pace. The educational preparation of nurses as consumers and producers of research has been better delineated, the number of nursing journals devoted to the dissemination of research findings has increased, nursing leaders have identified priorities for nursing research, and increasing numbers of nurses are investigating problems of a clinical nature.

The establishment of the National Center for Nursing Research at the National Institutes of Health attests to the growth and importance of nursing research. The future direction of nursing research seems sure to continue in the area of nursing practice and theory development. The establishment of a scientific base of nursing knowledge will permit nurses to make more informed decisions in their practice and will have implications for the education of future nursing students.

≡ STUDY SUGGESTIONS

1. What are some of the current changes occurring in the health-care delivery system and how could these changes influence nursing research?
2. Read the list of priorities identified by the ANA Cabinet on Nursing Research (1985) that appear in Box 1-1. How many of the articles published in a recent issue of *Nursing Research* address these priorities?
3. How would collaborative research efforts among health professionals benefit nursing?

≡ SUGGESTED READINGS

Abdellah, F.G., & Levine, E. (1978). *Better patient care through nursing research* (2nd ed.). New York: Macmillan. (Chapter 1).

American Nurses' Association. (1974). Resolutions of priorities in nursing research. *American Nurse, 6,* 5.

American Nurses' Association. (1980). *Nursing: A social policy statement.* Kansas City: Author.

American Nurses' Association Cabinet on Nursing Research. (1985). *Directions for nursing research: Toward the twenty-first century.* Kansas City, MO: Author.

American Nurses' Association Commission on Nursing Research. (1976). *Preparation of nurses for participation in research.* Kansas City, MO: Author.

American Nurses' Association Commission on Nursing Research. (1980). Generating a scientific basis for nursing practice: Research priorities for the 1980s. *Nursing Research, 29,* 219.

American Nurses' Association Commission on Nursing Research. (1981). *Guidelines for the investigative function of nurses.* Kansas City, MO: Author.

American Nurses' Association Congress for Practice. (1973). *Standards of nursing practice.* Kansas City, MO: Author.

Bates, B. (1983). *A guide to physical examination* (3rd ed.). Philadelphia: J.B. Lippincott.

Bauknecht, V.L. (1986). Congress overrides veto, nursing gets center for nursing research. *American Nurse, 18,* 1, 24.

Brower, H.T., & Crist, M.A. (1985). Research priorities in gerontologic nursing for long-term care. *Image: The Journal of Nursing Scholarship, 17,* 22–27.

Brown, E.L. (1948). *Nursing for the future.* New York: Russell Sage.

Carnegie, M.E. (1978). Quo vadis? *Nursing Research, 27,* 277–278.

Elliott, J.E., Krueger, J.C., & Kearns, J.M. (1980). Update on nursing research in the West. *Nursing Research, 29,* 184–188.

Federal Register. (1985, September 26). *Grants programs for baccalaureate degree-granting institutions: Academic Research Enhancement Award* (p. 39046).

Glaser, B.C., & Strauss, A.L. (1966). *Awareness of dying.* Chicago: Aldine.

Gordon, M. (1982). *Nursing diagnosis: Process and applications.* New York: McGraw-Hill.

Gostner, S.R. (1974). Scientific accountability in nursing. *Nursing Outlook, 22,* 764–768.

Hall, L.E. (1963). A center for nursing. *Nursing Outlook, 11,* 805–806.

Henry, B., Moody, L.E., Pendergast, J.F., O'Donnell, J., Hutchinson, S.A., & Scully, G. (1987). Delineation of nursing administration research priorities. *Nursing Research, 36,* 309–314.

Hinshaw, A.S. (1988). The new National Center for Nursing Research patient care research programs. *Applied Nursing Research, 1,* 2–4.

Hughes, E.C. (1958). *Twenty thousand nurses tell their story.* Philadelphia: J.B. Lippincott.

Jones, D., Lepley, M., & Baker, B. (1984). *Health assessment across the life span.* New York: McGraw-Hill.

Lewandowski, L.A., & Kositsky, A.M. (1983). Research priorities for critical care nursing: A study by the American Association of Critical Care Nurses. *Heart and Lung, 12,* 35–44.

Lindeman, C.A. (1975). Delphi survey of priorities in clinical nursing research. *Nursing Research, 24,* 434–441.

Lysaught, J. (1970). *An abstract for action.* New York: McGraw-Hill.

Merritt, D.H. (1986). The National Center for Nursing Research. *Image: The Journal of Nursing Scholarship, 18,* 84–85.

Montag, M. (1954). Experimental programs in nursing education. *Nursing Outlook, 2,* 620–621.

Raff, B.S., & Paul, N.W. (Eds.). (1985). Research priorities established at the NAACOG invitational conference, July 27–28, 1984. *NAACOG invitational research conference: Birth defects: Original article series, 21,* 105–110.

Sands, O., & Belcher, H. (1958). *An experience in basic nursing education.* New York: G.P. Putnam's Sons.

Simmons, L.W., & Henderson, V. (1964). *Nursing research: Survey and assessment.* New York: Appleton-Century-Crofts. (Chapters 2 & 8).

Solomon, S. (1985). *Important dated news.* New York: National League for Nursing.

Thomas, B.S. (1984). Identifying priorities for prepared childbirth research. *Journal of Obstetric, Gynecologic, and Neonatal Nursing, 13,* 400–408.

Werley, H. (1972). *Nursing and research.* Paper presented at the National Commission for the Study of Nursing and Nursing Education, Atlanta, GA.

2
The Scientific Approach

The human experience in this world of physical, chemical, biologic, social, and psychologic forces is a complex affair, defying total comprehension. In our daily private lives and in our work, we strive to make sense of our experience, to understand regularities, and to predict future circumstances. The scientific researcher, similarly, endeavors to understand, explain, predict, or control phenomena. The scientist, however, goes about this task in a more orderly and systematic fashion than is typical of most of our everyday efforts to solve problems. The scientific method involves the formal application of systematic, logical procedures that guide the investigation of phenomena of interest. In this chapter, we discuss the rationale, characteristics, goals, assumptions, and limitations of the scientific method of inquiry.

≡ SOURCES OF HUMAN KNOWLEDGE

Human knowledge has many roots. Think for a moment about some "facts" you have learned relating to the practice of nursing. For example, as nursing students we learn facts such as "washing hands between patients reduces the spread of bacteria" and "the output of fluids for a patient should be comparable in amount to the intake of fluids per day." What is the source of this and other similar information? Some of the "facts" we learn are derived from scientific research, but some probably are not. A brief discussion of some alternative sources of understanding shows how scientific information is different.

Tradition

Many questions are answered and problems solved on the basis of inherited customs or tradition. Within our culture, certain "truths" are accepted as givens. For example, as citizens of the United States, most of us accept, without demanding "proof," that democracy is the highest form of government. This type of knowledge often is so much a part of our heritage that few of us seek verification. The discipline of nursing, like other disciplines, also has its store of information passed on to us by tradition or custom. For example, one of the tasks traditionally performed by nurses is the "change of shift" report for each and every patient, whether the patient's condition has changed or not. The question of whether it might be more productive or effective under certain circumstances to make a report for only those patients whose conditions have changed has not been seriously addressed.

Tradition offers some advantages as a source of knowledge. It is efficient in the sense that each individual is not required to begin anew in an attempt to understand the world or certain aspects of it. Tradition or custom also facilitates communication by providing a common foundation of accepted "truth." Nevertheless, tradition poses some problems for human inquiry. Many traditions have never been evaluated for their validity. Indeed, by their very nature, traditions may interfere with the ability to perceive alternatives. Walker's (1967) research on ritualistic practices in nursing suggests that some traditional nursing practices, such as the routine taking of a patient's temperature, pulse, and respirations, may be dysfunctional. The Walker study illustrates the potential value of critical appraisal of custom and tradition before accepting them as truth.

Authority

In our complex society, there are "authorities," or people with specialized expertise, in every field. We are constantly faced with making decisions about matters with which we have had no direct experience and, therefore, it seems natural to place our trust in the judgment of people who are authoritative on an issue by virtue of specialized training or experience. As a source of understanding, however, authority has shortcomings. Authorities are not infallible, particularly if their expertise is based primarily on personal experience; yet, like tradition, their knowledge often goes unchallenged. Although nursing practice would flounder if every piece of advice from nursing educators were challenged by students, nursing education would be incomplete if students never had occasion to pose such questions as: How does the authority (the instructor) *know*? What evidence is there that what I am learning is true?

Experience and Trial and Error

Our own experiences represent a familiar and functional source of knowledge. The ability to generalize, to recognize regularities, and to make predictions based on observations is an important characteristic of human behavior. Despite the obvious utility of experience, it has limitations as a basis of understanding. First, each individual's experience may be too restricted to develop generalizations. A nurse may notice, for example, that two or three cardiac patients follow very similar postoperative sleep patterns. This observation may lead to some interesting discoveries with implications for nursing interventions, but does the one nurse's observation and experience justify widespread changes in nursing care? A second limitation of experience as a source of knowledge lies in the fact that the same objective event generally is experienced or perceived differently by two individuals. Whose experience constitutes truth?

Closely related to experience is the method of trial and error. In this approach, alternatives are tried successively until we find one that answers our questions or solves our problems. Probably we have all used the trial and error method at some time in our lives, including in our professional work. For example, many patients dislike the taste of potassium chloride solution. Nurses try to disguise the taste of the medication in various ways until one method meets with the approval of the patient. Trial and error may offer a practical means of securing knowledge, but it is fallible and inefficient. This method is haphazard and unsystematic, and the knowledge obtained is often unrecorded and, hence, inaccessible to subsequent problem solvers.

Logical Reasoning

The solutions to many of our perplexing problems are developed by means of logical thought processes. Logical reasoning as a method of knowing combines experience, our intellectual faculties, and formal systems of thought. *Inductive reasoning* is the process of developing generalizations from specific observations. For example, a nurse may observe the anxious behavior of (specific) hospitalized children and conclude that children's separation from their parents is (in general) very stressful. *Deductive reasoning* is the process of developing specific predictions from general principles. For example, if we assume that separation anxiety does occur in hospitalized children (in general), then we might predict that the children in Hospital X whose parents do not room-in (a specific) would manifest symptoms of stress.

Both systems of reasoning are useful as a means of understanding and organizing phenomena, and both play a role in the scientific approach. Neither system of thought, however, is without limitations when used alone as a basis of knowledge. The quality of knowledge arrived at through inductive reasoning depends highly on *which* specific examples are used as the basis for generalization. The reasoning process itself offers no mechanism for evaluating whether the examples are really "typical" and has no built-in checks for self-correction. Deductive reasoning is not itself a source of new information; it is, rather, an approach to illuminating relationships as one proceeds from the general (an assumed truth) to the specific. Deductive logic depends, furthermore, on the truth of the generalizations (called *premises*) to arrive at valid conclusions.

Scientific Method

The scientific approach is the most sophisticated method of acquiring knowledge that humans have developed. The scientific method combines important features of induction and deduction, together with several other characteristics, to create a system of obtaining knowledge that, though fallible, is generally more reliable than tradition, authority, experience, or inductive or deductive reasoning alone. One important aspect that distinguishes the scientific approach from other methods of understanding is its capacity for self-evaluation. That is, scientific research uses checks and balances that minimize the possibility that the researcher's emotions or biases will affect the conclusions.

☰ CHARACTERISTICS OF THE SCIENTIFIC APPROACH

The *scientific approach* to inquiry refers to a general set of orderly, disciplined procedures used to acquire dependable and useful information. *Research* is the application of this scientific approach to the study of a question of interest. Kerlinger (1973), a leader in the field of research methodology, has defined scientific research as the "systematic, controlled, empirical, and critical investigation of hypothetical propositions about the presumed relations among natural phenomena" (p. 11). This definition is complex, so let us briefly examine some characteristics to provide a firmer basis for understanding.

Order and Control

The scientific method is a *systematic* approach to problem solving and to the expansion of knowledge. In a scientific study, the researcher moves in an orderly and systematic fashion from the definition of a problem, through the design of the study and collection of information, to the solution of the problem. By "systematic," we mean that the investigator progresses logically through a series of steps, according to a prespecified plan of action. An overview of the steps taken in a scientific study is provided in Chapter 4.

Control is another critical characteristic of the scientific approach. Control involves imposing conditions on the research situation so that biases and confounding factors are minimized. The problems that are of interest to scientists— for example, lung cancer, obesity, compliance with a regimen, or perceptions of pain—are highly complicated phenomena, often representing the effects of various forces. In trying to isolate relationships between phenomena, the scientist must attempt to control factors that are not under direct investigation. For example, if a scientist is interested in exploring the relationship between diet and heart disease, steps must be taken to control other potential contributors to coronary disorders, such as stress and cigarette smoking, as well as additional factors that might be relevant, such as a person's age and sex. The mechanisms of scientific control are the subject of a large part of this book.

Empiricism

Empiricism refers to the process whereby evidence rooted in objective reality and gathered directly or indirectly through the human senses is used as the basis for generating knowledge. This requirement causes findings of a scientific investigation to be grounded in reality rather than in the personal beliefs of the researcher. Empirical inquiry imposes a certain degree of objectivity on the research situation because ideas or hunches are exposed to testing in the real world.

Empirical evidence, then, consists of observations made known to us by way of our sense organs. The observations are verified through sight, hearing, taste, touch, or smell. Observations of the presence or absence of skin inflammation, the heart rate of a patient, or the weight of a newborn infant are all examples of empirical observations.

Generalization

An important goal of science is to understand phenomena. This pursuit of knowledge, however, is focused not on isolated events or situations but rather on a more generalized understanding of phenomena and how they are in-

terrelated. For example, the scientific researcher is typically not as interested in understanding why Ann X has cervical cancer as in understanding what general factors led to this form of carcinoma in Ann and in others. Of course, a health practitioner would want to take advantage of the general knowledge obtained in the course of scientific research in an effort to assist a particular individual. The ability to go beyond the specifics of the situation at hand is an important characteristic of the scientific approach. *Generalizability* of research findings is an important criterion for assessing the quality of an investigation.

≡ ASSUMPTIONS OF THE SCIENTIFIC APPROACH

Assumptions refer to basic principles that are accepted on faith, or assumed to be true, without proof or verification. This section extends our discussion of the characteristics of the scientific approach by paying specific attention to the assumptions upon which science is founded.

The Nature of Reality

The scientist assumes that there is an objective reality that exists independent of human discovery or observation. That is, the world is assumed to be real and not a creation of the human mind; the processes of the universe would continue to exist even if humans were incapable of observing or recording them.

A related assumption is the belief that nature is basically orderly and regular. Events in nature are assumed to be, at least to a certain extent, consistent. If this principle were not assumed, it would make little sense to conduct scientific research.

Determinism

The assumption of *determinism* refers to the belief that all phenomena have antecedent (preceding) causes. Natural events or conditions are assumed to not be haphazard, random, or accidental. Given the presumed orderliness of nature, events must have causes. If a pregnant woman has a premature delivery, there must be a reason that can potentially be identified and understood. If an individual has a cerebral vascular accident, there must be a cause or perhaps several causes.

Much of the activity in which a scientific researcher engages is directed toward an understanding of cause-and-effect relationships. Scientists believe that antecedent factors relating to all phenomena exist and can be discovered. Science does, however, accept the concept of multiple causation. A particular phenomenon may have several different causes. For example, heart disease may be caused by smoking habits, diet, stress, and additional factors or combinations of factors. The identification of these causes, that is, the search for an explanation of *why* things are the way they are, is one of the chief goals of science.

☰ *PURPOSES OF SCIENTIFIC RESEARCH*

The scientific approach has been discussed in a general way as a method of problem solving or a system for acquiring knowledge. In this section, we examine some of the more specific reasons for conducting research in the context of the nursing profession.

Description

Many nursing research studies have as their main objective the description of phenomena relating to the nursing process. The researcher who conducts a descriptive investigation observes, describes, and, perhaps, classifies. Descriptive studies can be of considerable value to the nursing profession. The phenomena that nursing researchers have been interested in describing are varied: stress in patients, grieving behavior, sleep patterns, nutritional habits, health beliefs, time patterns of temperature readings, to mention only a few.

Exploration

Exploratory research is an extension of descriptive research that focuses more directly on the discovery of relationships. In descriptive studies, the researcher selects a specific event, condition, or behavior and makes observations and records of the phenomenon. The final result of such an investigation is a list, a catalog, a classification, or some other type of description. Exploratory research also focuses on a phenomenon of interest, but pursues the question: What factor or factors influence, affect, cause, or relate to this phenomenon? For example, a descriptive study might examine patients' satisfaction with the nursing care they received. Such a study might reveal that 75% of the hospitalized patients who were questioned indicated that they were satisfied with the quality of nursing care. The purpose of such a descriptive study would probably be to document the need (or the absence of a need) to improve the quality of care currently available in hospitals. An exploratory study, on the other hand, would try to identify important relationships. What kinds of factors are related to a patient's degree of satisfaction? Is the patient's diagnosis an important factor? Do the patient's age, sex, or prior hospitalization record play a role? Or is patient satisfaction related to characteristics of the hospital, such as size, geographic location, or staff traits?

Researchers may engage in exploratory research for two basic reasons. First, the investigator may desire a richer understanding of the phenomenon of interest than a straightforward descriptive study could provide. This reason is particularly salient when a new area or topic is being investigated. Second, exploratory studies are sometimes conducted to estimate the feasibility and cost of undertaking a more rigorous or extensive research project on the same topic. When large-scale studies are anticipated, it is usually wise to explore potential difficulties with a smaller version of the study.

Explanation

The third basic purpose for conducting research is to provide explanations. Formal explanations of natural phenomena are *theories*. Theories represent a method of organizing, integrating, and deriving abstract conceptualizations about the manner in which phenomena are interrelated. In its aim to understand and explain phenomena, the scientific approach unites empirical observations, logical reasoning, order, and control to formulate systematic, abstract, and generalized interpretations concerning natural phenomena. Theories, then, offer an opportunity for bringing together observed events and relationships, for explaining how and why phenomena are associated with one another, and for predicting the occurrence of future events and relationships.

Many writers on the scientific process argue that theory formation is the ultimate aim of science. It might be said that, whereas descriptive and exploratory research provide new information, theoretical or explanatory research offers us understanding. Reinforcement theory, for example, asserts that when a behavior is positively reinforced, that is, rewarded in some way, then that behavior will tend to be repeated. This generalized explanation of human behavior offers the possibility of understanding a broader range of behavior than would the more specific proposition that children who are praised (reinforced) for taking their medications tend to be more compliant in following a medications regimen. A theory gets us much closer to the "why" of phenomena.

Prediction and Control

Although the goal of explanation epitomizes the spirit of scientific inquiry, there are unfortunately numerous problems that, with our current level of knowledge and technology, defy absolute comprehension. Yet it is frequently possible to use the scientific approach to make reliable predictions and to develop control mechanisms in the absence of total understanding. For example, various scientific studies have demonstrated an association between the age of mothers and the incidence of Down's syndrome in their infants. Such an association makes it possible to predict that women beyond the age of 35 are at a greater risk of bearing infants with Down's syndrome than are younger women. The ability to predict, in turn, offers the possibility of control. That is, through appropriate education, women can learn to have an amniocentesis performed after they turn 35. Note that the ability to predict and control in this example does not depend on the scientist's complete explanation of *why* older women are at a higher risk of having an abnormal child than younger women. There are many examples of medical and nursing research investigations in which prediction and control are key objectives.

Each of these purposes corresponds to different types of questions that the researcher might pose, as shown in Table 2-1. This table also gives an example of an actual research study for each of these four major purposes.

Basic Versus Applied Research

We have seen that scientific research strives to describe, explore, explain, predict, or control phenomena. A second approach to classifying the functions of research is based on the degree to which the findings have direct practical utility or application. *Basic research* is concerned with making empirical observations that can be used to accumulate information or to formulate or refine a theory. Basic research is not designed to solve immediate problems but, rather, to extend the base of knowledge in a discipline for the sake of knowledge and understanding itself. Of course, many of the findings from basic research endeavors are ultimately applied to practical problems. For example, advances in the practice of nursing have resulted from basic research in biochemistry, psychology, and nursing itself. But basic research is not directly concerned with the social utility of its findings, and many years may pass before a relevant application is developed.

Whipple, who studied the bleeding tendency in liver disease, and Dam, who studied cholesterol metabolism, probably could not have envisioned that their independent and seemingly unrelated basic research endeavors would combine for the practical application of treating bleeding tendencies with vitamin K.

Researchers who engage in *applied research* concentrate on finding a solution to an immediate problem. Applied research has as its final goal the scientific planning of induced change in a troublesome situation. We need basic research for the discovery of general laws about human behavior and bodily functioning, but applied research tells how these laws operate in, say, a hospital environment. Just as the possibility of practical application is not ruled out in basic research, applied research may also contribute to general knowledge in a field. It is perhaps more meaningful to think of applied and basic research

as two end points on a continuum, because in a given study there may be multiple goals and multiple lessons.

Much of the research conducted in nursing tends to be more applied in nature. For example, the question of how long a rectal, oral, or axillary thermometer must be in place to record accurately is a problem for which the solution has immediate application in practice. Yet nursing researchers are demonstrating increasing interest in the conduct of theory-based research designed to enhance a general understanding of the nursing process and the role of nurses. In nursing, as in medicine, the feedback process between basic and applied research seems to operate more freely than in the case of other disciplines. The findings from applied research almost immediately pose questions for basic research, and the results of basic research many times suggest clinical application to an immediate problem.

Table 2-1, *Research Purposes and Research Questions*

PURPOSE	*TYPE OF QUESTIONS*	*NURSING RESEARCH EXAMPLE*
DESCRIPTION	How prevalent is the phenomenon? What are the characteristics of the phenomenon? What has happened? What is the process by which some phenomenon is experienced?	What are the characteristics of maternal behavior in response to the reflexive urge to bear down during the expulsive phase of labor? (Roberts et al., 1987)
EXPLORATION	What is the full nature of the phenomenon? What is going on? What factors are related to the phenomenon?	What is the nature and type of support provided to women experiencing chronic illness? (Primomo et al., 1990)
EXPLANATION	What is the underlying cause? What does the occurrence of the phenomenon mean? Why does the phenomenon exist? Why are two phenomena related?	What are the causes of job satisfaction among registered nurses? (Blegen & Mueller, 1987)
PREDICTION AND CONTROL	If phenomenon X occurs, will phenomenon Y follow? Can the occurrence of the phenomenon be controlled? Does an intervention result in the intended effect?	What factors predict the incidence and duration of diarrhea associated with tube feeding in mechanically ventilated patients? (Smith et al., 1990)

≡ LIMITATIONS OF THE SCIENTIFIC METHOD

The scientific approach to inquiry is regarded by many as the highest form of attaining knowledge that humans have devised. This is not to say, however, that scientific research can solve all human problems or that scientists are immune from making mistakes. There are a number of limitations of applying the scientific approach to nursing problems that should be mentioned lest the impression be given that scientific research is infallible. Some of the limitations discussed here are common to all scientific endeavors, whereas others are more prevalent in the social science disciplines (psychology, sociology, and education), with which nursing research sometimes overlaps.

General Limitations

Perfectly designed and executed studies are unattainable. Virtually every research study contains some flaw. Every research question can be addressed in an almost infinite number of ways. The researcher must make decisions about how best to proceed. Invariably, there are trade-offs. The best methods are often very expensive and time-consuming. Even when tremendous resources are expended, there are bound to be some flaws. This does not mean that small, simple studies are worthless. It means that *no single study can ever definitively prove or disprove our hunches*. Each completed study adds to a body of accumulated knowledge. If the same question is posed by several researchers, each of whom obtains the same or similar results, increased confidence can be placed in the answer to the question. This is especially true if the researchers' studies have different types of shortcomings.

Moral or Ethical Issues

Moral or ethical issues create limitations for scientific research in two respects. The first concerns constraints on what is considered acceptable in the name of science with regard to the rights of living organisms. Research ethics are discussed in greater detail in Chapter 3.

The second issue concerns the kind of problems that can be solved using the scientific method. Questions that focus on ethical or value-laden matters cannot be empirically tested. Many of our most persistent and intriguing questions about the human condition fall into the category of moral/ethical problems. Consider, for example, the issue of euthanasia. Descriptive research concerning how nurses feel about euthanasia is certainly possible. Studies concerning the characteristics of nurses with different points of view are also feasible. Similarly, a researcher could explore the extent to which nurses' attitudes concerning euthanasia affect their behavior toward terminally ill patients. All of these hypothetical studies lend themselves to a scientific approach. But no specific investigation could be expected to answer the question "Should euthanasia be practiced?" The nursing process may increasingly incorporate scientific knowledge into its problem-solving strategies. However, it is probable that the nursing process will never completely rely on scientific information because some decisions involve moral, ethical, or value issues that cannot be addressed by scientific research.

Human Complexity

One of the major obstacles to conducting nursing studies using the scientific paradigm is the complexity of the central topic of investigation—humans. This problem is much less troublesome in clinical research dealing with bodily processes than in research concerning human behavior or attitudes. Biologic and physical functioning is considerably more regular and consistent and less susceptible to external influences than is psychologic functioning. Each human being is essentially unique with respect to his or her personality, social environment, mental capacities, values, and life style. Thus, it is relatively more difficult to detect regularities in, say, human eating behavior than to make generalizations concerning the functioning of, say, the pancreas. In other words, there appear to be fewer individual biologic/chemical differences than there are individual social/psychologic differences. Thus, it has been impossible to achieve the same level of order and discipline over the research situation in studies focusing on human behavior and thought than is the case in studies dealing with biologic or physical phenomena.

The inability of the traditional scientific approach to meaningfully capture the human experience holistically has led a growing number of nurse researchers to adopt an alternative approach of investigation. This emerging school of thought, which has as its intellectual roots the tradition known as *phenomenology,* offers an alternative to the scientific method, whose philosophical underpinnings are *logical positivism.* The phenomenological approach rests on different assumptions about the nature of humans and how that nature is to be understood. Phenomenologists emphasize the complexity of humans, the ability of humans to shape and create their own experiences, and the idea that "truth" is a composite of realities. Investigations in the phenomenological tradition place a heavy emphasis on understanding the human experience as it is actually experienced, generally through the careful collection and analysis of narrative, subjective materials. According to phenomenologists, a major limitation of the classical scientific approach is that it is *reductionist,* that is, it reduces human experience to only the few concepts under investigation, and those concepts are defined in advance by the researcher rather than emerging from the experience of those under study.

In this book, we take the view that both the phenomenological and scientific approaches represent valid and important paradigms for the study of nursing problems. We have devoted more attention to methods normally associated with the scientific approach because the vast majority of nursing research studies have adopted this approach. However, there is some overlap in the activities undertaken in phenomenological and scientific research, and so much of the discussion is applicable to both approaches.

Measurement Problems

Another limitation of the scientific approach that is related to the issue of human complexity concerns problems of measurement. To study, for example, patient morale, we must be able to observe or measure it; that is, we must be able to assess whether a patient's morale is high or low, or higher under certain conditions than under others. Although there are reasonably accurate measures of such physiologic phenomena as blood pressure, temperature, and cardiac activity, comparably accurate measures of such psychologic phenomena as anxiety, pain, self-confidence, or body image have not been developed. The problems associated with measurement are often the most perplexing in the research process.

Control Problems

In discussing the characteristics of the scientific approach, we pointed out that the scientist attempts to control the research situation to have confidence in the outcomes. Because scientists accept the principle of multiple causation, and because all potential causes of a phenomenon generally cannot be studied simultaneously, scientists generally attempt to control factors that are not under direct investigation. For example, a researcher focusing on the link between prenatal care and low birthweight might want to control—that is, remove the influence of—maternal diet and smoking behavior, both of which have been implicated as contributing to low birthweight.

Adequate control, however, is often difficult to achieve. Confounding factors may be difficult to even identify, let alone control, if the phenomenon of interest is complex. Control over confounding factors is especially problematic in research with humans in naturalistic settings.

Despite the various obstacles mentioned above, nurse researchers have made outstanding progress in contributing knowledge and understanding about the practice and theory of nursing. Even further progress can be anticipated in the years to come as information accumulates and forms a foundation for more sophisticated theories, as data collection methods and research design become more refined, and as nurses integrate findings from phenomenological and scientific studies.

≡ METHODS FOR NURSING RESEARCH

The methods that nurse researchers use to study problems of interest in the development of a scientific basis for nursing are quite diverse. This diversity, in our view, is critical to the spirit of science, the basic aim of which is the discovery of knowledge. There is no single "right" way to understand our complex world. Throughout this book, we discuss alternative ways of asking questions, identifying sources of information, and gathering and analyzing that information. Scientific knowledge would be slim, indeed, if there were not a rich array of alternative approaches available to us.

A distinction is often made between two broad types of research methods: qualitative and quantitative. *Quantitative research* involves the systematic collection of numerical information, often under conditions of considerable control, and the analysis of that information using statistical procedures. *Qualitative research* involves the systematic collection and analysis of more subjective narrative materials, using procedures in which there tends to be a minimum of researcher-imposed control. Although most nursing research studies are quantitative, there are a growing number of qualitative investigations. There has also been an increase recently in the number of studies using both qualitative and quantitative methods.

In our view, the selection of an appropriate method depends to some degree on the researcher's personal taste and "philosophy," but also depends in large part on the nature of the research question. If a researcher asks what the effects of surgery are on circadian rhythms (bio-

logic cycles), the researcher really needs to express the effects through the careful quantitative measurement of various bodily processes subject to rhythmic variation. On the other hand, if a researcher inquires about the process by which parents learn to cope with the death of a child, the researcher may be hard pressed to quantify such a process. Personal world views of the researchers generally help to shape the types of questions they ask.

There is a tendency to attach convenient labels to emphasize the distinction between qualitative and quantitative research. For example, the logical positivist paradigm is most frequently associated with quantitative methods. However, many researchers who would consider themselves squarely in the logical positivist tradition also collect and analyze qualitative data. Ethnographers, who conduct in-depth studies of specific cultures or subcultures, rely heavily on qualitative data but may also use available quantitative data on the members of the culture to provide a context for their inquiry. Similarly, historical researchers often blend qualitative and quantitative information, although historical research has traditionally been qualitative.

Although we think that the distinctions between qualitative and quantitative methods have sometimes been exaggerated, it is nevertheless true that there tend to be some important differences in these two types of research. Quantitative research, which is referred to by some as a "hard" science, tends to emphasize deductive reasoning, the rules of logic, and the measurable attributes of the human experience. Thus, quantitative research does have its roots in logical positivism. Research that uses a quantitative approach *generally*

- focuses on a relatively small number of specific concepts
- begins with preconceived ideas about how the concepts are interrelated
- uses structured procedures and formal "instruments" to collect information
- collects the information under conditions of control

- emphasizes objectivity in the collection and analysis of information
- analyzes numerical information through statistical procedures

Qualitative research, on the other hand, has sometimes been referred to as a "soft" science. Qualitative researchers tend to emphasize the dynamic, holistic, and individual aspects of the human experience and attempt to capture those aspects in their entirety, within the context of those who are experiencing them. Phenomenological research is almost always exclusively qualitative (although not all qualitative research is phenomenological). Research that uses a qualitative approach *generally*

- attempts to understand the entirety of some phenomenon rather than focus on specific concepts
- has few preconceived ideas and stresses the importance of people's interpretation of events and circumstances, rather than the researcher's interpretation
- collects information without formal, structured "instruments"
- does not attempt to control the context of the research but, rather, attempts to capture it in its entirety
- attempts to capitalize on the subjective as a means for understanding and interpreting human experiences
- analyzes narrative information in an organized, but intuitive, fashion

Both qualitative and quantitative approaches have strengths and weaknesses, which are identified throughout this book. It is precisely because the strengths of one approach complement the weaknesses of the other that both are essential to the further development of nursing science.

≡ *SUMMARY*

Nurse researchers are increasingly utilizing the scientific approach to extend their knowledge about nursing theory and practice. The scientific approach may be contrasted with other sources of truth and understanding. Certain "truths" are passed on to us by tradition or custom—that is, they are accepted as cultural givens without demands for verification. Authority figures or specialists are another common source of information or knowledge. Our own experiences, together with trial and error procedures, are familiar to all of us as a method of acquiring understanding. Some of our problems can be dealt with by logical reasoning. *Inductive reasoning* is the process of establishing generalizations from specific observations, and *deductive reasoning* is the process of developing specific predictions from general principles. These approaches suffer various limitations as techniques for solving problems. The scientific method offers several advantages as a method of inquiry.

The *scientific approach* may be described in terms of a number of characteristics. It is, first of all, a systematic, disciplined, and controlled process. Scientists base their findings on *empirical* observations, which means that evidence is rooted in objective reality and collected by means of the human senses. Unlike many other problem-solving techniques, the scientific approach strives for *generalizability* and for the development of conceptual explanations or *theories* concerning the relationships among phenomena.

The scientist assumes that there is an objective reality that is not dependent on human observation for its existence. A related belief is that natural phenomena are basically regular and orderly. The assumption of *determinism* refers to the belief that events are not haphazard but, rather, are the consequence of prior causes. The search for an understanding of cause-and-effect relationships is an activity basic to many scientific endeavors.

Scientific research can be categorized in terms of its functions or objectives. Description, exploration, explanation, prediction, and control of natural phenomena represent the most common goals of a research investigation. It is also possible to describe research in terms of the direct practical utility that it aspires to achieve. *Basic research* is designed to extend the base of knowledge in a discipline for the sake of knowl-edge itself. *Applied research* focuses on discover-ing solutions to immediate problems.

Although the *scientific approach* offers a number of distinct advantages as a system of in-quiry, it is not without its share of limitations. In general, researchers must make compromises in the face of limited time and resources so that no single study can ever definitively answer a given question. The design of studies with humans is constrained not only by resources but also by standards of professional ethics. In addition, there are numerous questions of interest to nurse re-searchers that are difficult to study because they deal with complex social or psychologic function-ing, such as pain, fear, guilt, anxiety, motivation, and the like. Such phenomena are difficult to accurately measure (in comparison with aspects of biologic functioning such as blood pressure) and difficult to control in a natural setting. In fact, *phenomenologists* have argued that the scientific approach, which has its roots in the tradition of *logical positivism,* is overly reductionist and can-not adequately capture the human experience in all of its complexity.

Problems of interest to nurse researchers can be addressed using a wide range of available methods. A distinction is often made between two broad types of methods. *Quantitative research* involves the systematic collection and analysis of numerical information, generally under con-trolled conditions. *Qualitative research,* which involves the collection and analysis of more sub-jective, narrative materials, generally attempts to view the experiences of those being studied through their own eyes. Both qualitative and quantitative research have complementary strengths and limitations; both play important roles in the advancement of nursing science.

☰ *STUDY SUGGESTIONS*

1. Consider one or two nursing "facts" that you possess and then trace the facts back to some source. Is the basis for your knowledge tradi-tion, authority, experience, or scientific re-search?

2. Explain the ways in which scientific knowl-edge differs from knowledge based on tradi-tion, authority, trial and error, and logical rea-soning.

3. How does the assumption of scientific deter-minism conflict with or coincide with super-stitious thinking? Take, as an example, the superstition associated with four-leaf clovers or a rabbit's foot.

4. How does the ability to predict phenomena offer the possibility of their control?

5. Below are a few research problems. For each problem, specify whether you think it is es-sentially a basic or applied research question. Justify your response.
   a. Is the stress level of patients related to the level of information they possess about their medical status?
   b. Do students who get better grades in nursing school become more effective nurses than students with lower grades?
   c. Does the early discharge of maternity patients lead to later problems with breast-feeding?
   d. Can the incidence of decubitus ulcers be affected by a certain massaging tech-nique?
   e. Is individual contraceptive counseling more effective than group-based instruc-tion in minimizing unwanted pregnan-cies?

6. Consider the following research questions. For each, indicate whether you think the question would best lend itself to a qualitative or quantitative research study.
   a. What is the process by which nursing students acquire a professional nursing identity?
   b. What are the effects of prenatal instruc-tion on the labor and delivery outcomes of pregnant women?
   c. What are the health care needs of the homeless? What are the barriers they face in having those needs met?

d. What are the psychological consequences of having acquired immunodeficiency syndrome virus?

☰ *SUGGESTED READINGS*

METHODOLOGICAL/THEORETICAL REFERENCES

Braithwaite, R. (1955). *Scientific explanation.* Cambridge, England: Cambridge University Press.

Hacking, I. (1981). *Scientific revolutions.* Oxford, England: Oxford University Press.

Hesse, M.B. (1974). *The structure of scientific inference.* Berkeley: University of California Press.

Kerlinger, F. (1973). *Foundations of behavioral research* (2nd ed.). New York: Holt, Rinehart and Winston. (Chapter 1).

Kuhn, T.S. (1970). *The structure of scientific revolutions* (2nd ed.). Chicago: University of Chicago Press.

Madden, E.H. (Ed.). (1974). *The structure of scientific thought.* Boston: Houghton Mifflin.

Meyers, S.T. (1982). The search for assumptions. *Western Journal of Nursing Research, 4,* 91–98.

Newton, D.E. (1974). *Science and society.* Boston: Holbrook Press.

Oiler, C. (1982). The phenomenological approach in nursing research. *Nursing Research, 31,* 178–181.

Popper, K.R. (1959). *The logic of scientific discovery* (rev. ed.). New York: Harper & Row.

Simon, H.M. (1968). Panel discussion: The position of the pure and applied scientist. Conference on the nature of science and nursing. *Nursing Research, 17,* 507–509.

Walker, V.H. (1967). *Nursing and ritualistic practice.* New York: Macmillan.

Wysocki, A.B. (1983). Basic versus applied research: Intrinsic and extrinsic considerations. *Western Journal of Nursing Research, 5,* 217–224.

SUBSTANTIVE REFERENCES

Blegen, M.A., & Mueller, C.W. (1987). Nurses' job satisfaction: A longitudinal analysis. *Research in Nursing and Health, 10,* 227–237.

Primomo, J., Yates, B.C., & Woods, N.F. (1990). Social support for women during chronic illness. *Research in Nursing and Health, 13,* 153–161.

Roberts, J.E., Goldstein, S.A., Gruner, J.S., Maggio, M., & Mendiz-Bauer, C. (1987). A descriptive analysis of involuntary bearing-down efforts during the expulsive phase of labor. *Journal of Obstetric, Gynecologic, and Neonatal Nursing, 16,* 48–55.

Smith, C.E., Marien, L., Brogdon, C., Faust-Wilson, P., Lohr, G., Gerald, K., & Pingleton, S. (1990). Diarrhea associated with tube feeding in mechanically ventilated critically ill patients. *Nursing Research, 39,* 148–152.

3
Ethics and Scientific Research

In nursing research, humans are usually the source of information to the investigators—that is, humans are usually the *subjects* under study. When humans are used as subjects, great care must be exercised in ensuring that the rights of those humans are protected. The requirement for ethical conduct may strike the reader as so self-evident as to require no further comment, but the fact is that investigators sometimes fail to fully consider the ethical dimensions of a study. Moreover, conflicts sometimes arise in designing research that is both ethical and scientifically rigorous. This chapter is designed to acquaint researchers with major principles and procedures for protecting the rights of human subjects.

≡ THE NEED FOR ETHICAL GUIDELINES

Within the past few decades, the protection of the rights of human subjects has become a high priority among members of the scientific and health-care communities. However, ethical considerations have not always been given adequate attention. In this section, we consider some of the reasons that the development of ethical guidelines became imperative.

Historical Background

As modern "civilized" humans, we might like to think that systematic violations of moral principles within the context of research occurred centuries ago rather in recent times, but this is not the case. The Nazi medical experiments of the 1930s and 1940s are the most famous example of recent disregard for ethical conduct. The Nazi program of research involved the use of prisoners of war and racial "enemies" in numerous experiments designed to test the limits of human endurance and human reaction to diseases and untested drugs. The studies were unethical, not only because they exposed the human subjects to permanent physical harm and even death, but also because the subjects were not given an opportunity to refuse participation.

There are, unfortunately, recent examples that are closer to home. For instance, between 1932 and 1972, a study (known as the Tuskegee Syphilis Study) sponsored by the U.S. Public Health Service investigated the effects of syphilis among 400 men from a poor black community. Medical treatment was deliberately withheld to study the course of the untreated disease. Another well-known case of unethical research involved the injection of live cancer cells into elderly patients at the Jewish Chronic Disease Hospital in Brooklyn, without the consent of those patients. Many other examples of studies with ethical transgressions—often much more subtle than these examples—have emerged to give ethical concerns the high visibility they have today.

Ethical Dilemmas in Conducting Research

Research that violates ethical principles is rarely done specifically to be cruel or immoral, but more typically occurs out of a conviction that knowledge is important and potentially life-saving or beneficial (usually to others) in the long run. There are, unfortunately, research problems in which the rights of subjects and the demands of science are put in direct conflict. Here are some examples of situations in which the scientist's need for rigor can be compromised by ethical considerations:

> *Research problem:* How empathic are nurses in their treatment of patients in intensive care units?
>
> *Ethical dilemma:* Ethical research generally involves having subjects be fully cognizant of their participation in a study. Yet if the researcher informs the nurses serv-

ing as subjects that their treatment of patients will be under scrutiny, will their behavior be "normal"? If the nurses' behavior is distorted, the entire value of the study could be undermined.

> *Research problem:* What are the feelings and coping mechanisms of parents whose children have a terminal illness?
>
> *Ethical dilemma:* To fully answer this question, the researcher may need to intrusively probe into the psychologic state of the parents at a highly vulnerable time in their lives; such probing could be painful and even traumatic. Yet knowledge of the parents' coping mechanisms could help to design more effective ways of dealing with parents' grief and anger.
>
> *Research problem:* Does a new medication prolong life in cancer patients?
>
> *Ethical dilemma:* The best way to test the effectiveness of interventions is to administer the intervention to some subjects but withhold it from others to see if differences between the groups emerge. However, if the intervention is untested (e.g., a new drug), the group receiving the intervention may be exposed to potentially hazardous side effects. On the other hand, the group not receiving the drug may be denied a beneficial treatment.
>
> *Research problem:* What are the familial characteristics that are predictive of child sexual abuse?
>
> *Ethical dilemma:* In identifying factors that place children at high risk of sexual exploitation, the researcher would ideally like to study a typical sample of families with child victims. However, ethical considerations might restrict the sample to families who volunteer to participate in the study, and these volunteering families might be highly atypical, in which case the results might be inaccurate and misleading.

As these examples suggest, researchers involved with human subjects are often in a bind:

they are obligated to advance knowledge, using the most scientifically rigorous procedures available, but they must also adhere to the dictates of ethical rules that have been developed to protect the rights of subjects. It is precisely because of such conflicts that codes of ethics are so important in guiding the efforts of researchers.

Codes of Ethics

Over the past four decades, largely in response to the human rights violations described earlier, various codes of ethics have been developed. One of the first internationally recognized efforts to establish ethical standards is referred to as the Nuremberg Code, developed after the Nazi atrocities were made public in the Nuremberg trials. Several other international standards have followed, the most notable of which is the Declaration of Helsinki, which was adopted in 1964 by the World Medical Assembly, and then later revised in 1975.

Most disciplines have established their own code of ethics. The American Nurses' Association (1975) has put forth a document entitled *Human Rights Guidelines for Nurses in Clinical and Other Research.* The American Sociological Association published its *Code of Ethics* in 1984. Guidelines for psychologists were published by the American Psychological Association (APA, 1982) in *Ethical Principles in the Conduct of Research With Human Participants.* Although there is considerable overlap in the basic principles articulated in these documents, each deals with problems of particular concern to their respective disciplines.

An especially important code of ethics was adopted by the National Commission for the Protection of Human Subjects of Biomedical and Behavioral Research (1978). The commission, established by the National Research Act (Public Law 93-348), issued a report in 1978 that served as the basis for regulations affecting research sponsored by the federal government. The report, sometimes referred to as the Belmont Report, also served as a model for many of the guidelines adopted by specific disciplines.

The Belmont Report articulated three primary ethical principles upon which standards of ethical conduct in research are based: (1) beneficence, (2) respect for human dignity, and (3) justice.

☰ THE PRINCIPLE OF BENEFICENCE

One of the most fundamental ethical principles in research is that of *beneficence,* which encompasses the maxim of "above all, do no harm." Most ethicists and researchers consider that this principle contains multiple dimensions.

Freedom From Harm

Clearly, exposing research participants to experiences that result in serious or permanent harm is unacceptable. Research should only be conducted by scientifically qualified persons, especially if potentially dangerous technical equipment or specialized procedures are used. The researcher must be prepared at any time during the study to terminate the research if there is reason to suspect that continuation would result in injury, disability, undue distress, or death to study participants. When a new medical procedure or drug is being tested, it is usually important to first experiment with animals or tissue cultures before proceeding to tests with humans.

Although protecting study participants from physical harm is in many cases clear-cut, some psychologic consequences of participating in a study may be subtle and, thus, require closer attention and sensitivity. Sometimes, for example, people are asked questions about their personal views, weaknesses, or fears. Such queries might require individuals to admit to aspects of themselves that they dislike and would perhaps rather forget. The point is not that the researcher should refrain from asking any questions but, rather, that it is necessary to think very carefully about the nature of the intrusion upon people's psyches. Researchers strive to avoid inflicting psychologic harm by carefully considering the phrasing of questions, by providing *debriefing* sessions following the research to permit participants to ask questions and by providing subjects with written information on how they may later contact the researchers.

Freedom From Exploitation

Involvement in a research study should not place subjects at a disadvantage or expose them to situations for which they have not been explicitly prepared. Subjects need to be assured that their participation, or the information they might provide to the researcher, will not be used against them in any way. For example, a subject describing his or her economic circumstances to a researcher should not be exposed to the risk of losing Medicaid benefits; the person reporting drug abuse should not fear exposure to criminal authorities.

The subject enters into a very special relationship with the researcher, and it is critical that that relationship not be exploited in any way. Exploitation might be overt and malicious (e.g., sexual exploitation, using subjects' identifying information to create a mailing list, and the use of donated blood for the development of a commercial product), but it may also be more subtle. For example, subjects may agree to participate in a study requiring 30 minutes of their time. The researcher may then decide one year later to go back and talk to the subjects to follow their progress or circumstances. Unless the researcher had previously warned the subjects that there might be a follow-up study, the researcher might be accused of not adhering to the agreement previously reached with subjects and of exploiting the researcher–subject relationship. Because nurse researchers may have a nurse–patient (in addition to a researcher–subject) relationship, special care may need to be exercised to avoid exploitation of people's vulnerabilities.

Benefits From Research

Subjects agree to participate in scientific investigations for a number of reasons. They may perceive that there are some direct benefits to themselves. More often, however, any benefits from the research would accrue to society in general or to other individuals. Thus, many subjects may participate in a study out of a desire to be helpful. The researcher should strive insofar as possible to maximize benefits and to candidly communicate the potential benefits to subjects.

The Risk/Benefit Ratio

In deciding to conduct a study, the researcher must carefully assess the risks and benefits that would be incurred. The assessment should weigh the direct costs and benefits that individual subjects might experience, and the assessment should be shared with the subjects so that they can evaluate whether it is in their best interest to participate. Box 3-1 summarizes some of the more salient benefits and costs to which research subjects might be exposed. In evaluating the anticipated costs and benefits, the researcher might want to consider how comfortable he or she would feel about the risk/benefit ratio if it were family members participating in the study.

The risk/benefit ratio should also be considered in terms of whether the risks to research subjects are commensurate with the benefit to society and the nursing profession in terms of the knowledge produced. The general guideline is that the degree of risk to be taken by those participating in the research should never exceed the potential humanitarian benefits of the knowledge to be gained. Thus, the selection of a significant topic for study is the first step in ensuring that research is ethical.

All research involves some risks, but in many cases the risk is minimal. *Minimal risk,* according to federal guidelines, is defined as anticipated risks that are no greater than those ordinarily encountered in daily life or during the performance of routine physical or psychologic tests or procedures. When the risks are not minimal, the researcher must proceed with great caution, taking every step possible to reduce risks and maximize benefits. If the perceived risks and costs to subjects outweigh the anticipated benefits of the research, the research should be either abandoned or redesigned.

BOX 3-1 POTENTIAL BENEFITS AND COSTS OF RESEARCH TO PARTICIPANTS

Major Potential Benefits

- Access to an intervention to which they might otherwise not have access
- Comfort in being able to discuss their situation or problem with an objective and nonjudgmental researcher
- Increased knowledge about themselves or their conditions, either through opportunity for introspection or through direct interaction with the researcher
- Enhanced self-esteem resulting from special attention or treatment
- Escape from normal routine, excitement of being part of a scientific study, and satisfaction of curiosity about what it is like to participate in a study
- Knowledge that the information subjects provide may help others with similar problems or conditions
- Direct monetary or material gains

Major Potential Costs

- Physical harm, including unanticipated side effects
- Physical discomfort, fatigue, or boredom
- Psychologic or emotional distress resulting from self-disclosure, introspection, fear of the unknown or interacting with strangers, fear of eventual repercussions, anger at the type of questions being asked, and so on
- Loss of privacy
- Loss of time
- Monetary costs (e.g., for transportation, baby-sitting, time lost from work, or charges for additional procedures and tests associated with the research)

≡ *THE PRINCIPLE OF RESPECT FOR HUMAN DIGNITY*

Respect for the human dignity of subjects is the second ethical principle articulated in the Belmont Report. This principle includes the right to self-determination and the right to full disclosure.

The Right to Self-determination

Humans should be treated as autonomous agents, capable of controlling their own activities and destinies. The principle of *self-determination* means that prospective subjects have the right to voluntarily decide whether or not to participate in a study, without the risk of incurring any penalties or prejudicial treatment. It also means that subjects have the right to decide at any point to terminate their participation, to refuse to give information, or to ask for clarification about the purpose of the study or specific questions.

A person's right to self-determination includes freedom from coercion of any type. *Coercion* involves explicit or implicit threats of penalty from failing to participate in a study, or excessive rewards from agreeing to participate. The obligation to honor and protect individuals from coercion may require careful thought when the researcher is in a position of authority, control, or influence over potential subjects, as might often be the case in a nurse–patient relationship. The ideal of noncoercion may also require intense scrutiny even when there is not a pre-established relationship. For example, a monetary incentive offered to an economically disadvantaged group—such as the homeless—might be considered mildly coercive; its acceptability might have to be evaluated in terms of the risk/benefit ratio. That is, if risks are high relative to any benefits and the group of subjects is vulnerable, monetary incentives (sometimes referred to as *subject stipends*) may place undue pressure on prospective subjects.

The Right to Full Disclosure

The principle of respect for human dignity encompasses people's right to make informed voluntary decisions about their participation in a study. Such decisions cannot be made without full disclosure. *Full disclosure* means that the researcher has fully described the nature of the study, the subject's right to refuse participation, the researcher's responsibilities, and the likely risks and benefits that would be incurred. The right to self-determination and the right to full disclosure are the two major elements upon which informed consent is based. Procedures for obtaining informed consent from research subjects are discussed in a later section of this chapter.

Although full disclosure is normally provided to subjects before their participation in a study, there is often a need for further disclosure after the subjects have participated, either in debriefing sessions or in written communications. For example, issues that arise during the course of collecting information from subjects may need to be clarified, or the participant may want aspects of the study explained once again. Many investigators also offer to send participants summaries of the research findings after the information has been analyzed.

Issues Relating to the Principle of Respect

Although most researchers would, in the abstract, endorse subjects' right to self-determination and full disclosure, there are circumstances that make these standards difficult to adhere to in practice. One issue concerns the inability of certain individuals to make well-informed judgments about the costs and benefits associated with participation. Children, for example, may be unable to give truly informed consent. The issue of groups that are vulnerable within a research context is discussed in a subsequent section of this chapter.

There are other circumstances in which the researcher may feel that the right to full disclosure and self-determination must be violated for the research to yield meaningful information. Researchers concerned with the validity of the study findings are sometimes worried that full disclosure might result in two types of biases: (1) the bias resulting from distorted information and (2) the bias resulting from failure to recruit a representative sample.

Let us suppose that a researcher were studying the relationship between men's drinking patterns and spouse abuse. That is, the researcher wanted to know if men who abused their wives were heavier users and more regular users of alcohol than men who did not abuse their wives. If the researcher approached potential subjects and fully explained the purpose of the study, certain people might refuse to participate. The problem is that nonparticipation would be highly selective; one would expect, in fact, that the type of person least likely to volunteer for such a study would be men who had abused their wives or men who were heavy drinkers—the very groups of primary interest in the research. Moreover, by knowing the focus of the study, those who did volunteer to participate might be less inclined to give candid responses. The researcher in such a situation might argue that full disclosure would totally undermine his or her ability to conduct the study productively.

Researchers who feel that full disclosure is incompatible with the conduct of rigorous scientific research sometimes use two techniques. The first is *covert data collection* or *concealment,* which means the collection of information without the subjects' knowledge and, thus, obviously without their consent. This might happen, for example, if a researcher wanted to observe naturalistic behavior in a real-world setting and was concerned that doing so openly would result in changes in the very behavior of interest. In such a situation, the researcher might obtain the information through concealed methods, such as by audiotaping or videotaping subjects through hidden equipment, observing through a one-way mirror, or observing while pretending to be engaged in other activities. As another example of covert data collection, hospital patients might unwittingly become subjects in a study through the researcher's use of existing hospital records. In general, covert data collection may be acceptable as long as the risks to the subjects are negligible and the subjects' right to privacy has not been violated. Covert data collection is least likely to be ethically acceptable if the research is focused on sensitive aspects of the subjects' behavior, such as drug use, sexual conduct, or illegal acts.

The second, and more controversial, technique is the researcher's use of *deception.* Deception can involve either withholding information about the study or providing subjects with false information. For example, the researcher studying spouse abuse might describe the research as a study of marital relationships, which is a mild form of misinformation.

The practice of deception is clearly problematic from an ethical standpoint because it interferes with the subjects' right to make a truly informed decision regarding the personal costs and benefits of participation. Some people argue that the use of deception is never justified. Others, however, believe that if the study involves minimal risk to subjects and if there are anticipated benefits to science and society, then deception may be justified to enhance the validity of the findings. APA's (1982) code of ethics offers the following guideline regarding the use of deception and concealment:

> Methodological requirements of a study may make the use of concealment or deception necessary. Before conducting such a study, the investigator has a special responsibility to (1) determine whether the use of such techniques is justified by the study's prospective scientific, education, or applied value; (2) determine whether alternative procedures are available that do not use concealment or deception; and (3) ensure that the participants are provided with sufficient explanation as soon as possible. (pp. 35–36)

≡ THE PRINCIPLE OF JUSTICE

The third broad principle articulated in the Belmont Report concerns justice. This principle includes the subjects' right to fair treatment and their right to privacy.

The Right to Fair Treatment

Subjects have the right to fair and equitable treatment both before, during, and after their participation in the study. Fair treatment includes the following aspects:

- the fair and nondiscriminatory selection of subjects such that any risks and benefits will be equitably shared; subject selection should be based on research requirements and not based on the convenience, gullibility, or compromised position of certain types of people
- the nonprejudicial treatment of individuals who decline to participate or who withdraw from the study after agreeing to participate
- the honoring of all agreements made between the researcher and the subject, including adherence to the procedures outlined in advance and the payment of any promised stipends
- subjects' access to research personnel at any point in the study to clarify information
- subjects' access to appropriate professional assistance if there is any physical or psychologic damage
- debriefing, if necessary, to divulge information that was withheld before the study or to clarify issues that arose during the study
- respectful and courteous treatment at all times

The Right to Privacy

Virtually all research with humans constitutes some type of intrusion into the subjects' personal lives. Researchers need to ensure that their research is not more intrusive than it needs to be and that the subjects' privacy is maintained throughout the study.

Subjects have the right to expect that any information collected during the course of a study will be kept in strictest confidence. This can occur either through anonymity or through other confidentiality procedures. *Anonymity* occurs when even the researcher cannot link a subject with the information for that subject. For example, if questionnaires were distributed to a group of nursing home residents and the questionnaires were returned without any identifying information on them, the responses would be considered anonymous. As another example, if a researcher reviewed hospital records from which all identifying information (e.g., name, address, social security number, and so forth) had been expunged, anonymity would again protect the subjects' right to privacy. Whenever it is possible to achieve anonymity, the researcher should strive to do so.

In situations in which anonymity is impossible, appropriate confidentiality procedures need to be implemented. A *promise of confidentiality* to subjects is a guarantee that any information that the subject provides will not be publicly reported or made accessible to parties other than those involved in the research. This means that research information should not be shared with strangers nor with people known to the subjects, such as family members, counselors, physicians, and other nurses, unless the researcher has been given explicit permission to share the information.

Researchers can take a number of steps to safeguard the confidentiality of subjects, including the following:

- Obtain identifying information from subjects only when it is essential to do so.
- Assign an identification (ID) number to each subject and attach the ID number rather than other identifiers to the actual research information.
- Maintain any identifying information and lists of ID numbers with corresponding identifying information in a locked file.
- Restrict access to identifying information to a small number of individuals, on a "need-to-know" basis.
- Enter no identifying information onto computer files.
- Destroy identifying information as quickly as feasible.
- Have all research personnel who have contact with the research information or identifiers sign pledges of confidentiality.
- Report research information in the aggregate; if information for a specific subject is reported, take steps to disguise the person's identity, such as the use of a fictitious name together with sparing use of descriptors of the individual.

≡ INFORMED CONSENT

Potential subjects who are fully informed about the nature of the research, the demands that it will make on them, and potential costs and benefits to be incurred are in a position to make thoughtful decisions regarding participation in the study. *Informed consent* means that subjects have adequate information regarding the research; are capable of comprehending the information; and have the power of free choice, enabling them to voluntarily consent to participate in the research or decline participation. This section discusses procedures for obtaining informed consent.

The Content of Informed Consent

Fully informed consent involves the disclosure of the following pieces of information to prospective subjects:

1. Subject status. Prospective subjects should be informed that the information they provide will be used in a research investigation. Patients should be told which health-care activities are routine and which are implemented specifically for the purposes of the research.
2. Study purpose. The overall purpose of conducting the research should be stated, preferably in lay rather than technical terms. The use to which the research information will be put should also be described.
3. Type of information. Prospective subjects should be told the type of information that will be obtained from them during the course of the study.
4. Nature of the commitment. Information regarding the duration of the study should be provided, together with an estimated time commitment at each point of contact.
5. Sponsorship. Information on who is sponsoring or funding the research should be mentioned; if the study is a course or degree requirement, this information should be shared.
6. Subject selection. The researcher should ex-

plain how the prospective subjects came to be selected for recruitment into the study; the explanation may also indicate how many subjects will be involved in the study.

7. Procedures. Prospective subjects should be given a description of the procedures that will be used to collect research information and of the procedures involved in any special or experimental treatment.

8. Potential risks or costs. Prospective subjects should be informed of any potential foreseeable risks (physical, psychologic, or economic) or costs that might be incurred as a result of participation. The possibility of unforeseeable risks should also be discussed, if appropriate. If injury or damage is possible, treatments that will be made available to subjects should be described.

9. Potential benefits. Specific benefits to subjects, if any, should be described, together with information on possible benefits to others. If subject stipends are to be paid, they should be discussed.

10. Confidentiality pledge. Prospective subjects should be assured that their privacy will at all times be protected.

11. Voluntary consent. The researcher should clearly indicate that participation is strictly voluntary and that failure to comply will not result in any penalties or loss of benefits.

12. Right to withdraw. Prospective subjects should be informed that even after consenting to cooperate they will have the right to withdraw from the study and to refuse to provide any specific piece of information. Additionally, researchers may, in some cases, need to provide subjects with a description of circumstances under which the researcher will terminate their participation or the overall study.

13. Alternatives. If appropriate, the researcher should provide information regarding alternative procedures or treatments that exist, if any, that might be advantageous to subjects.

14. Contact information. The researcher should provide information on whom the subjects could contact in the event of further ques-

tions, comments, or complaints relating to the research or to the subjects' rights.

Comprehension of Informed Consent

The information just described is normally presented to prospective subjects orally while they are being recruited to participate in a study. As discussed in the next section, researchers often present information to prospective subjects in writing as well. However, a written form should not take the place of an oral explanation of critical information about the study (unless the study does not involve face-to-face contact with subjects). Oral presentations provide opportunities for greater elaboration and for subject questioning. Because informed consent is based on a person's evaluation of the potential costs and benefits of participation, it is important that the critical information be not only communicated but also understood.

Researchers preparing statements for prospective subjects should be careful to use simple language, avoiding jargon and technical terms whenever possible. Written statements should be consistent with the subjects' reading levels and educational levels. For subjects from a general population (e.g., patients in a hospital), the statement should be written at about the seventh- or eighth-grade reading level.

For studies involving more than minimal risk, researchers need to make special efforts to ensure that prospective subjects understand what participation in the research will involve. In some cases, this might involve "testing" the subjects for their comprehension of the informed consent material before ruling them eligible for participation.

Documentation of Informed Consent

In most cases, researchers should document the informed consent process by having subjects sign a consent form. Federal regulations covering studies conducted under the sponsorship of government agencies require written consent, except under two circumstances: (1) when the consent document would be the only record linking the subject and the research information, and subjects agree that documentation can be foregone in the interest of protecting their privacy; or (2) when the study involves minimal risk and involves no procedures for which written consent would normally be needed. For example, for studies involving the completion of a questionnaire, informed consent documentation is normally optional.

The consent form should contain all of the information essential to informed consent, as described in a previous section. An example of a written consent form is presented in Figure 3-1. The prospective subject should have ample time to review the written document before signing it. The document should also be signed by the researcher, and a copy should be maintained by both parties.

If the informed consent information is lengthy, government regulations give researchers whose study is funded by federal agencies the option of presenting the full information orally and then summarizing essential information in a "short form." However, if a short form is used, the oral presentation must be witnessed by a third party, and the signature of the witness must appear on the short consent form. The signature of a third-party witness is also advisable in studies involving more than minimal risk, even when a long and comprehensive consent form is used.

≡ *VULNERABLE SUBJECTS*

Adherence to ethical standards such as those discussed thus far may, in most cases, be straightforward. However, the rights of special vulnerable groups may need to be protected through additional procedures and heightened sensitivity on the part of the researcher. Vulnerable subjects may be incapable of giving fully informed consent (e.g., mentally retarded people) or may be at high risk of unintended side effects because of

their circumstances (e.g., pregnant women). Researchers interested in studying high-risk groups should become acquainted with laws and guidelines governing informed consent, risk/benefit assessments, and acceptable procedures for research involving the group of interest. In general, research with vulnerable groups should be undertaken only when the researcher has determined that the benefit-to-risk ratio is very high.

Among the groups that nurse researchers should consider as being especially vulnerable are the following:

- Children. Legally and ethically, children do not have the competence to give their informed consent. Generally, the informed consent of children's parents or legal guardians should be obtained. If the child is developmentally mature enough to understand the basic information involved in informed consent (e.g., a 13-year-old), it is advisable to obtain written consent from the child as well, as evidence of respect for the child's right to self-determination.
- Mentally or emotionally disabled people. Individuals whose disability makes it impossible for them to weigh the risks and benefits of participation and make an informed decision (e.g., people affected by mental retardation, senility, mental illness, unconsciousness, and so on) also cannot legally or ethically be expected to provide informed consent. In such cases, the researcher should obtain the written consent of each person's legal guardian. However, the researcher should be sensitive to the fact that the legal guardian may not necessarily have the person's best interests in mind. In such cases, informed consent should also be obtained from a person whose primary interest is the person's welfare. As in the case of children, informed consent from prospective subjects themselves should be sought to the extent possible, in addition to consent from the guardian.
- Physically disabled people. For certain physical disabilities, special procedures for obtain-

In signing this document, I am giving my consent to be interviewed by an employee of Human-alysis, Inc., a nonprofit research organization based in Saratoga Springs, New York. I understand that I will be part of a research study that will focus on the experiences and needs of mothers of young children in the United States. This study, supported by a grant from the U.S. Department of Health and Human Services, will provide some guidance to people who are trying to help mothers and their children.

I understand that I will be interviewed in my home at a time convenient to me. I will be asked some questions about my experiences as a parent, my feelings about how to raise children, the health and characteristics of my oldest child, and my use of community services. I also understand that the interviewer will ask to have my oldest child present during at least some portion of the interview. The interview will take about 1½ to 2 to hours to complete. I also understand that the researcher may contact me for more information in the future.

I understand that I was selected to participate in this study because I was involved in a study of young mothers at the time of my oldest child's birth. At that time, I was recruited into the study, along with about 500 other young mothers, through a hospital or service agency.

This interview was granted freely. I have been informed that the interview is entirely voluntary, and that even after the interview begins I can refuse to answer any specific questions or decide to terminate the interview at any point. I have been told that my answers to questions will not be given to anyone else and no reports of this study will ever identify me in any way. I have also been informed that my participation or nonparticipation or my refusal to answer questions will have no effect on services that I or any member of my family may receive from health or social services providers.

This study will help develop a better understanding of the experiences of young mothers and the services that can be most helpful to them and their children. However, I will receive no direct benefit as a result of participation. As a means of compensating for any fatigue, inconvenience or monetary costs associated with participating in the study, I have received $25 for granting this interview.

I understand that the results of this research will be given to me if I ask for them and that Dr. Denise Polit is the person to contact if I have any questions about the study or about my rights as a study participant. Dr. Polit can be reached through a collect call at (518) 587-3994.

_____   _____
Date   Respondent's Signature

                                         _____
                                         Interviewer's Signature

Figure 3-1. *Sample consent form.*

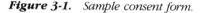

ing consent may be required. For example, with deaf subjects, the entire consent process may need to be in writing. For people who have a physical impairment preventing them from writing (or for subjects who cannot read and write), alternative procedures for documenting informed consent (such as audiotap-ing or videotaping the consent proceedings) should be used.

- Institutionalized people. Nurses often conduct studies using hospitalized or institutionalized people as subjects. Special care may be required in recruiting such subjects, because they often depend on health-care personnel and may feel pressured into participating or may feel that their treatment would be jeopardized by their failure to cooperate. Inmates of prisons and other correctional facilities, who have lost their autonomy in many spheres of activity, may similarly feel constrained in their ability to give free consent. The government has issued special regulations for the additional protection of prisoners as subjects (see Code of Federal Regulations, 1983). Researchers studying institutionalized groups need to emphasize the voluntary nature of participation.

- Pregnant women. The government has issued stringent additional requirements governing research with pregnant women (Code of Federal Regulations, 1983). These requirements reflect a desire to safeguard both the pregnant woman, who may be at heightened physical and psychologic risk, and the fetus, who cannot give informed consent. The regulations stipulate that a pregnant woman cannot be involved in a study unless the purpose of the research is to meet the health needs of the pregnant woman and risks to her and the fetus will be minimized or there is only a minimal risk to the fetus.

≡ REVIEWING THE PROTECTION OF HUMAN RIGHTS

Researchers may not be objective in their assessment of the risk/benefit ratio or in their development of procedures to protect the rights of subjects. Biases may arise as a result of the researchers' commitment to an area of knowledge and their desire to conduct a study with as much scientific rigor as possible. Because of the risk of a biased evaluation, the ethical dimensions of a study should normally be subjected to external review.

Institutional Review Boards

Most hospitals, universities, and other institutions where research is conducted have estab-

lished formal committees and protocols for reviewing research plans and proposed research procedures. These committees are sometimes called "human subjects committees" or "research advisory panels."* If the institution receives federal funds that help to pay for the costs of research, it is likely that the committee will be an *Institutional Review Board* (IRB).

Research involving human subjects that is sponsored through federal funds (including federally sponsored fellowships) is subject to strict guidelines for evaluating the treatment of human subjects. Before undertaking such a study, the researcher must submit research plans to the IRB.† The duty of the IRB is to ensure that the proposed plans meet the federal requirements for ethical research. An IRB can approve the proposed plans, require modifications, or disapprove the plans. IRB decisions are usually documented on an approval form, such as the one shown in Figure 3-2. The main requirements governing IRB decisions may be summarized as follows (Code of Federal Regulations, 1983):

- Risks to subjects are minimized.
- Risks to subjects are reasonable in relation to anticipated benefits, if any, to subjects, and the importance of the knowledge that may reasonably be expected to result.
- Selection of subjects is equitable.
- Informed consent will be sought, as required.
- Informed consent will be appropriately documented.
- Adequate provision is made for monitoring the research to ensure the safety of subjects.

* Many clinical agencies have specific protocols and forms for submitting human subjects' protection information. Because nursing students are often under fairly stringent time constraints to complete course-related research projects, they should consult with the nurse researcher or nursing administration personnel at the agency as quickly as possible to determine the appropriate procedures to follow. Additionally, it is advantageous to ascertain the time sequence for proposal submission, the schedule of Institutional Review Board (IRB) or human subjects committee meetings, and when the researcher may expect to receive information regarding the committee's decision.

† See Appendix A for an example.

- Appropriate provisions are made to protect the privacy of subjects and the confidentiality of data.
- When vulnerable subjects are involved, appropriate additional safeguards are included to protect the rights and welfare of these subjects.

Many research projects require a full review by the IRB. For a full review, the IRB convenes meetings at which a majority of IRB members must be present. An IRB must consist of five or more members, at least one of whom is not a researcher (e.g., a member of the clergy or a lawyer might be appropriate). One member of the IRB must also be a person who has no affiliation with the institution and is not a family member of a person affiliated with the institution. The IRB cannot comprise entirely men (or women) or members from a single profession. These requirements are designed to safeguard against the possibility of various biases.

For certain kinds of research involving no more than minimal risk to human subjects, the IRB can use expedited review procedures, which do not require that a meeting be convened. In an *expedited review,* a single IRB member (usually the IRB chairperson or another member designated by the chairperson) carries out the review. Examples of the kinds of research activities that qualify for an expedited IRB review include the following:

- recording of information from subjects 18 years old or older using noninvasive procedures routinely employed in clinical practice (e.g., weighing, testing sensory acuity, electrocardiography, and thermography)
- collection of blood samples by venipuncture, in amounts not exceeding 450 milliliters, in an 8-week period from subjects at least 18 years old, in good health, and not pregnant
- collection of excreta and external secretions, including sweat, uncannulated saliva, placenta removed at delivery, and amniotic fluid at the time of rupture of the membrane before or during delivery
- the study of existing documents, records, pathologic specimens, or diagnostic specimens
- research on individual behavior or characteristics where the researcher does not manipulate the subjects' behavior and where the study will not involve stress to the subjects

The federal regulations also allow certain types of research to be totally exempt from IRB review. These are studies in which there are no apparent risks to human subjects. Box 3-2 summarizes the types of research for which investigators could request an exemption from the IRB review process.

Other External Reviews

Not all research is subject to federal guidelines, and so not all studies are reviewed by IRBs or other formal committees. Nevertheless, researchers have a responsibility to ensure that their research plans are ethically acceptable. APA's (1982) code of ethics stipulates that investigators should seek the advice of others with issues relating to the protection of human subjects: "That investigators cannot rely on their own judgements to be unbiased underlies the recommendation that investigators turn to the advice of others.... The investigator should seek advice with respect to the potential costs of the research procedures to the participants, even if there is no legal requirement to do so" (p. 20). "Advisers" could include faculty members, the clergy, representatives from the group that would be asked to participate in the research, or advocates for that group.

≡ *RESEARCH EXAMPLES*

Because researchers generally attempt to report the results of their research as succinctly as possible, they rarely describe in much detail the efforts they have made to safeguard the rights of their subjects. (The absence of any mention of such safeguards does not, of course, imply that no precautions were taken.) Researchers are espe-

REVIEW OF SAFEGUARDS FOR HUMAN SUBJECTS

Proposal/Project Number: Internal _____ Sponsor: _____

Proposal/Project Title: _____

_____

Type of review:

____ Determination of Exemption ____ Full Board Proposal Review
____ Expedited Review ____ Ongoing research in certifi-
cation of change

____ Other (Specify): _____

_____

After reviewing the above proposal/project:

Exemption ____ The institutional official has determined that the research is exempt under 45 CFR 46.101 (b) or

Safeguards ____ This Institutional Review Board (or member signing below in the case of expedited review) has determined by unanimous vote of the members present that:

____ Risks to subjects are minimized and are reasonable in relation to anticipated benefits. Selection of subjects is equitable, and the privacy of the subjects and confidentiality of the data are adequately protected. Approval is given.

____ Approval is given under the following conditions:

____ Approval is not given, for the following reasons:

Where applicable, attach summary of controverted issues and their resolution.

_____

Date: _____

Names of Members Present: *Signatures of Members Present:*

_____   _____

_____   _____

_____   _____

_____   _____

_____   _____

Figure 3-2. *Sample IRB review/approval form.*

BOX 3-2 TYPES OF RESEARCH EXEMPT FROM IRB REVIEW

Research activities in which the only involvement of human subjects will be in one or more of the following categories are ordinarily exempt from IRB review:

1. Research conducted in established or commonly accepted educational settings, involving normal educational practices.
2. Research involving the use of educational tests (cognitive, diagnostic, achievement), if information taken from these sources is recorded such that the identity of subjects is not divulged.
3.* Research involving survey or interview procedures, *except* where all the following conditions are met:
    a. responses are recorded in such a way that the human subjects can be identified
    b. the subject's responses, if they became known, could place the subject at risk of criminal or civil liability or financial loss
    c. the research deals with sensitive aspects of the subject's own behavior, such as illegal conduct, sexual behavior, or use of alcohol
4. Research involving the observation of public behavior, except when all of the three conditions described above in (3) exist.
5. Research involving the collection or study of existing data, documents, records, pathological specimens, if the sources are publicly available or if the information is recorded such that the subject cannot be identified.
6. Unless specifically required by statute, research and demonstration projects that are conducted or approved by the U.S. Department of Health and Human Services that are designed to study or evaluate the following:
    a. programs under the Social Security Act or other public benefit or service programs
    b. procedures for obtaining benefits or services under those programs
    c. possible changes in or alterations to those programs or procedures
    d. possible changes in methods or levels of payment for benefits or services under those programs

*The exemption does not apply when the subjects are minors. Also, all survey research is exempt, without exception, when the subjects are elected or appointed public officials or are candidates for public office.

These exemptions are based on guidelines appearing in the Code of Federal Regulations, revised as of March 8, 1983.

cially likely to discuss their adherence to human subjects guidelines when the study involves more than minimal risk or when the group of people being studied is a vulnerable one. Table 3-1 outlines the procedures used in several studies in which the authors did describe some of the steps taken to protect human rights. Below is one example of a study in which safeguards were described in considerable detail.

Engle (1986) was interested in studying movement (as measured by a person's walking cadence, or the number of steps walked per minute) and time (as measured by a person's perceived duration of a fixed interval of clock time) in relation to functional health in older women. She believed that women who were healthy would exhibit faster movement and shorter perception of time.

A sample of 114 women older than age 60, who were able to speak English and give informed consent, was drawn at random from residents of federally subsidized housing for the aged. Permission to do the study was obtained from both the resident council and the administration of the housing units.

Potential participants received a letter explaining the study, followed by a telephone call to obtain verbal consent and to set up an appointment. The person collecting the information met with the participants in their apartment for approximately 1 hour, during which time informed consent was obtained. A letter was sent to participants within 1 week to thank them, and within 1 year to give them the results of the study. Engle found that functional health was higher among those women whose movement was faster, and concluded that movement, as measured by walking cadence, may be a useful measure of older adults' health.

Engle took a number of steps in her study to ensure that the research was conducted ethically. The researcher excluded from participation any potential subjects who could not give informed consent because of language barriers. She obtained consent from each individual participant, as well as from groups overseeing the housing units. She selected subjects fairly (i.e., at random, rather than on the basis of some arbitrary traits)

Table 3-1.   *Examples of Procedures to Protect Human Rights*

PRINCIPLE	STUDY QUESTION	PROCEDURES
Informed consent IRB review	What are the effects of non-oscillating waterbed flotation on energy expenditure in preterm infants?	Parents of the infants signed an informed consent form allowing infants to participate. Approval for the conduct of the study was obtained from appropriate committees for the protection of human subjects. (Deiriggi, 1990)
Anonymity Informed consent	What are the smoking practices of critical-care nurses?	Questionnaires were distributed and instructions given to place completed questionnaires in a collection box. Information was obtained anonymously, and potential subjects were informed that completion and return of the questionnaire would be considered as voluntary informed consent. (Haughey et al., 1989)
Informed consent of minors	What is the effect of backrest elevation on central venous pressure readings in children after cardiac surgery?	The researcher met with each child's parent or legal guardian, explained the study, and obtained informed consent. (Callow & Pieper, 1989)
Anonymity Informed consent IRB review Risk reduction	What are patients' attitudes about, desired knowledge of, and involvement in clinical research in a tertiary medical care setting?	Subjects volunteered to participate after being informed of the study purpose, and completed an anonymous questionnaire. Vulnerable subjects (e.g., mentally retarded or confused persons) were excluded from the study. The study was approved by an IRB. (Larson & McGuire, 1990)
Informed consent Confidentiality/ anonymity	Does the communication style of nursing students change as a result of increased education or experience?	All respondents signed an informed consent form and were assured of the confidentiality of their responses. Special coding procedures were undertaken to ensure anonymity. (Harrison et al., 1989)
IRB review Risk reduction	Which measurement site is optimal for temperature monitoring in hypothermic postcardiac surgery patients?	Following approval by the appropriate IRBs, a sample of 55 patients was studied on admission to a cardiac surgery intensive care unit. Patients were excluded from the study if they had a recent history of rectal bleeding or surgery. (Mravinac et al., 1989)

and treated them with courtesy before, during, and after the study was completed.

≡ *SUMMARY*

Research involving humans requires a careful consideration of the procedures to be used to protect the rights of human *subjects*. Because scientific research has not always been conducted ethically, and because of the genuine dilemmas that researchers often face in designing studies that are both ethical and scientifically rigorous, codes of ethics have been developed to guide researchers. The three major ethical principles that are incorporated into most guidelines are beneficence, respect for human dignity, and justice.

Beneficence encompasses the maxim of "above all, do no harm." This principle involves the protection of subjects from physical and psychologic harm, protection of subjects from exploitation, and the performance of some good. In deciding to conduct a study, the researcher must carefully weigh the costs and benefits of participation to individual subjects and must also weigh the risks to the subjects against the potential benefits to society.

The principle of respect for human dignity includes the subjects' *right to self-determination,* which means that subjects have the freedom to control their own activities, including their voluntary participation in the study. The respect principle also includes the subjects' right to full disclosure. *Full disclosure* means that the researcher has fully described to prospective subjects the nature of the study and subjects' rights. Because full disclosure can lead to potentially misleading and distorted study findings, researchers sometimes feel that this principle can be violated in the name of good science. When full disclosure poses the risk of biased results, researchers sometimes use *covert data collection* or *concealment,* which means the collection of information without the subjects' knowledge or consent. In other research situations, researchers have used *deception* (either withholding information from subjects or providing false information) to avoid biases. When deception or concealment are necessary, extra precautions are usually needed to minimize risks and protect the other rights of subjects.

The third principle, *justice,* includes the *right to fair treatment* (both in the selection of subjects and during the course of the study) and the *right to privacy.* Privacy of subjects can be maintained through *anonymity* (wherein not even the researcher knows the identity of the subjects) or through formal *confidentiality procedures.* Whenever possible, researchers should strive to collect information anonymously.

Most studies should involve *informed consent* procedures designed to provide prospective subjects with sufficient information to make a reasoned decision about the potential costs and benefits of participation. Informed consent normally involves having the subject sign a consent form, which documents the subject's voluntary decision to participate after receiving a full explanation of the research.

Certain people, sometimes referred to as *vulnerable subjects,* require additional safeguards to protect their rights. These subjects may be vulnerable because they are not competent with regard to making an informed decision about participating in a study (e.g., children or mentally retarded people); because their circumstances make them feel that free choice is constrained (e.g., an institutionalized group of subjects); or because their circumstances heighten their risk for physical or psychologic harm (e.g., pregnant women).

External review of the ethical aspects of a study is highly recommended and, in many cases, is required by either the agency funding the research or the organization from which subjects would be recruited or within which the research would be conducted. Most institutions have special review committees for such purposes. Research funded through the federal government is normally reviewed by the *Institutional Review Board* (IRB) of the institution with which the researcher is affiliated. In studies in which risks to subjects are minimal, an *expedited review* (review by a single member of the IRB) may be substituted for a full board review; in cases where there are no anticipated risks, the research may be exempted from review. However, researchers are always advised to consult with at least one external adviser whose perspective allows him or her to evaluate objectively the ethics of a proposed study.

≡ STUDY SUGGESTIONS

1. Point out the ethical dilemmas that might emerge in the following studies:
   a. a study of the relationship between sleeping patterns and acting-out behaviors in hospitalized psychiatric patients
   b. a study of the effects of a new drug on human subjects
   c. an investigation of an individual's psychologic state following an abortion
   d. an investigation of the contraceptive decisions of adolescents (minors) using a family planning clinic
2. For each of the studies described in question 1, indicate whether you think the study would require a full IRB review or an expedited review, or whether it would be totally exempt from review.
3. For the study described in the research example section (the study by Engle, 1986), prepare an informed consent form that includes required information, as described in the section on informed consent.
4. Read "Conceptual models used in clinical practice" by M.G. Wardle and C.L. Mandle (1989, *Western Journal of Nursing Research, 11*, 108–114). Discuss the ethical aspects of this study.

≡ SUGGESTED READINGS

REFERENCES ON RESEARCH ETHICS

American Nurses' Association. (1975). *Human rights guidelines for nurses in clinical and other research*. Kansas City, MO: Author.

American Nurses' Association. (1985). *Code for nurses with interpretive statements*. Kansas City, MO: Author.

American Psychological Association. (1982). *Ethical principles in the conduct of research with human participants*. Washington, DC: Author.

American Sociological Association. (1984). *Code of ethics*. Washington, DC: Author.

Arminger, B., Sr. (1977). Ethics of nursing research: Profile, principles, perspective. *Nursing Research, 26,* 330–336.

Bower, R.T., & De Gasparis, P. (1978). *Ethics in social research: Protecting the interests of human subjects*. New York: Praeger Press.

Burns, N., & Grove, S.K. (1987). *The practice of nursing research: Conduct, critique, and utilization*. Philadelphia : W.B. Saunders. (Chapter 12).

Code of Federal Regulations. (1983). *Protection of human subjects: 45CFR46* (revised as of March 8, 1983). Washington, DC: Department of Health and Human Services.

Cowles, K.V. (1988). Issues in qualitative research on sensitive topics. *Western Journal of Nursing Research, 10,* 163–179.

Damrosch, S.P. (1986). Ensuring anonymity by use of subject-generated identification codes. *Research in Nursing and Health, 9,* 61–63.

Davis, A.J. (1985). Informed consent: How much information is enough? *Nursing Outlook, 33,* 40–42.

Davis, A.J. (1989a). Clinical nurses' ethical decision-making in situations of informed consent. *Advances in Nursing Science, 11,* 63–69.

Davis, A.J. (1989b). Informed consent process in research protocols: Dilemmas for clinical nurses. *Western Journal of Nursing Research, 11,* 448–457.

Davis, A.J., & Krueger, J.C. (1980). *Patients, nurses, ethics*. New York: American Journal of Nursing Co.

Diener, E., & Crandall, R. (1978). *Ethics in social and behavioral research*. Chicago: University of Chicago Press.

Jacobson, S.F. (1973). Ethical issues in experimentation with human subjects. *Nursing Forum, 12,* 58–71.

Levine, R.J. (1981). *Ethics and the regulation of clinical research*. Baltimore: Urban & Schwarzenberg, Inc.

May, K.A. (1979). The nurse as researcher: Impediment to informed consent? *Nursing Outlook, 27,* 36–40.

Munhall, P.L. (1988). Ethical considerations in qualitative research. *Western Journal of Nursing Research, 10,* 150–162.

National Commission for the Protection of Human Subjects of Biomedical and Behavioral Research. (1978). *Belmont report: Ethical principles and guidelines for research involving human subjects.* Washington, DC: U.S. Government Printing Office.

Packard, J.S. (1981). Human subjects protection in hospital field studies. *Western Journal of Nursing Research, 3,* 216–230.

Purtillo, R.B., & Cassel, C.K. (1981). *Ethical dimensions in the health profession.* Philadelphia: W.B. Saunders Co.

Ramos, M.C. (1989). Some ethical implications of qualitative research. *Research in Nursing and Health, 12,* 57–64.

Reynolds, P.D. (1979). *Ethical dilemmas and social science research.* San Francisco: Jossey-Bass.

Robb, S.S. (1983). Beware of the informed consent. *Nursing Research, 32,* 132–135.

Silva, M.C., & Sorrell, J.M. (1984). Factors influencing comprehension of information for informed consent. *International Journal of Nursing Studies, 21,* 233–240.

Watson, A.B. (1982). Informed consent of special subjects. *Nursing Research, 31,* 43–47.

Wilson, H.S. (1985). *Research in nursing.* Menlo Park, CA: Addison-Wesley. (Chapter 3).

SUBSTANTIVE REFERENCES*

Callow, L.B., & Pieper, B. (1989). Effect of backrest on central venous pressure in pediatric cardiac surgery. *Nursing Research, 38,* 336–338.

Deiriggi, P.M. (1990). Effects of waterbed flotation on indicators of energy expenditure in preterm infants. *Nursing Research, 39,* 140–146.

Engle, V.F. (1986). The relationship of movement and time to older adults' functional health. *Research in Nursing and Health, 9,* 123–129.

Harrison, T.M., Pistolessi, T.V., & Stephen, T.D. (1989). Assessing nurses' communication: A cross-sectional study. *Western Journal of Nursing Research, 11,* 75–91.

Haughey, B.P., Methewson, M.K., Dittmar, S.S., & Wu, Y.B. (1989). Smoking practices of critical care nurses. *Heart and Lung, 18,* 29–35.

Hinds, P.S., & Martin, J. (1988). Hopefulness and the self-sustaining process in adolescents with cancer. *Nursing Research, 38,* 336–339.

Larson, E., & McGuire, D.B. (1990). Patient experiences with research in a tertiary care setting. *Nursing Research, 39,* 168–171.

Mahon, N.E., & Yarcheski, A. (1988). Loneliness in early adolescents: An empirical test of alternate explanations. *Nursing Research, 37,* 330–335.

Moen, J.E., Chapman, S., Sheehan, A., & Carter, P. (1987). Axillary versus rectal temperatures in preterm infants under radiant warmers. *Journal of Obstetric, Gynecologic, and Neonatal Nursing, 16,* 48–55.

Morse, J.M., & Park, C. (1988). Home birth and hospital deliveries: A comparison of the perceived painfulness of parturition. *Research in Nursing and Health, 11,* 175–181.

Mravinac, C.M., Dracup, K., & Clochesy, J.M. (1989). Urinary bladder and rectal temperature monitoring during clinical hypothermia. *Nursing Research, 38,* 73–76.

Nuttall, P. (1988). Maternal responses to home apnea monitoring of infants. *Nursing Research, 37,* 354–357.

Walden, J., Stevenson, L., Dracup, K., Wilmarth, J., Kobashigawa, J., & Morigushi, J. (1989). Heart transplantation may not improve quality of life for patients with stable heart failure. *Heart and Lung, 18,* 497–506.

Zimmerman, L., Pozehi, B., Duncan, K., & Schmitz, R. (1989). Effects of music in patients who had chronic cancer pain. *Western Journal of Nursing Research, 11,* 298–309.

*In this chapter and in subsequent chapters, studies that illustrate the concepts discussed in the text are listed in the section designated as "Substantive References." The inclusion of a study is not intended to imply that it is technically excellent in all respects but rather that it contains a concept or methodological element that has relevance for the issues discussed in the chapter. The research reports listed here include an explicit reference to some of the precautions taken to protect the rights of human subjects, such as the use of informed consent procedures, the review of research plans by an IRB, and so on.

4
Overview of the Research Process

Scientific research, though complex, generally proceeds in an orderly fashion through a number of steps. In this chapter an overview of the major steps in research is presented so that the reader can gain some understanding of how a research study is planned and executed. In a sense, this chapter represents an outline of the issues that will be addressed in the remainder of the book.

Like any other discipline, scientific research has its own language and terminology. Therefore, before turning to the description of the steps involved in research, some important ideas and terms that will be discussed throughout this book are introduced here. Although a more thorough familiarization with research terminology will be acquired as the reader progresses through this book, it is recommended that this section be read with particular care before proceeding to more advanced chapters.

Scientific Concepts, Constructs, and Theories

Conceptualization refers to the process of developing and refining abstract ideas. Scientific research almost always is concerned with abstract rather than tangible phenomena. For example, the terms "illness," "pain," "emotional disturbance," "patient care," and "grieving" are all abstractions that are formulated by generalizing from particular manifestations of certain behaviors or characteristics. These abstractions are referred to as *concepts*.

The term construct is also encountered frequently in the scientific literature. Like the term concept, a *construct* refers to an abstraction or a mental representation inferred from situations, events, or behaviors. Kerlinger (1973) distinguished concepts from constructs by noting that constructs are terms that are deliberately and systematically invented (or constructed) by researchers for a specific scientific purpose. For example, "self-care" in Dorothea Orem's model of health maintenance may be considered a construct. In practice, the terms concept and construct are often used interchangeably.

A *theory* is an abstract generalization that presents a systematic explanation about the interrelationships among phenomena. Concepts are the building blocks of theories. In a theory, concepts (or constructs) are knitted together into an orderly system to explain the way in which our world and the people in it function.

Variables

Within the context of a research investigation, concepts are generally referred to as variables. A *variable* is, as the name implies, something that varies. Weight, height, body temperature, blood pressure readings, and preoperative anxiety levels all are variables. That is, each of these properties varies or differs from one individual to another. When one considers the variety and complexity of humans and their experiences, it becomes clear that nearly all aspects of individuals and the environment can be considered variables. If everyone had black hair and weighed 125 pounds, hair color and weight would not be variables. If it rained continuously and the outdoor temperature was a constant 70°F, weather would not be a variable. But it is precisely because individuals and conditions *do* vary that most research is conducted. The bulk of all research activity is aimed at trying to understand how or why things vary and to gain insights into how differences in one variable are related to differences in another. For example, lung cancer research is concerned with the variable of lung cancer, which is a variable because not everybody has lung cancer. Researchers in this area are concerned with learning what other variables can be linked to lung cancer. They have discovered that cigarette smoking appears to be related to lung

cancer. Again, this is a variable because not everyone smokes. A variable, then, is any quality of an organism, group, or situation that takes on different values.

CONTINUOUS VERSUS CATEGORICAL VARIABLES

Sometimes a variable can take on a range of different values. Age, for instance, can take on values from zero to more than 100 when we are referring to the age in years of humans. Such variables are sometimes referred to as *continuous variables,* because their values can be represented on a continuum. Continuous variables can meaningfully take on values that are not whole numbers. For example, a person's weight (another continuous variable) could be designated to the nearest tenth or hundredth of a pound.

Other variables, however, take on a much smaller range of values, representing discrete categories rather than incremental placement along a continuum. The variable "gender," for example, has only two values (male/female). Variables of this type, which take on only a handful of discrete values, are referred to as *categorical variables.* Other examples of categorical variables include race/ethnicity (e.g., white, black, Hispanic, other) and marital status (single, married, divorced/widowed, other). When categorical variables take on only two values, they are sometimes referred to as *dichotomous variables.* Some additional examples of categorical variables that are dichotomous include smoker/nonsmoker, presence of allergic reaction/absence of allergic reaction, alive/dead, and pregnant/nonpregnant.

ACTIVE VERSUS ATTRIBUTE VARIABLES

Variables are not restricted to preexisting attributes of individuals, organisms, events, or environments. In many research situations, the investigator creates or designs a variable. For example, if a researcher is interested in testing the effectiveness of ice chips as opposed to effervescent ginger ale to refresh the mouth after vomiting, some individuals might be given ice chips and others would receive ginger ale. For the purpose of this study, the type of mouth care may be considered a variable because different individuals receive ice chips or ginger ale. Kerlinger (1973) referred to these variables that the researcher creates or designs as *active variables. Attribute variables,* on the other hand, are preexisting characteristics that the researcher simply observes and measures.

DEPENDENT VERSUS INDEPENDENT VARIABLES

An important distinction is generally made between two types of variables in a research study, and it is a distinction that needs to be mastered before proceeding to later chapters. Many research studies are aimed at unraveling and understanding the causes underlying phenomena. Does a drug *cause* improvement of a medical problem? Does a nursing intervention *cause* more rapid recovery? Does smoking *cause* lung cancer? The presumed cause is referred to as the *independent variable* and the presumed effect is referred to as the *dependent variable.* Variability in the dependent variable is presumed to *depend* on variability in the independent variable. For example, the researcher investigates the extent to which lung cancer (the dependent variable) depends on smoking behavior (the independent variable). In another study, a researcher might examine the effects of two special formulas (the independent variable) on premature infants' weight gain (the dependent variable). Or, an investigator may be concerned with the extent to which patients' perception of pain (the dependent variable) depends on different types of nursing approaches (the independent variable).

The terms independent variable and dependent variable are frequently used to indicate directionality of influence rather than a causal connection. For example, let us say that a researcher is studying nurses' attitudes toward abortion and finds that older nurses hold less favorable opinions about abortion than younger nurses. The researcher might be unwilling to infer that the nurses' attitudes were *caused* by their age. Yet the direction of influence clearly runs from age to attitudes. That is, it would make little sense to suggest that the attitudes caused or influenced age. Even though in this example the researcher does not infer a causal relationship between age and attitudes, it is appropriate to conceptualize attitudes toward abortion as the dependent variable and age as the independent variable.

The dependent variable usually is the variable the researcher is interested in understanding, explaining, or predicting. In lung cancer research, it is the carcinoma that is of real interest to the research scientist, not smoking behavior per se. In studies of the effectiveness of therapeutic treatments for alcoholics, it is the drinking behavior of the subjects that is the dependent variable. Although a great deal of time, effort, and resources may be devoted to designing new therapies (the independent variable), they are of interest primarily as they relate to improvements in drinking behavior and overall functioning of alcoholics.

Many of the dependent variables that are studied by researchers have a multiplicity of causes or antecedents. If we are interested in studying the factors that influence people's weight, for example, we might consider their age, height, physical activity, and eating habits as the independent variables. Note that some of these independent variables are attribute variables (age and height), and others (activity and eating patterns) can be influenced by the investigator. Just as a study may examine more than one independent variable, two or more dependent variables may be of interest to the researcher. For example, an investigator may be concerned with comparing the effectiveness of two methods of nursing-care delivery (primary versus functional) for children with cystic fibrosis. Several dependent variables could be designated as measures of treatment effectiveness, such as length of stay in the hospital, number of recurrent respiratory infections, presence of cough, dyspnea on exertion, and so forth. In short, it is quite common to design studies with multiple independent and dependent variables.

The reader should not get the impression that variables are inherently dependent or independent. A variable that is classified as dependent in one study may be considered an independent variable in another study. For example, a researcher may find that the religious background of a nurse (the independent variable) has an effect on his or her attitude toward death and dying (the dependent variable). Another study, however, may analyze the extent to which nurses' attitudes toward death and dying (the independent variables) affect their job performance (the dependent variable). To illustrate this point with another example, consider a study that examines the relationship between contraceptive counseling (the independent variable) and unwanted pregnancies (the dependent variable). Yet another research project could study the effect of unwanted pregnancies (the independent variable) on the incidence of child abuse (the dependent variable). In short, the designation of a variable as independent or dependent is a function of the role the variable plays in a particular investigation. Table 4-1 presents some additional examples of research questions and specifies the dependent and independent variables.

It should be pointed out that some researchers use the term *criterion variable* (or criterion measure) rather than dependent variable. In studies that analyze the consequences of a treatment, therapy, or some other type of intervention, it is usually necessary to establish criteria against which the success of the intervention can be assessed and, hence, the origin of the expression criterion variable. The term dependent variable, however, is broader and more general in its implications and applicability. Therefore, we use the term dependent variable more frequently than criterion variable, although, in many situations, the two are equivalent and interchangeable.

A term that is frequently used in connection with variability is heterogeneity. When an attribute is extremely varied in the group under investigation, the group is said to be *heterogeneous* with respect to that variable. If, on the other hand, the amount of variability is limited, the group is described as relatively *homogeneous*. For example, with respect to the variable height, two-year-old

Table 4-1.   *Examples of Independent and Dependent Variables*

RESEARCH QUESTION	INDEPENDENT VARIABLE	DEPENDENT VARIABLE
What are the effects of alternatively worded messages regarding the results of a Pap test on women's follow-up visits to clinics? (Lauver & Rubin, 1990)	Messages with alternative wordings	Follow-up visits
What is the effect of a comprehensive discharge planning protocol by a gerontological nurse specialist on the postdischarge morbidity of hospitalized elderly? (Naylor, 1990)	Discharge planning protocol	Postdischarge morbidity
Do visits by family members affect a hospitalized patient's intracranial pressure? (Prins, 1989)	Family visits	Intracranial pressure
What is the effect of a parent-recorded story (vs. stranger-recorded story vs. no story) on the incidence of distress in hosptialized children? (White et al., 1990)	Story presentation	Incidence of distress
Do alcoholic women experience more menstrual distress than nonalcoholic women? (Shelley & Anderson, 1986)	Alcohlic status	Menstrual distress

children are generally more homogeneous than 18-year-old adolescents. The degree of variability of a group has implications for the design of a study.

Operational Definitions

Before a study progresses, the researcher usually clarifies and defines the variables under investigation. This is especially likely to be the case in quantitative studies. For the definition to be precise, the researcher should specify how the variable will be observed and measured in the actual research situation. Such a definition of a concept, an *operational definition,* is a specification of the operations that the researcher must perform to collect the required information.

Variables differ considerably in the facility with which they can be operationalized. The variable weight, for example, is easy to define and measure. We may use as our definition of weight "the heaviness or lightness of an object in terms of pounds." Note that this definition designates that weight will be determined according to one measuring system (pounds) rather than another (grams). The operational definition might specify that the weight of subjects in a research study would be measured to the nearest pound using a spring scale with the subjects fully undressed after ten hours of fasting. This operational definition spells out what the investigator must do to measure weight in such a way that a person not associated with the study would know precisely what the term "weight" meant.

Unfortunately, many of the variables of interest in nursing research are not operationalized as easily and straightforwardly as weight. Often there are multiple methods of measuring a variable, and the researcher must choose the method that best captures the variable as he or she conceptualizes it. For example, "patient well-being" may be defined in terms of either physiologic or psychologic functioning. If the researcher chooses to emphasize the physiologic aspects of patient well-being, the operational definition would involve a measure such as heart rate, white blood cell count, blood pressure, vital capacity,

and so forth. (Furthermore, the definition should clarify what is meant by "patient.") If, on the other hand, well-being is conceptualized for the purposes of research as primarily a psychologic phenomenon, the operational definition would need to identify the method by which emotional well-being would be assessed, as for example the responses of the patient to certain questions or the behavior of the patient as observed by the researcher.

Not all readers of a research report may agree with the way that the investigator has conceptualized and operationalized the concepts. Nevertheless, precision in defining the terms conceptually and operationally has the advantage of communicating exactly what the terms mean. If the researcher is reluctant to be explicit, it will be impossible for others to gauge the full meaning and implications of the research findings. Table 4-2 presents some operational definitions from several nursing research studies.

Researchers operating in a phenomenological framework generally do not define in operational terms the concepts in which they are interested before gathering information. This is because of their desire to have the meaning of concepts defined by those being studied themselves. Nevertheless, in summarizing the results of a study, all researchers should be careful in describing the conceptual and methodological basis of key research concepts.

Relationships

Researchers are rarely interested in single, isolated variables, except perhaps in some descriptive studies. As an example of a descriptive study, a researcher might focus on the percentage of women who elect to breast-feed their babies. In this example, there is only one variable: breast-feeding versus bottle-feeding. Usually, however, researchers study two or more variables simultaneously. What scientists are most often interested in is the *relationship* between the independent and dependent variables of a study.

But what exactly is meant by the term "relationship" in scientific terms? Generally speaking, a *relationship* refers to a bond or connection between two entities. Let us consider as a possible dependent variable a person's body weight. What variables are related to (associated with) a person's weight? Some possibilities include height, bone structure, metabolism, caloric intake, and exercise. For each of these five independent variables, we can make a tentative "relational" statement:

Height: Tall people, in general, weigh more than short people.
Bone structure: The finer the bone structure, the lower the person's weight.
Metabolism: The lower a person's metabolic rate, the more he or she weighs.
Caloric intake: People with high caloric intake are heavier than those with lower caloric intake.
Exercise: The greater the amount of exercise, the lower the person's weight.

Each of these statements expresses a presumed relationship between weight and an independent variable. The terms "more than" and "lower than" imply that as we observe a change in one variable, we are likely to observe a corresponding change in the other. If Jane were taller than Jean, we would expect (in the absence of any other information) that Jane would be also heavier than Jean.

Research is often conducted to determine whether relationships exist among variables, as suggested by the following research questions. Is there a relation between nursing shift assignments and absentee rates? Is there a relation between the frequency of turning patients and the incidence and severity of decubiti? Is prematurity related to the incidence of nosocomial viral infections? The scientific method can be used to answer questions about whether and to what degree variables are related.

Variables can be related to one another in different ways. Scientists are often interested in what is referred to as *cause-and-effect relationships*. As noted in Chapter 2, the scientist assumes that natural phenomena are not random or haphazard, but rather that all phenomena have antecedent factors or causes, and that these causes are generally discoverable. If variable X causes the occurrence or manifestation of variable Y, then it can be said that those variables are causally related. For instance, in the previous example, we might say that there is a causal relationship between caloric intake and weight: eating more calories causes increased weight.

Table 4-2. *Examples of Operational Definitions*

SOURCE	CONCEPT	OPERATIONAL DEFINITION
Naylor, 1990	Postdischarge morbidity	Number of rehospitalizations that patients reported during the 12-week period following initial hospital discharge; number and type of infections following discharge
Prins, 1989	Family visit	Ten minutes or more spent with a patient in the neurological intensive care unit by any people describing themselves as family members.
Ailinger, 1988	High blood pressure	A systolic blood pressure above 140 mm Hg or a diastolic pressure of above 90 mm Hg.
Shelley & Anderson, 1986	Menstrual distress	The degree of disequilibrium attributed to menstruation that is experienced by an individual and measured by the Menstrual Distress Questionnaire.
Lauver & Rubin, 1990	Follow-up attendance at clinic	Coming or not coming for colposcopy within 6 weeks after contact by nurse

Not all relationships between variables can be inferred as cause-and-effect relationships. There is a relationship, for example, between a person's gender and weight; men tend to be heavier than women, on the average. The relationship is not perfect; some women are heavier than some men. Nevertheless, if we had to guess whether Mike Stewart or Gina Stewart were heavier, we would be likely to say Mike, because men generally weigh more than women. However, we cannot really say that a person's gender causes his or her weight, despite the relationship that exists between the two variables. This type of relationship is sometimes referred to as a *functional relationship* rather than a causal relationship.

Control

The concept of research control is central to scientific inquiry, especially in studies that are quantitative. It is a topic to which much of this book is devoted. Chapter 12, in particular, discusses methods of achieving control in scientific research. The concept is so important, however, that some basic ideas about control are presented here.

Essentially, *research control* is concerned with holding constant the possible influences on the dependent variable under investigation so that the true relationship between the independent and dependent variables can be understood. In other words, research control attempts to eliminate any contaminating factors that might otherwise obscure the relationship between the variables that are really of interest. A detailed example should clarify this point. Let us suppose that a researcher is interested in studying whether teenage women are at higher risk of having low-birthweight infants than are older mothers because of their age. In other words, the researcher wants to test whether there is something about the physiologic development of women that causes differences in the birthweights of their babies. Existing studies have shown that, in fact, teenagers have a higher rate of low-birthweight babies than women in their twenties. The question, however, is whether age

itself causes this difference or whether there are other factors that can account for the relationship between maternal age and infant birthweight. The researcher in this example must design the study in such a way that these other factors are controlled. But what are the other factors? To answer this, one must ask the following critical question:

> *What variables could affect the dependent variable under study while at the same time be related to the independent variable?*

In the current study, the dependent variable is infant birthweight and the independent variable is maternal age. Two variables are prime candidates for concern as contaminating factors (although there are several other possibilities): the nutritional habits of the mother and the amount of prenatal care received. Teenagers are not always as careful as older women about their eating patterns during pregnancy and are also less likely to obtain adequate medical care. Both nutrition and the amount of care could, in turn, affect the baby's birthweight. Thus, if these two factors are not controlled, then any observed relationship between the mother's age and her baby's weight at birth could be caused by the mother's age itself, her diet, or her prenatal care. It would be impossible to know what the underlying cause really is.

These three possible explanations are shown schematically as follows:

1. mother's age → infant birthweight
2. mother's age → prenatal care → infant birthweight
3. mother's age → nutrition → infant birthweight

The arrows here symbolize a causal mechanism or an influence. The researcher's task is to design a study in such a way that the true explanation is made clear. Both nutrition and prenatal care must be controlled to see if explanation 1 is valid.

How can the researcher impose such control? There are a number of ways, as discussed in Chapter 12, but the general principle underlying each alternative is the same: the competing influences—often referred to as *extraneous variables*—must be held constant. The extraneous variables to be controlled must somehow be handled in such a way that they are not related to the independent or dependent variable. Again, an example should help make this point more clear. Let us say we want to compare the birthweights of infants born to two groups of women: (1) those aged 15 to 19 and (2) those aged 25 to 29. We must then design a study in such a way that the nutritional and prenatal health-care practices of the two groups are comparable, even though, in general, the two groups are not comparable in these respects. Some information from a fictitious study (Table 4-3) illustrates how a researcher deliberately selected subjects for the study in such a way that both older and younger mothers had similar eating habits and amounts of prenatal attention. By building this comparability into the two groups of mothers, the researcher was holding nutrition and prenatal care constant. If the babies' birthweights in the two groups differ (as they, in fact, did in Table 4-3), then the researcher would be in a position to infer that age (and not diet or prenatal care) influenced the birthweight of the infants. If the two groups do not differ, however, then the researcher would be left to tentatively conclude that it is not the mothers' age per se that causes young women to have a higher percentage of low-birthweight babies, but rather some other variable or set of variables, such as nutrition or prenatal care.

By exercising research control in this example, we have taken a step toward one of the most fundamental aims of science, which is to explain the relationship between variables. Control is essential in firmly establishing cause-and-effect relationships because the world is extremely complex and many variables are interrelated in complicated ways. When studying a particular problem, it is difficult to examine this complexity directly: the researcher must generally be content to analyze a couple of relationships at a time and put the pieces together like a jigsaw puzzle. That is why even modest research studies can make important contributions to science. The extent of the contribution, however, is often directly related to how well a researcher is able to control contaminating influences. A controlled study allows a researcher to understand the nature of the relationship between the dependent and independent variables.

In the current example, we identified three variables that could affect a baby's birthweight, but dozens of others could have been suggested, such as maternal stress, mothers' use of drugs or alcohol during pregnancy, sonogram testing, and so on. Researchers need to isolate the independent and dependent variables in which they are interested and then pinpoint from the dozens of possible candidates those extraneous variables that need to be controlled. It is often impossible to control all the variables that affect the dependent variable and not necessary to do so. It is essential to control a variable only if it is simultaneously related to both the dependent and independent variables.

Table 4-3. *Fictitious Example of Controlling Two Variables in a Research Study*

AGE OF MOTHER	RATING OF NUTRITIONAL PRACTICES	NUMBER OF PRENATAL VISITS	INFANT BIRTHWEIGHT
15–19	33% Good 33% Fair 33% Poor	33% 1–3 visits 33% 4–6 visits 33% >6 visits	20% ≤2500 g 80% >2500 g
25–29	33% Good 33% Fair 33% Poor	33% 1–3 visits 33% 4–6 visits 33% >6 visits	9% ≤2500 g 91% >2500 g

Figure 4-1 illustrates this notion. In this figure, each circle represents the variability associated with a particular variable. The large circle in the center represents the dependent variable, infant birthweight. Overlapping variables indicate the degree to which the variables are related to each other. In this hypothetical example, four variables are shown as being related to infant birthweight: the mother's age, the amount of prenatal care she receives, her nutritional practices, and her smoking practices during pregnancy. The first three variables are also related to each other; this is shown by the fact that these three circles overlap not only with infant birthweight but also with each other. That is, younger mothers tend to have different patterns of prenatal care and nutrition than older mothers. The mother's prenatal use of cigarettes, however, is unrelated to these three variables. In other words, women who smoke during their pregnancies (according to this hypothetical representation) are as likely to be young as old, to eat properly as not, and to get a lot of prenatal care as not. If this representation is accurate, then it would not be essential to control smoking in a study of the effect of maternal age on infant birthweight. If this scheme is incorrect—if teenage mothers smoke more or less than older mothers—then the mother's smoking practices should be controlled.

Figure 4-1 does not represent infant birthweight as being totally determined by the four other variables. The darkened area of the birthweight circle designates unexplained variability in infant birthweight. That is, other "circles" or determinants of birthweight are needed in order for us to fully understand what causes babies to be born weighing different amounts. Genetic characteristics, events occurring during the pregnancy, and medical treatments administered to the pregnant woman are examples of other factors contributing to an infant's weight at birth. Dozens, and perhaps hundreds, of circles would need to be sketched onto Figure 4-1 in order for us to fully understand the complex interrelationships between infant birthweight and other phenomena. In designing a study, we might be interested in the effect of only one variable (such as maternal age) on the dependent variable. This is perfectly respectable—indeed, often necessary. However, researchers should attempt to control those variables that overlap with both the independent and dependent variables to fully understand the rela-

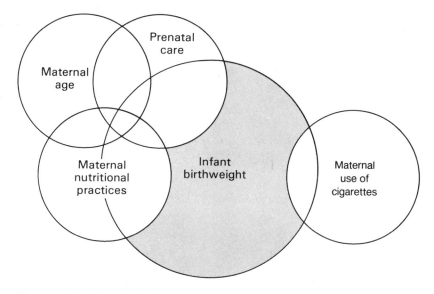

Figure 4-1. *Hypothetical representation of factors affecting infant birthweight.*

tionship between the main variables of interest. In Figure 4-1, if there are other variables that belong in the darkened area that are also related to maternal age, then those extraneous variables ideally should be controlled. Because uncontrolled extraneous variables can lead to erroneous or misleading conclusions, the researcher designing a study must plan how best to control these extraneous variables to maximize the usefulness and validity of the research.

Research rooted in the phenomenological paradigm is usually less concerned with the issue of control. With its emphasis on a holistic perspective and the individuality of human experience, the phenomenological approach holds that to impose controls on a research setting is to irrevocably remove some of the meaning of reality. However, critics of the phenomenological approach argue that lack of control often makes it impossible to rule out numerous alternative explanations to the findings, in which case firm conclusions about critical relationships among variables cannot be reached.

Data

The *data* (singular, datum) of a research study are the pieces of information obtained in the course of the investigation. The researcher identifies the variables of interest, develops operational definitions of those variables, and then collects the necessary data. The variables, because they vary, take on different values. The *actual* values of the study variables constitute the data for a research project. In quantitative research, those values are numbers.

For example, suppose we were interested in studying the relationship between sodium consumption and blood pressure. That is, we want to learn if people who consume more sodium are particularly susceptible to high blood pressure, or whether these variables are unrelated. The data for the study might consist of three pieces of information for all participants: (1) their average daily intake of sodium (in milligrams); (2) their diastolic blood pressure; and (3) their systolic blood pressure. Some hypothetical data for ten subjects are shown in Table 4-4. These numerical values associated with the variables of interest represent the data for a research project. The collection and analysis of data are typically the most time-consuming parts of a study.

In qualitative studies, the pieces of data are usually narrative descriptions rather than numerical values. Narrative descriptions can be obtained by having conversations with subjects, by making detailed notes of how subjects behave in naturalistic settings, or by obtaining narrative records from subjects, such as diaries.

Table 4-4.   *Hypothetical Data for Blood Pressure Study*

SUBJECT NUMBER	DAILY SODIUM INTAKE (MG)	SYSTOLIC BLOOD PRESSURE	DIASTOLIC BLOOD PRESSURE
1	8125	130	90
2	7530	126	80
3	1000	140	90
4	4580	118	78
5	2810	114	76
6	4150	112	78
7	6000	120	80
8	2250	110	70
9	5240	114	76
10	3330	116	74

☰ *MAJOR STEPS IN THE RESEARCH PROCESS*

A researcher typically moves from the beginning point of a study (the posing of a question) to the end point (the obtaining of an answer) in a fairly logical progression. True, in some studies the steps in this progression overlap. Sometimes the steps are interchangeable and in yet other cases some of the steps are unnecessary. Still, there is a general flow of activities that is typical of a scientific investigation. This section briefly describes the major phases of a research project and the steps that are typical of each. The remainder of the book provides more detail about these research activities in roughly the same sequential order.

Phase 1: The Conceptual Phase

The early steps in a research project typically involve activities with a strong conceptual or intellectual element. These activities involve thinking, reading, rethinking, theorizing, and reviewing ideas with colleagues or advisers. During this phase, the researcher calls upon such skills as creativity, deductive reasoning, insightfulness, and a firm grounding in knowledge on a topic of interest. The four main steps in the conceptual phase are briefly described below.

STEP 1: FORMULATING AND DELIMITING THE PROBLEM

Good research depends to a great degree on good questions. Sometimes the importance of securing an interesting and meaningful topic gets lost in the concern for utilizing appropriate and sophisticated research procedures. Yet without a significant, interesting topic, the most carefully and skillfully designed research project will be of no value.

Researchers generally proceed from the selection of broad topic areas of interest to the development of specific questions that are amenable to empirical inquiry. One of the most common difficulties for beginning researchers is the development of a manageable, researchable problem statement. In developing research problems to be studied, the researcher must consider its substantive dimensions (is this research question of theoretical or practical significance?); its methodological dimensions (how can this question be studied?); its practical dimensions (are adequate resources available to conduct the study?); and its ethical dimensions (can this question be studied in a manner that is consistent with guidelines for the protection of human subjects?).

STEP 2: REVIEWING THE RELATED LITERATURE

Good research does not exist in a vacuum. For research findings to be useful, they should be an extension of previous knowledge and theory as well as a guide for future research activity. For a researcher to build on existing work, it is essential to understand what is already known about a topic. A thorough review of the literature provides a foundation upon which to base new knowledge.

A familiarization with previous studies can also be useful in suggesting research topics or in identifying aspects of a problem about which more research is needed. Thus, in some cases a literature review precedes the delineation of the problem.

STEP 3: DEVELOPING A THEORETICAL FRAMEWORK

Theory is the ultimate aim of science in that it transcends the specifics of a particular time, place, and set of individuals and aims to identify regularities in the relationships among variables. When research is performed in the context of a theoretical framework, it is more likely that its findings will have long-lasting significance and utility.

STEP 4: FORMULATING HYPOTHESES

A *hypothesis* is a statement of the researcher's expectations concerning relationships between the variables under investigation. In other words, a hypothesis is a prediction of expected outcomes; it states the relationships that the researcher expects to find as a result of the study. The problem statement identifies the phenomena under investigation; a hypothesis predicts how those phenomena will be related. For example, a problem statement might be phrased as follows: "Is preeclamptic toxemia in pregnant women associated with stress factors present during pregnancy?" This might be translated into the following hypothesis or prediction: "Pregnant women with preeclamptic toxemia will report a higher incidence of emotionally disturbing or stressful events during pregnancy than asymptomatic pregnant women." Problem statements represent the initial effort to give a research project direction; hypotheses represent a more formalized focus for the collection and interpretation of data.

Phase 2: The Design and Planning Phase

In the second major phase of a research project, the investigator must make a number of decisions about the methods to be used to address the research question and test the hypotheses and must carefully plan for the actual collection of data. Sometimes the nature of the question dictates some of the methods to be used, but more often than not the researcher has considerable flexibility to be creative and to make many decisions.

These methodological decisions generally have crucial implications for the validity and credibility of the study findings. If the methods used to collect and analyze the research data are flawed, then little confidence can be put in the conclusions. Much of this book is designed to acquaint readers with a range of methodological options and to give them skills to evaluate their appropriateness for various research problems.

STEP 5: SELECTING A RESEARCH DESIGN

The *research design* is the overall plan for how to obtain answers to the questions being studied and how to handle some of the difficulties encountered during the research process. The design specifies which of the various types of research approach will be adopted and, as appropriate, how the researcher plans to implement a number of scientific controls to enhance the interpretability of the results.

For studies using traditional scientific methods, a wide variety of research designs are available. A basic distinction is the difference between *experimental* designs in which the researcher actively introduces some form of intervention and *nonexperimental* designs in which the researcher passively collects data without trying to make any changes or introduce any treatments. For example, if a researcher gave bran flakes to one group of subjects and prune juice to another over a fixed period to evaluate which method facilitated elimination more effectively, then the study would involve an intervention and would be considered experimental. If the researcher compared elimination patterns of two groups of people whose regular eating patterns differed (for example, some normally took foods that stimulated bowel elimination while others did not), then the study would not involve an intervention and would be considered nonexperimental. Experimental designs generally offer the possibility of greater control over extraneous variables than nonexperimental designs. However, if the researcher's primary interest is understanding some human behavior in naturalistic contexts (as in the case of phenomenological research), the design will inevitably be nonexperimental.

STEP 6: IDENTIFYING THE POPULATION TO BE STUDIED

The term *population* refers to the aggregate or totality of all the objects, subjects, or members that conform to a designated set of specifications. For example, we may specify "nurses," that is, registered nurses (RNs), and "living in the United States" as the attributes of interest: our study population would then consist of all licensed RNs who reside in the United States. We could in a similar fashion define a population consisting of *all* children under 10 years of age with muscular dystrophy in the state of California, or *all* the patient records in a particular hospital, or *all* the individuals who had a fatal coronary during a particular year.

The requirement of defining a population for a research project arises from the need to specify the group to which the results of a study can be applied. It is seldom possible to study an entire population, unless it is quite small. Research studies typically involve only a small fraction of the population, referred to as a *sample*. Before one selects actual study participants, it is essential to know what characteristics the subjects should possess.

STEP 7: SELECTING MEASURES FOR THE RESEARCH VARIABLES

To meaningfully address a research problem, some method must be developed to observe or measure the research variables as accurately as possible. In most situations, the researcher begins by carefully defining the research variables to clarify exactly what each one means. Then the researcher needs to select or design an appropriate method of measuring the variables—that is, of collecting the data. A variety of measurement approaches exist. *Biophysiologic measurements* often play an important role in nursing research. Another popular form is *self-reports,* wherein subjects are directly asked about their feelings, behaviors, attitudes, and personal traits. Another method of measuring variables is through *observational techniques*. Here, the researcher collects data by observing people's behavior and recording relevant aspects of it. The task of measuring research variables is a complex and challenging process that permits a great deal of creativity and choice.

Data collection methods vary in the structure imposed on the research subjects. Qualitative methods tend to be loosely structured, permitting subjects full opportunity to express themselves and behave in naturalistic ways. Quantitative approaches are more structured and con-

trolled and generally involve the use of a formal instrument that obtains exactly the same information from every subject. Before finalizing the data collection plan, the researcher must carefully evaluate whether the chosen approach is likely to accurately capture the concepts under study.

STEP 8: DESIGNING THE SAMPLING PLAN

Data are generally collected from a sample rather than from an entire population. The advantage of using a sample is that it is more practical and less costly than collecting data from the population. The risk is that the sample selected might not adequately reflect the behaviors, traits, symptoms, or beliefs of the population.

Various methods of obtaining a sample are available to the researcher. These methods vary in cost, effort, and level of skills required, but their adequacy is assessed by the same criterion: the representativeness of the selected sample. That is, the quality of the sample is a function of how typical, or representative, the sample is of the population under study with respect to the key research variables. Sophisticated sampling procedures can produce samples that have a high likelihood of being representative. The most sophisticated sampling methods are referred to as *probability sampling,* which uses random procedures for the selection of the sample. In a probability sample, every member of the population has the possibility of being included in the sample. With *nonprobability sampling* techniques, by contrast, there is no way of ensuring that each member of the population could be selected; consequently, the risk of a biased (unrepresentative) sample is greater. The design of a sampling plan includes the selection of a sampling method, the specification of the sample size, and the selection of procedures for recruiting the subjects.

STEP 9: FINALIZING AND REVIEWING THE RESEARCH PLAN

Normally, researchers have their research plan reviewed by several individuals or groups before proceeding with the actual implementation of the plan. When a researcher is seeking financial support for the conduct of a study, the research plan is generally presented as a formal proposal to a funding source. Even when proposed projects are considered to be of sufficiently high quality for funding, the reviewers generally offer suggestions for improving the study design. Students conducting a study as part of a course or degree requirement must also have their plans reviewed by faculty advisers. Even under other circumstances, however, the researcher is well advised to have individuals external to the project check the preliminary plans. An experienced researcher with a fresh perspective on a research problem can often be invaluable in identifying pitfalls and shortcomings that otherwise might not have been recognized. Finally, before proceeding with a study, researchers often need to have their research plan approved by Institutional Review Boards to ensure that the plan does not violate ethical principles, as discussed in Chapter 3.

STEP 10: CONDUCTING THE PILOT STUDY AND MAKING REVISIONS

Unforeseen problems often arise in the course of a project. The effects of such problems may be negligible but, in other cases, may be so severe that the study has to be stopped so that modifications can be introduced. For this reason, it is often advisable to carry out a *pilot study,* which is a small-scale version, or trial run, of the major study. The function of the pilot study is to obtain information for improving the project or for assessing its feasibility. The pilot study may reveal that revisions are needed in one or more aspects of the project. For example, the pilot study may provide information suggesting that the target population was defined too broadly. Or it may reveal that the initial conceptualization was somehow inadequate or that the hypotheses as stated cannot really be put to a test. From a more practical point of view, a trial run may reveal that it will be impossible to secure the cooperation of people by the intended procedures or that the study

is more costly than anticipated. Very often, the principal focus of a pilot study is the assessment of the adequacy of the data collection plan. The researcher may need to know, for example, if technical equipment is functioning properly. If questionnaires are used, it is important to know whether respondents understand the questions and directions, or if they find certain questions objectionable in some way.

A pilot study should be carried out with as much care as the major study so that any weaknesses that are detected will be truly representative of inadequacies inherent in the major study. Subjects for a pilot study should possess the same characteristics as individuals who will compose the main sample. That is, pilot subjects should be chosen from the same population as subjects for the major study. It is often useful to question the individuals who participate in a pilot study concerning their reactions to, and overall impressions of, the project.

When the data from the test run have been collected and scrutinized, the researcher should make the revisions and refinements that in her or his judgment would eliminate or reduce problems encountered during the pilot study. If extensive revisions are required, it may prove advisable to have a second trial run that incorporates those revisions.

Phase 3: The Empirical Phase

The empirical portion of a research study involves the actual collection of research data and the preparation of those data for analysis. In many studies, the empirical phase is the most time-consuming part of the investigation, although the actual amount of time spent varies considerably from project to project. If data are collected by distributing a written questionnaire to intact groups, this task may be accomplished in a day or so. More often, however, the data collection requires several weeks, or even months, of work.

STEP 11: COLLECTING THE DATA

The actual collection of data normally proceeds according to a preestablished plan to minimize confusion, delays, and mistakes. The researcher's plan typically specifies procedures for the actual collection of data (e.g., where and when will the data be gathered?); for describing the study to participants; for obtaining the necessary informed consents; and, if necessary, for training those who will be involved in the collection of the research data.

A considerable amount of both clerical and administrative work is required in the data collection task. The investigators must be sure, for example, that enough materials are available to complete the study; that participants are informed of the time and place that their presence may be required; that research personnel (such as interviewers) are conscientious in keeping their appointments; that schedules do not conflict; or that a suitable system of assigning an identification number to maintain subject anonymity has been implemented.

Data collection can occur in a variety of settings that vary in terms of their naturalism. In studies that are done "in the field," the data are collected in the natural settings in which the subjects work and live in their daily lives. At the opposite extreme, some studies are conducted in highly contrived and controlled laboratory settings. Many nursing studies are conducted in settings that fall in between these two extremes (e.g., a hospital setting). Research settings may influence the quality—and quantity—of the data being gathered.

STEP 12: PREPARING THE DATA FOR ANALYSIS

After the data are collected, a few preliminary activities must be performed before the actual analysis of the data can begin. For instance, it is normally necessary to look through questionnaires to determine if they are usable. Sometimes such forms are left almost entirely blank or contain other indications of misinterpretation or noncompliance. Another step that should be taken at this point is to assign identification numbers to the responses or observations of different subjects, if this has not been done previously.

Frequently, a step known as coding is required. *Coding* refers to the process of "translating" verbal data into categories or numerical form. For example, patients' responses to a question about the quality of nursing care they received during hospitalization might be coded into positive reactions, negative reactions, neutral reactions, and mixed reactions. Another preliminary step that is increasingly common is transferring research information from written documents onto computer files so that the data can be analyzed by computer.

Phase 4: The Analytic Phase

The data gathered in the empirical phase are not reported in "raw" form. They are subjected to various types of analysis and interpretation, which occurs in the fourth major phase of a project.

STEP 13: ANALYZING THE DATA

The data themselves do not provide us with answers to our research questions. Ordinarily the amount of data collected in a study is rather extensive and, therefore, needs to be processed and analyzed in some orderly, coherent fashion so that patterns and relationships can be discerned. *Qualitative analysis* involves the integration and synthesis of narrative, nonnumerical data. Quantitative information is generally analyzed through statistical procedures.

Statistical analyses cover a broad range of techniques, from some very simple procedures to complex and sophisticated methods. The underlying logic of statistical tests, however, is relatively simple and should, therefore, be no cause for concern to the beginning researcher. Computers and pocket calculators have virtually eliminated the need to get bogged down with detailed arithmetic operations.

STEP 14: INTERPRETING THE RESULTS

Before the results of a study can be communicated effectively, they must be organized and interpreted in some systematic fashion. By *interpretation* we refer to the process of making sense of the results and of examining the implications of the findings within a broader context. The process of interpretation begins with an attempt to explain the findings.

If the research hypotheses have been supported, an explanation of the results is usually straightforward, because the findings fit into a previously conceived argument. If the hypotheses are not supported, then the investigator must develop some possible explanations. Is the underlying conceptualization wrong or perhaps inappropriate for the research problem? Or do the findings reflect problems with the research methods rather than the theory (e.g., was the measuring tool inappropriate)? To provide sound explanations for obtained findings, then, the researcher must not only be familiar with the literature on a topic and with the conceptual underpinnings of the problem, but must also be able to understand the methodological weaknesses of the study design. A researcher should be in a position to critically evaluate the decisions that he or she made in designing the study and to recommend alternatives to others interested in the same research problem.

Phase 5: The Dissemination Phase

Phase 4 brings the researcher full circle: it provides the answers to the questions posed in the first phase of the project. However, the researcher's job is not complete until the results of the study are disseminated.

STEP 15: COMMUNICATING THE FINDINGS

The results of a research investigation are of little utility if they are not communicated to others. Even the most compelling hypothesis, the most careful and thorough study, and the most dramatic results are of no value to the nursing community if they are unknown. Another—and

often final—task of a research project, therefore, is the preparation of a research report.

There are various forms of research reports: term papers, dissertations, journal articles, papers for presentation at professional conferences, books, and so on. Journal articles—that is, short reports appearing in such professional journals as *Nursing Research*—are generally the most useful because such reports are available to a broad audience. Nurse researchers currently have many journals available for publishing their research reports.

STEP 16: UTILIZING THE FINDINGS

Many interesting studies have been conducted by nurses without having any effect on nursing practice or nursing education. Ideally, the concluding step of a high-quality study is to plan for its utilization in the real world. Although nurse researchers are often not themselves in a position to implement a plan for utilizing research findings, they can contribute to the process by including in their research reports recommendations regarding how the results of the study could be incorporated into the practice of nursing.

≡ ORGANIZATION OF A RESEARCH PROJECT

The steps described in the preceding section represent an idealized conception of what researchers do. The research process rarely follows a neatly prescribed pattern of sequential procedures. Developments in one step, for example, may require alterations in a previously completed activity. This fact does not eliminate the need for careful planning in advance; indeed, it makes careful organization even more important.

Almost all research projects are conducted under some time pressure. Students in research courses may have end-of-term deadlines; government-sponsored research involves funds granted for a specified time. Those who may not have such formal time constraints—such as graduate students working on dissertations—normally have their own goals for project completion. Setting up a timetable in advance may be an important step toward meeting such goals. This means that the investigator should make projections about which tasks should be completed by what point in time. Of course, initial projections often have to be modified, but estimates made at the outset of a project often help in setting intermediary goals. Having deadlines for tasks—even tentative ones— helps to impose some structure and delimits tasks that might otherwise continue indefinitely, such as the selection of a problem and review of the literature.

Unfortunately it is not possible for us to give even approximate figures for the relative percentage of time that should be spent on each task.

Some projects require many months to develop and pilot test the measuring instruments whereas other studies use previously existing instruments. The write-up of the study may take many months or only a few days. Clearly, however, not all of the steps will be equally time-consuming. If the researcher knew that there was a specified final deadline, it would make little sense to simply divide the time available by the total number of tasks.

Let us suppose that during a 12-month period we were studying the problem, "Does the presence of fathers in the delivery room affect the mothers' perception of pain?" Figure 4-2 presents a hypothetical time schedule for the research tasks to be completed. The selection of the problem is not included because the research topic

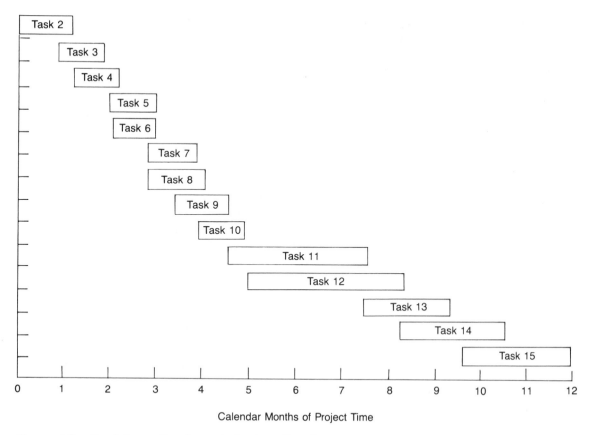

Figure 4-2. *Breakdown of project tasks by time allotted.*

has already been identified. Note that many activities overlap and that some tasks are projected to involve very little time in terms of time elapsed on the calendar.

In developing a time schedule of this sort, a number of considerations should be kept in mind, including the level of knowledge and competence of the researcher. Resources available to the researcher, in the form of research funds and personnel, will greatly influence the time estimates. It is also important to consider the practical aspects of performing the study, which were not all enumerated in the preceding section. Obtaining supplies, securing the necessary permissions, having forms or instruments approved by granting agencies or supervisors, holding meetings, and the like are all time-consuming, but often necessary, activities.

Individuals differ in the kinds of tasks that are appealing to them. Some people greatly enjoy the preliminary phase, which has a strong intellectual component, whereas others are more eager to collect the data, a task that is often more interpersonal in nature. The researcher should attempt, however, to allocate a reasonable amount of time to do justice to each activity. Inadequately conceived and hastily designed studies are doomed to failure, or at best mediocrity, no matter how much care and time are given to the collection and analysis of data. On the other hand, the person who lingers too long in the library may never reach the final goal.

≡ *RESEARCH EXAMPLE*

Moenning and Hill (1987) conducted a study to test the efficacy of two alternative methods of breast stimulation during pregnancy for inducing uterine activity. Their independent variable was the method of breast stimulation and their dependent variables included uterine response, fetal-placental function, exaggerated uterine activity, and hyperstimulation. The operational definitions for these variables, which were clearly described in the research report, were as follows:

INDEPENDENT VARIABLE

Method of breast stimulation
> Breast stimulation tactile method—application of the method of breast stimulation using touch by rolling or tugging the nipple.
> Breast stimulation warm compress method—application of the method of breast stimulation using moist, warm compresses in addition to nipple rolling or tugging.

DEPENDENT VARIABLES

Uterine response
> Frequency and duration of contractions during the breast stimulation stress test; three contractions should be obtained within ten minutes. These contractions should last at least 40 seconds, be felt by the patient, and palpated by the nurse.

Fetal-placental function
> Response of the fetal heart rate to uterine contractions during the breast stimulation stress test. Stable fetal heart rate should range from 120 to 160 beats per minute without persistent deceleration.

Exaggerated uterine activity
> Contractions that last longer than 90 seconds or occur more frequently than every two minutes.

Hyperstimulation
> The occurrence of fetal heart rate deceleration during a contraction that lasts longer than 90 seconds or occurs more frequently than every two minutes.

≡ *SUMMARY*

Scientific research focuses on *concepts* or *constructs,* which are abstractions or mental representations inferred from behavior or events. Concepts are the building blocks of *theories,* which present a systematic explanation about the way in which phenomena are interrelated.

In research studies, the concepts under investigation are referred to as *variables.* A variable is a characteristic or quality that takes on different values; that is, a variable is something that varies from one person or object to another. The blood type, blood pressure, grip strength, and hair color of a person are variables. These variables, which are inherent characteristics of a person that the researcher only measures or observes, are referred to as *attribute variables*. When a researcher actively creates or manipulates a variable, as when a special intervention or treatment is introduced, the variable may be referred to as an *active variable*. Variables that can take on a range of values along a specified continuum are referred to as *continuous variables* (e.g., height and weight), whereas variables that consist of only several discrete values are *categorical variables* (e.g., gender and blood type).

An important distinction for researchers is differentiation between the dependent and independent variables of a study. The *dependent variable* is the behavior, characteristic, or outcome that the researcher is interested in understanding, explaining, predicting, or affecting. The dependent variable (or *criterion variable*) is the presumed consequence or effect of the *independent variable*. The independent variable is the presumed cause of, antecedent to, or influence on the dependent variable. Groups that are highly varied with respect to some attribute are described as *heterogeneous;* groups with limited variability are described as *homogeneous*.

In an actual investigation, the variables are generally clarified and defined in such a way that they are amenable to observation or measurement. The *operational definition* of a concept is the specification of the procedures and tools required to make the needed measurements.

Except in rare cases, researchers are not interested in studying variables in isolation but rather are interested in learning about the *relationship* between two or more variables simultaneously. A relationship refers to a bond or connection between two variables. Researchers focus on the relationship between the independent and dependent variables. When the independent variable causes the occurrence, manifestation, or alteration of the dependent variable, a *cause-and-effect relationship* is said to exist. Variables that are not causally related can be linked by a *functional relationship.*

In attempting to understand how variables are related, researchers generally attempt to design a study that controls contaminating factors. *Research control* involves holding constant contaminating influences, known as *extraneous variables,* that might otherwise mask the true relationship between the independent and dependent variables.

Data are the pieces of information collected during the course of a study. Because variables take on different values, the record of those values for the subjects in the study constitutes the data. In qualitative studies, the data are generally narrative descriptions rather than numerical values.

Although the steps involved in conducting a research project and the sequencing of those steps may vary somewhat from one study to another, many of the activities are fairly standard. The research tasks can be organized into five major phases:

1. *The conceptual phase*—the phase in which the researcher develops the formal question to be studied and places it into some larger context; this phase includes such activities as
   - formulating and delimiting the problem to be studied
   - reviewing the literature relevant to the problem
   - developing a theoretical framework to place the problem in a broader context
   - formulating hypotheses to be tested
2. *The design and planning phase*—the phase in which the researcher makes a number of methodological decisions regarding the strategies to be used to collect and analyze the data to address the research question and evaluates those decisions before implementing them; this phase includes such activities as
   - selecting a research design appropriate for the study problem
   - specifying the population on which the study will focus
   - selecting measures for the research variables under study

- designing the plan for selecting and recruiting the sample
- finalizing and reviewing all aspects of the research plan
- conducting a pilot study and making revisions

3. *The empirical phase*—the phase in which the data are gathered by the researcher according to a carefully established plan, and data are prepared for later analysis; this phase includes
  - collecting the research data
  - preparing the data for analysis through coding and computer preparation

4. *The analytic phase*—the phase in which the researcher organizes, integrates, and makes sense of the data and tests the research hypotheses, encompassing the following tasks:
  - analyzing, through appropriate qualitative or quantitative methods, the research data
  - interpreting the results of the analyses

5. *The dissemination phase*—the phase in which the findings from the study are communicated to others and steps taken to integrate the findings into the practice of nursing; this phase includes
  - communicating the findings through written or oral presentation
  - undertaking steps to utilize the findings or to promote their utilization

The conduct of research requires careful planning and organization. The preparation of a timetable with expected deadlines for task completion can be extremely useful in establishing subgoals and in helping the researcher to be more realistic in the allocation of time to different tasks.

≡ *STUDY SUGGESTIONS*

1. Suggest ways of operationally defining the following concepts: nursing competency, patients' time to first voiding after surgery, aggressive behavior, patients' level of pain, home health hazards, postsurgical recovery, social class, and body image.

2. Name five categorical and five continuous variables; identify which, if any, are dichotomous.

3. Identify which of the following variables could be active variables and which are attribute variables (some might be both): height, degree of fatigue, cooperativeness, noise level on hospital units, length of stay in hospital, educational attainment, self-esteem, nurses' job satisfaction.

4. In the following research problems, identify the independent and dependent variables:
  a. How do nurses and physicians differ in the way they view the extended role concept for nurses?
  b. Does problem-oriented recording lead to more effective patient care than other recording methods?
  c. Do elderly patients have lower pain thresholds than younger patients?
  d. How are the sleeping patterns of infants affected by different forms of stimulation?
  e. Can home visits by nurses to released psychiatric patients reduce readmission rates?

5. Suppose that you were planning to study the following question: "Does a patient's body position affect the measurement of vital bodily signs?" You would like to collect data for at least five physiologic measurements and four body positions from 100 subjects. The project must be completed in 9 months. Prepare a time schedule such as the one shown in Figure 4-2 for the completion of the required research steps.

≡ *SUGGESTED READINGS*

METHODOLOGICAL REFERENCES

Burns, N., & Grove, S.K. (1987). *The practice of nursing research: Conduct, critique, and utilization.* Philadelphia:W.B. Saunders. (Chapter 3).

Kerlinger, F. (1973). *Foundations of behavioral research* (2nd ed.). New York: Holt, Rinehart & Winston. (Chapter 3).

Prescott, P.A., & Soeken, K.L. (1989). The potential uses of pilot work. *Nursing Research, 38,* 60–62.

Wilson, H.S. (1989). *Research in nursing* (2nd ed.). Menlo Park, CA: Addison-Wesley. (Chapter 1).

Woods, N.F., & Catanzaro, M. (1988). *Nursing research: Theory and practice.* St. Louis: C.V. Mosby. (Chapter 1).

SUBSTANTIVE REFERENCES*

Ailinger, R.L. (1988). Folk beliefs about high blood pressure in Hispanic immigrants. *Western Journal of Nursing Research, 10,* 629–636.

Broom, B.L. (1984). Consensus about the marital relationship during transition to parenthood. *Nursing Research, 33,* 223–228.

Derdiarian, A.K., & Forsyth, A.B. (1983). An instrument for theory and research development using the Behavioral Systems Model for nursing. *Nursing Research, 32,* 260–266.

Fehring, R.J. (1983). Effects of biofeedback-aided relaxation on the psychological stress symptoms of college students. *Nursing Research, 32,* 362–366.

Keller, E., & Bzdek, V.M. (1986). Effects of therapeutic touch on tension headache pain. *Nursing Research, 35,* 101–106.

Kovner, C.T. (1989). Nurse–patient agreement and outcomes after surgery. *Western Journal of Nursing Research, 11,* 7–19.

Kurzuk-Howard, G., Simpson, L., & Palmieri, A. (1985). Decubitus ulcer care: A comparative study. *Western Journal of Nursing Research, 7,* 58–79.

Lauver, D., & Rubin, D. (1990). Message framing, dispositional optimism, and follow-up for abnormal Papanicolau tests. *Research in Nursing and Health, 13,* 199–207.

Moenning, R.K., & Hill, W.C. (1987). A randomized study comparing two methods of performing the breast stimulation test. *Journal of Obstetric, Gynecologic, and Neonatal Nursing, 16,* 253–257.

Munro, B.H. (1983). Job satisfaction among recent graduates of schools of nursing. *Nursing Research, 32,* 350–355.

Naylor, M.D. (1990). Comprehensive discharge planning for hospitalized elderly. *Nursing Research, 39,* 156–161.

Prins, M.M. (1989). The effect of family visits on intracranial pressure. *Western Journal of Nursing Research, 11,* 281–297.

Richards, K.C., & Bairnsfather, L. (1988). A description of night sleep patterns in the critical care unit. *Heart and Lung, 17,* 35–42.

Shelley, S., & Anderson, C. (1986). The influence of selected variables on the experience of menstrual distress in alcoholic and nonalcoholic women. *Journal of Obstetric, Gynecologic, and Neonatal Nursing, 15,* 484–491.

White, M.A., Williams, P.D., Alexander, D.J., Powell-Cope, G., & Conlon, M. (1990). Sleep onset latency and distress in hospitalized children. *Nursing Research, 39,* 134–139.

*These are examples of studies with explicit operational definitions of variables or identification of independent and dependent variables.

Part II

Preliminary Research Steps

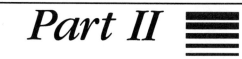

5
Selecting and Defining a Nursing Research Problem

For many beginning researchers, the selection of a problem for study is the most difficult task of the research endeavor. The difficulty of selecting a problem for study does not stem from a shortage of study topics. Nothing has been researched in its entirety. Rather, sometimes researchers find it difficult to select a particular topic for study because there are so many things to be known and it is perplexing to choose only one. Other researchers may experience difficulty in selecting a topic because they are unfamiliar with previous research. Beginning researchers may experience an additional dilemma of having to choose a problem for study at a time when they are unsure of what the research process entails and what constitutes a researchable problem.

Ideally, the selection of a problem should not be hurried. Many hours will be devoted to investigating the chosen problem and the time will be more profitably spent if the researcher is devoting his or her efforts to a problem that is of real interest. The identification of a researchable problem is not an easy matter, but it is a crucial one. It is simply impossible to proceed in an orderly, intelligent fashion on a research project unless a clear notion of the problem has been developed. Much as health professionals do not administer medications or perform surgery without some understanding of a person's ailment, so a researcher should not attempt to solve a research problem until it has been unambiguously stated. Researchers must know what they are trying to do before they can succeed at doing it.

≡ SOURCES OF PROBLEMS

Beginning researchers often are puzzled and perhaps even threatened by a requirement to develop a research problem. Where do ideas for research problems come from? How can a topic be selected? In this section we will suggest some sources for locating a problem or topic. The four most common sources are (1) experience, (2) the nursing literature, (3) theories, and (4) ideas from others.

Experience

The nurse's everyday experience provides a rich supply of problems for investigation. Whether you are a student nurse, practicing nurse, nurse educator, or nursing administrator, there are sure to be occurrences or situations that you have found puzzling or problematic. If you have ever asked such questions as, "Why are things done this way?" "I wonder what would happen if . . . ?" "What approach would work better?" or "Who is most likely to benefit from this?" you may be well along the way to developing a research idea. For the beginning researcher in particular, experience is often the most compelling source for topics. Immediate problems that are in need of solution or that excite the curiosity are relevant and interesting and, thus, may generate more enthusiasm than abstract and distant problems inferred from a theory.

An important ingredient for a successful research project is the investigator's curiosity. If you look around as you are performing your nursing functions, you are bound to find a wealth of research ideas if you are curious about why things are the way they are, or how things could be improved if something were to change. Here are a few hints:

- Watch for recurring problems and see if you can discern a pattern in situations that lead to the problem.
  Example: Why do many patients complain of being tired after being transferred from a coronary care unit to a progressive care unit?
- Think about aspects of your work that are irksome, frustrating, or do not result in the intended outcome—then try to identify factors contributing to the problem that could be changed.
  Example: Why is supper-time so frustrating in a nursing home?
- Critically examine some of the decisions you make in the performance of your functions. Are these decisions based on tradition or are they based on scientific evidence that supports their efficacy? Many practices in nursing that have become custom might be challenged.
  Example: What would happen if visiting hours in the intensive care unit were changed from ten minutes every hour to the regularly scheduled hours existing in the rest of the hospital?

Nursing Literature

Ideas for research projects often come from reading the nursing literature. The beginning nurse researcher would profit from regularly reading nursing journals, especially ones that report the results of nursing studies, such as *Nursing Research, Advances in Nursing Science, Applied Nursing Research in Nursing and Health,* and the *Western Journal of Nursing Research.* Many nursing specialty journals (e.g., *Heart and Lung* and *Oncology Nursing*) also publish research studies. Reading published reports may help the neophyte researcher to find a problem amenable to scientific investigation and may also help to familiarize the beginning researcher with the wording of research problems and the actual conduct of research studies.

Published research reports may suggest problem areas indirectly by stimulating the reader's imagination or interest in a topic and directly by specifying further areas in need of investigation. For example, Brandt (1984) found that stress and social support influenced maternal discipline of young children with a developmental delay. Her findings led her to suggest further study of the type and amount of social support that enables parents to cope with acute and chronic stresses and to provide optimal caretaking. She also suggested observation of caretaking and limit-setting interactions between the parent and child.

Inconsistencies in the findings reported in nursing literature often generate ideas for research studies. For example, there are inconsistencies regarding which irrigation fluid (e.g., water, cranberry juice, or cola) is most effective in maintaining the patency of patients' feeding tubes. Such discrepancies could lead to the design of a rigorous study to resolve the matter.

A researcher may also wonder whether a study similar to one reported in a journal article would yield comparable results if applied in a different setting or with different subjects. A deliberate duplication of a previous study with a new sample of subjects is often referred to as a *replication*. Replications are needed to establish the validity and generalizability of previous findings.

Sometimes problems can be identified not by what is in the literature but rather by what is not. That is, gaps in the research literature may provide a rich area for research. For example, many articles have appeared in relation to the nursing process as a method of clinical practice. The *Standards of Nursing Practice* published by the American Nurses' Association (ANA, 1973) for evaluating the quality of nursing care are formulated according to the steps of the nursing process, as discussed in Chapter 1. A large number of nursing educators teach students according to these steps. Yet, few studies have actually investigated the effectiveness of the nursing process as a method of clinical practice, as a way of evaluating nursing care, or as a method of teaching nursing.

In sum, a familiarity with existing research, or with problematic and controversial nursing issues that have yet to be understood and investigated scientifically, is an important route to developing a research topic. The student who is actively seeking a problem to study, such as the student required to do an empirical thesis, will find it useful to read widely in areas of interest. In the next chapter we deal more extensively with the procedures of doing a research literature review.

Theory

The third major source of problems lies in the theoretical systems and conceptual schemes that have been developed in nursing and other related disciplines. As explained in Chapter 4, a theory is an abstract, generalized explanation of phenomena. Because theories are abstract and nonspecific, they must be translated into real-world conditions and scientifically tested. To be useful in nursing practice, research must be conducted to test the applicability of the theory to the hospital unit, the emergency room, the classroom, and other nursing environments.

If a researcher decides to base a research project on an existing theory, deductions from the theory must be developed. This deductive process is explained in greater detail in Chapters 7 and 8. Essentially, the researcher must ask the questions, "If this theory is correct, what kind of behavior would I expect to find in certain situations or under certain conditions?" and "What kind of evidence would support this theory?" This process would eventually result in a specific problem that could be subjected to scientific investigation.

Let us look at an example of how a problem can be derived from a conceptual system. Levine (1973) has postulated a conceptual framework for nursing that concerns conservation. She explains nursing as conserving the patient's energy, structural integrity, personal integrity, and social integrity. From this theory, the researcher could formulate specific predictions about expected findings. For example, it might be hypothesized that primary nursing is more effective in conserving the patient's energy and social integrity than team nursing. By developing measures of energy expenditure and social integration, this hypothesis could be tested scientifically.

The 1970s and 1980s have witnessed a proliferation of conceptual frameworks and theories of nursing. Few studies have been conducted to substantiate whether the theories or conceptual frameworks hold up in actual nursing practice. It seems likely that these theoretical systems will play a growing role in the formulation of future nursing research problems.

Ideas from External Sources

External sources can sometimes provide the impetus for a research idea. In some cases, a research topic may be given as a direct suggestion. For example, a faculty member may give students a list of topics from which to choose or may actually assign a specific topic to be studied. Entities that sponsor funded research, such as the federal government, often identify broad or specific topics on which research proposals are encouraged. For example, in recent years there has been considerable interest in research relating to acquired immunodeficiency syndrome (AIDS), and various government agencies have requested a variety of AIDS-related research projects. For beginning students, it is often useful to have some guiding suggestions on the development of a research problem. However, even when a research area is designated, it is preferable for the researcher to identify the aspect of the problem that is of greatest interest, because curiosity is a critical ingredient in successful research.

Research ideas sometimes represent a response to priorities that are established within the nursing profession. For example, the ANA Cabinet on Nursing Research (1985) identified 11 broad areas in which research is perceived to be especially needed. These priorities are presented in Table 1-1 in Chapter 1. Also, as indicated in Chapter 1, priorities for nursing research have been established by many nursing specialty practices. These priorities are published from time to time in the specialty journals. Priority lists can often serve as a useful starting point for exploring research topics.

Often, ideas for studies emerge as a result of a brainstorming session. It is quite useful to interact with others to discuss and refine potential ideas. By discussing possible research topics with peers, advisers, or researchers with advanced skills, ideas often become clarified and sharpened, or enriched and more fully developed. Research or other professional conferences often provide an excellent opportunity for such discussions.

☰ *DEVELOPING AND REFINING A RESEARCH TOPIC*

Unless a research problem is developed on the basis of theory or an explicit suggestion from an external source, the actual procedures for developing a research topic are difficult to describe. The process is rarely a smooth and orderly one; there are likely to be many false starts, several inspirations, and several disappointments in the first efforts to devise a problem statement. The few suggestions offered here are not intended to imply that there are techniques for making this first step easy but, rather, to encourage the beginning researcher to persevere in the absence of instant success.

Selecting a Topic

The development of a research problem is essentially a creative process that depends on imagination, insight, and ingenuity. Research on creativity has revealed that the creative process can be impeded or stifled by tension and by a too-early evaluation of ideas. In the early stages, when research ideas are being generated, it is wise not to be critical of them immediately. It is much better to begin by just relaxing and jotting down general areas of interest as they come to mind. At this point it matters very little if the terms used to remind you of your ideas are abstract or concrete, broad or specific, technical or colloquial—the important point is to put some ideas on paper. Examples of some broad topics that may come to mind include "communication with patients," "reducing stress in hospitalized children," "needs of a grieving spouse," "styles of leadership of nurse administrators," and "postoperative loss of orientation."

After this first step, the ideas can be sorted

in terms of interest, the researcher's knowledge of the areas, and the perceived promise that they hold as a research topic. When the most fruitful idea has been selected, the rest of the list should not be discarded; it may be necessary to return to it.

Narrowing the Topic

Once you have identified one or more general topics of interest, you will need to begin asking questions that will lead to a researchable problem statement. Some examples of question stems that may help you focus your inquiry include the following:

- What causes . . . ?
- What is the extent of . . . ?
- Why do . . . ?
- When do . . . ?
- What factors lead to . . . ?
- What influences . . . ?
- How intense are . . . ?
- What conditions prevail before . . . ?
- What characteristics are associated with . . . ?
- What are the consequences of . . . ?
- What is the relationship between . . . ?
- How effective is . . . ?
- How do you know when . . . ?
- What differences exist . . . ?

Here again, early criticism of ideas is often inappropriate and counterproductive in this basically creative endeavor. Try not to jump to the conclusion that an idea sounds "silly" or "trivial" without giving it more careful consideration or without exploring it with fellow students, colleagues, or advisers. Not too much energy should be wasted in concern over whether some other researcher has already done a similar study. Totally original and unique problems are rare, despite the almost infinite range of possible topics. At the same time, no two studies are ever identical, so that every study has the potential of making some contribution to knowledge.

Beginning researchers typically develop problems that are too broad in scope or too complex and unwieldy for their level of meth-

odological expertise. The transformation of the general topic into a workable problem is typically accomplished in a number of uneven steps, involving a series of successive approximations. Each step should result in progress toward the goals of narrowing the scope of the problem and sharpening and defining the concepts.

As the researcher moves from a general topic of interest to more specific researchable problems, it is likely that more than one potential problem area will emerge. Let us consider the following example. Suppose you were working on a medical unit and observed that some patients always complained about having to wait for pain medication when certain nurses were assigned to them and, yet, these same patients offered no complaints when other nurses were assigned to them. You wonder why this phenomenon occurs. The general problem area is discrepancy in complaints from patients regarding pain medications administered by different nurses. You might ask, "What accounts for this discrepancy?" or "How can I improve the situation?" Such questions are not actual research questions because they are too broad and vague. They may, however, lead you to ask other questions such as, "How do the two groups of nurses differ?" or "What characteristics are unique to each group of nurses?" or "What characteristics do the group of complaining patients share?" At this point, you may observe that the cultural background of the patients and nurses appears to be a relevant factor. This may direct you to a review of the literature for studies concerning ethnic subcultures in relation to nursing interventions or it may provoke you to discuss the observations with peers. The result of these efforts may be several researchable problems, such as the following:

Is there a relationship between the ethnic background of nurses and the frequency with which they dispense pain medication?
Is there a relationship between the ethnic background of patients and their complaints of having to wait for pain medication?
Does the number of patient complaints increase when the patients are of dissimilar ethnic back-

grounds as opposed to when they are of the same ethnic backgrounds as the nurse?

Do nurses' dispensing behaviors change as a function of the similarity between their own ethnic background and that of the patients?

All of these problems have a similar theme, yet each would be studied in a different manner. How does one choose the final problem to be studied? Tentative problems usually vary considerably in their feasibility and worth. It is at this point that a critical evaluation of ideas is appropriate. The factors that should be considered in the final selection of a problem are discussed in the next section.

≡ CRITERIA FOR EVALUATING RESEARCH PROBLEMS

There are no fixed rules for making a final selection of a research problem. There are, however, some criteria that should be kept in mind in the decision process. The four most important considerations are the significance, researchability, and feasibility of the problem, and its interest to the researcher.

Significance of the Problem

A crucial factor in selecting a problem to be studied is its significance to nursing. The research question should have the potential of contributing to the body of knowledge in nursing in a meaningful way. The researcher should pose the following kinds of questions: Is the problem an important one? Will patients, nurses, or the broader health-care community or society benefit by the knowledge that will be produced? Will the results lead to practical applications? Will the results have theoretical relevance? Will the findings challenge (or lend support to) untested assumptions? Will the study help to formulate or alter nursing practices or policies? Will anyone *care* what the findings are? If the answer to all of these questions is "no," then the problem should be abandoned.

The problem does not need to be of Nobel Prize caliber to be useful, but trivial questions should be avoided. It would be technically possible to study, for example, the relationship between surgical patients' hair color and their length of stay in a hospital, but who would be interested in learning the results of such a study? If blondes as a group were found to have a longer hospital stay, on the average, than brunettes, would this finding have any implications for nursing care? The problem is trivial because it has little significance for nursing practice and does not have any theoretical relevance.

Researchability of the Problem

Not all questions are amenable to study through scientific investigation. Problems or issues of a moral or ethical nature, although provocative, are incapable of being researched. An example of a philosophically oriented question is, "Should nurses join unions?" The answer to such a question is ultimately based on a person's values. There are no right or wrong answers, only points of view. The question as stated is more suitable to a debate than to scientific research. To be sure, it is possible to modify the question so that aspects of the issue could be researched. For instance, each of the following questions could be investigated in a research project:

What are nurses' attitudes toward unionization? Do younger nurses hold more favorable opinions of unions than older nurses?

Does a person's role (nurse versus nursing administrator versus hospital administrator) affect his or her perceptions of the consequences of unions on the delivery of health care?

Is opposition to unionization for nurses based primarily on perceived outcomes to patients and clients or on outcomes to the nursing profession?

The findings from these hypothetical projects would have no bearing, of course, on the answer to the original question of whether or not nurses *should* join unions, but the information could be useful in developing a comprehensive understanding of the issues and in facilitating decision making.

Generally, researchable problems are ones that involve variables capable of being precisely defined and measured. For example, suppose the researcher was trying to determine what effect early discharge had on the general well-being of patients. General well-being is too broad and fuzzy a concept to measure as it is stated. The researcher would have to find a means of sharpening the concept so that it could be observed and measured before proceeding to subsequent steps in the research process. One would have to establish criteria against which the patients' progress toward well-being would be assessed. In other words, the researcher would need to answer the question, "How will I be able to distinguish those who have a positive 'general well-being' from those who do not?"

However, when a new area of inquiry is being pursued, it may be impossible to define the concepts of interest in precise terms. In such cases, it may be appropriate to address the problem using in-depth qualitative research. The problem may then be stated in fairly broad terms to permit full exploration of the concept of interest.

Feasibility of the Problem

Problems that are both significant and researchable may still be inappropriate if they are not feasible. The issue of feasibility is a complex one and encompasses a variety of considerations. Not all of the following seven factors are relevant for every problem, but most of them should be kept in mind in making a final decision.

1. TIME AND TIMING

As pointed out in Chapter 4, most studies have deadlines or at least informal goals for their completion. The problem must, therefore, be one that can be adequately studied within the time allotted. This means that the scope of the problem should be sufficiently restricted that enough time will be available for the various steps reviewed in

Chapter 4. It is usually wise to allocate more time to the performance of the tasks than originally anticipated. Research activities almost always require more time to accomplish than one thinks.

A related consideration is the timing of the project. Some of the research steps are more readily performed at certain times of the day, week, or year than at other times. This consideration is particularly relevant for the data collection task. For example, if the problem focused on patients with peptic ulcers, the research might be more easily conducted in the fall and spring because of the increase in the number of patients with peptic ulcers during these seasons than in the summer or winter months. When the timing requirements of the tasks do not match or overlap with the periods available for their performance, the feasibility of the project may be seriously jeopardized.

2. AVAILABILITY OF SUBJECTS

In any study involving humans, the researcher needs to consider whether individuals with the desired characteristics will be available *and* willing to cooperate. Securing people's cooperation may be relatively easy, as in the case of studies conducted in classrooms. Other situations may pose more difficulties for the researcher: some people may not have the time or interest to participate in a study that has little personal relevance or benefit, and others may be suspicious of the researcher's motives or even hostile to research in general.

Fortunately, people are usually willing to cooperate with a researcher if the demands on their time and comfort are minimal. However, if the research is time consuming, additional effort may be necessary to obtain a sufficiently large and representative sample of subjects. For example, it may be necessary to offer a stipend (typically $10 to $25) in compensation for the time subjects commit to a study.

An additional problem may be that of identifying and locating subjects with the needed characteristics. For example, suppose we were interested in studying the health-care needs of individuals who had lost an intimate friend or relative through suicide. Such individuals may not present themselves for treatment—indeed, that is precisely the reason that such an investigation might be necessary. There are procedures for locating individuals with specialized attributes, but these methods are often time consuming and expensive.

3. COOPERATION OF OTHERS

Often it is insufficient to obtain the cooperation of prospective subjects alone. If the sample includes children, mentally retarded or mentally incompetent people, or senile individuals, it is almost always necessary to secure the permission of parents or guardians. In institutional settings, such as hospitals, clinics, public schools, or industrial firms, access to clients, members, personnel, or records usually requires administrative approval. As mentioned in Chapter 3, many health-care facilities require that any project be presented to a panel of reviewers for approval before permitting the study to be conducted.

4. FACILITIES AND EQUIPMENT

All research projects have some resource requirements, although in some cases the needs may be quite modest. It is prudent to consider what facilities and equipment will be needed, and whether or not they will be available, before embarking on a project, so that disappointments and frustration can be prevented. The following is a partial list of considerations that fall into this category:

Will space be required and can it be obtained?
Will telephones, typewriters, or other office supplies be required?
If technical equipment and apparatus are needed, can they be secured and are they functioning properly?
Are duplicating or printing services available and are they reliable?
Will transportation needs pose any difficulties?
Will a computer be required for the collection or analysis of the data and are computing facilities easily obtainable?

The researcher who has given some thought to the feasibility of the study in terms of these requirements usually will be rewarded for his or her efforts.

5. MONEY

Monetary requirements for research projects vary widely, ranging from $10 to $20 for small student projects to hundreds of thousands of dollars for large-scale, federally sponsored research. The investigator on a limited budget should think very carefully about projected expenses before making the final selection of a problem. Some major categories of research-related expenditures include the following:

- literature costs—index cards, books and journals, reproduction of articles, and computerized literature search service charges
- personnel costs—payments to individuals hired to help with the interviewing, coding, keypunching, typing, and so forth
- subject costs—payment to subjects as an incentive for their cooperation, or to offset their own expenses (e.g., transportation or baby-sitting costs)
- supplies—paper, envelopes, typewriter ribbons, pens, and so forth
- equipment—laboratory apparatus, typewriters, calculators, and the like
- computer service charges
- laboratory fees, for the analysis of biophysiologic data
- other service charges, such as the costs of printing and duplicating materials
- transportation costs

In assessing the feasibility of a study in terms of monetary considerations, researchers should ask themselves not only, "Will I have enough money to complete this project?" but also, "Does the anticipated cost outweigh the value of the expected findings?"

6. EXPERIENCE OF THE RESEARCHER

The problem should be chosen from a field about which the investigator has some prior knowledge or experience. The researcher will have a difficult time in adequately preparing and designing a study on a topic that is totally new and unfamiliar. In addition to substantive knowledge of existing concepts, findings, or theories, the issue of technical expertise should not be overlooked. A beginning researcher usually has limited methodological skills and should, therefore, avoid research problems that require the development of sophisticated measuring instruments or that involve complex statistical analyses.

7. ETHICAL CONSIDERATIONS

A research problem may not be feasible because the investigation of the problem would pose unfair or unethical demands on the participants. The ethical responsibilities of researchers should not be taken lightly. Persons engaged in research activities should be thoroughly knowledgeable about the rights of human or animal subjects. An overview of major ethical considerations concerning human subjects was presented in Chapter 3 and should be reviewed in considering the feasibility of a prospective project.

Interest to the Researcher

If the tentative problem passes the tests of researchability, significance, and feasibility, there is still one more criterion for its selection, and that is the researcher's own interest in the problem. Genuine interest in and curiosity about the chosen research problem are important prerequisites to a successful study. A great deal of time and energy are expended in any scientific investigation and interest as well as enthusiasm ebb and flow throughout the time required for completion of the project. The problem selected should extend the researcher's personal knowledge as well as the base of knowledge for others.

Personal interest in a research problem is least likely to be high when the topic has been suggested or assigned to the researcher by others. Beginning research students often seek out suggestions and may be grateful for assistance in selecting a topic area; often such assistance can be helpful in getting started. Nevertheless, it is rarely wise to be talked into a research topic toward which you are not personally inclined. If you do not find a problem attractive or stimulating during the beginning phases of a study—when the opportunity for creativity and intellectual reasoning is at its highest—then you are bound to regret your choice later in the project.

≡ STATEMENT OF THE RESEARCH PROBLEM

It is clear that a study cannot progress without the choice of a problem; it is less clear, but nonetheless true, that the problem should be carefully stated in written form before proceeding with the design of the study. Putting one's ideas in writing is often sufficient to illuminate ambiguities and uncertainties.

A good statement of the problem should serve as a guide to the researcher in the course of designing the study. The problem statement should identify the key study variables, which should be amenable to observation or measurement, and the nature of the population of interest.

Form of the Statement

Researchers differ in their opinions concerning the form of the problem statement. The two basic alternatives are (1) declarative and (2) interrogative. The following example illustrates these two options:

Declarative: The purpose of this research is to investigate the relationship between the dependency level of renal transplant patients and their rate of recovery.

Interrogative: What is the relationship between the dependency level of renal transplant patients and their rate of recovery?

The question (interrogative) form has the advantage of simplicity and directness. Questions invite an answer and help psychologically to focus the researcher's attention on the kinds of data that would have to be collected to provide that answer. Therefore, we recommend the interrogative form for the statement of the problem.

To familiarize the reader with researchable problem areas and appropriate forms for the problem statement, a number of examples are presented in Table 5-1. The left column of this table gives examples of the original topics and the right-hand column presents the more formal statements of the problem. In real-life situations, the transition from the broad topic to the final statement usually requires many intermediary attempts. Note that each of these problem statements identifies one or more measurable variables as well as the population to be studied.

Defining Terms in a Problem Statement

The problem statements in Table 5-1 would be incomplete without an accompanying set of definitions of the variables involved. Sometimes the definition and clarification of concepts can be inserted into the statement of the problem itself, but it is likely that this practice would make the statement inordinately complex and clumsy.

Without further clarification, many of the concepts in Table 5-1 are inadequate for precise and unambiguous communication. For instance, what exactly does the researcher mean by "early discharge" in the first example? Dictionary definitions of terms and concepts are almost always inadequate for research purposes. The definition provided by the researcher must imply or specify a method of operationalizing (observing and measuring) the variables. To pursue the same example, "early discharge" might be defined as "discharged on the first postoperative day"; "post-

Table 5-1. *Hypothetical Examples of Problem Statements*

GENERAL TOPIC	FORMAL PROBLEM STATEMENT
1. Early discharge	Is early discharge for hemorrhoidectomy patients related to postoperative problems?
2. Chloasma gravidarum	Are women who have chloasma gravidarum more likely to have premature infants than those who do not?
3. Bladder catheterization	Is there a relationship between bladder catheterization and urinary infection in patients?
4. Decubitus ulcers	Is there a relationship between the incidence of decubitus ulcers in comatose patients and the frequency of turning?
5. Blood pressure variations	Are month-to-month blood pressure variations predictive of cerebral vascular accidents in the elderly?
6. Effects of visitors	Do hospitalized patients who have daily visitors express fewer somatic complaints than patients who do not have daily visitors?
7. Attitudes toward the mentally ill	Are nurses' attitudes toward the mentally ill related to the nurses' length of experience in working with them?
8. Nursing diagnoses	Do nursing diagnoses for surgical patients differ from those for medical patients?
9. Malpractice risks	How aware are nurses of their liabilities with respect to malpractice?
10. Children's hospital adjustment	Do children who are instructed about pain manifest better adjustment to hospitalization than those who are not?

operative problems" might be defined, in part, as "the patient's inability to have a bowel movement within three postoperative days." If adequate definitions are appended to a well-formulated problem statement, there should be little confusion about what is being studied.

≡ RESEARCH EXAMPLES

Research reports, unfortunately, do not always identify the problem under investigation in a concise, articulate fashion. When the study problem is carefully stated, as in the following research examples, the reader is generally in a good position to judge the adequacy of the research methods.

First, let us consider a quantitative study.

Chang and colleagues (1984) tested preferences for different types of nursing care among elderly ambulatory women. The researchers presented alternatives by showing simulated patient–nurse encounters on videotape. The subjects consisted of a sample of women at senior citizen nutrition sites. Three aspects of nursing care were systematically varied in the videotaped presentations: (1) medical-technical care, (2) psychosocial aspects of care, and (3) patient involvement through self-care. The research report carefully delineated the problem statements and the definition of terms used in the investigation. One of the research questions was the following:

"What are the effects of different levels (high and low) of three components of care (technical quality, psychosocial, patient participation) on patients' global satisfaction?"

In other words, is patient satisfaction affected when the technical quality of care is high or low, when the psychosocial aspects of nursing are high or low, or when patient involvement in self-care is high or low? The investigators increased the precision of their problem by presenting clear definitions of terms. For example, patients' global satisfac-

tion "was measured by adaptations of Section III of the Patient Satisfaction Questionnaire (PSQ)" (p. 371). Seven items designed to capture the subject's satisfaction with the nursing care depicted on the videotape were used to measure the dependent variable.

A study by Allan (1989) provides a good example of a problem statement in a qualitative nursing study.

Allan used in-depth interviews to explore factors associated with successful weight loss in a sample of 21 women. Each woman was interviewed on multiple occasions over a 7-month period. The research questions guiding this primarily descriptive study were as follows:

What methods for weight management are used by women who successfully manage their weight?
What factors influence the selection of particular methods?

The key concept here, successful weight management, was defined as having maintained a weight within the biomedically normal range for a period of at least one year.

Some additional examples of research problems that have been studied by nurse researchers are presented in Table 5-2.

The care that a researcher takes in carefully and methodically stating a problem and defining the concepts is often a good index of the thoroughness of the overall design and conceptualization. It is extremely difficult to evaluate the methods used to collect research data if one does not have a clear picture of what the study was attempting to accomplish in the first place.

≡ SUMMARY

The selection of a problem in a scientific investigation frequently is an arduous task, particularly for novice researchers. The most common sources of ideas for research questions are experience, relevant literature, theory, and external sources such as peers and advisers. Nurses, nursing students, nurse educators, and nurse administrators are likely to have an abundance of experiences in their daily activities that are puzzling, problematic, or provoke curiosity. Any situation that is poorly understood or any condition that gives you cause to wonder if a better method could be devised represents a potential research topic. Readings in areas of interest constitute a second method of generating ideas for a scientific study. Theories and conceptual frameworks often serve as a springboard for empirical studies: the utility and viability of any theory ultimately depend on its ability to withstand tests in real-life situations. Finally, research ideas are often generated in interactions with peers or experienced researchers or may be identified by a funding source, faculty member, or by the nursing profession through the issuance of research priority statements.

The process of developing a research problem is not a smooth and direct one. The researcher usually starts with the identification of several topics of broad interest. The researcher should be open-minded about the possibilities that are developed at this early phase because a hasty evaluation may result in the rejection of several potentially valuable ideas. After the researcher has tentatively selected a topic, he or she must begin the task of successively narrowing the scope of the problem. This task begins by posing a series of questions linked to the topic of interest.

A number of criteria should be considered in making the final selection of the problem. First, the problem should be a significant one. That is, the research question should contribute to nursing practice or nursing theory in a meaningful way. Second, the problem should be researchable. Questions of a moral or ethical nature are inappropriate, and concepts that defy precise definition and measurement should usually be avoided. Third, a problem may have to be abandoned if the investigation is not feasible.

Table 5-2. *Actual Examples of Nursing Research Problem Statements*

RESEARCH PROBLEM	SOURCE
What differences, if any, are there between mother and father interactions with term and preterm infants?	Harrison, 1990
What variables are predictive of physiologic adaptation in adults with insulin-dependent diabetes mellitus?	Pollock, 1989
Is there a difference between men and women in functional disability and psychosocial adjustment to a burn injury?	Brown et al., 1988
What is the effect of backrest position on mixed venous oxygen saturation in patients after coronary artery bypass surgery?	Noll & Fountain, 1990
In response to neonatal intensive care unit stressors, do nurses use a variety of coping strategies and do they consider problem-oriented strategies?	Rosenthal et al., 1989
Is there a relationship between individuals' responses on the Health Risk Appraisal and their tendency to respond to questions in a socially desirable manner?	Killeen, 1989
Is there a relationship between blood glucose symptom belief accuracy and metabolic control in individuals with Type II diabetes?	O'Connell et al., 1990
What differences exist in the health self-concepts of handicapped versus able-bodied children?	Natapoff & Essoka, 1989
Are adolescent mothers more likely than adult mothers to underestimate infant developmental rate?	Becker, 1987
Will patients report less pain intensity, less disruption in daily activities, and less emotional upset if they manage their own pain medication after surgery?	King et al., 1987

Feasibility involves the issues of timing, availability of subjects, cooperation of other individuals, availability of facilities and equipment, monetary requirements, experience and competencies of the researcher, and ethical considerations. Finally, the research question should be one that is of interest to the researcher.

The selected problem should be stated formally (in writing) before proceeding to the design of the study. A good statement of the problem will serve as a guide throughout the study. The problem may be stated in either declarative or interrogative form; the interrogative form is preferred because it is more simple and concise and because it leads more directly to a solution. The statement of the problem should identify the major variables under consideration and specify the characteristics of the population being studied. The problem statement should be accompanied by a set of clear definitions of the concepts involved to facilitate communication of the research ideas and to help bridge the gap between abstract phenomena and measurable variables.

≡ STUDY SUGGESTIONS

1. Think of a frustrating experience you have had as a nursing student or as a practicing nurse. Identify the problem area. Ask yourself a series of questions until you have one that you feel is researchable. Evaluate the problem in terms of the criteria of a researchable problem discussed in this chapter.
2. Examine the following five problem statements. Are they researchable problems as stated? Why or why not? If a problem statement is not researchable, modify it in such a way that the problem could be studied scientifically.
   a. What are the factors affecting the attrition rate of nursing students?
   b. What is the relationship between atmospheric humidity and heart rate in humans?
   c. Should nurses be responsible for inserting nasogastric tubes?

   d. How effective are walk-in clinics?
   e. What is the best approach for conducting patient interviews?
3. Identify a researchable problem from one of the conceptual frameworks or theories of nursing. Of what relevance is the problem to scientific nursing knowledge?
4. Examine one issue of the journal *Nursing Research*. Find an article that does not present a formal, well-articulated problem statement. Write a problem statement for that study in both declarative and interrogative form.
5. Below are three general topics that could be investigated. Develop at least one problem statement for each. Assess the adequacy of the problems in terms of their researchability and feasibility.
   a. nurse–patient interaction
   b. sleep disturbances
   c. preoperative anxiety

≡ SUGGESTED READINGS

METHODOLOGICAL REFERENCES

American Nurses' Association Congress for Practice. (1973). *Standards of nursing practice.* Kansas City, MO: Author.

American Nurses' Association Cabinet on Nursing Research. (1985). *Directions for nursing research: Toward the twenty-first century.* Kansas City, MO: Author.

Burns, N., & Grove, S.K. (1987). *The practice of nursing research: Conduct, critique, and utilization.* Philadelphia: W.B. Saunders. (Chapter 5).

Campbell, J.P., Daft, R.L., & Hulin, C.L. (1982). *What to study: Generating and developing research questions.* Beverly Hills: Sage Publications.

Fuller, E.O. (1982). Selecting a clinical nursing problem for research. *Image: The Journal of Nursing Scholarship, 14*(2), 60–61.

Gordon, M. (1980). Determining study topics. *Nursing Research, 29,* 83–87.

Lewandowski, L.A., & Kositsky, A.M. (1983). Research priorities for critical care nursing. *Heart and Lung, 12,* 35–44.

Lindeman, C.A., & Schantz, D. (1982). The research

question. *Journal of Nursing Administration, January,* 6–10.

Moody, L., Vera, H., Blanks, C., & Visscher, M. (1989). Developing questions of substance for nursing science. *Western Journal of Nursing Research, 11,* 393–404.

Valiga, T.M., & Mermel, V.M. (1985). Formulating the researchable question. *Topics in Clinical Nursing, 7*(2), 1–14.

Wilson, H.S. (1989). *Research in nursing* (2nd ed.). Menlo Park, CA: Addison-Wesley. (Chapters 7 & 8).

Woods, N.F., & Catanzaro, M. (1988). *Nursing research: Theory and practice.* St. Louis: C.V. Mosby. (Chapters 3 & 5).

*SUBSTANTIVE REFERENCES**

Allan, J.D. (1989). Women who successfully manage their weight. *Western Journal of Nursing Research, 11,* 657–675.

Anderson C.J. (1981). Enhancing reciprocity between mother and neonate. *Nursing Research, 30,* 89–93.

Becker, P.T. (1987). Sensitivity to infant development and behavior: A comparison of adolescent and adult single mothers. *Research in Nursing and Health, 10,* 119–127.

Brandt, P.A. (1984). Stress-buffering effects of social support on maternal discipline. *Nursing Research, 33,* 229–234.

Brown, B., Roberts, J., Browne, G., Byrne, C., Love, B., & Streiner, D. (1988). Gender differences in variables associated with psychosocial adjustment to a burn injury. *Research in Nursing and Health, 11,* 23–30.

Chang, B.L., Uman, G.C., Linn, L.S., Ware, J.E,, & Kane, R.L. (1984). The effect of systematically varying components of nursing care on satisfaction in elderly ambulatory women. *Western Journal of Nursing Research, 6,* 367–379.

Haack, M.R. (1988). Stress and impairment among nursing students. *Research in Nursing and Health, 11,* 125–134.

Harrison, M.J. (1990). Comparison of parental interactions with term and preterm infants. *Research in Nursing and Health, 13,* 173–179.

Juhl, N. (1989). Formalization, control and satisfaction

Killeen, M.L. (1989). What is the health risk appraisal telling us? *Western Journal of Nursing Research, 11,* 614–620.

King, K.B., Norsen, L.H., Robertson, R.K., & Hicks, G.L. (1987). Patient management of pain medication after cardiac surgery. *Nursing Research, 36,* 145–150.

McKeever, P., & Galloway, S.C. (1984). Effects of non-gynecological surgery on the menstrual cycle. *Nursing Research, 33,* 42–46.

Nakagawa-Kogan, H., Garber, A., Jarrett, M., Egan, K.J., & Hendershot, S. (1988). Self-management of hypertension. *Research in Nursing and Health, 11,* 105–115.

Natapoff, J.N., & Essoka, G.C. (1989). Handicapped and able-bodied children's ideas of health. *Journal of School Health, 59,* 436–440.

Noll, M.L., & Fountain, R.L. (1990). Effect of backrest position on mixed venous oxygen saturation in patients with mechanical ventilation after coronary artery bypass surgery. *Heart and Lung, 19,* 243–251.

O'Connell, K.A., Hamera, E.K., Schorfheide, A., & Gurthrie, D. (1990). Symptom beliefs and actual blood glucose in Type II diabetes. *Research in Nursing and Health, 13,* 145–151.

O'Rourke, M.W. (1983). Subjective appraisal of psychological well-being and self-reports of menstrual and nonmenstrual symptomatology in employed women. *Nursing Research, 32,* 288–292.

Pollock, S.E. (1989). Adaptive responses to diabetes mellitus. *Western Journal of Nursing Research, 11,* 265–280.

Rosenthal, S.L., Schmid, K.D., & Black, M.M. (1989). Stress and coping in a NICU. *Research in Nursing and Health, 12,* 257–265.

Uphold, C.R., & Susman, E.J. (1985). Childrearing, marital, recreational, work role integration and climacteric symptoms in midlife women. *Research in Nursing and Health, 8,* 73–81.

Walker, L.O., Crain, H., & Thompson, E. (1986). Maternal role attainment and identity in the postpartum period. *Nursing Research, 35,* 68–71.

OTHER REFERENCE CITED IN CHAPTER 5

Levine, M.E. (1973). *Introduction to clinical nursing* (2nd ed.). Philadelphia: F.A. Davis.

*The references cited were chosen because they include a clearly labeled problem statement.

6

Locating and Summarizing Existing Information on a Problem

There are two ways in which the term literature review is used by the research community. The first refers to the activities involved in identifying and searching for information on a topic, and developing a comprehensive picture of the state of knowledge on that topic. A researcher may thus say that he or she is "doing a literature review" before conducting a study.

The term is also used to designate a written report that is a critical summary of the "state-of-the-art" on a research problem. In research reports, researchers generally summarize the relevant literature in the introductory section or in an early section specifically labeled "Review of the Literature." Both the search and the write-up are important in the research process.

This chapter discusses several aspects of a literature review: first, the functions that a literature review can play in a research project; second, the kinds of materials covered in a literature review; third, suggestions concerning where to find appropriate references and how to record the information once it is located; fourth, tips on how to read research reports; and finally, the organization and presentation of a written literature review.

≡ *PURPOSES OF A LITERATURE REVIEW*

Usually beginning researchers are required by their instructors to read materials related to their research topic before actually conducting a study. The fact that a literature review is a standard requirement may obscure the purposes and importance of this task. By examining some specific functions of a literature review, we hope to clarify its value.

Source for Research Ideas

Familiarizing oneself with practical or theoretical issues relating to a problem area often helps the researcher to generate ideas or focus on a research topic. A review of the literature may, in some cases, precede the identification of a topic. Readings in areas of general interest to the researcher can be extremely useful in alerting him or her to unresolved research problems or to new applications suitable for a project. When a general topic has already been selected, readings on that topic help to bring the problem into sharper focus and aid in the formulation of appropriate research questions.

Orientation to What is Already Known

One of the major functions of the literature review is to ascertain what is already known in relation to the problem of interest. Acquaintance with the current state of knowledge should enable the researcher to avoid unintentional duplication of effort and may also lead the researcher to explore aspects of the problem about which there is relatively little knowledge. Of course, there are situations in which a deliberate decision to replicate a study is made but, here too, the researcher needs to be thoroughly familiar with existing research to make that type of decision.

A search of related research is also useful in identifying truths or assumptions about certain aspects of the phenomena being studied. An *assumption* is a proposition or statement whose truth is either considered self-evident or has been satisfactorily (at least tentatively) established by earlier research. Research studies necessarily build on a series of assumptions. Without a foundation of accepted knowledge and theory, little scientific progress would be possible. However, the beginning researcher needs to be extremely careful not to assume that a fact is proved or established simply because one researcher or author has reported it.

Provision of a Conceptual Context

Reviewing the literature is important for developing a broad conceptual context into which a problem will fit. It is only within such a context that the findings of a project can make a contribution to a body of knowledge. The more one's study is linked with other research, the more of a contribution it is likely to make. The accumulation of scientific knowledge is very much analogous to the fitting together of a jigsaw puzzle. Your piece of the puzzle, small though it may be, may help to join together other parts of the puzzle.

The review also serves the essential function of providing the individual researcher with a perspective on the problem necessary for interpreting the results of his or her study. The comparison of the results of a study with earlier findings is often a good point of departure for suggesting new research to either resolve conflicts or extend the base of knowledge.

Finally, a written review included in a research report is useful to the nursing community in that it makes explicit to readers the context within which the study was conducted.

Information on Research Approach

A very important role of the literature review, particularly for students engaged in their first research project, is to suggest ways of going about the business of conducting a study on a topic of interest. In other words, the review can be useful in pointing out the research strategies and specific procedures, measuring instruments, and statistical analyses that might be productive in pursuing one's problem. Research reports differ considerably in the amount of detail they include concerning specific procedures, but it is not unusual for a report to provide complete documentation for the investigator's methods, including a description of the measuring instruments used. When the actual instrument is not published with the report, it is almost always possible to obtain a copy by writing to the author.

☰ *SCOPE OF A LITERATURE REVIEW*

Most readers are undoubtedly familiar with locating library documents and organizing them. However, a review of research literature differs in a number of respects from other kinds of term papers or summaries that students are called upon to prepare. In this section the type of information that should be sought in conducting a research review is examined, and other issues relating to the breadth and depth of the review are considered.

Types of Information to Seek

Written materials vary considerably in their quality, their intended audience, and the kind of information they contain. The researcher performing a review of the literature ordinarily comes in contact with a wide range of materials and, thus, has to be selective in deciding what to examine or include. How are such decisions to be made? There is, unfortunately, no easy answer to this question, but we can offer a number of suggestions that might prove useful.

The first step in selecting appropriate materials is to make sure that you have been thorough in tracking down all (or most) of the relevant references. It is annoying to learn of good references *after* the completion of a study. The next main section of this chapter addresses the issue of locating good source materials.

The type of information included in academic or other nonfictional documents can be classified roughly into five categories: (1) facts, statistics, or findings; (2) theory or interpretation; (3) methods and procedures; (4) opinions, beliefs, or points of view; and (5) anecdotes, clinical impressions, or narrations of incidents and situations. Table 6-1 summarizes the functions that each type of information normally serves in a literature review. A brief description of the utility of the various kinds of information follows.

1. Research findings. This category of information represents the results of research investigations; it clearly constitutes one of the most important types of information for a research review. Research findings provide information on what is already known on a topic, based on empirical investigations using the scientific approach. As Table 6-1 indicates, published studies can also inspire new research ideas and can help in the development of the conceptualization and design of new research. Normally, research findings are available in a variety of sources including textbooks, encyclopedias, reports, conference proceedings, and, especially, scholarly jour-

Table 6-1. *Summary of the Uses of Various Types of Information*

TYPE OF INFORMATION	REVIEW FUNCTION			
	Source of Research Ideas	*Information on What Is Known*	*Conceptual Context*	*Research Approach*
Research findings	✓	✓	✓	✓
Theoretical explications	✓		✓	
Methodology				✓
Opinions	✓			
Clinical anecdotes	✓			

nals such as *Nursing Research*. Depending on the topic, it is usually useful to review research findings in the nursing literature, as well as in the literature of related disciplines, such as sociology, psychology, medicine, or physiology. Because research reports are often difficult for beginning students to understand, a section of this chapter is devoted to suggestions on reading published research studies.

2. Theory. The second type of information deals with broader, more conceptual issues of relevance to the topic of interest. Descriptions of theory are useful in providing a conceptual context for a research problem but may also be useful for suggesting a research topic. Sometimes discussions of a body of theory are briefly presented in research reports and journal articles, but they are more likely to be found in developed form in books.

3. Methodological information. The third type of information that should be sought in a literature review concerns the methods of conducting a study on the topic of interest. That is, in reviewing the literature, the researcher should pay attention not only to what has been found but also *how* it was found. What approaches have other researchers used? How have they operationalized or measured their variables? How have they controlled the research situation to enhance interpretation? What statistical procedures have they used to analyze their data? Although we may have to greatly modify existing approaches and instruments, it usually is possible to find techniques that can serve as a foundation for our research activities. Articles and reports concerning similar research problems should be useful in this regard. Articles and texts on methods and statistics may be helpful. Several references that deal exclusively with various tests, measures, and instruments also may be useful. Several of these sources are cited in the bibliographies of the chapters in Part IV.

4. Opinions and viewpoints. The general and specialty nursing literature contains numerous papers and articles that focus on an author's opinions or attitudes concerning a topic of interest. Such articles are inherently subjective, presenting the suggestions and points of view of the authors. Opinion articles are often an important source of ideas for studies that focus on controversial or emerging issues in nursing.

5. Anecdotes and clinical descriptions. There are numerous reports of an anecdotal nature that appear frequently in nursing, medical, and health-related literature. These articles relate the experiences and clinical impressions of the authors. For instance, Calarco (1989), in an article that appeared in the *American Journal of Nursing,* discussed her experience in dealing with a difficult psychiatric patient diagnosed with chronic paranoid schizophrenia and described the "mutual withdrawal" that occurred when both the patient and her caretakers withdrew from each other. Anecdotes or other types of non-research literature (such as opinion articles) may serve to broaden the researcher's understanding of the problem, particularly if the researcher is relatively unfamiliar with the underlying issues. Such sources may also illustrate a point or demonstrate a need for rigorous research. However, these two categories have limited utility in literature reviews for research studies because of their highly subjective nature. Beginning researchers should avoid the temptation of relying very heavily on such sources in their review of the literature, particularly if they are preparing a written review. This is not to say that such materials are uninteresting or unimportant, but generally they are inappropriate in summarizing scientific knowledge and theories concerning a research question.

Depth and Breadth of Literature Coverage

Beginning students often are troubled by the question of how limited or broad their literature review should be. Once again, there is no convenient formula giving a precise number of references to be tracked down. The extensiveness of the literature review depends on a number of factors. For written reviews, one determinant is the nature of the document being prepared. Doctoral dissertations often include a very thorough and extensive review that covers materials directly and indirectly related to the problem area. Reports in research journals, on the other hand, tend to have a much more selective bibliography covering only highly pertinent findings from other studies. Another factor to consider is the researcher's own level of knowledge and expertise. Inexperienced researchers who are relatively unfamiliar with a topic may have to cover more materials than more experienced researchers to feel secure about their level of understanding.

The breadth of a literature review depends quite heavily on how well-researched the topic is. If there have been 30 published studies on a specific problem, it would be difficult for the researcher to come to conclusions about the current state of knowledge on a topic without reading all 30 reports. However, it is not necessarily true that the literature task is more easily accomplished if the topic has not been heavily researched. Literature reviews on new topics or little-researched problems may need to involve reviews of a broad spectrum of peripherally related studies to develop a meaningful context.

Students embarking on their first research review should strive for relevancy and quality rather than quantity in selecting references for a written review of the literature. A common misconception is that the quality of the review depends on the number of references included. A small review covering pertinent studies and organized in a coherent fashion is of more value than a rambling presentation of questionably relevant information.

With respect to the depth of coverage in a written review, the most important criterion is, once again, relevancy. Research that is highly related to the problem or theory usually merits rather detailed coverage, including a description of the purpose, research approach, instruments, sample, target population, findings, and conclusions. Studies that are only indirectly related can often be summarized in a sentence or two.

☰ *SOURCES FOR A LITERATURE REVIEW*

The ability to identify and locate documents on a topic of interest is an important skill that is not as easily acquired as one might suspect. It is, nevertheless, a skill worth cultivating because it is clearly indispensable for a researcher or scholar to know how to access previous work on a topic. In this section some general issues concerning the mechanics of locating references are discussed, and some specific major sources commonly used by nurse researchers are presented.

Primary and Secondary Sources

References can be categorized as being either primary or secondary sources. Although this distinction probably is familiar to most readers, it is sufficiently important to merit a comment here. A *primary source,* from the point of view of the research literature, is the description of an investigation written by the person who conducted it. For example, most of the articles appearing in the journals *Nursing Research, Research in Nursing and Health, Applied Nursing Research,* and the *Western Journal of Nursing Research* are original research reports and, therefore, are primary sources. A *secondary source* is a description of a study or studies prepared by someone other than the original researcher. Review articles that summarize the literature on a topic are secondary sources. When you have completed and written up a review of the literature on a topic, your presentation will be considered a secondary reference. If you go on to collect new data on the same topic, however, your description of the hypotheses, methods, and results of the study will be a primary source reference for others doing a literature review.

Both primary and secondary sources play

important, but different, roles in the literature review task. Secondary sources are useful in providing bibliographical information on relevant primary sources. However, secondary descriptions of studies should not be considered substitutes for the primary sources. Secondary sources typically fail to provide sufficient detail about research studies. An even more serious limitation of secondary sources is that it is rarely possible to achieve complete objectivity in summarizing and reviewing written materials. We must accept our own values and biases as one filter through which information passes (although we should certainly make every effort to control such biases). However, we should not have to accept as a second filter the biases of the person who prepared a summary of research studies. The literature review task should utilize primary sources whenever possible.

Bibliographical Aids for Nursing Research Problems

The number of individual books, journals, and reports that could be consulted in compiling information on a nursing research topic is overwhelming. Fortunately, there are various indexes, abstracting services, and other retrieval mechanisms that facilitate the process of locating pertinent references. Several major sources that can be consulted in performing the review of the literature are identified here. However, these materials by no means exhaust the possibilities. Librarians are a particularly valuable resource inasmuch as they are knowledgeable about the literature, literature retrieval tools, and services in their own and other libraries.

Table 6-2 is designed to assist students in the selection of an appropriate literature retrieval source for locating references from books, periodicals, government documents, and abstracts. The table indicates whether the source can be searched by computer. The table is not meant to imply that these are the only sources but, rather, its intent is to aid the beginning researcher who is initiating a literature search. Two additional aids that serve as detailed guides to the nursing litera-

ture are *Lippincott's Guide to Nursing Literature: A Handbook for Students, Writers and Researchers* (Binger & Jensen, 1980) and *Guide to Library Resources for Nursing* (Strauch & Brundage, 1980).

INDEXES

Health sciences indexes are the key to the vast health sciences literature. It is a wise practice in using any index to begin the search for relevant references with the most recent issue of the index and proceed backward, keeping a careful record of the indexes and issues already consulted to avoid duplication or gaps in the search. Several indexes particularly useful to nurse researchers are the *International Nursing Index, Cumulative Index to Nursing and Allied Health, Nursing Studies Index, Index Medicus, Hospital Literature Index,* and *Current Index to Journals in Education.* Additional sources of information may be found in "References Sources for Nursing," prepared by a committee of the Interagency Council on Library Resources for Nursing and published in *Nursing Outlook* every two years.

1. The *International Nursing Index* is one of the major sources for locating references from both nursing and non-nursing journals. Articles from more than 270 nursing journals as well as nursing articles appearing in more than 2700 non-nursing journals are listed alphabetically by subject heading and author. Foreign journal articles appear at the end of each subject heading and are enclosed in brackets.

    Although the *International Nursing Index* is primarily a periodical index, it also lists in special appendixes publications of professional organizations and agencies, nursing books published during the year, and doctoral dissertations by nurses. It is published quarterly with an annual cumulative index and covers articles beginning with 1966 to the present.

    The procedure for locating references through an index is described in the prelimi-
    (text continues on page 96)

Table 6-2. A Quick Guide to Selected Abstracts and Indexes for Nursing and Related Subjects

Title	Type of Index: Index	Type of Index: Abstract	Frequency	Date coverage	Subject Coverage: Medicine	Nursing	Hospital	Materials: Other	Books	Studies	Technical report	Periodical	ANA/NLN Publ.	Gov't Publ.	Pamphlet	Dissert.	Book review	Data Base: Name	Data Base: Date
Books																			
Card catalog of the library	●								●										
National Library of Medicine Current Catalog @	●		Qa	1880	●	●	●		●	●	●		X	X	X	X		CATLINE	1801 +
Catalog—Sophia F. Palmer Memorial Library, AJN Co	●		2 vol	1922–1973		●			●				●						
Medical Books in Print	●		A	1986	●	●	●	H	●									Books in Print	Current
Periodicals																			
Annual or cumulative indexes to individual periodical titles (e.g., AJN, Public Health Nursing)	●					●						●							
INI (International Nursing Index)	●		Qa	1966	●	●			O			●	O	O	O	O	X	MEDLINE	1966 +
CINAHL (Cumulative Index to Nursing and Allied Health Literature) @	●		B-Ma	1956		●			O			●	+	O	O			CINAHL	1983 +

(continued)

Table 6-2. A Quick Guide to Selected Abstracts and Indexes for Nursing and Related Subjects (continued)

TITLE	Index	Abstract	Frequency	Date coverage	Medicine	Nursing	Hospital	Other	Books	Studies	Technical report	Periodical	ANA/NLN Publ.	Gov't Publ.	Pamphlet	Dissert.	Book review	Data Base Name	Data Base Date
Periodicals																			
Nursing Studies Index (V. Henderson)	●		4 vol	1900–1959		●			●	●		●	+	+	+	+			
Index Medicus/Cumulated Index Medicus @	●		Ma	1927+	●	+	+				○	●						MEDLINE	1966+
Hospital Literature Index/Cumulative Index of Hospital Literature	●		Qa	1945		+	●	H	○			●			+			HEALTH	1975+
History of Nursing. Index to Adelaide Nutting, Teachers' College, Columbia U. Collection.	●		1 vol			●			●										
Bibliography of Bioethics	●		A	1973/75+		●		M	●	+	+	+	+	+	+			BIOETHICS	1973+
Bibliography of the History of Medicine	●		Aa	1965+	●	●		e	●	+		●	X	+				HISTLINE	1970+
Gov't.																			
NTIS—SRIM INDEX to HEALTH PLANNING	●		Qa	1978+	+	+	+	H		●	●	●		+	+			NTIS	1964+
MEDOC	●		Qa	1968+				H						●				MEDOC	1976–1979
Monthly Catalog—U.S. Government Publications	●		Msa	1895+	+	+	+	M						●				Monthly Catalog	1976+

Abstracts

Title	@	Frequency	Dates	col1	col2	col3	Subject: col4	H	SC	SO	SP	col9	col10	col11	e	Online name	Online dates
Annual Review of Nursing Research		A	1983+		•				+	+		+	X	X				
Nursing Abstracts	•	B-Ma	1979+		•							•	X	X				
Abstracts of Reports of Studies in Nursing (in each issue of Nursing Research)	•	B-M	1960–1978		•				+	•		+	+					
Abstracts of Studies in Public Health Nursing (in Nursing Research 8 Spring, 1957)	•		1924–1957		•				+	•		+	+					
Nursing Research Abstracts (England)	•	Qa	1979+		•				•	•	•							
Abstracts of Health Care Management Studies @	•	Qa	1965+	+		•			•	•				+		PARADEX (offline)		
ERIC (Educational Resources Information Center)	•	Qa	1966+	+			E		•	•			•			ERIC	1966+	
Psychological Abstracts	•	Msaa	1927+				P	•				•		+		Psyc INFO	1967+	
Dissertation Abstracts International @	•	Ma	1938+				M							•		DISS ABS	1861+	
Excerpta Medica	•	Msa	1947+	•				•				•				EXCERPTA MEDICA	1974+	

Key
@—title varies
●—primary focus
+—some coverage included
○—included in special appendices, etc.
X—may be included

Frequency
A—annual
M—monthly
B-M—bi-monthly
Q—quarterly
a—with annual or multiyear cumulation
sa—with semiannual cumulation

Subject Coverage
e—ethics
E—education
H—health
M—multidiscipline
P—psychology/psychological aspects
SC—science
SO—social science
SP—special subject

Some titles listed in this chart under periodical indexes also include books and other materials. This table is printed with the permission of its author, ML Pekarski, Coordinator, Special Projects, O'Neill Library (which contains Nursing collection), Boston College, Chestnut Hill, MA 02167.

nary pages of each volume. Because the procedures tend to be similar for various indexes, only those for accessing information in the *International Nursing Index* are described here. The *International Nursing Index* begins with a thesaurus, which lists commonly used terms, not all of which are actual subject headings. The thesaurus directs the reader to the actual subject heading by means of a "see" reference if the term is not one used. For example, suppose you are looking for references on "nursing care plans." This phrase, although common in nursing, is not one of the subject headings. "Nursing Care Plans" would be listed and followed by a "see" reference directing you to look under the subject headings of "Nursing Process" and "Patient Care Planning."

In addition to "see" references, the thesaurus also suggests, at times, other subject headings that are pertinent to your particular topic. It does this by means of a "see also" reference. Sometimes both "see" and "see also" references appear for a particular term.

The researcher proceeds to the subject section of the index following use of the thesaurus. The subject heading lists the actual references. Each reference contains the following information: title of the article, author, journal, volume number, issue number, page numbers, and date of issue. A recent reference found under "Patient Care Planning" is:

title
↓
Spiritual care: An element
in nursing care planning. Labin, E. ←—— author
J Adv Nurs 1988 May; 13(3): 314–320.
↑   ↗   ↑   ↖
journal date of issue volume issue page numbers

A list of journal abbreviations cited in the references appears in the section "Journals Indexed" at the beginning of each issue of the *International Nursing Index*. In the above example, "J Adv Nurs" represents the *Journal of Advanced Nursing*.

If the researcher is seeking articles published by a particular author, the procedure would be to go directly to the author section of the index. Each researcher must decide, based on the title of the articles, whether the references cited might be pertinent to the topic under study. Once relevant references are identified, the particular articles can be obtained and reviewed.

2. *CINAHL,* the Cumulative Index to Nursing and Allied Health Literature, is published bimonthly with an annual cumulation. It indexes more than 300 nursing, allied health, and health-related journals published in English and also the publications of the American Nurses' Association and the National League for Nursing. It includes pertinent articles from the biomedical journals indexed in *Index Medicus* and relevant material from popular journals. *CINAHL* started publication in 1956, before the *International Nursing Index,* and is the only index to nursing journals from 1960 to 1965. Articles unavailable through local sources or the Regional Medical Library and its area libraries may be obtained for a fee from the CINAHL or American Journal of Nursing Libraries.

3. The *Nursing Studies Index* is a four-volume index prepared by Virginia Henderson and others. It is an annotated guide to reported studies, research methods, and historical and biographical materials in periodicals, books, and pamphlets published in English. The *Nursing Studies Index* constitutes the only means of access to nursing literature for the 1900 to 1959 period. Originally published by J.B. Lippincott, this index is now available in reprint format from Garland Publishing.

4. The *Index Medicus* is one of the most well-known biomedical indexes. More than 3000 worldwide biomedical journals are indexed. A small number of nursing journals are also indexed. It is published monthly and cumulated annually. Foreign language articles appear at the end of a subject and are enclosed in brackets. An additional feature included as a separate entity in both the monthly and annual cumulated volumes is the *Bibliography of Medical Reviews,* an index to the latest

review articles that have appeared in bio-medical journals.

5. The *Hospital Literature Index* is published four times annually, with the final issue containing an annual cumulation of listings. This index, which covers primarily administrative aspects of health-care delivery, has been published since 1945. It includes citations from more than 1000 English language journals.

6. Educational Resources Information Center (ERIC) was established in 1964 by the U.S. Office of Education and is useful to the researcher concerned with educational issues. Access to ERIC is by *The Thesaurus of ERIC Descriptors* found in most libraries. The *Current Index to Journals in Education* is a monthly publication produced by ERIC. The index references articles, by subject and author, from more than 500 educational journals.

ABSTRACTS

Abstract journals summarize articles that have appeared in other journals. Abstracting services are generally more useful than indexes in that they provide a summary (abstract) of a study rather than just a title. The title of an article often does not fully indicate its contents. Having an abstract helps in deciding whether a particular reference is worth pursuing.

1. *Nursing Abstracts* is a bimonthly publication that was first published in 1979. The periodical presents abstracts of articles from 63 nursing journals. Entries in *Nursing Abstracts* are indexed by subject, author, and journal. Examples of three entries from *Nursing Abstracts* is presented in Box 6-1.

2. Each issue of *Nursing Research* for the 1960 to 1978 period contains abstracts of research studies having relevance to nursing. The articles are classified alphabetically by author under alphabetical subject headings. The subject headings are listed at the beginning of the abstract section. The journals from which articles were abstracted are listed in each September–October issue. Sometimes only

the title of a particular article is given, and the reader is referred to the journal in which the original article appears. There is an author–subject guide to these abstracts in the annual index.

3. Abstracts of books and journal articles in the field of psychology and other behavioral and social sciences appear in *Psychological Abstracts*. Articles from selected nursing journals (e.g., *Nursing Research*) that are psychologically oriented are abstracted. To use this tool, the researcher first looks up the appropriate subject heading in the cumulative index. Under each subject heading are listed, in alphabetical order, the titles of research reports pertaining to the subject area of interest and an abstract number. The abstract number can then be located in the abstract section of this periodical.

4. *Sociological Abstracts* covers more than 1000 publications in the field of sociology and related behavioral and social sciences. This abstract periodical is published five times a year, with an annual cumulative index. Because the fields of medical sociology and the sociology of illness are growing, there may be many relevant references in this abstract journal.

5. *Research in Education,* another monthly publication of ERIC, abstracts reports of research projects funded by the U.S. Office of Education. These abstracts are indexed by subject and author.

Computer Searches

As an alternative to searching indexes or abstracts manually, computerized literature searches have become increasingly popular. A computer search provides the researcher with a list of references with complete bibliographic information and, in many cases, abstracts as well. References to new literature may be available by way of the computer up to one month before their appearance in the printed index or abstract. In addition, computer searches may save some of the researcher's time and energy, thereby providing more time for reading the original publications.

No knowledge of computers is necessary for requesting a computer literature search. The researcher typically fills out a request form indicating the topic of interest and any limitations on the search, such as dates of publication. If the researcher has done some manual searching of the literature, subject headings found to be useful can be indicated. The librarian confers with the researcher, devises the best search strategy, and then performs the actual search.

Most computer searches are able to produce an immediate search, generating references at the same time the request is received. This is called an *on-line search*. Generally, if more than a small number of citations is obtained, the bulk of them will be printed *off-line* because this process is less expensive. The off-line printout is sent by mail and usually arrives three to five days after the computer search is conducted. The cost of a computer search varies depending on the type of search (the extensiveness of the bibliography requested) and the data base used in the search.

Table 6-2 includes a selected listing of data bases available for computer literature searches relevant for nursing. MEDLINE, the data base most commonly used by nurse researchers, is one of the largest data bases in the world. MEDLINE centers are located at the libraries of major research centers, medical schools, nursing schools, and hospitals. MEDLINE covers all areas

---

BOX 6-1 EXAMPLES OF ENTRIES FROM *NURSING ABSTRACTS*

#886029
LIFE STYLE AND PATTERNS OF HEALTH AND SOCIAL BEHAVIOR IN HIGH-RISK ADOLESCENTS.
Kulbok, Pamela P., et al.
Adv Nurs Sci, 11:1, Oct 88, pp 22–35
This article examines the life style of young people aged 14 to 19 years to describe the interrelations among social and health-related modes of behavior. A broad range of health habits, risk behaviors, and social activities are examined, including leisure activities, social relations, sexual behavior, substance use behavior, violent social behavior, seat belt use, etc. The analyses show two major modes of behavior, health-promoting and health compromising, while a third pattern can be interpreted as group or social activity. Implications of these life-style distinctions are discussed in relation to health promotion.

#881232
INFLUENCE OF ADMINISTRATION TIME ON CHEMOTHERAPY-INDUCED NAUSEA AND VOMITING.
Headley, Judith A.
Oncol Nurs For, 14:6, Nov/Dec 87, pp 43–47
This is a paper on the relationship between nausea and vomiting experienced by cancer patients receiving chemotherapy and the time of day that chemotherapy was given. No statistically significant difference between administration time and these symptoms was noted, but there was a trend for the evening group to report less frequency of distress from nausea and vomiting.

#886018
CHARACTERISTICS OF MEDICARE-ELIGIBLE HOME CARE CLIENTS
Pasquale, Debra K.
Pub Hl Nurs, 5:3, Sept 88, pp 129–134
This study was designed to identify Medicare-eligible home care clients' characteristics, and define the scope and complexity of health-related problems of this group. Findings showed that chronic health care problems predominated. Over half of the sample had at least moderate functional impairment, female recipients tended to be older and to rely on informal care givers, females were usually more functionally impaired than males, and wives usually provided care to male clients.

*All entries are from Volume 10 (1988) of *Nursing Abstracts*.

of biomedical literature and corresponds to *Index Medicus* with added coverage of nursing, hospital, and dental literature. All journals currently indexed in the *International Nursing Index* are included in MEDLINE. Several subfiles relating to specific subject areas or types of materials are also included. For example, CANCERLINE contains literature on all aspects of cancer, and AIDSLINE cites references relating to acquired immunodeficiency syndrome.

CINAHL, the resource mentioned earlier in the section on indexes, is also a bibliographic retrieval system available for on-line searching. The Combined Health Information Database is a combination of files of books, periodicals, and other materials from various clearinghouses on arthritis, diabetes, health, digestive diseases, and high blood pressure.

The PSYCHOLOGICAL ABSTRACTS data base provides worldwide coverage of the literature of psychology and other behavioral sciences, including journals monographs, dissertations, and some technical reports and treatises. The SOCABS data base, corresponding to *Sociological Abstracts,* provides international coverage of sociological references.

ERIC is another data base that may be of great help to the nurse researcher. It contains the complete file of educational materials from the U.S. Office of Education and corresponds to the publications, *Current Index to Journals in Education* and *Research in Education.*

SOCIAL SCISEARCH and SCISEARCH are data bases that correspond to the printed *Social Science Citation Index* and the *Science Citation Index,* respectively. These data bases may be useful to nurse researchers in obtaining references in scientific and social scientific disciplines.

Finally, the NTIS data base covers all publications contained in the weekly *Government Reports Announcements.* This service covers technical reports released by more than 240 government and other agencies and encompasses completed research in a wide range of disciplines, including nursing and health planning.

Although the traditional data base search systems generally require the services of a li-

brarian, a new and intensifying trend is end-user searching.

End-user systems are designed to allow researchers without computer expertise to conduct their own computer search in the library or in other locations with a personal computer (PC) or terminal without the assistance of a search specialist. Selected examples of end-user systems include BRS AFTER DARK, BRS COLLEAGUE, BRS BRKTHRU, DIALOG KNOWLEDGE, DIALOG MEDICAL CONNECTION, SILVERPLATTER, and GRATEFUL MED. These commercial systems can be used to access many data bases, including MEDLINE and CINAHL. Many data bases are now available in CD-ROM (compact disc-read only memory) format. They are identified in Table 6-2.

A recent innovation is NurseSearch, a unique bibliographic retrieval system. NurseSearch can be used to search a list of citations from 60 nursing journals from the CINAHL data base. This system provides subscribers with both the computer program that provides the searching (which can be used on PCs) and the actual data base on floppy diskettes. This means that the users of NurseSearch do not incur any on-line costs to access the data base.

BOOKS

Books should not be overlooked by the researcher conducting a literature search. Although periodicals contain more up-to-date information than books, books do provide more extensive coverage of a particular topic by treating more than one facet or aspect of the issue in depth. Books are a particularly valuable resource for locating discussions of theoretical issues. Books are also useful in that they usually contain numerous references to other sources of information. Books can be identified through library card catalogs and the computerized data bases corresponding to those catalogs.

BIBLIOGRAPHIES

Bibliographies are compilations of references found in books, periodicals, and reports on some particular topic. Annotated bibliographies provide comments concerning the purposes or findings of the references and, sometimes, concerning their quality. Examples of bibliographies include *Bibliography on Bioethics, Bibliography on Suicide and Suicide Prevention, International Bibliography of Studies on Alcoholism, Selected Bibliography on Death and Dying,* and *A Classified Bibliography of Gerontology and Geriatrics.*

≡ *READING RESEARCH REPORTS*

Once the researcher has identified potential references, he or she must proceed to locate the actual references. Academic libraries (i.e., libraries in colleges and universities) are likely to contain many of the references identified in the initial literature search. If a reference cannot be located, it is wise to check with a librarian, because most academic libraries have interlibrary loan capabilities that make it possible to obtain a reference from another cooperating library.

For research literature reviews, most relevant information will be found in research reports, which constitute the primary sources. The most common source of research reports is professional journals such as *Nursing Research* or *Research in Nursing and Health.* Before discussing how to prepare a written review, we briefly present some suggestions on how to read a research report.

What Are Journal Articles?

Research journal articles are reports that summarize the highlights of a scientific investigation. Because journal space is limited, the typical research article is relatively brief, which means that the researcher must condense a lot of information about the study into a very short space.

Research reports are accepted by journals on a competitive basis and are critically reviewed before acceptance for publication. Readers of research journal articles thus have some assurance that the studies have already been scrutinized for their scientific merit. Nevertheless, the publication of an article does not mean that the research findings can be uncritically accepted as true, because the validity of the findings depends to a large degree on how the study was conducted; this is why both producers and consumers of research can profit from gaining some knowledge about research methods.

Research reports in journals tend to follow a certain format for the presentation of material and tend to be written in a particular style. The next two sections discuss the content and style of research reports.

The Content of Research Reports

Research reports in professional journals typically consist of six major sections: (1) abstract, (2) introduction, (3) methods, (4) results, (5) discussion, and (6) references. These sections are briefly described below to provide some guidelines for what to look for and expect in a scientific report.

ABSTRACT

The *abstract* is a brief description of the study and is generally placed at the beginning of the journal article. Because researchers know that many people will read the abstract only, they generally strive to include only the essentials that allow readers to grasp what the study was all about. The abstract (or a summary, often placed at the end of an article as a substitute for the abstract) should be carefully read by the reviewer to determine the study's relevance to the topic being reviewed. (The author's abstract is generally the source for the entries appearing in abstract journals, discussed in the previous section.)

INTRODUCTION

The purpose of the introductory section of a research report is to acquaint readers with the research problem and with the context within which it was formulated. Generally, the introduction consists of following elements:

- the problem statement, research questions, or hypotheses to be tested
- a review of the related literature
- the theoretical framework
- an explanation of the significance of and need for the study

METHODS

The purpose of the methods section is to communicate to readers the researcher's methodological decisions—that is, exactly what he or she did to solve the research problem or answer the research questions. Generally, the methods section describes the following:

- the study population and sampling plan
- the research design
- methods of data collection and measurement of variables
- study procedures, including descriptions of any interventions

The methods section is usually enhanced by the researcher's discussion of not only *what* was done, but *why* it was done. That is, the researcher may defend his or her methodological decisions by clearly articulating a rationale.

RESULTS

The results section presents the key research findings and is therefore the core focus of the article for the person doing a literature review. Tables are used to summarize extensive pieces of statistical information, and the text usually highlights the most noteworthy results.

In quantitative studies, the results section typically reports the following three types of information:

1. Descriptive information. Descriptive procedures are used to summarize in a few simple numbers the average values of important research variables. For example, the report may tell us about average temperature readings of subjects or the percentage of infants in the sample who weighed less than 2500 grams at birth.

2. The name of the statistical test used. A *statistical test* is a procedure for evaluating the believability of the findings. For example, if the percentage of low-birthweight infants in a sample is computed, how likely is it that the percentage is accurate? Dozens of statistical tests exist, but they are all based on common principles; readers do not have to know the names of all statistical tests to comprehend the findings.

3. The significance of the statistical test. Perhaps the most important piece of information in the results section is whether the results are "significant," which does not mean "important." If a researcher reports that the results are statistically significant, it means that, according to the statistical test, the findings are likely to be valid and replicable with a completely new sample of subjects.

In qualitative studies, the results section generally presents a summary of the researcher's integration of narrative materials, often with direct excerpts from the data to illustrate important points.

DISCUSSION

In the discussion section of a journal article, the researcher draws conclusions about the meanings and implications of the study. This section tries to unravel what the results mean and why things turned out the way they did. The discussion typically incorporates the following elements:

- an interpretation of the results
- a discussion of study limitations
- implications of the study for research and practice

REFERENCES

Research journal articles conclude with a list of the books, reports, and other journals articles that were referenced in the text of the report. For those interested in pursuing additional reading on a substantive topic, the reference list of a current research study is an excellent place to begin.

The Style of a Research Report

The style in which most research journal articles is written often makes it difficult for beginning researchers to become interested in the "story" that the researcher is communicating. To unaccustomed audiences, research reports often sound stuffy and pedantic. Three factors contribute to this impression:

1. Compactness. Because journal space is limited, authors must try to compress as many ideas and concepts into the short space available. Some of the interesting, personalized aspects of the investigation cannot be reported. Furthermore, the need for efficiency means that tables must be used rather than text to present an array of information.
2. Jargon. The authors often use complex scientific terms that are assumed to be part of the reader's vocabulary. Often the jargon can be translated into everyday terms, but at the expense of inefficiency and, in some cases, reduced precision.
3. Objectivity. The writer of a research report generally strives to present findings in a manner that suggests neutrality and the absence of personal biases. The scientist is primarily an observer and recorder of natural phenomena and, therefore, researchers often take pains to avoid any impression of subjectivity. Because of this, research "stories" are often told in a way that makes them sound impersonal. Typically, for example, a research article is written in the passive voice—that is, personal pronouns such as "I" and "we" are avoided. Use of the passive voice tends to make a report less inviting and lively than the use of the active voice and tends to give the impression that the researcher did not actually "do" anything.

What can beginning students do about these issues? First, it is important that you recog-

nize the underlying rationale for the style of research reports. Second, we recommend that, at least initially, you read research journal articles rather slowly; it may be useful to first skim the article to get the major points and then re-read the article more carefully a second time. Finally, until you become more accustomed to the style and jargon of scientific writing, you may want to mentally "translate" research articles by translating compact paragraphs into looser constructions, by translating jargon into more familiar phrases and terms, and by re-casting the report into an active voice to get a better sense of the researcher's dynamic role in the research process. As an example of such a translation, Box 6-2 presents a brief summary of a fictitious study.

The top panel is written in the style that is typically found in research journal articles. The bottom panel presents a "translation" of the summary that recasts the information into language that is more digestible to students or beginning researchers.

Reading Research Reports Critically

Although it is certainly important to read research reports with understanding, it is also important to read them critically, especially when you are preparing a written literature review. A critical reading involves an evaluation of the researcher's major conceptual and methodological decisions. Unfortunately, it is difficult for students to criticize these decisions before they have gained some conceptual and methodological skills themselves. These skills will be strengthened as you progress through this book, but sometimes common sense and thoughtful analysis will suggest to beginning students flaws in a study. Some of the key questions to ask include the following: Does the way the researcher conceptualized the problem make sense—for example, do the hypotheses seem sensible? Did the researcher design the study in such a way that the relationship between the independent and dependent variables could be understood? Were the major research variables measured in an adequate way or would an alternative method have been better? Did the researcher choose subjects in such a way that they are representative of the group being studied, and was the sample large enough that the results seem believable? Additional guidelines for critiquing various aspects of a research report are presented in Chapter 28.

BOX 6-2 SUMMARY OF A FICTITIOUS STUDY AND A "TRANSLATION"

Original Version

The potentially negative sequelae of having an abortion on the psychologic adjustment of adolescents has not been adequately studied. The current study sought to determine whether alternative pregnancy resolution decisions have different long-term effects on the psychologic functioning of young women.

Three groups of low-income pregnant teenagers attending an inner-city clinic were the subjects in the study: (1) those who delivered and kept the baby, (2) those who delivered and relinquished the baby for adoption, and (3) those who had an abortion. There were 25 subjects in each group. The study instruments included a self-administered questionnaire and a battery of psychologic tests measuring depression, anxiety, and psychosomatic symptoms. The instruments were administered upon entry into the study (when the subjects first came to the clinic) and then 1 year after termination of the pregnancy.

The data were analyzed using analysis of variance (ANOVA). The ANOVA tests indicated that the three groups did not differ significantly in terms of depression, anxiety, or psychosomatic symptoms at the initial testing. However, at posttest, the abortion group had significantly higher scores on the depression scale and were signficantly more likely than the two delivery groups to report severe tension headaches. There were no significant differences on any of the dependent variables for the two delivery groups.

The results of the study suggest that young women who elect to have an abortion may experience a number of long-term negative consequences. It would appear that appropriate efforts should be made to follow-up abortion patients to determine their need for suitable treatment.

"Translated" Version

We wondered whether young women who had an abortion had any emotional problems in the long run. It seemed to us that not enough research had been done to really know whether there was any psychologic harm resulting from an abortion.

We decided to study this question by comparing the experiences of three types of teens who became pregnant: (1) girls who delivered and kept their babies, (2) those who delivered the babies but gave them up for adoption, and (3) those who elected to have an abortion. All of the teens in the sample were poor, and all were patients at an inner-city clinic. Altogether we studied 75 girls: 25 in each of the three groups. We evaluated the teens' emotional states by asking them to fill out a questionnaire and several psychologic tests. These tests allowed us to assess things like the girls' degree of depression and anxiety and whether or not they had had any complaints of a psychosomatic nature. We asked the teens to fill out the forms twice: once when they came into the clinic, and then again a year after the abortion or the delivery.

We learned that the three groups of teens looked pretty much alike in terms of their emotional states when they first filled out the forms. But when we compared how the three groups looked a year later, we found that the abortion group teens were more depressed and were more likely to say they had severe tension headaches than teens in the other two groups. The teens who kept their babies and those who gave their babies up for adoption looked pretty similar 1 year after their babies were born, at least in terms of things like depression, anxiety, and psychosomatic complaints.

Thus, it seems that we may be right in being concerned about the emotional effects of having an abortion. Nurses should be aware of these long-term effects, and it even might be advisable to institute some type of procedure of following these young women up to find out if they need additional help.

≡ PREPARING AND WRITING A LITERATURE REVIEW

There are a number of steps involved in preparing a written review; these steps are summarized in Figure 6-1. As the figure shows, after identifying potential sources, the reader must locate the references and screen them for their relevancy to the topic being reviewed. References that appear appropriate are read and notes are taken, and inappropriate references can be discarded. Frequently, one reference will provide citations to many other relevant references, which sends the reader back to locate additional sources. After all relevant references have been reviewed, the researcher can proceed to organize, analyze, and integrate the body of literature. The written review can then be prepared. This section provides some advice on the last few steps in preparing a written review.

Abstracting and Recording Notes

Once a document has been determined to be relevant, the entire report should be read carefully and critically, identifying material that is sufficiently important to warrant note-taking as well as observing flaws or gaps in the report. Notes should be made on index cards and should synthesize the contents of the reference. If the reference is a research report, the following kinds of information should usually be recorded: the *full* citation for inclusion in your bibliography, the problem statement or hypotheses, the theoretical framework, the research methods, and the key findings. It is a good idea to note any of the researcher's own criticisms or comments while reading the article. If the article is not a research report but is a discussion of theory or opinion, the main points of the author's arguments should be abstracted and recorded together with collaborating or supporting evidence.

Organizing the Review

If the end product of your literature search is to be a written review, a critical task is the organization of the gathered information. Most writers find it helpful to work from an outline. If the review is lengthy, it will be useful to write out the outline on paper. For shorter reviews, a mental outline might be sufficient. The important point is to sit back for a minute before starting to write and work out a structure so that the presentation has a meaningful and understandable organization. Lack of organization is perhaps the most common weakness of students' first attempts at writing a literature review.

Once the main topics and their order of presentation have been determined, a review of the notes is in order. This will not only help recall materials read earlier but will also lay the groundwork for decisions about where (if at all) a particular reference fits in terms of the outline.

Another aid to organization and integration of results is the preparation of a chart summarizing key aspects of studies. A chart is often useful for bringing inconsistencies to the reviewer's at-

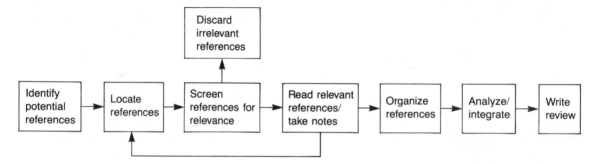

Figure 6-1. *Flow of tasks in a literature review.*

tention or highlighting differences in the way that key variables are measured. An example of such a chart, using fictitious studies of the effects of therapeutic touch on pain, is presented in Table 6-3.

Content of the Written Literature Review

A written review of the literature should be neither a series of quotes nor a series of abstracts. The central task is to organize and summarize the references to lay a systematic foundation for new research (or sometimes for implementing changes in a practice setting). The review should point out both consistencies and contradictions in the literature as well as offer possible explanations for the inconsistencies in terms of, say, different conceptualizations or methods.

Studies that are particularly relevant should be described in detail. However, reports that result in comparable findings can often be grouped together and briefly summarized, as in the following fictitious example: "A number of studies have found that the incidence of phlebitis is directly related to the method of administering intravenous infusions and to certain parameters of materials used in the infusions (Baum & Schwerin, 1989; Gendron, 1990)."

It is important to paraphrase, or summarize,

a report in one's own words. The review should demonstrate that thoughtful consideration has been given to the materials. Stringing together quotes from various documents fails to show that previous research and thought on the topic have been assimilated and understood.

Another point to bear in mind is that the review should be as objective as possible. Studies that conflict with personal values should not be omitted. It is not unusual to find studies with contradictory results. The review should not deliberately ignore a study simply because its findings contradict other studies. Analyze inconsistent results and evaluate the supporting evidence as objectively as possible.

The literature review should conclude with a summary or overview of the "state of the art" of the problem under consideration. The summary should point out not only what has been studied and how adequate the investigations have been but should also make note of any gaps or areas of research inactivity. The summary requires some critical judgment concerning the extensiveness and dependability of information on a topic. If the literature review is conducted as part of a research project, this critical summary should demonstrate the need for the new study and should clarify the context within which the hypotheses will be developed.

Table 6-3. *Chart Synthesizing (Fictitious) Studies on Therapeutic Touch (TT)*

CITATION	SAMPLE	MEASUREMENT OF PAIN	FINDINGS
Benton, 1990	50 patients in TT group; 50 in non-TT control group	McGill Pain Questionnaire	No differences between groups
Roth, 1989	22 patients measured before and after TT	10-point visual analogue scale	Reduced pain before versus after TT
Springer, 1987	15 women with migraines	Observations over a 5-hour period	Decreased manifestations of severe pain
Lucas, 1988	42 patients in TT group; 38 in non-TT comparison group	McGill Pain Questionnaire	No differences between groups
Hentze, 1984	35 clients in high pain group; 35 clients in low pain group	McGill Pain Questionnaire	Reduced pain scores in high pain but not low pain group before versus after TT

Style of a Research Review

One of the most frequent problems for the student researcher preparing a written review for the first time is adjusting to the style of writing that is appropriate for research reviews. There is a tendency, for example, for students to accept the results of previous research as a fact or as proof that a finding is conclusive or a theory is correct. This tendency is understandable; it is the style of presentation commonly used in many texts, opinion articles, and other nonresearch papers. This style may derive from a desire for clarity and unambiguity for pedantic purposes, but it is also, in part, the result of a common misunderstanding about the degree of conclusiveness that results from empirical research. *No hypothesis or theory can be definitively proved or disproved by empirical testing.* This statement may come as a surprise to most individuals who, throughout their education, have been taught to accept as given many research findings. The fact that theories and hypotheses cannot be ultimately proved or disproved does not, of course, mean that we must disregard evidence or challenge every idea we encounter. The problem is partly a semantic one: hypotheses are not proved—they are supported by research findings; theories are not verified, but they may be tentatively accepted if there is a substantial body of evidence demonstrating their legitimacy. The researcher must learn to adopt this language of tentativeness in presenting the review of the literature.

A related stylistic problem is the inclination of beginning researchers to liberally intersperse opinions (their own or someone else's) with the findings of research investigations. The review should use statements of opinions sparingly, if at all, and should be explicit about the source of the opinion. A description of the point of view of a knowledgeable or influential individual may be useful in establishing the need to investigate the problem or in providing a perspective on the topic, but it should occupy a relatively small section of the review. The researcher's own opinions do not belong in a review section, with the exception of an assessment of the quality of existing studies.

The left-hand column of Table 6-4 presents several examples of the kinds of stylistic diffi-

Table 6-4. *Examples of Stylistic Difficulties for Research Reviews*

INAPPROPRIATE STYLE OR WORDING	RECOMMENDED CHANGE
1. It is known that unmet expectations engender anxiety.	1. A number of commentators have asserted that unmet expectations engender anxiety. (Bradford, 1986; Thompson, 1990)*
2. The woman who does not undertake preparation for childbirth classes tends to manifest a high degree of stress during labor.	2. Previous studies have demonstrated that women who participate in preparation for childbirth classes manifest less stress during labor than those who do not. (Andrew, 1991; Chase, 1988)
3. Studies have proved that doctors and nurses do not fully understand the psychobiologic dynamics of breast-feeding.	3. The studies by O'Hara (1990) and Jenkins (1985) suggest that doctors and nurses do not fully comprehend the psychobiologic dynamics of breast-feeding.
4. Attitudes cannot be changed overnight.	4. Attitudes, presumably, are enduring attributes that cannot be changed overnight.
5. Responsibility is an intrinsic stressor.	5. Responsibility is an intrinsic stressor, according to Doctor A. Cassard, an authority on stress. (Cassard, 1989)

*All references are fictitious.

culties we have been discussing in this section. The right-hand column offers some recommendations for rewording the sentences to conform to a more generally acceptable form for a research literature review. Many alternative phrasings are possible.

≡ *RESEARCH EXAMPLES*

Table 6-5 contains brief excerpts from the literature review sections of five research reports. These examples will help to acquaint beginning researchers with the style and content considered appropriate for written literature reviews, as well as illustrate the range of research problems in which nurse researchers have been interested. In addition, we present an expanded excerpt below.

Frank-Stromberg (1989) developed a special questionnaire to assess the initial reactions of individuals diagnosed as having cancer. The questionnaire contained 27 questions that were developed on the basis of a literature review and a pilot study. The following excerpt represents essentially the entire literature review section of Frank-Stromberg's research report, which appeared in *Nursing Research.**

> The diagnosis of cancer frequently arouses feelings of anger and hostility (Hamera & Shontz, 1978). Fear of the unknown is thought to be especially anxiety producing (Cain et al., 1983). Fear and panic are so common that they may even be considered normal (Novotny et al., 1984). Helplessness, regression, depression, withdrawal, hypochondriasis, or exaggerated dependency have also been described (Cooper, 1984; Krant, 1981; Westbrook & Nordholm, 1986). . . .
>
> Four mutually exclusive categories of psychological responses to the diagnosis of cancer have been identified, based on pa-

tients' descriptions of their moods: fighting spirit, helpless/hopeless, stoic acceptance, and denial (Greer et al., 1979; Morris et al. 1985). In a follow-up, multidisciplinary study of 69 women with early breast cancer, significant differences in survival at 5 and 10 years were found when the women were compared by initial responses to cancer. Women who had initially reacted with denial or a fighting spirit had a more favorable outcome than did those who showed stoic acceptance or helpless/hopeless responses (Pettingale et al., 1985).

Gotay (1984) found that the most frequently mentioned initial coping reactions were taking firm action, seeking additional information, and finding something favorable about the situation. Highes (1982) reported that many women with early breast cancer demonstrated a philosophical acceptance or an active determination to recover. Mages et al. (1981), in their study of 66 cancer patients of varying ages and diagnoses, identified three main responses. The largest group of responses were positive and optimistic, but a minority of responses indicated bearing up despite being quite ill or reflected lack of adjustment to the illness. Furthermore, patterns of adaptation responses among these patients three and four months after diagnosis did not change unless a marked alteration in the patients' medical condition occurred. Westbrook and Viney (1982) studied 126 patients with chronic illness (including cancer) and found that patients expressed many positive feelings in addition to emotions indicating distress. Similarly, Hamera and Shontz (1978) reported that their sample of 42 cancer patients identified positive aspects (social, familial, and emotional) of their disease.

Some degree of denial has been seen as necessary for patients to maintain the hope needed for participation in social and work-related activities (Forester et al., 1978), maintain emotional equilibrium (Tiendt, 1975), and defend against the fear of death (Peck, 1972). Four major aspects of denial identified in a study of Wool and Goldberg (1986) included denial of physical manifestations of the illness, diagnosis, implications of the illness, and affective responses to the illness. . . . In general, the literature tends to support the

* (Reprinted from Frank-Stromberg, M. (1989). Reaction to the diagnosis of cancer questionnaire: Development and psychometric evaluation. *Nursing Research, 38,* 364–369, copyright © 1989 by American Journal of Nursing Company, with permission.) The reader is referred to this source for the full article and references in the literature review.

Table 6-5.   *Excerpts from Published Literature Reviews in Research Reports*

SOURCE	PROBLEM STATEMENT FOR NEW STUDY	LITERATURE REVIEW EXCERPT
Frank, 1990	Do men and women hold different perceptions about the factors they consider important in making infertility treatment decisions?	Research findings suggest that women experience greater emotional turmoil than men in response to infertility. In a study of 107 infertility-clinic patients, McEwan et al. (1) reported that 37% of 62 women and only 1% of 45 men showed psychological disturbance in relation to their own or their partner's infertility... Similar findings were reported in a study of the emotional response of 200 couples seen in a pre-treatment program for in-vitro fertilization (2).
Coreil & Murphy, 1988	How strongly does prenatal intent influence breast-feeding duration?	According to several studies, most women choose between breast-feeding and bottle-feeding during pregnancy (1–5).* However, little is known about how closely a mother's intended length of breast-feeding corresponds to actual duration. Some researchers suggest that anticipated duration has a significant influence on lactation success because it reflects maternal confidence and motivation (6–7).
Bliss-Holtz, 1989	What is the mean time of thermometer placement necessary to reach maximum temperature in three sites in full-term newborns?	In their studies of preterm infants, several researchers (1–3) presented findings that support the supposition that this population has little difference between rectal and axillary temperature readings.... In contrast, findings in full-term infant samples are not in agreement (4–6).
Henneman, 1989	What is the effect of direct nursing contact on the stress response of patients being weaned from mechanical ventilation?	Several researchers have examined the effect of staff interaction on critically ill patients. One team (1) studied family and staff interaction with surgical intensive care patients in an effort to examine the effects of these visits on the "stress arousal" level. They reported no significant increase in heart rate, blood pressure, or vocal micrometer suppression. In contrast, another team (2) found that the simple act of taking a critically ill patient's radial pulse produced significant increases in heart rate and the frequency of ectopic beats.
MacVicar et al., 1989	What is the effect of aerobic interval training on cancer patients' functional capacity?	A number of studies on other chronically ill populations have used aerobic exercise as an intervention technique. The earliest and most extensive research was conducted on medically and surgically treated cardiac patients. Data from these studies showed improved functional capacity evidenced by increased cardiac output with associated increased oxygen uptake (1, 2).

*The numbers in parentheses refer to the researchers' references, which are not included here because of space constraints.

assumption that denial is an important mechanism for the psychological adaptation to the stress of cancer. This assumption is supported in the work of Watson et al. (1984), who found that denial of the implication of breast cancer was an effective method of dealing with stress for 24 newly diagnosed patients. The use of denial among these patients was not related to an increased delay in seeking treatment.

From the literature, it can be concluded that patients exhibit a range of responses to a diagnosis of cancer. Some responses may be helpful in that they enable the patient to confront the disease. Others may be harmful, promoting undue distress that interferes with adaptation.

≡ SUMMARY

The task of reviewing literature involves the identification, selection, critical analysis, and reporting of existing information on the topic of interest. It is almost always necessary to examine previous literature on a subject before actually undertaking a research project. Such a review can play a number of important roles. First, in the start-up phase of a project, a review of work conducted in an area of general interest can help in the formulation or clarification of a research problem. Second, a study of previous work acquaints the researcher with what has been done in a field, thereby minimizing the possibility of unintentional duplication. Third, the review provides a conceptual context or framework for the researcher and for the research community, thereby facilitating the cumulation of scientific knowledge. Fourth, the researcher may be in a better position to assess the feasibility of a proposed study by becoming familiar with related work. Finally, the review can be highly useful in providing methodological suggestions for the actual conduct of the investigation.

The kinds of information available in written documents can be categorized into five broad classes: (1) facts, findings, or results; (2) theory; (3) research procedures or methods; (4) opinions, points of view, or personal commentaries; and (5) anecdotes or impressions of a particular event or situation. Another way of categorizing literature is in terms of its being either a primary or secondary source. A *primary source* with respect to the research literature is the original description of a study prepared by the researcher who conducted it; a *secondary source* is a description of the study by a person unconnected with the investigation. Primary sources should be consulted whenever possible in performing the literature review task.

The search for existing writings on a topic is greatly facilitated by the use of various abstracting and indexing services, such as *CINAHL* or *Index Medicus*. An important bibliographic development to emerge in recent years is the increasing availability of various computerized information retrieval systems, such as MEDLINE. *End-user systems*, which allow individuals to do their own search rather than rely on a librarian, have become more popular with the widespread availability of personal computers.

After the researcher has identified and located references, he or she must screen them for relevance and then read them critically. For research reviews, most references are likely to be found in professional journals. Research journal articles, which present concise descriptions of scientific investigations, typically contain six sections: (1) abstract (or summary); (2) introduction; (3) methods; (4) results; (5) discussion; and (6) references. The compactness of research journal articles, the use of technical scientific terms, and the impersonal style in which they are written often make research articles difficult for students to read without an intermediary step of "translation."

Skillful note-taking and organization can greatly simplify the task of analyzing, summarizing, and evaluating literature on a given topic. In preparing a written review, it is important to organize materials in a logical, coherent fashion. The preparation of an outline is recommended, and the development of summary charts often helps in integrating diverse studies. The written review should not be a succession of quotes or abstracts. The role of the reviewer is to point out what has been studied to date, how adequate and dependable those studies are, what gaps there seem to be in the existing body of research, and what contribution a new study would make. The reviewer should present "facts" and "findings" in the tentative language that befits scientific inquiry and should remember to identify the source of opinions, points of view, and generalizations.

≣ STUDY SUGGESTIONS

1. Read Susan Kelley's (1990) study entitled, "Parental stress response to sexual abuse and ritualistic abuse of children in day-care centers," *Nursing Research, 39*, 25–29. Write a summary of the problem, methods, findings, and conclusions of the study. Your summary should be capable of serving as notes for a review of the literature.
2. Suppose that you were planning to study counseling practices and programs for rape trauma victims. Make a list of several key words relating to this topic that could be used with indexes or information retrieval systems for identifying previous work.
3. Below are five sentences from literature reviews that require stylistic improvements. Rewrite these sentences to conform to considerations mentioned in the text. (Feel free to give fictitious references if desired.)
    a. Children are less distressed when immunized when their parents are present.
    b. Young adolescents are unprepared to cope with complex issues of sexual morality.
    c. More structured programs to use part-time nurses are needed.
    d. Intensive care nurses need so much emotional support themselves that they can provide insufficient support to patients.
    e. Most nurses have not been adequately educated to understand and cope with the reality of the dying patient.
4. Suppose you are studying factors relating to the discharge of chronic psychiatric patients. Obtain five bibliographical references for

this topic. Compare your references and sources with those of other students.

≣ SUGGESTED READINGS

METHODOLOGICAL REFERENCES

American Psychological Association. (1983). *Publication manual* (3rd ed.). Washington, DC: Author.

Binger, J.L., & Jensen, L.M. (1980). *Lippincott's guide to nursing literature: A handbook for students, writers and researchers.* Philadelphia: J.B. Lippincott.

Burns, N., & Grove, S.K. (1987). *The practice of nursing research: Conduct, critique and utilization.* Philadelphia: W.B. Saunders. (Chapter 6).

Cooper, H.M. (1984). *The integrative research review.* Beverly Hills, CA: Sage.

Fox, R.N., & Ventura, M.R. (1984). Efficiency of automated literature search mechanisms. *Nursing Research, 33,* 174–177.

Light, R.J., & Pillemer, D.B. (1984). *Summing up: The science of reviewing research.* Cambridge, MA: Harvard University Press.

Saba, V.K., Oatway, D.M., & Rieder, K.A. (1989). How to use nursing information sources. *Nursing Outlook, 37,* 189–195.

Smith, L.W. (1988). Microcomputer-based bibliographic searching. *Nursing Research, 37,* 125–127.

Strauch, K.P., & Brundage, D.J. (1980). *Guide to library resources for nursing.* New York: Appleton-Century-Crofts.

Taylor, S.D. (1975). Bibliography on nursing research, 1950–1974. *Nursing Research, 24,* 207–225.

Turabian, K.L. (1973). *A manual for writers of term papers, theses, and dissertations* (4th ed.). Chicago: University of Chicago Press.

Woods, N.F., & Catanzaro, M. (1988). *Nursing research: Theory and practice.* St. Louis: C.V. Mosby. (Chapter 4).

SUBSTANTIVE REFERENCES*

Beckman, C.A. (1990). Postterm pregnancy: Effects on temperature and glucose regulation. *Nursing Research, 39,* 21–24.

*These studies are cited because they include an explicitly labeled "Literature Review" section.

Bliss-Holtz, J. (1989). Comparison of rectal, axillary, and inguinal temperatures in full-term newborn infants. *Nursing Research, 38,* 85–87.

Cahill, C.A. (1989). Beta-endorphin levels during pregnancy and labor: A role in pain modulation? *Nursing Research, 38,* 200–203.

Coreil, J., & Murphy, J. (1988). Maternal commitment, lactation practices, and breastfeeding duration. *Journal of Obstetric, Gynecologic, and Neonatal Nursing, 17,* 273–278.

Dougherty, M., Bishop, K., Mooney, R., & Gimotty, P. (1989). The effect of circumvaginal muscle (CVM) exercise. *Nursing Research, 38,* 331–335.

Flaskerud, J.H. (1984). A comparison of perceptions of problematic behavior by six minority groups and mental health professionals. *Nursing Research, 33,* 190–197.

Frank, D. (1990). Gender differences in decision making about infertility treatment. *Applied Nursing Research, 3,* 56–62.

Frank-Stromberg, M. (1989). Reaction to the diagnosis of cancer questionnaire: Development and psychometric evaluation. *Nursing Research, 38,* 364–369.

Henneman, E. (1989). Effect of nursing contact on the stress response of patients being weaned from mechanical ventilation. *Heart and Lung, 18,* 483–489.

MacVicar, M.G., Winningham, M.L., & Nickel, J.L. (1989). Effects of aerobic interval training on cancer patients functional capacity. *Nursing Research, 38,* 348–351.

Medoff-Cooper, B., Weininger, S., & Zukowsky, K. (1989). Neonatal sucking as a clinical assessment tool: Preliminary findings. *Nursing Research, 38,* 162–165.

Ventura, J.N. (1986). Parental coping, a replication. *Nursing Research, 35,* 77–80

OTHER REFERENCE CITED IN CHAPTER 6

Calarco, M.M. (1989). Managing Myra's madness. *American Journal of Nursing, 89,* 346–349.

7

Placing the Problem in a Theoretical Context

The term theory is used in many ways. For example, nursing instructors and students frequently use the term theory to refer to the content covered in classrooms, as opposed to the actual practice of performing nursing activities. Sometimes the term is used to refer to someone's hunches or ideas, as in "My theory is that if you smile at people and establish rapport with them, they will be more compliant." Whatever the usage, the term theory usually connotes an abstraction or a generalization.

Scientists use *theory* to refer to an abstract generalization that presents a systematic explanation about how phenomena are interrelated. Scientists are fact-finders, but they are rarely content with the accumulation of isolated facts. Scientific researchers strive to integrate the findings into an orderly, coherent system. Theories and conceptual frameworks constitute the mechanisms by which researchers organize empirical findings into a meaningful pattern. Theories embody principles for explaining, predicting, and controlling phenomena. Thus, theory construction and testing are intimately related to the advancement of scientific knowledge, and it may even be claimed that theory is the ultimate goal of science. Theoretical and conceptual systems represent the highest and most advanced efforts of humans to understand the complexities of the world in which they live.

≡ PURPOSES OF THEORIES

The development of theories is not an end in and of itself; theories must ultimately be of some utility. Theory plays several interrelated roles in the progress of a science. The overall purpose of theory is to make scientific findings meaningful and generalizable. Several subgoals are subsumed under this broader objective—summarization, explanation, and stimulation.

Summarization of Existing Knowledge

Theories allow scientists to knit together observations and facts into an orderly system. They are efficient mechanisms for drawing together and summarizing accumulated facts from separate and isolated investigations. The linkage of findings into a coherent structure makes the body of accumulated knowledge more accessible and, thus, more useful both to practitioners who seek to implement findings and to researchers who seek to extend the knowledge base. The summarizing aspects of a theory are critical to the organization and advancement of scientific knowledge. For example, consider the theory of hypertension in renal disease. This theory states that the degree of renal hypertension varies directly with the degree of sodium retention, the degree of sodium retention varies with the amount of dietary sodium intake and, therefore, the degree of renal hypertension varies with the amount of sodium intake. This sequence of propositions represents a summary of previous observations concerning patients with renal hypertension.

Explanation of Observations and Prediction and Control of Outcomes

Theory guides the scientist's understanding of not only the "what" of natural phenomena but also the "why" of their occurrence. The power of theories to explain lies in their specification of which variables are related to one another and the nature of that relationship.

The explanatory principles embodied in a theory provide a framework for predicting the occurrence of phenomena. Although the summarization and explanation functions are concerned with what has occurred and has been established,

a theory is also expected to forecast facts and relationships that would be observed under specified circumstances. Prediction, in turn, has implications for the control of those phenomena. A theory should ideally provide the capacity to bring about desirable changes in people's behavior or the environment. To pursue the example of the theory of renal hypertension, the theory predicts conditions under which renal hypertension would be high. The theory also implies actions that would need to be taken to control renal hypertension and the degree of sodium retention.

Stimulation of New Discoveries

Theories help to stimulate research and the extension of knowledge by providing both direction and impetus. On the basis of a theory, scientists draw inferences (formulate hypotheses) about what will occur in specific situations. These hypotheses are then subjected to empirical testing in research studies. The outcome of the study may lend support to the theory or may suggest the need for modification. Theories, thus, serve as a springboard for scientific advances.

To illustrate this point, consider the theory of social facilitation proposed in the 1960s by social psychologist Robert Zajonc. The theory of social facilitation postulates that the presence of others in a performance situation facilitates well-learned responses or behavior but impairs the acquisition of new, yet-to-be learned responses. His theory integrated seemingly contradictory results from earlier research in which the presence of others was sometimes found to be debilitating to and other times enhancing of performance on a task. Zajonc's proposition has stimulated hundreds of investigations that have sought to refine, clarify, and extend social facilitation theory. For example, social facilitation effects have been extended to nonperformance situations. Davidson and Kelley (1973) used social facilitation theory as a basis for testing the effect of the presence of a nurse on anxiety levels in hospitalized psychiatric patients who watched a stressful film.

≡ *THE NATURE AND CHARACTERISTICS OF THEORY*

Scientific theories involve a series of propositions regarding the interrelationships among concepts, from which a large number of empirical observations can be deduced. In this section we describe the various aspects of a scientific theory. Although we will not discuss the formal calculus and deductive logic that have been developed in connection with theoretical systems, several references at the end of this chapter are recommended for the student who wishes to pursue theory development.

Origin of Theories

Theories are not discovered by scientists; they are created and invented by them. The building of a theory depends not only on the observable facts in our environment but also on the scientist's ingenuity in pulling those facts together and making sense of them. Theory construction, in short, is a creative and intellectual enterprise that can be engaged in by anyone with sufficient imagination. But imagination alone is not an adequate qualification; theories must be congruent with the realities of the world around us and with existing knowledge.

Components of a Theory

In the writings on scientific theory, one encounters a variety of terms such as "proposition," "postulate," "premise," "axiom," "law," "concept," "principle," and so forth, some of which are used interchangeably, and others of which introduce subtleties that are too complex for the beginning researcher. We, therefore, present a simplified analysis of the components of a theory for the sake of clarity.

Theories comprise, first of all, a set of concepts. As we noted in Chapter 4, concepts are abstract characteristics of the objects that are being studied. Examples of nursing concepts are adaptation, health, anxiety, nurse–client interaction, and social support. Concepts are the basic ingredients in the formulation of a theory. Second, theories comprise a set of statements or propositions, each of which indicates a relationship among the concepts. Relationships are denoted by such terms as "is associated with," "varies directly with," or "is contingent on." Third, the propositions must form a logically interrelated deductive system. This means that the theory must provide a mechanism for logically arriving at new statements from the original propositions.

Let us consider the following example, which illustrates these three points. Selye (1978) developed a theory of adaptation to stress. This theory postulates that a person's body responds to the nonspecific demands of stress by means of the General Adaptation Syndrome (GAS), which continues until adaptation occurs or death ensues. Stress may be internal or external to the individual and is manifested by the syndrome, which consists of nonspecifically induced changes occurring within the person's body. The GAS consists of three phases—(1) the alarm phase, (2) the phase of adaptation or resistance, and (3) the phase of exhaustion—all of which are reversible if adjustment to stress occurs. A greatly simplified construction of Selye's theory might consist of the following propositions:

1. Humans seek to attain a desired state (e.g., the reduction of stress) by mobilizing the body's general defense mechanisms to overact to maintain life.
2. When the specific defense mechanism is identified by the body for dealing with the sources of stress (such as increased muscular activity), the overactivity of the general mechanisms subsides and the specific mechanisms overact (such as increasing the oxygen supply in muscular activity).
3. If the specific defense mechanisms are unable to cope with the stress, then the general defense mechanisms reactivate to help the body adjust, or death ensues.
4. During the alarm and exhaustion phases, there is an increase in the production of adrenocortical hormones, which subsides during

the resistance phase when specific defense mechanisms come into play.

The concepts that form the basis of Selye's theory include stress, the GAS, the body's general defense mechanisms, and the body's specific defense mechanisms. His theory postulates that relationships occur between stress and the body's defense mechanisms, which are activated to cope with the stress. For example, the theory claims that the level of adrenocortical hormones varies with the stage of the GAS. Selye's propositions readily lend themselves to empirical verification by providing a mechanism for deductive hypothesis generation. We might hypothesize on the basis of Selye's theory that the level of adrenocorticotropic hormone (ACTH) will be greater before a meal than it is after a meal or that ACTH production is less during an intravenous infusion that it is immediately before its inception. On the basis of his theory, we should be able to identify how well the person is coping with the stress by measuring changes in ACTH production. Several nursing studies have been based on Selye's theory of stress and adaptation. For example, Erickson and Swain (1982) studied hospitalized medical-surgical patients to determine the relationship between their adaptive potential and length of hospital stay. Henneman (1989) used Selye's concepts of stress response to evaluate the effect of direct nursing contact on patients.

Types of Theories

Theories differ extensively in their level of generality. So-called grand theories or "macrotheories" purport to describe and explain large segments of the environment or of human experience. Some learning theorists, such as Clark Hull, or sociologists, such as Talcott Parsons, have developed highly general theoretical systems that claim to account for broad classes of behavior and social functioning. On the whole, macrotheories have not been shown to be particularly useful in the behavioral and applied sciences.

Within nursing and fields such as psychology, sociology, and education, theories are usually somewhat restricted in scope, focusing only on a narrow range of phenomena. Theories that focus on only a piece of reality or human experience and that incorporate a selected number of concepts are sometimes referred to as *middle-range theories*. For example, there are middle-range theories that attempt to explain such phenomena as decision-making behavior, leadership behavior, compliance, and attitude change. This limited scope is consistent with the state of scientific developments in many fields dealing with human behavior and is, therefore, appropriate and realistic. In the physical sciences, macrotheories such as the theory of mechanics are feasible and provide a goal toward which the younger social and applied sciences may aspire.

Theories also vary in their complexity. Here we refer to the number and intricacy of the concepts involved and the complexity of relationships presumed. Theories in the sciences dealing with humans often tend to be complex, not only because the subject matter is inherently complex but also because conditional relationships and multiple variables are required at the current level of understanding and conceptualization.

Tentative Nature of Theories

It cannot be stressed too strongly that a theory can never be "proved" nor "confirmed." A theory represents a scientist's best efforts to describe and explain phenomena; today's successful theory may be relegated to tomorrow's intellectual garbage dump. It is not only that new evidence or observations "disprove" a previously useful theory, but it is also possible that a new theoretical system can integrate new observations with the observations that the old theory "explained." There are also other reasons beside utility and parsimony for the rejection of a theory. Theories that are not congruent with a culture's values and philosophical orientation may be discredited. It is not unusual for a theory to lose supporters because its implications are not in vogue. For example, psychoanalytic and structural social theories, which had widespread support for decades, have come to be challenged and revised as a result of the emergence of feminism and changes in society's views about the roles of women. This link between theory and values may surprise those who think of science as being completely objective. It should be remembered, however, that theories are deliberately invented by humans; thus, they can never be freed totally from the human perspective, which is amenable to change over time.

In sum, no theory, no matter what its subject matter, can ever be considered final and verified. There always remains the possibility that a theory will be modified or discarded. Many theories in the physical sciences have received considerable empirical support, and their well-accepted propositions are often referred to as *laws,* such as Boyle's law of gases. Nevertheless, we have no way of knowing the ultimate accuracy and utility of any theory and should, therefore, treat all theories as tentative. This caveat is nowhere more relevant than in the emerging sciences such as nursing.

Relationship Between Theory and Research

The relationship between theory and research is a reciprocal and mutually beneficial one. A theory must be built inductively from observations, and there is no better source for those observations than scientific research. Concepts and relations that are validated in the empirical arena become the foundation for theory development. The theory, in turn, must be tested by subjecting deductions from it (hypotheses) to further scientific inquiry. Thus, research plays a dual and continuing role in theory building and testing. Theory guides and generates ideas for research; research assesses the worth of the theory and provides a foundation for new ones.

It would be unreasonable to assert that research without any theoretical underpinnings cannot make a contribution to knowledge. In nursing research, many "facts" still need to be accumulated, and descriptive inquiries may well form the basis for subsequent theoretical developments. Nontheoretical research can potentially be linked to theory at a later time. However, although it is not always easy to place one's research problems into a theoretical context, it is advantageous for the advancement of nursing science to do so. Although nursing theory *per se* is in its embryonic stages, there are useful conceptual frameworks from nursing that can be utilized in the conduct of nursing investigations.

≡ CONCEPTUAL FRAMEWORKS AND MODELS

The terms theory, theoretical framework, conceptual framework, conceptual scheme, conceptual model, and model are sometimes used synonymously in the research literature. We have been very careful in the preceding discussion to restrict our terminology to theory and theoretical framework and to use these terms to refer to a well-formulated deductive system of abstract formal statements. In this section we distinguish theories from conceptual frameworks and models.

Conceptual Frameworks

Conceptual frameworks, conceptual models, or *conceptual schemes* (we use the terms interchangeably here) represent a less formal and less well-developed attempt at organizing phenomena than theories. As the name implies, conceptual frameworks deal with abstractions (concepts) that are assembled by virtue of their relevance to a common theme. Both conceptual schemes and theories use concepts as building blocks. What is absent from conceptual schemes is the deductive system of propositions that assert a relationship between the concepts. As Fawcett (1989) observed, conceptual models also tend to be more global than theories. Homans (1964), in noting the virtual absence of formal theory in the field of sociology, pointed out the following with regard to conceptual schemes:

> Concepts and their definitions are certainly part of a theory, but they are not sufficient by themselves to constitute a theory. Concepts are names for properties of nature, and a theory does not

even begin to exist until propositions are stated about contingent relationships of the general form *x* varies as *y* between properties. (1964, p. 957)

Most of the conceptual work that has been done in connection with nursing practice is more rightfully designated as conceptual frameworks than as theories. This label in no way diminishes the importance and value of these endeavors. Indeed, many existing conceptual frameworks will undoubtedly serve as the preliminary steps in the construction of more formal theories. In the meantime, conceptual frameworks can serve to guide research that will further support theory development. Conceptual frameworks, like theories, can serve as a springboard for the generation of research hypotheses. A subsequent section of this chapter describes a few of the major conceptual models in nursing and illustrates how they have been used in nursing research.

Schematic and Statistical Models

The term model is sometimes used to denote a symbolic representation of conceptualizations of phenomena. Within a research context, the models that one is most likely to encounter are mathematical (or statistical) models and schematic models. These *models,* like conceptual frameworks, are constructed representations of some aspect of our environment. They use abstractions (i.e., concepts) as the building blocks, but they attempt to represent reality with a minimal use of words.

Language is, and probably always will be, a problem for scientists. A word or phrase that designates a concept can convey different meanings to different individuals, or to the same individual when used in different contexts. The creation of a dictionary of conceptual terms to accompany theoretical propositions does help some, but the definitions still consist of words whose imprecision can interfere with effective communication. A visual or symbolic representation of a theory or conceptual framework often helps to express abstract ideas in a more readily understandable or precise form than the original conceptualization.

Schematic models are quite common and undoubtedly are familiar to all readers. A schematic model or diagram represents the phenomena of interest figuratively. Concepts and the linkages between them are represented diagrammatically through the use of boxes, arrows, or other symbols. An example of a schematic model is presented in Figure 7-1. This model is described by its designer as "a human interaction diagram showing nurse and client interactions" (King, 1981, p. 145). The author noted that the perception, judgment, and reaction activities are not directly observable. However, the interactions are directly observable behaviors that can be recorded and analyzed to determine what transactions have occurred. Schematic models of this type can be quite useful in the research process in clarifying concepts and their associations, in enabling researchers to place a specific problem into an appropriate context, and in revealing areas where further inquiry is needed.

Statistical models are playing a growing role in research endeavors in nursing and related sciences. These models use symbols to express quantitatively the nature of relationships among variables. There are few relationships in the behavioral sciences that can be summarized as elegantly as in the mathematical model F = ma (force = mass × acceleration). Because human behavior is so complex and subject to so many influences as yet poorly understood, it is typically possible to model it only in a probabilistic manner. This means that we are not yet able (and probably never will be able) to develop equations, such as the example of force from mechanics, in which a human behavior can be simply described as the product of two other phenomena. What we can do, however, is describe the probability that a certain behavior or characteristic will exist, given the occurrence of other specified phenomena. This is the function of statistical models. An example of a statistical model is shown below:

$$Y = \beta_1X_1 + \beta_2X_2 + \beta_3X_3 + \beta_4X_4 + e$$

where Y = nursing effectiveness, as measured by a supervisor's evaluation

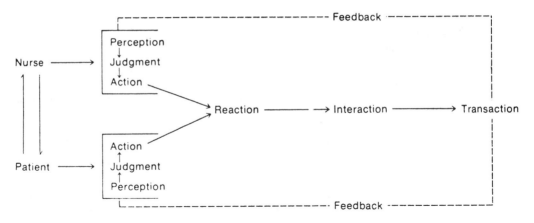

Figure 7-1. *Human interaction process. (After King, I.M. [1981]. A Theory for Nursing.* New York: John Wiley & Sons, p. 145. Used with permission.)

X_1 = nursing knowledge, as measured by the licensure examination

X_2 = past achievement, as measured by grades in nursing school

X_3 = decision-making skills, as measured by number of nursing diagnoses made

X_4 = empathy, as measured by timing between the patient's request for pain medication and actual administration of pain medication

e = a residual, unexplained factor

$\beta_1, \beta_2, \beta_3,$ and β_4 = weights indicating the importance of X_1, X_2, X_3, and X_4, respectively, in determining nursing effectiveness

Note that each term in this model is quantified or quantifiable; that is, every symbol can be replaced by a numerical value, such as an individual's score on the nursing licensure exam (X_1).

What does this equation mean and how does it work? This model constitutes a mechanism for understanding and predicting nursing effectiveness. The model proposes that on-the-job effectiveness is affected primarily by four factors:

the (1) nursing knowledge, (2) past achievement, (3) decision-making skill, and (4) empathy of the nurse. These influences are not presumed to be equally important. The weights (βs) associated with each factor represent a recipe for designating the relative importance of each. If empathy were much more important than past achievement, for example, then the weights might be 2 to 1, respectively (i.e., two parts empathy to one part past achievement). The "e" (or error term) at the end of the model represents all those unknown or unmeasurable other attributes that affect one's performance as a nurse. In the quantitative equation, "e" would be set equal to some constant value; it would not vary from one nurse to another, because it really constitutes an unknown element in the equation. Once the values of the weights and "e" have been established (through statistical procedures), the model can be used to predict the nursing effectiveness of any nurse for whom we have gathered information on the four Xs (licensure exam scores and so forth). Our prediction of who will make an especially effective nurse will not always be perfectly accurate, in part because of the influence of those unknown factors summarized by "e." Perfect forecasting is seldom attainable with probabilistic statistical models. However, such a model makes prediction of nursing effectiveness less haphazard than mere guesswork or intuition.

In summary, it may not always prove possible to identify a formal theory that is relevant to a nursing research problem, but conceptual schemes and models of the type discussed here can also be used to clarify concepts and to provide a context for findings that might otherwise be isolated and meaningless. Conceptual frameworks in nursing are very much in need of testing if theories for nursing are to be formulated.

≡ CONCEPTUAL FRAMEWORKS IN NURSING

In the past few decades, nurses have formulated a number of conceptual frameworks and models of nursing and for nursing practice. These models constitute formal explanations of what the nursing discipline is according to the model developer's point of view. As Fawcett (1989) has noted, there is general agreement that there are four central concepts of the nursing discipline: (1) person, (2) environment, (3) health, and (4) nursing. However, the various conceptual models define these concepts differently, link them in diverse ways, and give different emphasis to the relationships among them.

The conceptual models were not developed solely as a base from which nursing research could be launched. Indeed, these models have thus far had more impact on nursing education, administration, and clinical practice than on nursing research. Nevertheless, nurse researchers are turning increasingly toward these conceptual frameworks for their inspiration and theoretical foundations in formulating research questions and hypotheses. In this section we briefly examine some of the major conceptual frameworks in nursing and give examples of research that claimed their intellectual roots in these models.

Johnson's Behavioral System Model

Like other systems models, Johnson's (1980) model focuses on a system, its subsystems, and its environment. The system of central interest in Johnson's model is the patient as a behavioral system. According to this model, each individual behavioral system is a collection of seven interrelated subsystems, the response patterns of which form an organized and integrated whole. The seven subsystems are (1) attachment or affiliation, (2) dependency, (3) ingestion, (4) elimination, (5) sexuality, (6) aggression, and (7) achievement. Each subsystem carries out specialized tasks for the integrated system, and each is structured by four motivational elements: (1) goal, (2) set, (3) choice, and (4) action/behavior.

The model is concerned with behavioral functioning that results in the equilibrium of the integrated system. Behavioral system balance reflects adjustments and adaptations that are successful in the achievement of a steady state. Johnson indicates that the seven subsystems must be stimulated to grow and adapt but must also be protected from malfunctions and noxious influences. The function of nursing is to help restore the balance of each subsystem in the event of disequilibrium and to help prevent future system disturbances.

Several researchers have designated Johnson's Behavioral System Model as their conceptual basis. For example, Derdiarian and Forsythe (1983) described the development of an instrument (the Derdiarian Behavioral System Model Instrument) to measure the perceived behavioral changes of cancer patients. Holaday (1987) focused on Johnson's concept of "behavioral set" in her study of the vocal and visual interactions occurring between mothers and their chronically ill infants. Johnson's interrelated subsystems also guided Lovejoy's (1983) development of an assessment tool to measure leukemic children's perceptions of family functioning.

King's Interacting Systems Model

King's (1981) conceptual model includes three types of interacting systems. The first type of system, personal systems, is represented by individuals. The key concepts included in personal systems are perception, self, body image, growth and development, time, and space. Interpersonal systems are the second type in the network of interacting systems (Fig. 7-1). When individuals interact (e.g., client and nurse), they form interpersonal systems. Concepts relevant to interpersonal interactions include role, interaction, communication, transaction, and stress. The third major category in the framework is social systems. Any social system in which the nurse interacts with health-care consumers, such as a family or a hospital, belongs to this category of systems. Concepts relevant for functioning in social systems include organizations, role, power, authority, and decision making.

Within King's model, the domain of nursing includes promoting, maintaining, and restoring health. Nursing is viewed as "a process of action, reaction, and interaction whereby nurse and client share information about their perceptions of the nursing situation. Through purposeful communication they identify specific goals, problems, or concerns. They explore means to achieve a goal and agree to means to the goal" (King, 1981, p. 2).

King's model has not been used as the basis for many studies. However, King (1981) herself conducted a descriptive observational study of nurse–client encounters that yielded a classification of elements in nurse–client interactions. The study provided preliminary support for the proposition that goal attainment was facilitated by accurate nurse–client perceptions, satisfactory communication, and mutual goal setting.

Levine's Conservation Model

Levine's (1973) model focuses on individuals as holistic beings, and the major area of concern is maintenance of the person's wholeness. The model identifies adaptation as the process by which the integrity or wholeness of individuals is maintained.

Levine suggested four principles of conservation that aim to facilitate patients' adaptation processes:

1. conservation of patient energy, that is, the conservation of the individual's physiologic and psychologic energy resources
2. conservation of structural integrity, that is, the conservation of patients' body form and function
3. conservation of personal integrity, that is, the conservation of patients' self-esteem and psychologic identity
4. conservation of social integrity, that is, the conservation of patients' familial, community, and subcultural affiliations

Through these four conservation principles, the model emphasizes the nurse's responsibility to maintain the client's integrity in the threat of assault through illness or environmental influences.

Levine noted that her model is appropriate for investigating the interface between the internal and external environments of the person. Several researchers have used Levine's model as a conceptual base. For example, Levine's four conservation principles formed the basis of Yeates and Roberts' (1984) study comparing the effectiveness of two bearing-down techniques during the second stage of labor. Crawford-Gambel (1986) based her case study describing the perioperative clinical situation on Levine's conservation principles. Newport (1984), who investigated two alternative methods of conserving newborn thermal energy and social integrity, also linked her study to Levine's model.

Neuman's Health Care Systems Model

Neuman's (1989) model focuses on the person as a complete system, the subparts of which are interrelated physiologic, psychologic, sociocultural, spiritual, and developmental factors. These interacting variables determine the amount of resistance an individual can mount against stressors. The stressors may be intrapersonal, interpersonal, or extrapersonal.

The central core of protection the person has for his or her first-line defense against stressors is a flexible line of resistance—internal factors that help defend against the stressor. The next protective barrier is the normal line of defense, which includes such factors as the person's coping style, developmental stage, and so on. The final buffer against stressors is the flexible line of defense, which comprises dynamic factors that can fluctuate in response to circumstances.

In Neuman's model, the person maintains balance and harmony between internal and external environments by adjusting to stress and by defending against tension-producing stimuli. Wellness is equated with equilibrium, which is maintained when the person's flexible line of defense has prevented stressors from penetrating the normal line of defense. The primary goal of nursing is to assist in the attainment and maintenance of client system stability. Nursing interventions include activities to strengthen flexible lines of defense, to strengthen resistance to stressors, and to maintain adaptation.

The Neuman Health Care Systems Model has led to some applications in nursing research. For example, Craddock and Stanhope (1980) applied Neuman's scheme in a study of clients' and health-care providers' perceptions of stressors. Ziemer (1983) operationalized many of Neuman's concepts in a study of the effects of preoperative information on the postoperative outcomes of clients who have had abdominal surgery. Ross and Bourbonnais (1985) described the interpersonal, intrapersonal, and extrapersonal stressors identified in the home care of a man following a myocardial infarction. They developed nursing interventions directed toward strengthening the flexible lines of defense and resistance.

Orem's Self-Care Model

Orem's (1985) model focuses on each individual's ability to perform *self-care*—"the practice of activities that individuals initiate and perform on their own behalf in maintaining life, health, and well-being" (p. 35). One's ability to care for oneself is referred to as self-care agency, and the ability to care for others is referred to as dependent-care agency.

According to the model, there are three categories of self-care requisites, purposes to be attained through self-care actions: (1) universal requisites (associated with life processes and the maintenance of integrity of human structure and functioning); (2) developmental requisites (associated with developmental processes at various stages of the life cycle); and (3) health-deviation requisites (arising from structural/functional deviations or constitutional/genetic defects). Therapeutic self-care demand refers to the self-care actions needed to address these requisites. Self-care deficits are said to occur when a person does not have the capacity for continuous self-care.

In Orem's model, the goal of nursing agency is to help people meet their own therapeutic self-care demands. Orem identified three types of nursing systems: (1) wholly compensatory—wherein the nurse compensates for the patient's total inability to perform self-care activities; (2) partially compensatory—wherein the nurse compensates for the patient's partial inability to perform self-care activities; and (3) supportive-educative—wherein the nurse assists the patient in making decisions and acquiring skills and knowledge.

Orem's Self-Care Model has generated considerable interest among nurse researchers. For example, Chang and colleagues (1985) examined components of nurse practitioners' care in the context of Orem's model to determine what aspects of the care contributed most to the elderly patients' intentions to adhere to the care plan. Kearney and Fleischer (1979) undertook a study to develop an instrument measuring a person's exercise of self-care agency. This instrument was used in a study by Riesch (1988), who investigated the extent to which pregnant women and their coaches exercise self-care agency before and after childbirth-preparation activities. Patterson and Hale (1985) based their study of menstrual care practices on Orem's Self-Care Model. A fuller description of other research based on this model is provided in a subsequent section of this chapter.

Parse's Model of Man–Living–Health

Parse's (1987) model views a human being as an open system freely able to choose from among a series of options in giving meaning to a situation. Humans and the environment remain independent entities during interchanges, and together they co-create meaning and patterns. The three principles of Parse's model focus on the thematic elements of (1) meaning, (2) rhythmicity, and (3) cotranscendence. Meaning is multidimensional in nature. The three essential concepts for structuring meaning are (1) languaging, (2) imaging, and (3) valuing. Rhythmicity refers to the rhythmical patterns co-created by human-environment interchanges. Revealing–concealing, enabling–limiting, and connecting–separating are the three essential concepts for establishing rhythmicity. Cotranscendence is the process of reaching for the yet-to-be lived experiences. The three essential concepts enabling cotranscendence are (1) powering, (2) originating, and (3) transforming.

The goal of the Man–Living–Health model in nursing practice is to encourage a client to share his or her thoughts and feelings about the meaning of a situation. The explication of the meaning changes the situation and new meaning occurs. As new meanings arise, the rhythmical patterns co-created by client and environment change. Clients may then be guided to plan for the changing from the known health patterns to new health patterns.

The Parse model is a relatively young one, but has already generated several applications in the research literature, particularly among researchers with a phenomenological orientation. Banonis (1989) relied on the Parse model in her study of the experience of recovering from an addiction, and operationalized, for her sample, the themes of meaning, rhythmicity, and cotranscendence. Santopinto (1989) used Parse's model as a framework for her study of the lived experience of two women in their relentless drive to be thinner. Smith (1990) explored the experience of struggling through a difficult time for people who are unemployed, basing her study on Parse's framework.

Rogers' Model of the Unitary Human Being

Rogers' (1970) model focuses on individuals as a unified whole in constant interaction with the environment. The unitary person is viewed as an energy field that is more than, and different from, the sum of the biologic, physical, social, and psychologic parts. The environment constitutes another energy field. The human and environmental energy fields have pattern and organization, but are continuously and creatively changing.

Three principles of homeodynamics define the nature and direction of human change and development: (1) helicy—characterized by the diversity of the human and environmental field emerging from their interactions and manifesting nonrecurring rhythmicities; (2) resonancy—characterized by ongoing change from lower to higher frequency wave patterns in the human and environmental fields; and (3) integrality—the continuous, mutual, and simultaneous interaction between human and environmental fields.

In Rogers' model, nursing is concerned with the unitary person as a synergistic phenomenon. Nursing science is devoted to the study of the nature and direction of unitary human development. Nursing practice helps individuals achieve maximum well-being within their potential.

Several nursing studies have been based on Rogers' Model of the Unitary Human Being. For example, Benedict and Burge (1990), focusing on the principle of resonancy, studied the relationship between human field motion and preferred visible wavelengths. Smith (1986) based her study comparing the effectiveness of quiet and varied harmonic auditory inputs on perceived restfulness on Rogers' principle of integrality. Gaydos and Farnham (1988) also used this principle in studying human rhythms in response to environmental rhythms. Schodt (1989) applied Rogers' principle of integrality in her study of the nature of interactions between fathers and their unborn children.

Roy's Adaptation Model

In Roy's (1984) Adaptation Model, human beings are holistic adaptive systems who cope with environmental change through the process of adaptation. Within the human system are four subsystems: (1) physiologic needs, (2) self-concept, (3) role function, and (4) interdependence. These subsystems constitute adaptive modes that provide mechanisms for coping with environmental stimuli and change. The adaptive mode relating to physiologic needs is concerned with the need for physiologic integrity. The adaptive mode of self-concept addresses the need for psychic integrity. The adaptive modes of role function and interdependence focus on the need for social integrity.

The goal of nursing, according to this model, is to promote effective patient adaptation in all four modes. Nursing also regulates stimuli affecting adaptation. Nursing interventions generally take the form of increasing, decreasing, modifying, removing, or maintaining internal and external stimuli that affect adaptation.

Roy's Adaptation Model has been used as the conceptual framework in several nursing studies. For example, Tulman and her colleagues (1990) studied changes in functional status after childbirth according to Roy's four adaptive modes. Shannahan and Cottrell (1985) invoked Roy's concept of manipulation of contextual stimuli in their assessment of the effects of delivering in a birth chair versus a traditional delivery table. Henneman (1989) built on Roy's concepts of stress reduction and adaptation in her study of the effect of nurse contact on the stress response of patients being weaned from mechanical ventilation.

≡ TESTING, USING, AND DEVELOPING THEORY

In a previous section, we described the strong interrelationship between theory and research. The manner in which theory and conceptual frameworks are used by researchers is elaborated upon in the following section. In the discussion, the term "theory" will not be restricted to its narrow, formal connotation but will refer to its broader meaning as something conceptual, abstract, and general. In other words, the procedures discussed will almost always be equally applicable to conceptual frameworks and models as well as to formal theories.

Testing a Theory

As noted earlier, theories often stimulate new research investigations. For example, a nurse might read several papers relating to Orem's Self-Care Model. As the nurse's reading progresses, the following types of conjectures might arise: "If Orem's self-care model is valid, then one might expect that nursing effectiveness might be enhanced in environments more conducive to self-care (for example, a birthing room versus a delivery room)" or "Given this conceptual framework, it might be expected that the dependency level of patients (in terms of either their physical or psychologic characteristics) would affect the nature and intensity of effective interventions." These conjectures, derived from the theory or conceptual framework, can serve as a point of departure for testing the adequacy of the theory.

In testing a theory, the researcher deduces implications (as in the preceding example) and develops research hypotheses. These hypotheses are predictions about the manner in which variables would be related, if the theory were correct and useful. The hypotheses are then subjected to empirical testing through systematic research. A theory is never tested directly. It is the hypotheses deduced from a theory that are subjected to scientific investigations. Comparisons between the observed outcomes of research and the relationships predicted by the hypotheses are the major focus of the testing process. Through this process, the theory is continually subjected to potential disconfirmation. Repeated failures of research endeavors to disconfirm a theory result in increasing support for and acceptance of a theoretical position. The testing process continues until some piece of evidence cannot be interpreted within the context of the theory but *can* be explained by a new theory that also accounts for all previous findings. From the point of view of theory testing, the goal of a serviceable research project is to develop a research design that reduces the credibility of alternative explanations for observed relationships, to devise logically adequate deductions from theory, and to select methods that assess the theory's validity under maximally heterogeneous situations so that potentially competing theories can be ruled out. The theory-testing aspect of research is described in more detail in Chapter 8, which deals with hypotheses.

Before using a theory as a basis for a research study, the investigator should first evaluate the theory. Stevens (1984) and Chinn and Jacobs (1987) present useful criteria for assessing conceptual frameworks in nursing.

Testing Two Competing Theories

Researchers who directly test two competing theories to explain some phenomenon are in a particularly good position to advance scientific knowledge. Almost all phenomena can be explained in alternative ways, as suggested by the alternative conceptual models of nursing. There are also competing theories for such phenomena as stress, pain, child development, learning, and grieving. All of these phenomena are of great importance to nursing. Each competing theory for these phenomena suggests alternative approaches to facilitating a positive outcome or minimizing a negative one. It is therefore important to know which explanation has more validity, if we are to design maximally effective nursing interventions.

Typically, researchers have opted to test a single theory in a research investigation. Then, to evaluate the worth of competing theories, they must compare the results of different studies. However, such comparisons are often difficult to make because study designs rarely lend themselves to direct comparisons. For example, one study of stress might use a sample of college students, another might use military personnel in a combat situation, and yet another might use terminally ill cancer patients. Each of these studies might use an alternative approach to measuring stress. If the results of these studies support alternative theories of stress to different degrees, it would be difficult to know the extent to which the results reflected differences in the study design rather than differences in the validity of the theories.

The researcher who directly tests two (or more) competing theories, using a single sample of subjects and comparable measures of the key research variables, is in a position to make powerful and meaningful comparisons. Such a study typically requires considerable advance planning, and the inclusion of a wider array of measures than would otherwise be the case, but such efforts are to be commended. In recent years, a growing number of nursing investigators have used this approach to generate and refine our knowledge base and to provide promising new leads for further research. For example, Campbell (1989) tested a "grief model" and a "learned helplessness" model to explain women's responses to battering. She found that both theories had some support, but that the "learned helplessness" concepts had not been sufficiently operationalized in her study and required further investigation. Mahon and Yarcheski (1988) tested two alternative explanations for loneliness in adolescents: an explanation dependent on situational factors, and one linking loneliness to characterological or personality traits. The findings suggested that the situational explanation had substantially more support.

Fitting a Problem to a Theory

The preceding sections addressed the situation in which a researcher begins with one or more specific theories or conceptual frameworks and uses the theories as the basis for developing a research problem and design. Circumstances sometimes arise in which the problem is formulated before consideration is given to a theoretical framework. Even in such situations researchers may wish to (or may be required to) devise a theoretical context in an effort to enrich the value and interpretability of their inquiry. While we recognize that this situation sometimes occurs, we must nevertheless caution that an after-the-fact linkage of theory to a research question is usually considerably less meaningful than the testing of a particular theory of interest. This is especially true for neophyte researchers who may lack a thorough grounding in the theoretical positions of their own or related disciplines.

The search for relevant existing theories can be greatly facilitated by first conceptualizing on a sufficiently abstract level what the nature of the problem is. For example, take the problem statement, "Do daily telephone conversations between a psychiatric nurse and a patient for two weeks following discharge from the hospital result in lower rates of readmission by short-term psychiatric patients?" This is a relatively concrete research problem but might profitably be viewed as a subproblem for Orem's Self-Care Model, or a theory of reinforcement, or a theory of social influence, or a theory of crisis resolution. Part of the difficulty in finding a theory is that a single phenomenon of interest can be conceptualized in a number of ways and, depending on the manner chosen, may refer the researcher to conceptual schemes from a wide range of disciplines.

Once the researcher has conceptualized the research problem on an abstract level, the search for existing theories can proceed. Textbooks, handbooks, and encyclopedias in the chosen discipline usually are a good starting point for the identification of a theory. These sources usually summarize the status of a theoretical position and document the efforts to confirm and disconfirm it. Journal articles contain more current information but are usually restricted to descriptions of specific studies rather than to broad expositions or evaluations of theories. When a theoretical position has been developed at length or has been supported by extensive empirical observations, entire books may be devoted to their description.

Once a suitable conceptual framework has been identified, its utility should be carefully evaluated in terms of the framework's inherent merit,

using criteria such as those presented in Stevens (1984) and Chinn and Jacobs (1987); its congruity with the problem to be studied; and its congruity with the researcher's own philosophy and world view. If the framework is judged to be adequate on these grounds, it then becomes the researcher's job to design the study in such a way that it "fits" the framework.

The task of fitting a problem to a theory should be done with caution. It is true that having a theoretical context enhances the meaningfulness of a research study, but artificially cramming a problem into a theory is not the route to scientific utility. There are many published studies that purport to have a conceptual framework, when in fact the *post hoc* nature of the conceptualization is all too evident. If a conceptual framework is really linked to a research problem, then the design of the study, the selection of appropriate data collection strategies, the data analysis, and (especially) the interpretation of the findings *flow* from that conceptualization. We advocate a balanced and reasoned perspective on this issue: Researchers should not shirk their intellectual duties by failing to make an attempt to link their problem to broader theoretical concerns, but there is no point in fabricating such a link when it does not exist.

Developing a Theory

Many beginning researchers may think of themselves as unqualified to develop a theory or conceptual scheme of their own. But theory development depends much less on one's knowledge of research methods and experience in the conduct of investigations than on one's powers of observation, understanding of a problem, and readings about a substantive issue. There is, therefore, nothing to prevent an imaginative and sensitive person from formulating an original conceptual framework for a study. The conceptual scheme may or may not be a full-fledged formal theory with well-articulated postulates; the scheme should, however, place the issues of the study into some broader perspective. In the field of nursing research, where there has not yet been extensive theoretical work, the beginning researcher may have an easier task in devising an original framework than in finding one that is appropriate for the problem of interest.

The basic intellectual process underlying theory development is *induction,* which refers to the process of reasoning from particular observations and facts to generalizations. The inductive process involves integrating what one has experienced or learned into some concise and general conclusion. If one has observed that Morgan P., Brooke L., Shanley I., and Daniel S. (all of whom are tonsillectomy patients) have refused to eat their first postoperative meal, one might conclude that loss of appetite characterizes those who have just had a tonsillectomy operation. The "observations" used in the inductive process need not be personal observations; they may be (and often are in formal theories) the findings and conclusions from research investigations. When relationships among variables are arrived at this way, one has the makings of a theory that can be put to a more rigorous scientific test. The first step in theory development, then, is to formulate a generalized scheme of relevant concepts, that is, to perform a conceptual analysis. The product of

this step should be a conceptual framework, whose worth can be assessed through the collection of empirical information.

Let us consider the following simple example. Suppose that we were interested in understanding the factors influencing enrollment in a prenatal education program. We might begin by considering two basic sets of forces: (1) those that promote enrollment and (2) those that hinder it. After reviewing the literature, discussing the problem with colleagues, and developing ideas from our own experiences, we might arrive at a conceptual scheme such as the one presented in Figure 7-2. This framework is undoubtedly incomplete and imperfect, but it does allow us to study a number of research questions *and* to place those problems in perspective. For example, the conceptual scheme suggests that as the availability of social supports declines, the obstacles to participation in a prenatal education program increase. We might then make the following hypothesis: "Single pregnant women are less likely to participate in a prenatal education program than married pregnant women," on the assumption that husbands are an important source of social support to women in their pregnancy.

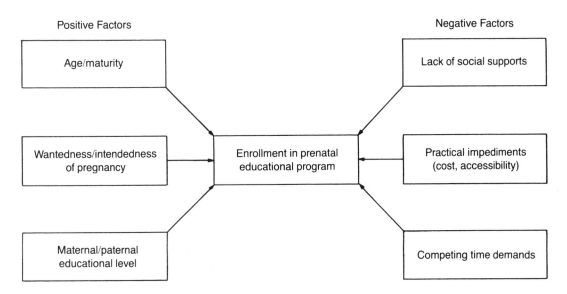

Figure 7-2. *Conceptual model—factors that influence enrollment in a prenatal education program.*

The translation of conceptual schemes into formal theories is considerably more complex and intellectually formidable than the initial conceptual analysis. To date, few formal theories have been devised in nursing and few have been subjected to rigorous confirmatory efforts. Theory development remains a critical challenge to this generation of nursing researchers.

≡ THEORETICAL CONTEXTS AND NURSING RESEARCH

Theory and research have reciprocal, beneficial ties. Fawcett (1978) described the relationship between theory and research as a double helix, with theory as the impetus of scientific investigations and findings from research shaping the development of theory. However, this relationship has not always characterized the progress of nursing science. Many have criticized nursing researchers for producing numerous pieces of isolated research that are not placed in a theoretical context.

This criticism was more justified a decade ago than it is today. Many researchers are developing studies on the basis of conceptual models of nursing. However, nursing science is still struggling to integrate accumulated knowledge within theoretical systems. This struggle is reflected, in part, in the number of controversies surrounding the issue of theoretical frameworks in nursing.

One of these controversies concerns whether there should be one single, unified model of nursing, or multiple, competing models. Fawcett (1989) has argued against combining different models, noting that "before all nurses follow the same path, the competition of multiple models is needed to determine the superiority of one or more of them" (p. 9). Research can play a critical role in testing the utility and validity of alternative nursing models.

Another controversy involves the desirability and appropriateness of developing theories unique to nursing. Some commentators argue that theories relating to humans developed within other disciplines (e.g., physiology, psychology, anthropology, and sociology) can and should be applied to nursing problems. Others advocate the development of unique nursing theories, claiming that only through such development can knowledge to guide nursing practice be generated.

Until these controversies are resolved, nursing research is likely to continue on its current path of conducting studies within a multidisciplinary and multitheoretical perspective. We are inclined to see the use of multiple frameworks as a healthy and unavoidable part of the development of nursing science. We conclude this chapter by presenting several nursing research applications using both "borrowed" and nursing-specific theoretical schemes.

≡ RESEARCH EXAMPLES

Example 1: The Health Belief Model

The Health Belief Model (HBM) has become a popular conceptual framework in nursing, especially in studies focusing on patient compliance and preventive health-care practices. The model integrates psychologic theories of goal setting, decision making, and social learning. The model postulates that health-seeking behavior is influenced by a person's perception of a threat posed by a health problem and the value associated with actions aimed at reducing the threat (Becker, 1978). The major components of the HBM include perceived susceptibility, perceived severity, perceived benefits and costs, motivation, and enabling or modifying factors. Perceived susceptibility refers to a person's perception that a health problem is personally relevant or that a diagnosis of illness is accurate. Even when one recognizes personal susceptibility, action will not occur unless the individual believes that becoming ill would have serious organic or social implications. Perceived benefits refer to the patients' beliefs that a given treatment will cure the illness or help prevent it, whereas perceived costs refer to the complexity, duration, and accessibility of the treatment. Motivation includes desire to comply with a treatment, belief that people should do what is prescribed by health-care personnel, concern about health matters in general, willingness to seek and accept health care, and engagement in positive health activities. Among the modifying factors that have been identified are personality variables, the patient–practitioner relationships, patient satisfaction, and sociodemographic factors.

DeVon and Powers (1984) used the HBM in their study of compliance and psychosocial adjustment in two groups of hypertensive patients. Subjects were classified as being either "controlled" or "uncontrolled" with respect to their hypertension, based on the clinical judgment of their physicians. The study sample involved 30 subjects (15 in each group). The subjects completed a compliance questionnaire (based on the HBM) and the Psychosocial Adjustment to Illness Scale. Blood pressure and hypertension-related information were obtained from the patients' records. Contrary to expectations, the two groups did not differ in their health beliefs affecting compliance, but differences were found with respect to psychosocial adjustment to illness. Uncontrolled hypertensives showed less illness-related adjustment and reported more psychologic distress. Lower adjustment to illness was found to be related to both lower compliance and to a more complex medication regimen. The investigators concluded that the findings supported the notion that psychosocial distress may be an important variable affecting the generalizability of the HBM and worthy of closer scrunity in other studies based on the model.

Several nurse researchers have used the HBM to study women's practice of breast self-examination. For example, Champion (1987) studied the relationship between frequency of breast self-examination and variables stipulated in the HBM in a sample of 588 women. The investigator measured such HBM variables as perceived susceptibility, seriousness, perceived benefits and barriers, health motivation, control, and knowledge about breast cancer. In this study, frequency of breast self-examination was found to be related to perceived barriers, perceived sus-

ceptibility, and the women's knowledge regarding breast cancer. Perceived barriers were especially strong predictors of the practice of breast self-examination. Champion also found that women taught about breast self-examination by a doctor or a nurse had a higher frequency of breast self-examination practice than women taught in other ways.

Example 2: The Health Promotion Model

The theoretical work of Becker has been extended by Pender (1987), whose model focuses on health promotion. According to Pender's model, *health promotion* is defined as activities directed toward the development of resources that maintain or enhance an individual's well-being. The Health Promotion Model (HPM) encompasses two phases: (1) a decision-making phase and (2) an action phase. In the decision-making phase, the model emphasizes seven cognitive-perceptual factors that compose primary motivational mechanisms for acquisition and maintenance of health-promoting behaviors (e.g., perceived barriers to health-promoting behaviors) and five modifying factors that indirectly influence patterns of health behavior (e.g., situational influences). In the action phase, both barriers and cues to action trigger activity in health-promoting behavior. According to the model, people move back and forth in a reciprocal fashion between the two phases.

Weitzel (1989) tested the HPM with a sample of 179 blue-collar workers. Four psychologic variables—(1) the importance of health, (2) perceived health locus of control, (3) health status, and (4) self-efficacy—and one modifying variable (selected demographics) were studied in relation to health-promoting behaviors (e.g., exercise, nutrition, and stress management). Each of the psychologic variables was found to be predictive of health-promoting behavior. In this sample, health status and self-efficacy were the most powerful predictors.

Volden and her colleagues (1990) studied differences in health and life style measures based on age, gender, and exercise involvement. Based on the HPM, the emphasis on this study was placed on two cognitive-perceptual factors—(1) the definition of health and (2) perceived health status; four modifying factors—(1) demographic characteristics, (2) biologic characteristics, (3) interpersonal influences, and (4) behavioral factors; and cues that lead to health-promoting activities. In their study of 478 adults from both urban and rural regions, the researchers found substantial gender differences on most of the variables studied, but age differences were less common. They concluded that the "data provided some support for Pender's Health Promotion Model and for the need of purposeful design of health-promoting classes and practices" (p. 25).

Example 3: Orem's Self-Care Model

Earlier in this chapter we reviewed the major features of Orem's Self-Care Model. In this section, we examine two studies that used this model as their conceptual framework.

Rothlis (1984) investigated whether people with reactive depression exposed to a self-help group experience a greater decrease in their feelings of hopelessness and helplessness than people not participating in a self-help group. Rothlis viewed reactive depression within Orem's framework as a health-deviation self-care deficit. Rothlis further identified the intervention (the introduction of the self-help groups) as a nursing activity within the educative–supportive–developmental domain. Self-help groups were conceptualized as a means of creating a milieu wherein therapeutic processes could occur. These processes were believed to increase the capacity for self-care agency and hasten the process of separating the patient from the health professional. The sample consisted of 28 patients with a primary diagnosis of reactive depression. Half of the subjects were assigned at random to participate in a self-help group and the other subjects did not participate. Subjects were administered a measure of hopelessness and helplessness before the implementation of the self-help groups and also four days later. The findings indicated that although the two groups were comparable at the beginning of the study, patients who participated in the self-help groups had significantly lower scores of helplessness and hopelessness at the end of the study.

Dodd (1984) studied the self-care behaviors of cancer patients in chemotherapy. She argued that because there is little information on how patients manage an illness, studies of self-care in disease are needed. The subjects in the study (48 cancer patients in chemotherapy) were assigned at random to four types of treatment that were hypothesized to influence patients' capabilities for self-care. The first group received drug information only; the second group received information on side-effect management techniques; the third group received both types of information; and the fourth group received no special intervention. Information on chemotherapy knowledge, self-care behavior, and overall psychologic well-being was obtained both before and after the completion of the interventions. Subjects who received the drug information scored higher than other subjects on the chemotherapy knowledge test. Subjects who received information on side-effect management techniques (either alone or with drug information) performed more self-care behaviors after the intervention than subjects who did not receive this information.

≡ SUMMARY

A *theory* is an abstract generalization that systematically explains the relationships among phenomena. The overall objective of theory is to make scientific findings meaningful and generalizable. In addition, theories help to summarize existing knowledge into coherent systems, stimulate new research by providing both direction and impetus, and explain the nature of relationships between or among variables, which provides a framework for predicting and, in turn, controlling the occurrence of the phenomena.

Theories are created or developed by scientists. Their creation requires imagination on the part of the scientist and congruence with reality and existing knowledge. The basic components of a theory are concepts. Theories consist of a set of statements, each of which expresses a relationship. The statements are arranged in a logically interrelated system that permits new statements to be derived from them.

Theories vary in their level of generality and level of complexity. Some theories attempt to describe large segments of the environment and are called *grand theories* or *macrotheories,* whereas other theories are more restricted in scope. Theories that are more specific to certain phenomena are sometimes referred to as *middle-range theories.* All theories are considered tentative and are never "proved."

Conceptual frameworks or *schemes* are less fully developed attempts at organizing phenomena than are theories. Concepts are the basic elements of a conceptual scheme, as in theories. However, in a conceptual framework, the concepts are not linked to one another in a logically ordered deductive system. Much of the conceptual work in nursing is more rightfully described as conceptual schemes than as theories. Conceptual frameworks are highly valuable in that they often serve as the springboard for theory development.

Models are symbolic representations of phenomena. Models depict a theory or conceptual scheme through the use of symbols or diagrams. The two types of models most frequently used in research are (1) mathematical or *statistical models* and (2) *schematic models.* Models are useful to scientists because they use a minimal amount of words, which tend to be ambiguous, in representing reality.

A number of conceptual models of nursing have evolved and have been used in nursing research. Among the major conceptual models of nursing are Johnson's Behavioral System Model, King's Interacting Systems Model, Levine's Conservation Model, Neuman's Health Care Systems Model, Orem's Self-Care Model, Parse's Model of Man-Living-Health, Rogers' Model of the Unitary Human Being, and Roy's Adaptation Model.

Conceptual schemes and theories can be integrated with empirical research in a number of ways. The investigator may design a scientific study specifically to test a theory of interest or to test two or more competing theories. In other situations, a problem may be developed first and a theory selected to "fit" the problem. An after-the-fact selection of a theory usually is more problematic and less meaningful than the systematic testing of a particular theory.

Nursing research is increasingly drawing on conceptual frameworks and models in its efforts to integrate accumulated knowledge and advance nursing science. Currently, many investigations are based on theories borrowed from other disciplines, but an increasing number of studies have conceptual models of nursing as their frameworks.

☰ *STUDY SUGGESTIONS*

1. Read the article by S.I. Laffrey (1985) entitled, "Health behavior choice as related to self-actualization and health conception." *Western Journal of Nursing Research, 7,* 279–300. What theoretical basis does the author develop for health conception and health behavior choice? Would you classify the theoretical basis as a theory or as a conceptual framework? Draw a schematic model of the major concepts used in the study.

2. Select one of the nursing conceptual frameworks or models described in the chapter. Formulate a research question and two hypotheses that could be used to empirically test the utility of the conceptual framework or model in nursing practice.

3. Four researchable problems are as follows:
   a. What is the relationship between angina pain and alcohol intake?
   b. What effect does rapid weight gain during the second trimester have on the outcome of pregnancy?
   c. Do multiple hospital readmissions affect the achievement level of children?

d. To what extent do coping mechanisms of individuals differ in health and illness?

Abstract a generalized issue or issues for each of these problems. Search for an existing theory that might be applicable and appropriate.

≡ SUGGESTED READINGS

THEORETICAL REFERENCES

Andrews, H.A., & Roy, C. (1986). *Essentials of the Roy Adaptation Model*. Norwalk, CT: Appleton-Century-Crofts.

Batey, M.V. (1977). Conceptualization: Knowledge and logic guiding empirical research. *Nursing Research, 26,* 324–329.

Becker, M. (1978). The Health Belief Model and sick role behavior. *Nursing Digest, 6,* 35–40.

Braithwaithe, R.B. (1962). Models in the empirical sciences. In E. Nagel, P. Suppes, & A. Tarski (eds.): *Logic methodology and philosophy of science* (pp. 224–231). Stanford, CA: Stanford University Press.

Chinn, P.L., & Jacobs, M. (1987). *Theory and nursing: A systematic approach* (2nd ed.). St. Louis: C.V. Mosby.

Craig, S.L. (1980). Theory development and its relevance for nursing. *Journal of Advanced Nursing, 5,* 349–355.

Fawcett, J. (1978). The relationship between theory and research: A double helix. *Advances in Nursing Science, 1,* 49–62.

Fawcett, J. (1989). *Analysis and evaluation of conceptual models of nursing* (2nd ed.). Philadelphia: F.A. Davis.

Flaskerud, J.H. (1984). Nursing models as conceptual frameworks for research. *Western Journal of Nursing Research, 6,* 153–155.

Flaskerud, J.H., & Halloran, E.J. (1980). Areas of agreement in nursing theory development. *Advances in Nursing Science, 3,* 1–7.

Hardy, M.E. (1974). Theories: Components, development, evaluation. *Nursing Research, 23,* 100–107.

Homans, G.C. (1964). Contemporary theory in sociology. In R.E.L. Farris (Ed.), *Handbook of modern sociology* (pp. 951–977). Chicago: Rand McNally.

Hurley, B.A. (1979). Why a theoretical framework in nursing research? *Western Journal of Nursing Research, 1,* 28–41.

Johnson, D.E. (1980). The Behavioral System Model for nursing. In J.P. Riehl & C. Roy (Eds.), *Conceptual models for nursing practice* (2nd ed.). Norwalk, CT: Appleton-Century-Crofts.

Kim, H.S. (1983). *The nature of theoretical thinking in nursing*. Norwalk, CT: Appleton-Century-Crofts.

King, I.M. (1981). *A theory for nursing: Systems, concepts, process*. New York: John Wiley and Sons.

Levine, M.E. (1973). *Introduction to clinical nursing* (2nd ed.). Philadelphia: F.A. Davis.

Marriner-Tomey, A. (1989). *Nursing theorists and their work* (2nd ed.). St. Louis: C.V. Mosby.

McFarlane, E.A. (1980). Nursing theory: The comparison of four theoretical proposals (King, Rogers, Roy, Orem). *Journal of Advanced Nursing, 5,* 3–19.

Neuman, B. (1989). *The Neuman systems model* (2nd ed.). Norwalk, CT: Appleton and Lange.

Orem, D.E. (1985). *Concepts of practice* (3rd ed.). New York: McGraw-Hill.

Parse, R.R. (1987). *Nursing science: Major paradigms, theories, and critiques*. Philadelphia: W.B. Saunders.

Pender, N. (1987). *Health promotion in nursing practice* (2nd ed.). Norwalk, CT: Appleton and Lange.

Rogers, M.E. (1970). *An introduction to the theoretical basis of nursing*. Philadelphia: F.A. Davis.

Roy, C. (1984). *Introduction to nursing: An adaptation model* (2nd ed.). Englewood Cliffs, NJ: Prentice-Hall.

Roy, C., Sr., & Roberts, S.L. (1981). *Theory construction in nursing: An adaptation model*. Englewood Cliffs, NJ: Prentice-Hall.

Selye, H. (1978). *The stress of life* (2nd ed.). New York: McGraw-Hill.

Stevens, B.J. (1984). *Nursing theory: Analysis, application, evaluation* (2nd ed.). Boston: Little, Brown.

SUBSTANTIVE REFERENCES*

Banonis, B.C. (1989). The lived experience of recovering from addiction. *Nursing Science Quarterly, 2,* 37–43. [Rogers' Model of the Unitary Human Being; Parse's Model of Man–Living–Health]

Benedict, S.C., & Burge, J.M. (1990). The relationship

* These studies have a formally stated conceptual framework, which is specified in brackets.

between human field motion and preferred visible wavelengths. *Nursing Science Quarterly, 3,* 73–80. [Rogers' Model of the Unitary Human Being]

Bush, J.P. (1988). Job satisfaction, powerlessness, and locus of control. *Western Journal of Nursing Research, 10,* 718–731. [Social learning theory]

Campbell, J.C. (1989). A test of two explanatory models of women's responses to battering. *Nursing Research, 38,* 18–24. [Testing two competing theories: the grief model and learned helplessness theory]

Champion, V.L. (1987). The relationship of breast self-examination to Health Belief Model variables. *Research in Nursing and Health, 10,* 375–382. [Health Belief Model]

Chang, B.L., Uman, G.C., Linn, L.S., Ware, J.E., & Kane, R.L. (1985). Adherence to health care regimens among elderly women. *Nursing Research, 34,* 27–31. [Orem's Self-Care Model]

Craddock, R.B., & Stanhope, M.K. (1980). The Neuman Health-Care Systems Model: Recommended adaptation. In J.P. Riehl & C. Roy (Eds.), *Conceptual models for nursing practice* (2nd ed.). New York: Appleton-Century-Crofts. [Neuman's Health Care Systems Model]

Crawford-Gamble, P. (1986). An application of Levine's conceptual model. *Perioperative Nursing Quarterly, 2,* 63–70. [Levine's Conservation Model]

Davidson, P.O., & Kelley, W.R. (1973). Social facilitation and coping with stress. *British Journal of Social Clinical Psychology, 12,* 130–136. [Social facilitation theory]

Derdiarian, A.K., & Forsythe, A.B. (1983). An instrument for theory and research development using the Behavioral Systems Model for Nursing: The cancer patient. *Nursing Research, 32,* 260–266. [Johnson's Behavioral System Model]

DeVon, H.A., & Powers, M.J. (1984). Health beliefs, adjustment to illness, and control of hypertension. *Research in Nursing and Health, 7,* 10–16. [Health Belief Model]

Dodd, M.J. (1984). Measuring informational intervention for chemotherapy knowledge and self-care behavior. *Research in Nursing and Health, 7,* 43–50. [Orem's Self-Care Model]

Erickson, H., & Swain, M.A. (1982). A model for assessing potential adaptation to stress. *Research in Nursing and Health, 5,* 93–101. [Selye's stress and adaptation theory]

Fawcett, J., & Burritt, J. (1985). An exploratory study of antenatal preparation for cesarean birth. *Journal of Obstetric, Gynecologic, and Neonatal Nursing, 14,* 224–230. [Roy's Adaptation Model]

Gaydos, L.S., & Farnham, R. (1988). Human–animal relationships within the context of Rogers' principle of integrality. *Advances in Nursing Science, 10,* 72–80. [Rogers' Model of the Unitary Human Being]

Gill, B.P., & Atwood, J.R. (1981). Reciprocity and helicy used to relate MEFG and wound healing. *Nursing Research, 30,* 68–72. [Rogers' Model of the Unitary Human Being]

Gulick, E.E. (1989). Model confirmation of the MS-related symptom checklist. *Nursing Research, 38,* 147–153. [Orem's Self-Care Model]

Hartley, L.A. (1988). Congruence between teaching and learning self-care. *Nursing Science Quarterly, 1,* 161–167. [Orem's Self-Care Model]

Henneman, E.A. (1989). Effect of nursing contact on the stress response of patients being weaned from mechanical ventilation. *Heart and Lung, 18,* 483–489. [Selye's stress and adaptation theory; Roy's Adaptation Model]

Holaday, B.J. (1974). Achievement behavior in chronically ill children. *Nursing Research, 23,* 25–30. [Social learning theory]

Holaday, B.J. (1981). Maternal response to their chronically ill infants' attachment behavior of crying. *Nursing Research, 30,* 343–348. [Johnson's Behavioral System Model]

Holaday, B.J. (1987). Patterns of interaction between mothers and their chronically ill infants. *Maternal-Child Nursing Journal, 16,* 29–45. [Johnson's Behavioral System Model]

Itano, J., Tanabe, P., Lum, J.L., Lamkin, L., Rizzo, E., Wieland, M., & Sato, P. (1983). Compliance of cancer patients to therapy. *Western Journal of Nursing Research, 5,* 5–16. [Health Belief Model]

Jones, S.L., Jones, P.K., & Katz, J.K. (1989). A nursing intervention to increase compliance in otitis media patients. *Applied Nursing Research, 2,* 68–73. [Health Belief Model]

Kearney, B.Y., & Fleischer, B.J. (1979). Development of an instrument to measure exercise of self-care agency. *Research in Nursing and Health, 2,* 25–34. [Orem's Self-Care Model]

LaMontagne, L.L. (1984). Children's locus of control beliefs as predictors of preoperative coping behavior. *Nursing Research, 33,* 76–79. [Social learning theory]

Lovejoy, M. (1983). The leukemic child's perceptions of

family behaviors. *Oncology Nursing Forum, 10,* 20–25. [Johnson's Behavioral System Model]

Mahon, N.E., & Yarcheski, A. (1988). Loneliness in early adolescents: An empirical test of alternate explanations. *Nursing Research, 37,* 330–335. [Testing two competing theories of loneliness: situational and characterological]

Muhlenkamp, A.F., & Broerman, N.A. (1988). Health beliefs, health value, and positive health behaviors. *Western Journal of Nursing Research, 10,* 637–646. [Social learning theory]

Neaves, J.J. (1989). The relationship of locus of control to decision making in nursing students. *Journal of Nursing Education, 28,* 12–17. [Social learning theory]

Newport, M.A. (1984). Conserving thermal energy and social integrity in the newborn. *Western Journal of Nursing Research, 6,* 175–188. [Levine's Conservation Model]

Patterson, E.T., & Hale, E.S. (1985). Making sure: Integrating menstrual care practices into activities of daily living. *Advances in Nursing Science, 7,* 18–31. [Orem's Self-Care Model]

Riesch, S.K. (1988). Changes in the exercise of self-care agency. *Western Journal of Nursing Research, 10,* 257–273. [Orem's Self-Care Model]

Ross, M.M., & Bourbonnais, F.F. (1985). The Betty Neuman Systems Model in nursing practice: A case study approach. *Journal of Advanced Nursing, 10,* 199–207. [Neuman's Health Care Systems Model]

Rothlis, J. (1984). The effect of a self-help group on feelings of hopelessness and helplessness. *Western Journal of Nursing Research, 6,* 157–168. [Orem's Self-Care Model]

Santopinto, M.D.A. (1989). The relentless drive to be ever thinner. *Nursing Science Quarterly, 2,* 29–36. [Parse's Model of Man–Living–Health]

Schodt, C.M. (1989). Parental–fetal attachment and couvade: A study of patterns of human–environment integrity. *Nursing Science Quarterly, 2,* 88–97. [Rogers' Model of the Unitary Human Being]

Shannahan, M.D., & Cottrell, B.H. (1985). Effect of the birth chair on duration of second-stage labor, fetal outcome, and maternal blood loss. *Nursing Research, 34,* 89–92. [Roy's Adaptation Model]

Small, B. (1980). Nursing visually impaired children with Johnson's model as a conceptual framework. In J.P. Riehl & C. Roy (Eds.), *Conceptual models for nursing practice* (2nd ed.). New York: Appleton-Century-Crofts. [Johnson's Behavioral System Model]

Smith, M.C. (1990). Struggling through a difficult time for unemployed persons. *Nursing Science Quarterly, 3,* 18–28. [Parse's Model of Man–Living–Health]

Smith, M.J. (1986). Human–environment process: A test of Roger's principle of integrality. *Advances in Nursing Science, 9,* 21–28. [Rogers' Model of the Unitary Human Being]

Toth, J.C. (1980). Effect of structured preparation for transfer on patient anxiety on leaving coronary care unit. *Nursing Research, 29,* 28–34. [Orem's Self-Care Model]

Tulman, L., Fawcett, J., Groblewski, L., & Silverman, L. (1990). Changes in functional status after childbirth. *Nursing Research, 39,* 70–75. [Roy's Adaptation Model]

Volden, C., Langemo, D., Adamson, M., & Oechsle, L. (1990). The relationship of age, gender, and exercise practices to measures of health, life-style, and self-esteem. *Applied Nursing Research, 3,* 20–26. [Health Promotion Model]

Watts, R.J. (1982). Sexual functioning, health beliefs, and compliance with high blood pressure medications. *Nursing Research, 31,* 278–283. [Health Belief Model]

Weitzel, M.H. (1989). A test of the Health Promotion Model with blue-collar workers. *Nursing Research, 38,* 99–103. [Health Promotion Model]

Wilson, V.S. (1987). Identification of stressors related to patients' psychologic responses to the surgical intensive care unit. *Heart and Lung, 16,* 267–273. [Neuman's Health Care Systems Model]

Yeates, D.A., & Roberts, J.E. (1984). A comparison of two bearing-down techniques during the second stage of labor. *Journal of Nurse-Midwifery, 29,* 3–11. [Levine's Conservation Model]

Ziemer, M.M. (1983). Effects of information on postsurgical coping. *Nursing Research, 32,* 282–287. [Neuman's Health Care Systems Model]

8
Formulating Hypotheses

A *hypothesis* is a tentative prediction or explanation of the relationship between two or more variables. A hypothesis, in other words, translates the problem statement into a prediction of expected outcomes. It is the hypothesis, rather than the problem statement, that is subjected to empirical testing through the collection and analysis of data.

The researcher normally formulates one or more hypotheses following identification of the problem, a review of the literature, the final conceptualization of the research variables, and identification of a suitable theoretical framework. Research problems, as we have seen, are typically phrased in the form of questions concerning how phenomena are related and interact. Hypotheses, on the other hand, are tentative solutions or answers to such research queries. For instance, the problem statement might ask: Does room temperature affect the optimal placement time of rectal temperature measurements in adults? As a tentative solution to this problem, the researcher might predict the following: "Cooler room temperatures will require longer placement times for rectal temperature measurements in adults than warmer rooms." Hypotheses should generally be developed *before* the conduct of the study itself because it is the hypothesis that gives direction to the gathering and interpretation of data. In the following section we briefly examine the role of the hypothesis in the research process.

☰ PURPOSES OF THE RESEARCH HYPOTHESIS

Generally speaking, the function of the hypothesis is to guide scientific inquiry. Various aspects of this function include unifying theory and reality, extending knowledge, and directing research.

Unifying Theory and Reality

Hypotheses often follow directly from a theoretical framework. The scientist reasons from theories to hypotheses and tests those hypotheses in the real world. Hypotheses are the conclusions that follow from the premises or assumptions inherent in the theory. Thus, hypotheses are the vehicle through which theories are linked to real-world situations.

Let us take as an example the general theory of reinforcement. This theory maintains that behavior or activity that is positively reinforced (rewarded) will tend to be learned or repeated. Because nurses play an important teaching and guiding role in hospitals or clinical settings, there are many opportunities for this general theory to be incorporated into the context of nursing practice. However, the theory itself is untestable. It makes no explicit prediction nor does it specify measurable or observable variables. In short, it is too abstract to be put to an empirical test. However, *if* the theory is valid, then it should be possible to make accurate predictions (hypotheses) about certain kinds of behavior in hospitals. For example, the following two hypotheses have been deduced from reinforcement theory: (1) Elderly patients who are praised (reinforced) by nursing personnel for self-feeding will require less assistance in feeding than patients who are not praised and (2) Hyperactive children who are given a reward (e.g., cookies or permission to watch television) when they perform a 15-minute motor task without disruption will tend to display less acting-out behavior during task performance than unrewarded peers. Both of these propositions can be put to a test in the real world. If the hypotheses are confirmed, the theory will be supported, and we can place more confidence in it.

Extending Knowledge

Not all hypotheses are derived from theory. Even in the absence of a theoretical framework, however, the researcher who proceeds to collect data without having made predictions about the outcome may jeopardize the contribution that the findings can make to human knowledge. Well-conceived hypotheses offer direction and suggest explanations.

Even when hypotheses fail to be confirmed, their presence provides a greater possibility for the advancement of understanding than the absence of hypotheses. Perhaps an example will clarify this point. Suppose we were to hypothesize that nurses who have received a baccalaureate education are more likely to experience stress in their first nursing job than nurses with diploma school education. We could justify our speculation on the grounds of theory (role conflict, cognitive dissonance theory, or reality shock theory); on the basis of earlier studies; on personal observations; on the basis of logic; or on the basis of some combination of these. *The need to develop justifications in and of itself forces the researcher to think logically, to exercise critical judgment, and to tie together earlier research findings.* Now let us suppose the above hypothesis is not confirmed by the evidence collected; that is, we find that baccalaureate and diploma nurses demonstrate an equal amount of stress in their first nursing assignment. *The failure of data to support a prediction forces the investigator to critically analyze theory or previous research, to carefully review the limitations of the study's methods, and to explore alternative explanations for the findings.* The use of hypotheses, in other words, induces critical thinking and, hence, promotes understanding.

To pursue the same example, suppose we conducted the investigation without formulating an explicit prediction and were guided only by a problem statement: "Is there a relationship between a nurse's basic preparation and the degree of stress experienced on the first job?" The investigator without a hypothesis is, apparently, prepared to accept any results. The problem is that it is almost always possible to explain something superficially after-the-fact, no matter what the findings are. Hypotheses guard against superficiality and minimize the possibility that spurious results will be misconstrued.

Directing Research

Problem statements typically are more vague than research hypotheses. A critical function of hypotheses is to provide direction to the research design and to the collection, analysis, and interpretation of data. Without a hypothesis (or, as is often the case, a set of hypotheses), there is sometimes a tendency for investigators to gather isolated pieces of information that are as unwieldy to analyze as they are meaningless. Hypotheses interconnect variables of interest through statements of formal relationships; it is these relationships that are subjected to an empirical test.

≡ *CHARACTERISTICS OF WORKABLE HYPOTHESES*

An essential characteristic of a workable research hypothesis is that it states the predicted relationship between two or more variables. The variables that are related to one another through the hypothesis are the *independent variable* (the presumed cause, antecedent, or influence) and the *dependent variable* (the presumed effect or phenomenon of primary interest). One of the most common flaws of the predictions of beginning researchers is the failure to make a relational statement. The prediction "Pregnant women who receive prenatal training will have favorable reactions to the labor and delivery experience" is not a hypothesis that can be tested using the scientific approach. This statement expresses no anticipated relationship; in fact, there is only one variable (the woman's reactions to the labor and delivery experience). A relationship by definition requires at least two variables. This prediction can, however, be altered to make it a suitable hypothesis with an independent and dependent variable: "Pregnant women who receive prenatal training will have *more* favorable reactions [the dependent variable] to the labor and delivery experience *than* pregnant women with no prenatal training." Here the second variable (the independent variable) is the woman's status with re-

spect to prenatal training: some will have received it and others will not have received it.

The relational aspect of the prediction is embodied in the phrase "more than." If a hypothesis lacks a phrase such as "more than," "less than," "greater than," "different from," "related to," or something similar, it is not amenable to scientific testing. As an example of why this is so, consider the original prediction: Pregnant women who receive prenatal training will have favorable reactions to the labor and delivery experience. How would we know whether the women's reactions are favorable? That is, what absolute standard could be used for deciding whether the women's reactions to their labor and delivery experiences were favorable or not? Perhaps this point will be clearer if we illustrate it more specifically. Suppose that we ask a group of women who have taken an 8-week prenatal training course to respond to the following question:*

On the whole, how would you describe your labor and delivery experience?

1. Very favorably
2. Rather favorably
3. Neither favorably nor unfavorably
4. Rather unfavorably
5. Very unfavorably

Based on this question, how could we compare the actual outcome with the predicted outcome that the women would have favorable responses? Would *all* of the women questioned have to respond "very favorably" for the hypothesis to be supported? Would our prediction be supported if the *majority* of the women said either "very favorably" or "favorably"? There is simply no adequate way of testing the accuracy of the prediction. If we modify the prediction, as suggested above, to "'Pregnant women who receive prenatal training will have more favorable reactions to the labor and delivery experience than

---

* This rather simple question is provided primarily for the sake of illustrating the need to have a relational statement in a hypothesis. Normally, a measure of a dependent variable would be somewhat more complex than this example suggests.

pregnant women with no prenatal training," then a test is straightforward. We could simply ask two groups of women with different prenatal training experiences to respond to the question and then compare the responses of the two groups. The absolute degree of favorability of either group would not be at issue.

Hypotheses, ideally, should be based on a sound, justifiable rationale. The most defensible hypotheses follow from previous research findings or are deduced from a theory. When a new area is being investigated, the researcher may have to turn to logical reasoning or personal experience to justify the predictions. There are, however, very few topics for which research evidence is totally lacking.

A good hypothesis should be consistent with an existing body of research findings. This requirement in some cases may be difficult to satisfy because it is not uncommon to find conflicting results on some topics in the research literature. For example, Clark and Clark (1984) critically reviewed the research literature relating to the effectiveness of therapeutic touch as a treatment modality and found inconsistent findings. Some investigators have found that therapeutic touch results in an increase of hemoglobin levels, increased relaxation, and reduced anxiety, and other investigators have found no differences among those treated and those not treated with therapeutic touch. Obviously, when the findings from previous research are inconsistent, it is impossible for the hypothesis to be consistent with all the findings. The researcher must then make a decision, and a good solid basis for such a decision is the critical evaluation of the methods used in earlier studies. The investigator should attempt to understand *why* conflicting results occurred through an examination of the research approach.

≡ *THE DERIVATION OF HYPOTHESES*

Many students ask the question, "How do I go about the task of developing hypotheses?" There are no formal rules for deriving hypotheses, but we can offer some suggestions by discussing two broad types of approach. Like the development of problem statements, the sources most likely to be fruitful as a basis for the formulation of hypotheses are theoretical systems, personal experience and observations, readings in related literature, and discussions with peers and advisers. However, two basic processes—induction and deduction—constitute the intellectual machinery involved in deriving hypotheses.

An *inductive hypothesis* is a generalization based on observed relationships. The researcher observes certain patterns, trends, or associations among phenomena and then uses these observations as a basis for a tentative explanation or prediction. Related literature should be examined to learn what is already known on a topic, but an important source of ideas for inductive hypotheses is the researcher's own experiences, combined with intuition and critical analysis. For example, a nurse may notice that presurgical patients who ask a lot of questions relating to pain or express many pain-related apprehensions have a more difficult time in learning appropriate postoperative procedures. The nurse could then formulate a hypothesis that could be tested through more rigorous scientific procedures. The following hypothesis might be derived: "Patients who are stressed by fears of pain will have more difficulty in deep breathing and coughing after their surgery than patients who are not stressed."

The other mechanism for deriving hypotheses is through deduction. Theories of how phenomena behave and interrelate cannot be tested directly. Through deductive reasoning, a researcher can develop scientific expectations or hypotheses based on general theoretical principles. Inductive hypotheses begin with specific observations and move toward generalizations; *deductive hypotheses* have as a starting point general "laws" or theories that are applied to particular situations.

Although a full explication of deductive logic is beyond the scope of this book, the following syllogism illustrates the reasoning process involved:

All human beings have red and white blood cells. John Doe is a human being.

Therefore, John Doe has red and white blood cells.

In this simple example, the "hypothesis" is that John Doe does, in fact, have red and white blood cells, a deduction that could be verified.

If a nurse researcher is familiar with a theory relating to phenomena of interest, the theory can serve as a valuable point of departure for the development of hypotheses. The researcher must ask the question, "If this theory is correct or valid, what would the logical consequences be in terms of a situation that interests me?" In other words, the researcher deduces that if the general law is true, specific outcomes or consequences can be expected. The specific predictions derived from general principles must then be subjected to further testing through the collection of empirical data. If these data are in fact congruent with hypothesized outcomes, then the theory is strengthened.

The advancement of scientific research depends on both inductive and deductive hypotheses. Ideally, a cyclical process is set in motion, wherein the researcher makes observations; formulates hypotheses inductively; makes systematic, controlled observations; develops theoretical systems; deduces hypotheses; seeks new systematic observations; rethinks the hypotheses or theories; modifies them inductively; and so forth. The scientific researcher needs to be an organizer of concepts (think inductively); a logician (think deductively); and, above all, a critic and a skeptic of resulting formulations.

≡ WORDING THE HYPOTHESIS

A workable hypothesis is one that is congruent with existing theory and research, states a relationship between two (or more) variables, and is testable. In this section we will look at how the hypothesis should be stated and provide examples of various kinds of hypotheses.

A good hypothesis is worded in simple, clear, and concise language and provides a definition of the variables in concrete, operational terms. These two requirements in some cases may be conflicting if the operational definition needs extensive explanation. If it is not too awkward to incorporate the operational definition of terms within the statement of the hypothesis itself, the researcher should attempt to do so. However, if the hypothesis is too unwieldy or unclear, the variables should be operationally defined separately, following the hypothesis statement. The hypothesis should, however, be specific enough so that the reader understands what the variables are and whom the researcher will be studying.

Simple Versus Complex Hypotheses

For the purpose of this book, we will define *simple hypotheses* as hypotheses that express an expected relationship between *one* independent and *one* dependent variable. A *complex hypothesis* refers to a prediction of a relationship between two (or more) independent variables and/ or two (or more) dependent variables. Sometimes complex hypotheses are referred to as *multivariate hypotheses* (because they involve multiple variables).

We give some concrete examples of both types of hypotheses, but let us first explain the differences in abstract terms. Simple hypotheses state a relationship between a single independent variable, which we will call X, and a single dependent variable, which we will label Y. Our Y variable is the predicted effect, outcome, or consequence of our X variable, which is the presumed cause, antecedent, or precondition. The nature of this relationship is presented in Figure 8-1 (A). In Figure 8-1 (A), the hatched area of the circles, representing variables X and Y, can be taken to signify the strength of the relationship between these two variables. If there were a one-to-one correspondence between variables X and Y, the two circles would completely overlap and the entire area would be hatched. If the variables were totally unrelated, the circles would not converge or overlap at all.

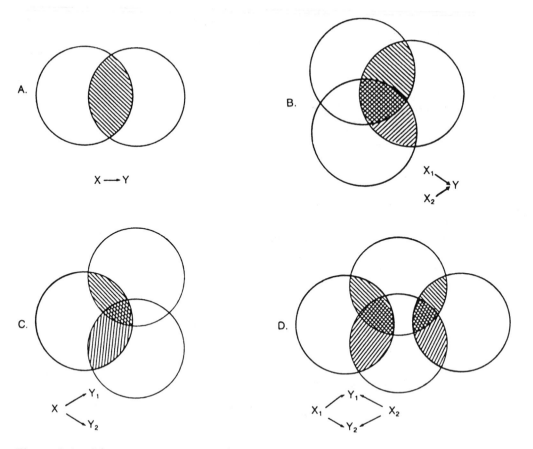

Figure 8-1. *Schematic representation of various hypothetical relationships.*

In the real world, the majority of phenomena are the result not of one variable, but of a complex network of many variables. A person's weight, for example, is affected simultaneously by such factors as the person's height, diet, bone structure, and metabolism. If the dependent variable—Y in Figure 8-1 (A)—were weight and the independent variable—X—were a person's caloric intake, we would not be able to completely explain or understand individual variation in weight. Knowing that Mr. A's daily caloric intake averaged 2500 calories would not allow us a precise prediction of his weight. Knowledge of other factors, such as Mr. A's height, would improve the accuracy with which his weight could be predicted.

Figure 8-1 (B) presents a schematic representation of a design that examines the simultaneous effect of two independent variables on a single dependent variable. The complex hypothesis would state the nature of the relationship between Y on the one hand and X_1 and X_2 on the other. To pursue the example above, the hypothesis might be "Taller people (X_1) and people with higher caloric intake (X_2) will weigh more (Y) than shorter people and individuals with lower caloric intake." As the figure shows, a larger proportion of the area of Y is hatched when there are two independent variables than when there is only one. This means that caloric intake *and* height do a better job in helping us understand weight (Y) than caloric intake alone. Complex hypotheses thus have the advantage of allowing researchers to capture some of the complexity of the real world. It is not always possible, of course, to design a study with complex hypotheses. A number of practical considerations, including the researcher's technical skills, resources, and time, may render the testing of complex hypotheses impossible or inadvisable. However, an important goal of research is to explain the dependent variable as thoroughly as possible and two or more independent variables are typically more successful than one alone.

Just as a phenomenon can be understood as resulting from more than one independent variable, so a single independent variable can have an effect on, or can be antecedent to, more than one phenomenon. Figure 8-1 (*C*) illustrates this type of relationship. A number of studies have found, for example, that cigarette smoking (the independent variable, *X*) can lead to both lung cancer (Y_1) and coronary disorders (Y_2). This type of complex hypothesis is common in studies that try to assess the impact of a nursing intervention on a variety of criterion measures of patient well-being. Finally, a more complex type of hypothesis,* which links two or more independent variables to two or more dependent variables, is shown in Figure 8-1 (*D*). An example might be a hypothesis that smoking *and* the consumption of alcohol during pregnancy might lead to lower birthweights *and* lower Apgar scores in infants.

Table 8-1 presents ten specific examples of simple and complex hypotheses. Most of these hypotheses would need further elaboration in terms of the specification of operational definitions, but each of these hypotheses is potentially testable and each delineates a predicted relationship. Beginning research students should carefully scrutinize this table to familiarize themselves with the language and style of scientific hypotheses. The first column specifies the hypotheses themselves and columns 2 through 4 indicate the independent and dependent variable for each hy-

pothesis and designate whether it is simple or complex.

Although researchers typically adopt a certain style in the phrasing of hypotheses, there is some degree of flexibility allowed. The same hypothesis can generally be stated in a variety of ways, so long as the researcher specifies (or implies) the relationship that will be tested. For example, hypothesis 3 from Table 8-1 can be reworded in the following six ways while still maintaining its integrity and usefulness:

1. Older nurses are less likely to express approval of the expanding roles of nurses than younger nurses.
2. There is a relationship between the age of a nurse and approval of the nurse's expanding role.
3. The older the nurse, the less likely it is that he or she will approve of the nurse's expanding role.
4. Older nurses will differ from younger nurses with respect to approval of the nurse's expanding role.
5. Younger nurses will tend to be more approving of the nurse's expanding role than older nurses.
6. Approval of the nurse's expanding role decreases as the age of the nurse increases.

A number of other variations of the wording of this hypothesis are also possible. The important point to remember is that the statement should specify the independent and dependent variables and the anticipated relationship between them.

Directional Versus Nondirectional Hypotheses

Sometimes hypotheses are described as being either directional or nondirectional. A *directional hypothesis* is one that specifies the expected direction of the relationship between variables. That is, the researcher predicts not only the existence of a relationship but also the nature of the relationship. In the six versions of the same hypothesis above, versions 1, 3, 5, and 6 are direc-

---

* A special kind of complex hypothesis, known as an *interaction hypothesis,* is described in Chapter 9.

Table 8-1. *Examples of Hypotheses*

HYPOTHESIS	INDEPENDENT VARIABLE	DEPENDENT VARIABLE	SIMPLE OR COMPLEX
1. Infants born to heroin-addicted mothers have lower birthweights than infants of nonaddicted mothers.	Addiction or nonaddiction of infant's mother	Birthweight	Simple
2. There is a relationship between tactile and auditory stimulation and heart rate response in premature infants.	a. Tactile stimulation; b. Auditory stimulation	Heart rate response	Complex
3. Older nurses are less likely to express approval of the expanding role of nurses than younger nurses.	Age of nurses	Approval of nurses' expanding role	Simple
4. Structured preoperative support is more effective in reducing surgical patients' perception of pain and requests for analgesics than structured postoperative support.	Timing of nursing intervention	a. Surgical patients' pain perception; b. Requests for analgesics	Complex
5. Teenage girls are better informed about the risks of venereal disease than teenage boys.	Gender of teenager	Knowledge about venereal disease	Simple
6. Nurses who are scheduled by the block rotation method will have a lower number of reported sick days and express a higher level of job satisfaction than nurses scheduled by a random rotation method.	Schedule method	a. Absenteeism; b. Level of job satisfaction	Complex
7. Nursing students who have been with a patient who dies will be more likely to report a physical complaint within 72 hours than students who have not had this experience.	Experiencing death of patient	Physical complaint	Simple
8. Patients who have a primary nurse assigned to them on admission report a more favorable impression of their nursing care than patients who do not have a primary nurse assigned on admission.	Assignment of primary nurse	Impression of nursing care	Simple
9. Patients who receive a copy of the "Patient's Bill of Rights" ask more questions about their treatment and diagnosis than those who do not receive this document.	Receipt of "Patient's Bill of Rights"	Number of questions asked by patients	Simple
10. Patients with a leg amputation who practice the prone lying position will develop fewer contractures than patients with a leg amputation who do not lie prone.	Type of position	Development of contractures	Simple

tional because there is an explicit expectation that older nurses will be less approving of the expanding role of nurses than younger nurses.

A *nondirectional hypothesis,* by contrast, does not stipulate the direction of the relationship. Such a hypothesis predicts that two or more variables are related but makes no projections concerning the exact nature of the association. Versions 2 and 4 in the example illustrate the wording of nondirectional hypotheses. These hypotheses state the prediction that a nurse's age and degree of approval of the nurse's changing role are related; they do not stipulate, however, whether the researcher thinks that older nurses or younger nurses will be more approving.

Deductive hypotheses derived from theory will almost always be directional, because theories attempt to explain phenomena and, hence, provide a rationale for expecting variables to behave in certain ways. Existing studies also supply, typically, a basis for directional hypotheses. When there is no theory or related research, when the findings of related studies are contradictory, or when the researcher's own experience results in ambivalent expectations, the investigator may use nondirectional hypotheses. Some people argue, in fact, that nondirectional hypotheses are generally preferable because they connote a degree of impartiality or objectivity. Directional hypotheses, it is said, carry the implication that the researcher is intellectually committed to a certain outcome, and such a commitment might lead to bias. This argument fails to recognize that researchers typically do have specific expectations or hunches concerning the outcomes, whether they state those expectations explicitly or not. Directional hypotheses have three distinct advantages: (1) they demonstrate that the researcher has thought critically and carefully about the phenomena under investigation, (2) they make clear to the readers of a research report the framework within which the study was conducted, and (3) they may permit a more sensitive statistical test of the hypothesis. This last point, which refers to whether the researcher chooses a one-tailed or two-tailed statistical test, is a rather fine point that is discussed in Chapter 21.

Research Versus Statistical Hypotheses

Hypotheses are sometimes classified as being either research hypotheses or statistical hypotheses. *Research hypotheses* (also referred to as substantive, declarative, or scientific hypotheses) are statements of expected relationships between variables. All of the hypotheses in Table 8-1 are research hypotheses. Such hypotheses indicate what the researcher expects to find as a result of conducting the study.

The logic of statistical inference operates on principles that are somewhat confusing to many beginning students. This logic requires that hypotheses be expressed such that *no* relationship is expected. *Statistical* or *null hypotheses* state that there is no relationship between the independent and dependent variables. The null form of hypothesis 1 in Table 8-1 would be as follows: "Infants born to heroin-addicted mothers have birthweights comparable to those of infants born to nonaddicted mothers." As another illustration, the null hypothesis for hypothesis 2 in Table 8-1 would read as follows: "There is no relationship between tactile and auditory stimulation and heart rate response in premature infants." The null hypothesis might be compared with the assumption of innocence of an accused criminal in our system of justice: the variables are assumed to be "innocent" of any relationship until they can be shown "guilty" through appropriate statistical procedures. The null hypothesis represents the formal statement of this assumption of innocence.

In designing a study, the researcher is typically concerned only with the research hypotheses. Although some research reports do express the hypotheses in null form, it is more common (and more desirable) to state the researcher's actual expectations. When statistical tests are performed, the underlying null hypothesis is usually assumed without being explicitly stated.

≡ *TESTING THE HYPOTHESIS*

The testing of hypotheses constitutes the heart of empirical investigations. It must again be emphasized, however, that neither theories nor hypotheses are ever proved in an ultimate sense through hypothesis testing. It is inappropriate to say that the data "proved" the validity of the hypothesis or that the conclusions "proved" the worthiness of the theory. Such statements are inappropriate not only because they are incongruent with the limitations of the scientific approach but also because they are inconsistent with the fundamentally skeptical attitudes of scientists. Scientists are basically doubters and skeptics, who are constantly seeking objective, replicable evidence as a basis for understanding natural phenomena. Findings are always considered tentative. Certainly, if the same results are repeatedly produced in a large number of investigations, then greater confidence can be placed in the conclusions. Hypotheses, then, come to be increasingly accepted or believed with mounting evidence, but ultimate proof is rarely possible nor, for that matter, is ultimate falsification of a hypothesis possible.

Let us look more closely at why this is so. Suppose we hypothesize that there is a relationship between height and weight. We predict that, on the average, tall people weigh more than short people. We would then take a sample of people, obtain height and weight measurements, and analyze the data. Now suppose we happened by chance to choose a sample that consisted of short, fat people, and tall, thin people. Our results might then indicate that there is no relationship between an individual's height and weight. Would we then be justified in stating that "this study proved that height and weight in humans are unrelated"?

A second example illustrates the converse principle. Suppose we hypothesize that taller people are better nurses than shorter people. This hypothesis is used here only to illustrate a point, because, in reality, one might suspect that there is no relationship between height and a nurse's job performance. Now suppose that, by chance again, we hit upon a sample of nurses in which the taller nurses happen to receive better job evaluations by their supervisors than short nurses. Could we conclude definitively that height is related to a nurse's performance? These two examples illustrate the difficulty of using observations from a sample to generalize to the broader group (the population) from which the sample has been taken. Other problems, such as the accuracy of our measures, the validity of underlying assumptions, the reasonableness of our logical deductions, and rapid changes in technologies and in society, prohibit us from concluding with finality that our hypotheses are proved.

≡ *ARE HYPOTHESES REQUIRED?*

In the first section of this chapter we reviewed the various important functions that scientific hypotheses play in the research process. The reader may be wondering if a hypothesis is always necessary. Most research that can be classified as descriptive proceeds without explicit hypotheses. *Descriptive research,* that is, research that aims predominantly at describing phenomena rather than explaining them, is common in the emerging field of nursing research. Examples of descriptive investigations include studies of the health needs of elderly citizens, studies of the coping patterns of mothers of handicapped children, and surveys of the nutritional status of low-income preschool children. This type of study is often extremely important in laying a foundation for later research. When a field is new, it may be quite difficult to provide adequate justification for the development of explanatory hypotheses because of a dearth of facts or previous findings. Also, studies that have a phenomenological perspective generally proceed without hypotheses because their aim is to provide an opportunity for the human experience to be revealed without preconceived restrictions. Thus, there are some studies of a descriptive or exploratory nature for which hypotheses may not be required.

However, initial efforts to investigate phenomena using the scientific approach are often strengthened by the formulation of hypotheses. Even when related literature on a topic is lacking, a nurse's experience is an extremely valuable source of ideas for predicting outcomes. Descriptive studies whose goal is to depict the status quo of some situation typically have some broader purpose in mind. A study that aims to describe nursing students' attitudes toward mentally ill people, for example, could have implications for nursing education. It seems likely that the ability to understand how attitudes toward mental illness are related to various characteristics of the students would have much more meaningful educational implications than a pure attitudinal description. Do nursing students in different specialty areas have more favorable attitudes than others? Does personal contact with a mentally ill person affect attitudes? What role does the student's age, social class, academic record, or emotional stability play? The answers to these questions might not only be interesting but also could lead to more useful approaches to making the student's attitudes toward mental illness more positive. These questions go beyond pure description; they deal with relationships. Where there is a relationship, there is a potential hypothesis.

≡ RESEARCH EXAMPLES

Table 8-2 presents hypotheses that have appeared in several different nursing research reports. These examples illustrate the proper wording of

Table 8-2. *Examples of Hypotheses from Actual Studies*

SOURCE	HYPOTHESIS
McPhail et al., 1990	Compared with the conventional method of team nursing, a primary nursing delivery system will show (1) an increase in patient satisfaction with nursing care; (2) a decrease in nurse absenteeism; and (3) an improvement in the nurses' perception of their work environment.
Johnson et al., 1989	Measurements of intracranial pressure will differ during a baseline (preconversation) period and during a conversation period among comatose patients in an intensive care unit.
Kolanowski, 1990	Elderly persons exposed to broad-spectrum fluorescent lighting will exhibit less motor activty than those exposed to warm white fluorescent lighting.
Shelley et al., 1987	"Do-not-resuscitate" orders reduce the aggressiveness of nursing care.
Hirsch, 1988	Catecholamine production, as measured by vanillymandelic acid excretion, will increase in all subjects when exposed to a stressful procedure.
Zimmerman et al., 1989	Cancer patients with chronic pain who listen to music with positive suggestion of pain reduction will have lower scores on the McGill Pain Questionnaire pain indices compared with those who do not listen to music.
Hollerbach & Sneed, 1990	The accuracy of radial pulse rate assessments per minute taken by nursing personnel palpating the right radial artery will differ from accuracy obtained by those palpating the left radial artery.
Forrester, 1988	Professional nurses holding androgynous sex-role identities will express lower levels of professional role discrepancy than nurses holding non-androgynous sex-role identities.
Broome & Endsley, 1989	Children whose mothers are present during an immunization will be less distressed than children whose mothers are not present.
Miller et al., 1990	Couple agreement regarding marital functioning following cardiac surgery of one of the spouses will increase as shared responsibility for compliance and reported compliance increase.

research hypotheses and illustrate areas in which nurses have launched scientific investigations. The following investigation, described in detail, is a more fully developed example of how hypotheses guided an actual study.

> Krouse and Roberts (1989) were interested in studying the effects of nurse–patient styles of interaction on patient satisfaction and compliance. Their study was based on the concept of self-care, which emphasizes greater responsibility for one's own health and illness and greater control over the initiation and increased individualization of care. The researchers designed a study to examine the difference between traditional patient–provider interaction and patient–provider interactions with greater opportunity for negotiation in terms of several indicators of patient well-being. Subjects in the study were put into one of three groups in which a health-care situation was simulated. The three groups were (1) a traditional approach group, (2) a partial negotiation group, and (3) an active negotiation group. The researchers' hypotheses were that individuals in the active negotiation group, in comparison with those in the other two groups, would

- perceive more control over their care and have fewer feelings of powerlessness
- express greater agreement with the recommended treatment plan
- demonstrate greater satisfaction with care

The investigators gave very clear definitions of all of the terms in their hypotheses. Three of the definitions are as follows:

> *Traditional approach:* An interactive process in which the practitioner decides on the appropriate treatment plan without involving the patient in the decision.
>
> *Active negotiation:* An interactive process in which the patient and provider decide on the prescribed treatment plan together.
>
> *Agreement with plan:* The patient's cooperation and willingness to adhere to the

prescribed treatment plan as evidenced by answers on the questionnaire.

The results of the study indicated that an actively negotiated process had a positive effect on patients' feelings of control and power.

☰ SUMMARY

A *hypothesis* is a statement concerning predicted relationships among variables. The successful progression from initial problem statement to the final collection and analysis of data is often intimately associated with the development of one or more clear, workable hypotheses. Hypotheses are important because they serve as a link between theory and real-world situations, they provide an effective mechanism for extending knowledge, and they offer overall direction for the investigation.

A workable hypothesis must specify the anticipated *relationship* between two or more variables. That is, the researcher must state the hypothesized association between the independent and dependent variables. A hypothesis that projects a result for only one variable is essentially untestable because there is typically no criterion for assessing absolute, as opposed to relative, outcomes. A good hypothesis should also be justifiable. It should be consistent with existing theory or knowledge (or with the researcher's own experiences) and with logical reasoning.

Knowledge and experience in an area and familiarity with related research and theory are important sources for the development of hypotheses. Hypotheses are derived either through *inductive*, observational processes or through *deductive*, theory-based processes.

Hypotheses can be classified according to various characteristics. *Simple hypotheses* express a predicted relationship between one independent and one dependent variable; *complex hypotheses* state an anticipated relationship between two or more independent and/or two or more dependent variables. Complex hypotheses are powerful because they offer the possibility of mirroring the complexity of the real world. A *directional hypothesis* specifies the expected direction or nature of a hypothesized relationship. *Nondirectional hypotheses* denote a relationship but do not stipulate the precise form that the relationship will take. Directional hypotheses are generally preferable. Sometimes a distinction between research and statistical hypotheses is made. *Research hypotheses* predict the existence of relationships; *statistical (null) hypotheses* express the absence of any relationships. The statistical or null hypothesis is related to the logic of statistical inference and is often assumed without being formally stated. These classifications illustrate the fact that there is some flexibility in the wording of hypotheses.

After hypotheses are developed and refined, they are subjected to an empirical test through the collection, analysis, and interpretation of data. It must be stressed, however, that hypotheses are never proved or disproved in an ultimate sense. Scientists say that hypotheses are "accepted" or "rejected," "supported" or "unsupported." Through replication of studies, hypotheses and theories can gain increasing acceptance, but scientists, who are essentially skeptics, avoid the use of the word "proof."

Not all investigations are designed to test hypotheses. Descriptive research, which focuses on a depiction of the status quo of some situation rather than on explanation, often proceeds without a hypothesis. Exploratory research and phenomenological research also may not require hypotheses.

☰ STUDY SUGGESTIONS

1. Below are five hypotheses. For each hypothesis, give a possible problem statement from which the hypothesis might have been developed.
   a. Absenteeism is higher among nurses in intensive care units than among nurses in other wards.
   b. Patients who are not told their diagnosis report more subjective feelings of stress than do patients who are told their diagnosis.
   c. Patients receiving intravenous therapy will report greater nighttime sleep pattern disturbances than patients not receiving intravenous therapy.
   d. Patients with roommates will call for a nurse less often than patients without roommates.
   e. Women who have participated in Lamaze classes will request pain medication less often than will women who have not taken these classes.

2. For each of the five hypotheses in suggestion 1, indicate whether the hypothesis is simple or complex and directional or nondirectional.

3. For each hypothesis in suggestion 1, state the independent and dependent variables.

4. State the five hypotheses in suggestion 1 in null form.

5. Below are five problem statements. Develop a hypothesis based on each one. Try to state each hypothesis in more than one way.
   a. Are verbalized feelings of helplessness by patients related to the amount of ambulation permitted by the patients' conditions?
   b. Is the clinical specialty of nurses related to their attitudes toward alcoholism?
   c. Are nutritional habits related to a person's age and sex?
   d. Is there a relationship between the prematurity of an infant and the mother's smoking behavior?
   e. Do nurse practitioners perform triage functions as well as physicians?

6. For each hypothesis in Table 8-2, do the following: identify the independent and dependent variables and indicate whether the hypothesis is simple or complex and directional or nondirectional.

7. Read one or more articles of the readings suggested for the "Substantive References." Discuss the adequacy of the hypotheses cited in terms of the existence of a relational statement and the justifiability of the hypotheses.

☰ *SUGGESTED READINGS*

METHODOLOGICAL REFERENCES

Armstrong, R.L. (1981). Hypothesis formulation. In S.D. Krampitz & N. Pavlovich (Eds.), *Readings for nursing research.* St. Louis: C.V. Mosby.

Burns, N., & Grove, S.K. (1987). *The practice of nursing research: Conduct, critique, and utilization.* Philadelphia: W.B. Saunders. (Chapter 8).

Kerlinger, F. (1973). *Foundations of behavioral research* (2nd ed.). New York: Holt, Rinehart & Winston. (Chapter 2).

Popper, K.R. (1959). *The logic of scientific discovery* (rev. ed.). New York: Basic Books. (Chapter 10).

Wilson, H.S. (1989). *Research in nursing* (2nd ed.). Menlo Park, CA: Addison-Wesley. (Chapter 9).

*SUBSTANTIVE REFERENCES**

Broome, M.E., & Endsley, R.C. (1989). Maternal presence, childrearing practices, and children's response to an injection. *Research in Nursing and Health, 12,* 229–235.

Brouse, S.H. (1985). Effect of gender role identity on patterns of feminine and self-concept scores from late pregnancy to early postpartum. *Advances in Nursing Sciences, 7,* 32–48.

Forrester, D.A. (1988). Sex role identity and perceptions of nurse role discrepancy. *Western Journal of Nursing Research, 10,* 600–612.

Hirsch, A.M. (1988). Type A behavior pattern and catecholamine excretion during cardiac catheterization. *Western Journal of Nursing Research, 10,* 307–316.

Hollerbach, A.D., & Sneed, N.V. (1990). Accuracy of radial pulse assessment by length of counting interval. *Heart and Lung, 19,* 258–264.

Johnson, S., Omery, A., & Nikas, D. (1989). Effects of conversation on intracranial pressure in comatose patients. *Heart and Lung, 18,* 56–63.

Kolanowski, A.M. (1990). Restlessness in the elderly:

* These studies are included here because they present clearly stated hypotheses.

The effect of artificial lighting. *Nursing Research, 39,* 181–183.

Krouse, H., & Roberts, S. (1989). Nurse–patient interactive styles: Power, control, and satisfaction. *Western Journal of Nursing Research, 11,* 717–725.

McPhail, A., Pikula, H., Roberts, J., Browne, G., & Harper, D. (1990). Primary nursing: A randomized crossover trial. *Western Journal of Nursing Research, 12,* 188–200

Miller, Sr. P., Wilkoff, R., McMahon, M., Garrett, M.J., & Ringel, K. (1990). Marital functioning after cardiac surgery. *Heart and Lung, 19,* 55–61.

Morse, J.M., & Park, C. (1988). Home birth and hospital deliveries: A comparison of the perceived painfulness of parturition. *Research in Nursing and Health, 11,* 175–181.

Norbeck, J.S., & Anderson, N.J. (1989). Psychosocial predictors of pregnancy outcomes in low-income black, Hispanic, and white women. *Nursing Research, 38,* 204–209.

Quinn, J.F. (1989). Therapeutic touch as energy exchange. *Nursing Science Quarterly, 2,* 79–87.

Randolph, G.L. (1984). Therapeutic and physical touch: Physiological response to stressful stimuli. *Nursing Research, 33,* 33–36.

Robinson, K.M. (1989). Predictors of depression among wife caregivers. *Nursing Research, 38,* 359–363.

Shelley, S.I., Zahorchak, R.M., & Gambril, C. (1987). Aggressiveness of nursing care for older patients and those with do-not-resuscitate orders. *Nursing Research, 36,* 157–162.

Vessey, J.A. (1988). Comparison of two teaching methods on children's knowledge of their internal bodies. *Nursing Research, 37,* 262–267.

Zimmerman, L., Pozehi, B., Duncan, K., & Schmitz, R. (1989). Effects of music in patients who had cancer pain. *Western Journal of Nursing Research, 11,* 298–309.

OTHER REFERENCE CITED

Clark, P.E., & Clark, M.J. (1984). Therapeutic touch: Is there a scientific basis for the practice? *Nursing Research, 33,* 37–41.

Part III

Designs for Nursing Research

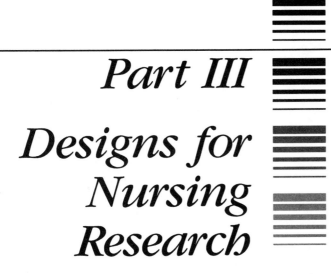

9
Experiments and Quasi-Experiments

The choice of an overall research approach constitutes one of the major decisions that must be made in conducting a research study. In some cases, the nature of the research problem dictates the approach to be taken. More often, however, there is considerable flexibility in the decision-making process. This flexibility provides researchers with opportunities to exercise their creativity, but it also means that they must be familiar with the options and must exercise judgment in the selection of an approach. Part III of this book examines some of the basic types of research strategies that have been used in nursing research; in this chapter, we discuss the types of research designs referred to as experiments and quasi-experiments.

≡ CHARACTERISTICS OF TRUE EXPERIMENTS

Experiments differ from nonexperiments in one very important respect: the researcher is an active agent in experimental work rather than a passive observer. Early physical scientists learned that although observation of natural phenomena is valuable and instructive, the complexity of the events occurring in the natural state often obscures understanding of important relationships. This problem was handled by isolating the phenomenon of interest in a laboratory setting and controlling the conditions under which it occurred. The procedures developed by physical scientists were profitably adopted by biologists during the nineteenth century, resulting in many achievements in physiology and medicine. The twentieth century has witnessed the utilization of experimental methods by scholars and researchers interested in human behavior and psychologic states.

The controlled experiment is considered

by many to be the ideal of science. Except for purely descriptive research, the aim of scientific research is to understand the nature of relationships among phenomena. For example, does a certain drug cause the cure of a certain disease? Do certain nursing techniques produce a decrease in patient anxiety? The strength of the true experiment over other methods lies in the fact that the experimenter can achieve greater confidence in the genuineness and interpretability of relationships because they are observed under carefully controlled conditions. As we have pointed out in Chapter 8, hypotheses are never ultimately proved or disproved by scientific methods, but true experiments offer the most convincing evidence concerning the effects one variable can have on another.

A true experiment is a scientific investigation characterized by the following properties:

- *manipulation*—the experimenter *does* something to at least some of the subjects in the study
- *control*—the experimenter introduces one or more controls over the experimental situation, including the use of a control group
- *randomization*—the experimenter assigns subjects to a control or experimental group on a random basis

Each of these properties is discussed more fully below.

Manipulation

Manipulation involves *doing* something to at least one group of subjects. The introduction of that "something" (often referred to as the *experimental treatment* or *experimental intervention*) constitutes the independent variable. The experimenter manipulates the independent variable by administering a treatment to some subjects and withholding it from others (or by administering some other treatment, such as a placebo). The experimenter, in other words, consciously *varies* the independent variable and observes the effect that the manipulation has on the dependent variable of interest.

For example, let us say we have hypothesized that the color of a pediatric nurse's uniform affects the degree to which children display positive affective behaviors such as smiling and laughing during hospitalization. The independent or presumed causative variable in this example is uniform color, which could be manipulated by assigning some nurses white uniforms (for instance) and other nurses brightly colored uniforms. Thus, in this study we might compare, 24 hours after hospitalization, the affective behaviors (the dependent variables) of two groups of children: (1) those cared for by white-uniformed nurses and (2) those cared for by nurses in colored uniforms. This simple design is sometimes referred to as an *after-only* or *posttest-only* experimental design because data on the dependent variable are only collected once—after the experimental treatment has been introduced.

A second example serves to illustrate a slightly more complex design. Let us suppose that we are interested in investigating the effect on heart rate of being physically restrained by posey belt. We might choose to begin our experimentation with some subhuman species such as the rat. We decide to use an experimental scheme such as the one shown in Figure 9-1. This design involves imposing restraint by posey belt on one group of rats (the experimental group) while imposing no restraint on another (the control group). In this design, the dependent variable is measured at two points in time, before and after the experimental intervention (physical restraint). This scheme permits us to examine what changes in heart rate were produced as a result of being physically restrained, which is our independent variable. This design, because of its two measurement points, is referred to as a *before–after* or *pretest–posttest* experimental design. In such designs, the initial measure of the dependent variable is often referred to as the *baseline measure*. (Some researchers involved in experimental research refer to the posttest measure of the dependent variable as the *outcome measure*—that is, the measure that captures the outcome of the experimental intervention).

Before   After

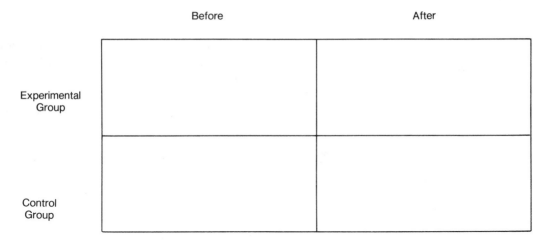

Experimental
Group

Control
Group

Figure 9-1. *Before–after experimental design.*

Control

The notion of control in an experimental context actually summarizes all of the major experimental activities: control is acquired by manipulating, by randomizing, by carefully preparing the experimental protocols, and by using a control group. This section focuses on the function of the control group in experiments.

Obtaining scientific evidence about relationships requires making at least one comparison. If we were to supplement the diet of a group of premature infants with a particular combination of vitamins and other nutrients every day for two weeks, the weight of those infants at the end of the two-week period would give us absolutely no information about the effectiveness of the treatment. At a bare minimum, we would need to compare their posttreatment weight with their pretreatment weight to determine if, at least, their weight had increased. But let us assume for the moment that we find an average weight gain of one pound. Does this finding support the conclusion that there is a causative relationship between the nutritional supplements (the independent variable) and weight gain (the dependent variable)? No, it does not. Babies normally gain weight as they mature. Without a control group—

a group that does *not* receive the nutritional supplements—it is impossible to separate the effects of maturation from those of the treatment. The term *control group,* in other words, refers to a group of subjects whose performance on a dependent variable is used as a basis for evaluating the performance of the *experimental group* (the group that receives the treatment of interest to the researcher) on the same dependent variable.

In some biologic, medical, and psychologic research, the experimenter administers the treatment of interest to the experimental group while the control group receives no treatment at all and is merely observed with respect to behavior on the dependent variable. This kind of situation probably is not feasible for many nursing research projects because it may be impossible to isolate a control group and do nothing to those subjects. For example, if we wanted to evaluate the effectiveness of some nursing intervention on hospital patients, it would be unlikely that we would devise an experiment in which the control group of patients received no nursing care at all. We would have to evaluate our new intervention not against the total absence of care but, rather, against a control group receiving conventional methods of care.

Randomization

Randomization involves the assignment of subjects to groups on a random basis. "Random" essentially means that every subject has an equal chance of being assigned to any group. If subjects are placed in groups randomly, there is no *systematic bias* in the groups with respect to attributes that may affect the dependent variable under investigation.

Before discussing the mechanics of random assignment, we should pause to consider the function of randomization. Suppose a researcher wishes to study the effectiveness of a hospital-based contraceptive counseling program for a group of multiparous women who have just given birth. Two groups of subjects are established, one of which will be counseled and the other of which will receive no counseling. The women in the sample may be expected to differ from one another on a number of characteristics, such as age, marital status, financial situation, attitudes toward childrearing, and the like. Any of these characteristics could have an effect on the diligence with which a woman practices contraception, quite independent of whether or not she receives counseling. The researcher naturally wants to have the "counsel" and "no counsel" groups equal with respect to these extraneous characteristics to adequately assess the impact of the counseling on the women's subsequent pregnancies. The random assignment of subjects to one group or the other is designed to perform this equalization function. One method might be to flip a coin for each woman (more elaborate procedures are discussed later). If the coin is "heads" the woman would be assigned to one group; if the coin is "tails" she would be assigned to the other group.

Although randomization is the preferred scientific method for equalizing groups, there is no guarantee that they will, in fact, be equal. Let us take as an extreme example the case in which only ten women, all of whom have given birth to at least four children, have volunteered to participate in the study. Five of the ten women are aged 35 or older and the remaining five are younger than 35. One would anticipate that a random assignment of women to a control and experimental group would result in approximately two or three women from the two age ranges in each group. But let us suppose that by chance the older five women ended up in the experimental group. Because these women are nearing the end of their childbearing years, the likelihood of their conceiving is diminished. Thus, follow-ups on their subsequent reproductive behavior (the dependent variable) might suggest that the counseling program was successful for the experimental group; however, a higher pregnancy rate for the control group may only reflect the age and, hence, fecundity difference and not the lack of exposure to counseling.

Despite this possibility, randomization remains the most trustworthy and acceptable method of equalizing groups. Unusual or deviant assignments such as this one are rare, and the likelihood of obtaining markedly unequal groups is reduced as the number of subjects increases.

Students often wonder why the researcher does not consciously control those characteristics of subjects that are likely to affect the experimental outcome. The procedure that is sometimes used to accomplish this is known as *matching*. For example, if matching were used in the contraceptive counseling study, the researcher might want to ensure that if there were a married, 38-year-old woman with six children in the "counsel" group, there would be a married, 38-year-old woman with six children in the control group as well. There are two serious problems with matching, however. First of all, to match effectively, we must know what the characteristics that are likely to affect the dependent variable are. This information is not always known. Second, even if we knew the relevant traits, the complications of matching on more than three or four characteristics are prohibitive. With random assignment, on the other hand, *all* possible distinguishing characteristics—age, sex, intelligence, blood type, religious affiliation, and so on—are likely to be equally distributed in all groups. Over the long run, the groups tend to be counterbalanced with respect to an infinite number of biologic, psychologic, economic, or social traits.

To demonstrate how random assignment is actually performed, we turn to another example. Suppose we have 15 children who are about to have a tonsillectomy and we are interested in testing the effectiveness of two alternative nursing interventions with regard to the child's level of preoperative anxiety. One intervention might focus on structured information regarding the activities of the surgical team (procedural information); the other might focus on structured information regarding what the child will feel (sensation information). A third group will receive no special intervention. Five children will be in each of the three groups. Because there are three groups, we can no longer use the flip of a coin to decide the group to which an individual will be assigned. One possibility would be to write the names of the individuals on slips of paper, put the slips into a hat, and then draw names. The first individuals whose names were drawn would be assigned to Group I, the second five would be assigned to Group II, and the remaining five would be assigned to Group III.

Pulling names from a hat involves considerable work, especially if there are many subjects. Researchers typically use a table of random numbers to facilitate the randomization process. A portion of such a table is reproduced in Table 9-1. A random number table is set up by using the digits from 0 to 9 in such a way that each number is equally likely to follow any other. These tables are often generated by computers. Going in any direction from any point in the table produces a random sequence.

In our example, we would number the 15 individuals from 1 to 15, as shown in the second column of Table 9-2 and then draw numbers between 1 and 15 from the random number table. A simple procedure for finding a starting point is to close your eyes and let your finger fall at some point on the table. For the sake of following the example, let us assume that we have followed this procedure and that the starting point is at number 52 as circled on Table 9-1. We can now move from that point in any direction on the table. Our task is to select the first five numbers that fall between 01 and 15. Let us move from the starting point to the

right, looking at two-digit combinations to be sure to get numbers from 10 to 15. The next number to the right of 52 is 06. The person whose number is 06, that is, Nathan O., is assigned to Group I. Moving along in the table, we find that the next number within the range of 01 to 15 is 11. Katy M., whose number is 11, is also assigned to Group I. When we get to the end of the row, we move down to the next row, and so forth. To find numbers in the required range, we may have to bypass a good many numbers. The next three numbers we find are 01, 15, and 14. Thus Kasia S., Nolan T., and Oliver E. are all put into Group I. The next five numbers between 01 and 15 that emerge in the random number table are used to assign five individuals to Group II in the same fashion, as shown in the third column of Table 9-2. The remaining five people are put into Group III. Note that numbers that have already been "used" often reappear in the table before our randomization task is completed. For example, the number 15 appeared four times before the assignment procedure was completed. This is perfectly normal because the numbers are random. After the first time a number appears and is used, subsequent appearances can be ignored.

It might be useful to look at the three groups to see if they are approximately equal with respect to one readily discernible characteristic, that is, the sex of the individual. We started out with eight females and seven males in the total group. The sex breakdown of the three groups is presented in Table 9-3. As this table shows, the randomization procedure did a good job of allocating the two sexes approximately equally across the three groups. We must accept on faith the probability that other characteristics are fairly well distributed in the randomized groups as well.

One more step in the randomization process must be completed before the experiment begins. Note that in the above discussion we did not state that Nathan O., Katy M., and the other three individuals in Group I would be assigned to the Procedural Information Group. This is because it is a good experimental strategy to randomly assign groups to experimental treatments, as well as individuals to groups. In fact, a general principle that is useful to remember is to randomize whenever possible. To continue with our example, we give the procedural information, sensation information, and control conditions the numbers 1, 2, and 3, respectively. Finding a new starting point in the random number table, we look for the numbers 1, 2, or 3. This time we can look at one digit at a time, because the range of values we are seeking does not include a two-digit number. Let us say that we start at number 8 in the ninth row of the table, which is indicated by a

rectangle. Reading *down* this time, we find the number 1. We, therefore, assign Group I to the procedural information condition. Further along in the same column we come to the number 3. Group III, therefore, is assigned to the second condition, sensation information, and the remaining group, Group II, is assigned to the control condition.

We now have fulfilled all three requirements for a true experiment: we have manipulated the independent variable (the different treatments); we have a control group; and we have

Table 9-1. *Small Table of Random Digits*

46 85 05 23 26	34 67 75 83 00	74 91 06 43 45
69 24 89 34 60	45 30 50 75 21	61 31 83 18 55
14 01 33 17 92	59 74 76 72 77	76 50 33 45 13
56 30 38 73 15	16 (52) 06 96 76	11 65 49 98 93
81 30 44 85 85	68 65 22 73 76	92 85 25 58 66
70 28 42 43 26	79 37 59 52 20	01 15 96 32 67
90 41 59 36 14	33 52 12 66 65	55 82 34 76 41
39 90 40 21 15	59 58 94 90 67	66 82 14 15 75
88 15 20 00 80	20 55 49 14 09	96 27 74 [82] 57
45 13 46 35 45	59 40 47 20 59	43 94 75 16 80
70 01 41 50 21	41 29 06 73 12	71 85 71 59 57
37 23 93 32 95	05 87 00 11 19	92 78 42 63 40
18 63 73 75 09	82 44 49 90 05	04 92 17 37 01
05 32 78 21 62	20 24 78 17 59	45 19 72 53 32
95 09 66 79 46	48 46 08 55 58	15 19 11 87 82
43 25 38 41 45	60 83 32 59 83	01 29 14 13 49
80 85 40 92 79	43 52 90 63 18	38 38 47 47 61
80 08 87 70 74	88 72 25 67 36	66 16 44 94 31
80 89 01 80 02	94 81 33 19 00	54 15 58 34 36
93 12 81 84 64	74 45 79 05 61	72 84 81 18 34
82 47 42 55 93	48 54 53 52 47	18 61 91 36 74
53 34 24 42 76	75 12 21 17 24	74 62 77 37 07
82 64 12 28 20	92 90 41 31 41	32 39 21 97 63
13 57 41 72 00	69 90 26 37 42	78 46 42 25 01
29 59 38 86 27	94 97 21 15 98	62 09 53 67 87
86 88 75 50 87	19 15 20 00 23	12 30 28 07 83
44 98 91 68 22	36 02 40 08 67	76 37 84 16 05
93 39 94 55 47	94 45 87 42 84	05 04 14 98 07
52 16 29 02 86	54 15 83 42 43	46 97 83 54 82
04 73 72 10 31	75 05 19 30 29	47 66 56 43 82

Reprinted from *A Million Random Digits with 100,000 Normal Deviates.* New York: The Free Press, 1955. Used with permission of the Rand Corporation, Santa Monica, CA.

Table 9-2. *Example of Random Assignment Procedure*

NAME OF SUBJECT	NUMBER	GROUP ASSIGNMENT
Kasia S.	1	I
John R.	2	III
Richard N.	3	III
Lauren C.	4	II
Diane B.	5	II
Nathan O.	6	I
Claire L.	7	III
Jesse R.	8	III
Thomas I.	9	II
Cassie F.	10	III
Katy M.	11	I
Brigitte N.	12	II
Evan W.	13	II
Oliver E.	14	I
Nolan T.	15	I

Table 9-3. *Breakdown of the Sex Composition of the Three Groups*

SEX	GROUP I	GROUP II	GROUP III
Male	3	2	2
Female	2	3	3

randomly assigned subjects to the treatments. If any one of these elements had been missing, we would not have had a true experimental design.

≡ EXPERIMENTAL DESIGNS

We have already described two of the most basic designs for experimental research—the posttest only and pretest–posttest designs. Three additional experimental designs are briefly described below; several others are described in Chapter 12.

Randomized Clinical Trials

Medical researchers and epidemiologists often evaluate an innovative treatment through the use of a randomized clinical trial (sometimes referred to simply as a clinical trial). *Clinical trials* typically use either a before–after or after-only design. The term "clinical trial," then, does not refer so much to a distinctive design as to an application of a design. Clinical trials always involve the testing of a clinical treatment; random assignment of subjects of experimental and one or more control condition; the collection of information on outcomes of the treatment from subjects in all groups, sometimes after a long period has elapsed; and generally, the use of a large and heterogeneous sample of subjects, frequently selected from multiple, geographically dispersed sites to ensure that the findings are not unique to a single setting.

When clinical trials involve the withholding of a potentially beneficial treatment from the control group or the administration of a potentially risky new treatment to the experimental group, researchers are sometimes reluctant to allocate subjects to groups on an equal basis. For example, for evaluating a promising new drug for the treatment of acquired immunodeficiency syndrome (AIDS), researchers may randomly allocate 75% of the subjects to the experimental group and 25% to the control group. This unequal allocation has obvious advantages from an ethical point of view, but (for reasons that are too complex to elaborate on here) it is generally more costly because when subjects are not equally divided among treatment groups, the total number of subjects needed is greater to achieve the same level of precision in performing statistical tests.

Solomon Four-Group Design

When data are collected both before and after an intervention, the pretest (initial) measure sometimes has the potential to distort the results. That is, the posttest measures may be affected not only by the treatment but also by exposure to the pretest. For example, if our intervention was a workshop to improve nurses' attitudes toward mentally ill people, a pretest attitudinal measure may in itself constitute a sensitizing "treatment" and could obscure an analysis of the workshop's effect. Such a situation might call for the *Solomon four-group design,* which consists of two experimental groups and two control groups. One experimental group and one control group would be administered the pretest and the other groups would not, thereby allowing the effects of the pretest measure and intervention to be segregated. Figure 9-2 illustrates the Solomon four-group design.

Factorial Design

The discussion to this point has considered designs in which the experimenter systematically varies or manipulates only one independent variable at a time. It is, however, possible to manipulate two or more variables simultaneously. Suppose that we are interested in comparing two therapeutic strategies for premature infants: one method involves tactile stimulation and the second approach involves auditory stimulation. At the same time, however, we are interested in learning if the daily amount of stimulation is related to the progress of the infant. The dependent variables for the study will be various measures of

	Data Collection	
Group	Before	After
Experimental — with pretest	X	X
Experimental — without pretest		X
Control — with pretest	X	X
Control — without pretest		X

Figure 9-2. *Solomon four-group experimental design.*

infant development, such as weight gain, cardiac responsiveness, and so forth. Figure 9-3 illustrates the structure of this experiment.

This type of study, which is known as a *factorial experiment,* offers a number of advantages to the researcher. In effect, factorial designs permit the testing of multiple hypotheses in a single experiment. In the current example, the three research questions being addressed are as follows:

TYPE OF STIMULATION

	Auditory A1	Tactile A2
DAILY EXPOSURE 15 min. B1	A1 B1	A2 B1
30 min. B2	A1 B2	A2 B2
45 min. B3	A1 B3	A2 B3

Figure 9-3. *Schematic diagram of a factorial experiment.*

1. Does auditory stimulation have a more beneficial effect on the development of premature infants than tactile stimulation?
2. Is the duration of stimulation (independent of modality) related to infant development?
3. Is auditory stimulation most effective when linked to a certain "dose" and tactile stimulation most effective when coupled with a different dose?

The third question demonstrates a major strength of factorial designs: they permit us to evaluate not only *main effects* (effects resulting from experimentally manipulated variables, as exemplified in questions 1 and 2) but also *interaction effects* (effects resulting from combining the treatment methods). We may feel that it is insufficient to say that auditory stimulation is preferable to tactile stimulation (or vice versa) and that 45 minutes of stimulation per day is more effective than 15 minutes per day. Rather, it is how these two variables interact (how they behave in combination) that is of interest. Our results may indicate that 15 minutes of tactile stimulation and 45 minutes of auditory stimulation are the most beneficial treatments. We could not have obtained these results by conducting two separate experiments that manipulated only one independent variable and held the second one constant.

In factorial experiments, subjects are assigned at random to a specific combination of conditions. In the example that Figure 9-3 illustrates, the premature infants would be assigned randomly to one of the six cells. A *cell* in experimental research refers to a treatment condition; it is represented in a schematic diagram as a box (cell) in the design.

Figure 9-3 can also be used to define some design terminology frequently encountered in the research literature. The two independent variables in a factorial design are referred to as the *factors*. The "type of stimulation" variable is factor A and the "amount of daily exposure" variable is factor B. Each factor must have two or more *levels* (if there were only one level, the factor would not be a variable). Level one of factor A is auditory and level two of factor A is tactile. When describing the

dimensions of the design, researchers refer to the number of levels. The design in Figure 9-3 would be described as a 2×3 design: two levels in factor A times three levels in factor B. If a third source of stimulation, such as visual stimulation, were added, and if a daily dosage of 60 minutes were also added, the design would be referred to as a 3×4 design.

Factorial experiments can be performed with three or more independent variables (factors). However, designs with more than four factors are rare, because the analysis becomes complex and because the number of subjects required would be prohibitive.

≡ ADVANTAGES AND DISADVANTAGES OF EXPERIMENTS

Controlled experiments are often considered the ideal of science. In this section, we will explore the reasons why experimental methods are held in high esteem. We will also examine some of the limitations of the experimental approach.

Experimental Strengths

True experiments are the most powerful method available to scientists for testing hypotheses of cause-and-effect relationships between variables. Because of its special controlling properties, the scientific experiment offers greater corroboration than any other research approach that, *if* the independent variable (e.g., diet, drug dosage, or teaching approach) is manipulated in a certain way, *then* certain consequences in the dependent variable (e.g., weight loss, recovery of health, or learning) may be expected to ensue. This "if–then" type of relationship is important to nursing and medical researchers because of its implications for prediction and control. The great strength of experiments, then, lies in the confidence with which causal relationships can be inferred.

Because the concept of causality is a controversial one, it is appropriate to briefly present our point of view. Some scholars take the position that the notion of causality among phenomena is untenable, on both metaphysical and empirical grounds. We would agree, as most scientists would, that causal laws can never be proved. Nevertheless, many scientists would support the assertion that "science was, is, and always will be, concerned ultimately with the causal genus of order" (Harre, 1970, p. 103). We will continue to use the concept of causality in this book in the sense suggested by Selltiz, Wrightsman, and Cook (1976). These authors avoid the issue of metaphysical causes and note that causation is instead a construct with useful properties for scientists: "Causes, like stories, are not discovered; they are invented. A causal sequence is a perspective we place on the world. It is proper, then, to speak of a causal hypothesis and develop criteria for testing the adequacy of the formulation" (p. 114). This view does not invoke mystical "forces" or "impulses" or notions of fate as a way of explaining phenomena. Here, causation between two variables only implies that when variable X occurs, there is a likelihood that variable Y will result.

Paul Lazarsfeld (1955), a sociologist, has identified three criteria for causality. The first criterion is temporal: a cause must precede an effect in time. If we were testing the hypothesis that saccharin causes bladder cancer, it would obviously be necessary to demonstrate that the subjects had not developed cancer before exposure to saccharin. The second requirement is that there be an empirical relationship between the presumed cause and the presumed effect. In the saccharin/cancer example, the researcher would have to demonstrate an association between the ingestion of saccharin and the presence of a carcinoma—that is, that a higher percentage of saccharin users than nonusers developed cancer. The final criterion in a causal relationship is that the relationship cannot be explained as being the result of the influence of a third variable. Suppose, for instance, that people who use saccharin tend also to drink more coffee than nonusers of saccharin. There is, thus, a possibility that any empirical relationship between saccharin use and bladder cancer in humans reflects an underlying causal relationship between a substance in coffee

and bladder cancer. It is particularly because of this third criterion that the experimental approach is so strong. Through the controls imposed by manipulation, comparison, and randomization, alternative explanations to a causal interpretation can often be ruled out or discredited.

Experimental Weaknesses

Despite the overwhelming advantages of experimental research, this approach has several limitations. First of all, there are a number of interesting variables that are simply not amenable to experimental manipulation. A large number of human characteristics, such as sex, metabolism, or intelligence, or environmental characteristics, such as weather, cannot be experimentally controlled. For example, we cannot randomly confer upon infants their weight at birth to observe the effect of birthweight on subsequent morbidity.

A second, but related, limitation is that there are many variables that could technically be manipulated except that ethical considerations prohibit such manipulation. For example, to date there have not been any experiments using human subjects to study the effect of cigarette smoking on lung cancer. Such an experiment would require us to randomly assign individuals to a smoking or nonsmoking group. Those in the first group would be required to smoke, and those in the second group would be prohibited from smoking. Experimentation with humans, therefore, is subject to a number of ethical constraints, as discussed in Chapter 3.

In many situations, experimentation may not be feasible simply because it is impractical. This often will be the case in hospital settings. It may, for instance, be impossible in the real world to secure the necessary cooperation to conduct an experiment from administrators or other key people. Cooperation may be withheld for many reasons, from a desire to avoid disruptions to a basic suspicion and uneasiness about the concept of experimentation.

A weakness of experiments that is sometimes mentioned is their artificiality. Part of the difficulty lies in the requirement for randomization and then equal treatment within groups. In ordinary life, the way in which we interact with people is not random. For example, within the nursing field certain aspects of the patient—his or her age, physical attractiveness, personality, or severity of illness—will cause us to modify our behavior and, hence, our care. The differences may be extremely subtle, but they undoubtedly are not random. Another aspect of experiments that is considered artificial by phenomenologists is the focus on only a handful of variables, while attempting to hold all else constant. This requirement is criticized as being reductionist and as artificially constraining human experience.

Another problem with experiments is the *"Hawthorne effect,"* which is a kind of placebo effect. The term is derived from a series of experiments conducted at the Hawthorne plant of the Western Electric Corporation in which various environmental conditions such as light and working hours were varied to determine their effect on worker productivity. Regardless of what change was introduced, that is, whether the light was made better or worse, productivity increased. Thus, it seems that the knowledge of being included in a study may be sufficient to cause people to change their behavior, thereby obscuring the effect of the variable of interest. In a hospital situation, the researcher might have to contend with a double Hawthorne effect. For example, if an experiment to investigate the effect of a new postoperative patient routine were conducted, nurses and hospital staff, as well as patients, might be aware of their participation in a study, and both groups could alter their actions accordingly. It is precisely for this reason that *double-blind experiments,* in which neither the subjects nor those who administer the treatment know who is in the experimental or control group, are so powerful. Unfortunately, the double-blind approach is not feasible for some types of nursing research because nursing interventions are more difficult to disguise than medications.

In sum, despite the clear-cut superiority of experiments in terms of their ability to test research hypotheses, they are subject to a number of limitations that make them difficult to apply to many real-world problems. Nevertheless, the fact that experimental conditions are difficult to establish does not mean that all attempts to achieve them should be abandoned. True experiments probably are possible in many situations in which nonexperimental methods are used.

≡ *RESEARCH EXAMPLES OF EXPERIMENTS*

Nurse researchers are increasingly using experimental designs to test their hypotheses. Table 9-4 summarizes some recent examples. An experimental study described in more detail follows.

> Geden and her colleagues (1985) were interested in examining which aspects of the Lamaze method of childbirth preparation are most effective as pain-coping strategies. Three components of Lamaze training were of special interest: (1) information, (2) breathing techniques, and (3) relaxation training. Because Lamaze-type preparation is so widely accepted as beneficial, the investigator recognized the potential ethical problem of randomly assigning women in labor to different components of the preparation, while denying them other components. Therefore, she used as subjects 80 nulliparous female undergraduates who were exposed to a laboratory pain stimulus that has been shown to be a good analogue of labor pain. The 80 subjects were randomly assigned to one of eight treatment conditions representing all possible combinations of the three major components of Lamaze preparation. That is, some subjects received information alone; others received information plus breathing techniques, and so on. One of the eight groups received no intervention. All subjects were exposed to a 1-hour session involving 20 exposures, each 80 seconds in length, to a pain stimulus, patterned to resemble labor contractions. The effectiveness of the various components in mediating pain was assessed by obtaining measures of the subjects' systolic and diastolic blood pressure, frontalis electromyogram, heart rate,

Table 9-4. *Examples of True Experimental Designs*

RESEARCH QUESTION	MANIPULATED VARIABLE	DESIGN	SUBJECTS	SOURCE
Does maternal position during the phase of maximum slope affect the length of labor and maternal comfort?	Maternal position—upright versus recumbent	After only	20 in upright position 20 in recumbent position	Andrews & Chrzanowski, 1990
What is the effect of nonnutritive sucking on the behavioral state of preterm infants before feeding?	Nonnutritive sucking on a pacifier for 5 minutes before feeding versus no sucking	Before–after	12 experimentals 12 controls	Gill et al., 1988
What is the effect of transcutaneous nerve stimulation on incisional pain caused by cleaning and packing an abdominal surgical wound?	Electrical stimulation before and during wound dressing versus placebo treatment (electrode placement without stimulation) versus no special treatment	After only	25 experimentals 25 placebos 25 controls	Hargreaves & Lander, 1989
Are relaxation and music therapy effective means of reducing stress in patients with acute myocardial infarction?	Exposure to three sessions of relaxation versus exposure to three sessions of music therapy versus no special treatment	Before–after	27 relaxation 26 music therapy 27 controls	Guzzetta, 1989
What are the heat loss prevention capabilities of three head treatment modalities for newborns?	Use of a fabric-insulated bonnet versus use of a stockinette versus use of no head covering	After only	30 bonnets 30 stockinettes 30 no covering	Greer, 1988
Do nurses' evaluations of rape victims in a simulated situation vary as a function of whether the victim locked her car or the time of day when the rape occurred?	Rape victim locked car versus did not lock car; incident occurred at 5:00 P.M. versus midnight	Factorial	20 in locked car, early episode 20 in unlocked car, early episode 20 in locked car, late episode 20 in unlocked car, late episode	Damrosch et al., 1987

R = Randomization	R	O_1	X	O_2
O = Observation or measurement				
X = Treatment or intervention	R	O_1		O_2

Figure 9-4. *Symbolic representation of a pretest-posttest experimental design.*

and self-reported pain. The findings suggested that the relaxation training is the most therapeutically active component of the Lamaze treatment.

Geden and her colleagues clearly used an experimental design. The experimental nature of the study should be obvious. The investigators manipulated the independent variable (the nature of the pain-coping strategy); had experimental and control groups; and randomly assigned subjects to groups. The fact that they were able to provide both the interventions and the pain stimulus in a laboratory setting ensured maximal control over the research conditions. Their conclusions were strengthened by having used multiple dependent variables that complemented each other.

≡ THE QUASI-EXPERIMENTAL APPROACH

Research that uses a quasi-experimental design often looks much like an experiment. *Quasi-experiments,* like true experiments, involve the manipulation of an independent variable, that is, the institution of an experimental treatment. However, quasi-experimental designs lack at least one of the other two properties that characterize true experiments, randomization or a control group.

The basic difficulty with the quasi-experimental approach is its weakness, relative to experiments, in allowing us to make causal inferences. We want to know if the experimental treatment does, in fact, cause the effect we observe in the dependent variable. Does the sensation information condition result in reduced anxiety in our group of subjects or was the anxiety reduction the result of some other factor or combination of factors? Evidence for cause-and-effect relationships is more convincing when true experimental designs rather than quasi-experimental designs are used.

Perhaps the following hypothetical examples will clarify the problems inherent in quasi-experiments. Before presenting these examples, however, it will be useful to introduce some notation that will facilitate our discussion.* Figure 9-4 presents a symbolic representation of a pretest–posttest experimental design, identical to the design shown in Figure 9-1. According to the notation used in Figure 9-4, *R* means that there has been a random assignment to separate treatment groups. *O* represents an observation—that is, the collection of data on the dependent variable. *X* stands for the exposure of a group to an experimental treatment. Thus the top line in Figure 9-4 represents the experimental group that has had subjects randomly assigned to it (R), has had both a pretreatment test (O_1) and a posttreatment test (O_2), and has been exposed to the experimental treatment of interest (X). The second row in the figure represents the control group, which differs from the experimental group only by the absence of exposure to the experimental treatment.

We are now equipped to examine a few quasi-experimental designs.

Nonequivalent Control Group Designs

Suppose that we wished to study the effect of introducing the problem-oriented method of charting on nursing staff morale. The system is to be implemented in a 600-bed hospital in a large metropolitan area. Because we anticipate that

---

* The notation, as well as most of the concepts in this section, are derived from Campbell and Stanley's (1963) classic monograph.

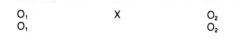

O₁   X   O₂
O₁   O₂

Figure 9-5. *Nonequivalent control group pretest–posttest design (quasi-experimental).*

there might be staff dissatisfaction problems, at least initially, we arrange to conduct a study. A number of alternative strategies are available in designing the investigation. However, It will be impossible to conduct an experiment. Hospital staff cannot be randomly assigned to different treatment groups because the new system will affect everyone. Therefore, we decide to find another hospital with similar characteristics (size, geographic location, and the like) that is not instituting the problem-oriented method of charting. We also decide to collect baseline data by administering a staff morale questionnaire in both hospitals before the change is made (the pretest). We would again collect data after the system is installed in the experimental hospital (the posttest).

Figure 9-5 depicts this hypothetical study symbolically. The top row is our experimental (problem-oriented charting) hospital; and the second row is the hospital using traditional methods. A comparison of this diagram with the one in Figure 9-4 shows that they are identical except that subjects have not been randomly assigned to treatment groups in the second diagram. The design in Figure 9-5 is the weaker of the two because *it can no longer be assumed that the experimental and comparison groups** are equal. Because of the inability to randomize subjects, our study is quasi-experimental rather than being truly experimental. The design is, nevertheless, a strong one because the collection of pretest data allows us to determine whether the groups were initially similar in terms of their morale. If the morale of the two groups were very different at the start, our interpretation of the posttest data would be difficult, although there are statistical procedures that help. If the comparison and ex-

perimental groups responded similarly, on the average, on their pretest questionnaire, then we could be relatively confident that any posttest group differences in self-reported morale were the result of the experimental treatment.

Suppose that we had not thought to or had been unable to collect pretest data before the new method of charting was introduced. The resulting study could be diagrammed to show the scheme in Figure 9-6. This design, which is not uncommon, has a flaw that is difficult to remedy. We have no basis on which to judge the initial equivalence of the two nursing staffs. If we find that, at the posttest, the morale of the experimental hospital staff is lower than that of the control hospital staff, can we conclude that the new method of charting *caused* a decline in staff morale? There could be several alternative explanations for the posttest differences. In particular, it might be that the morale of the employees in the two hospitals differed even at the outset. Campbell and Stanley (1963), in fact, would call the design shown in Figure 9-6 *pre-experimental* rather than quasi-experimental because of its essentially irreconcilable weaknesses. Thus, although quasi-experiments lack some of the controlling properties inherent in true experiments, the hallmark of the quasi-experimental approach is the effort to introduce other controls to compensate for the absence of either the randomization or control group component.

Time Series Designs

The designs reviewed in the previous section illustrate studies in which a control group was used but randomization was not. The designs we will examine in this section have neither a control group nor randomization. In some cases where both characteristics are absent, there are inherent weaknesses that seriously jeopardize the

* In quasi-experiments, the term "comparison group" is generally used in lieu of "control group" to refer to the group against which outcomes in the treatment group will be evaluated.

X   O
                     O

Figure 9-6. *Nonequivalent control group posttest only design (pre-experimental).*

validity of the findings. However, there are several designs that offer the researcher some measure of protection against these problems.

Let us suppose that a hospital decides to adopt a requirement that all its nurses accrue a certain number of continuing education units before being considered for a promotion or raise. The nursing administrators want to assess some of the positive and negative consequences of this mandate. Some of the indicators they might examine include turnover rate, absentee rate, qualifications of new employee applicants, number of raises and promotions awarded, and so on. For the purposes of this example, let us assume that there is no other comparable hospital that could reasonably serve as a comparison for this study. In such a case, the only kind of comparison that could be made is a before–after contrast. If the requirement were inaugurated in January, one could compare the turnover rate, for example, for the 3-month period before the new rule with the turnover rate for the subsequent 3-month period. The schematic representation for such a study is shown in Figure 9-7.

Although this design seems logical and straightforward, there actually are numerous problems with it. What if either of the 3-month periods is atypical, apart from any regulation? What about the effects of any other hospital rules inaugurated during the same period? What about the effects of external factors that influence employment, such as parking facilities, new employee benefits at other nearby hospitals, the availability of child care facilities, and the like? The design in Figure 9-7 offers no way of controlling for any of these problems. This design is also pre-experimental because it fails to control for so many possible extraneous factors.

A design that can assist us in this case is known as the *time series design* (sometimes referred to as the interrupted time series design) and is diagrammed in Figure 9-8. The basic no-

$$O_1 \qquad\qquad X \qquad\qquad O_2$$

Figure 9-7. *One group pretest–posttest design (pre-experimental).*

tion underlying the time series design is the collection of information over an extended period and the introduction of an experimental treatment during the course of the data collection period. In the figure, O_1 through O_4 represent four separate instances of observation or data collection on a dependent variable before treatment; X represents the treatment (the introduction of the independent variable); and O_5 through O_8 represent four posttreatment observations. In our present example, O_1 might be the number of nurses who left the hospital in January through March in the year before the new continuing education rule, O_2 the number of resignations in April through June, and so forth. After the rule is implemented, data on turnover are similarly collected for four consecutive 3-month periods, giving us observations O_5 through O_8.

Even though the time series design does not eliminate all of the problems of interpreting changes in turnover rate, the extended time perspective immensely strengthens our ability to attribute any change to our experimental manipulation, which in this case is the continuing education requirement. Figure 9-9 attempts to demonstrate why this is so. The two diagrams (*A* and *B*) in the figure show two possible outcome patterns for the eight measures of nurse turnover. The vertical dotted line in the center represents the time at which the continuing education rule was implemented. Both (*A*) and (*B*) reflect a feature that is common to most time series studies, and this is the fluctuation from one "observation" or measurement to another. These fluctuations are, of course, perfectly normal. One would not expect that, if 48 nurses resigned from a hospital in 1 year, the resignations would be spaced evenly

$$O_1 \qquad O_2 \qquad O_3 \qquad O_4 \qquad X \qquad O_5 \qquad O_6 \qquad O_7 \qquad O_8$$

Figure 9-8. *Time series design (quasi-experimental).*

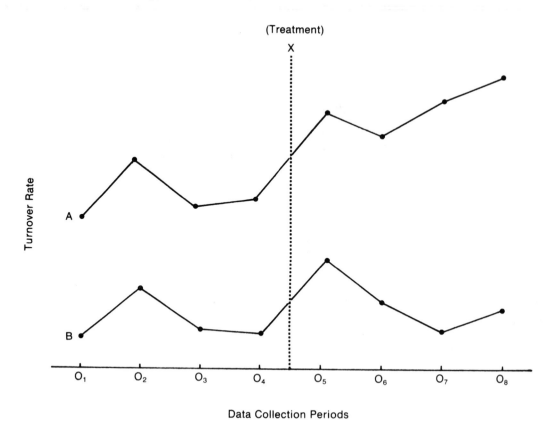

Figure 9-9. *Two possible time series outcome patterns.*

during the course of the year with exactly four resignations per month. It is precisely because of these fluctuations that the design shown in Figure 9-7, with only one observation before and after the experimental treatment, is so weak.

Let us compare the kind of interpretations that can be made for the outcomes reflected in Figure 9-9 (A) and (B). In both cases, the number of resignations increases between O_4 and O_5, that is, immediately after the introduction of the continuing education requirement. In (B), however, the number of resignations falls at O_6 and continues to decrease at O_7. The increase at O_5, therefore, looks similar to other apparently haphazard fluctuations in the turnover rate at other periods. Therefore, it probably would be erroneous to conclude that the treatment had had an effect on resignations. In (A), on the other hand, the

number of resignations increases at O_5 and remains relatively high for all subsequent periods of data collection. It is true, of course, that there may be other explanations for a change in turnover rate from one year to the next. The time series design, however, does permit us to rule out the possibility that the data reflect an unstable measurement of resignations made at only two points in time. If we had used the design in Figure 9-7 to study this problem, it would have been analogous to obtaining the measurements at O_4 and O_5 of Figure 9-9 only. The outcomes in both Figure 9-9 (A) and (B) look quite similar at these two points in time. Yet, the use of a broader time perspective leads us to draw different conclusions about the nature of the changes from one pattern of outcomes to the next.

A particularly powerful design results when

researchers are able to combine the time series and nonequivalent control group designs. Such a design is diagrammed in Figure 9-10. In the example just described, a *time series nonequivalent control group design* would involve the collection of data over an extended period from both the hospital introducing the continuing education mandate and another hospital not imposing the mandate. This use of information from another hospital with similar characteristics would make any inferences regarding the effects of the mandate more convincing because trends influenced by external factors would presumably be observed in both groups.

Numerous variations on the simple time series design are possible and are being used by nurse researchers. For example, additional evidence regarding the effects of a treatment can be achieved by instituting the treatment at several different points in time, strengthening the treatment over time, or instituting the treatment at one point in time and then reversing (withdrawing) the treatment at a later point, sometimes with reinstitution of treatment. These three designs are diagrammed in Figures 9-11 to 9-13. Nurse researchers are often in a good position to use such time series designs because measures of

patient functioning are generally routinely made at multiple points over an extended period.

≡ ADVANTAGES AND DISADVANTAGES OF THE QUASI-EXPERIMENTAL APPROACH

The great strength of quasi-experiments lies in their practicality, feasibility, and, to a certain extent, their generalizability. In the "real world," it is often quite impractical, if not impossible, to conduct true experiments. A good deal of the research that is of interest to nurses occurs in natural settings. Frequently, it is difficult to deliver an innovative treatment to only half of a group, and randomization may be even less feasible. The inability to randomize, or even to secure a control group, need not force a researcher to abandon all hopes of conducting a respectable investigation. Quasi-experimental designs are research plans that introduce some controls over extraneous variables when full experimental control is lacking.

However, it is precisely because the control inherent in true experiments *is* absent in quasi-experiments that the researcher needs to be acquainted with the weaknesses of this approach.

$$O_1 \quad O_2 \quad O_3 \quad O_4 \quad X \quad O_5 \quad O_6 \quad O_7 \quad O_8$$

$$O_1 \quad O_2 \quad O_3 \quad O_4 \quad \quad O_5 \quad O_6 \quad O_7 \quad O_8$$

Figure 9-10.   *Time series nonequivalent control group design (quasi-experimental).*

$$O_1 \quad O_2 \quad X \quad O_3 \quad O_4 \quad X \quad O_5 \quad O_6 \quad X \quad O_7 \quad O_8$$

Figure 9-11.   *Time series with multiple institutions of treatment (quasi-experimental).*

$$O_1 \quad O_2 \quad X \quad O_3 \quad O_4 \quad X+1 \quad O_5 \quad O_6 \quad X+2 \quad O_7 \quad O_8$$

Figure 9-12.   *Time series with intensified treatment (quasi-experimental).*

$$O_1 \quad O_2 \quad X \quad O_3 \quad O_4 \quad (-X) \quad O_5 \quad O_6 \quad X \quad O_7 \quad O_8$$

Figure 9-13.   *Time series with withdrawn and reinstituted treatment (quasi-experimental).*

When a researcher uses a quasi-experimental design, there may be several "rival hypotheses" competing with the experimental manipulation as explanations for observed results. Take as an example the case in which we administer certain medications to a group of babies whose mothers are heroin addicts. Suppose we are interested in whether this treatment will result in a weight gain in these typically low birthweight babies. If we use no comparison group or we use a nonequivalent control group and then observe a weight gain, we must ask the questions, Is it *plausible* that some other external factor caused or influenced the gain? Is it *plausible* that pretreatment differences between the experimental and comparison group of babies resulted in differential gain? Is it *plausible* that the babies could have gained the weight simply as a result of maturation? If the answer is "yes" to any of these questions, then the inferences we can make about the effect of the experimental treatment are weakened considerably. The plausibility of any one threat cannot, of course, be answered unequivocally. It is generally a situation in which judgment must be exercised. It is because quasi-experiments ultimately depend in part on human judgment rather than on more objective criteria that the validity of cause-and-effect inferences must be challenged. We must hasten to add that the quality of a study is not necessarily a function of its design. There are many excellent quasi-experimental investigations, as well as very poor experiments.

☰ *RESEARCH EXAMPLE OF A QUASI-EXPERIMENT*

Table 9-5 briefly summarizes the characteristics of several studies conducted by nurse researchers in which a quasi-experimental or pre-experimental design was used. A more detailed description of a quasi-experimental study follows.

Osguthorpe and colleagues (1983) tested the effectiveness of alternative methods of increasing medication knowledge among psychiatric patients. These investigators developed four alternative treatment conditions relating to how patients were instructed about their medications: (1) a drug information sheet condition, (2) a videotaped nurse explanation condition, (3) a combined drug information sheet/videotaped nurse explanation condition, and (4) a control condition (usual practices). Because the study was conducted in a psychiatric hospital, it was impractical to randomly assign patients to these four conditions. Instead, the investigators randomly assigned general psychiatric wards to conditions. Strictly speaking, even though the investigators used a random procedure to assign the wards to the treatment groups, this design is not experimental. This is because patients might have been assigned to different wards by some nonrandom procedure in the first place. Therefore, the groups could not be assumed to be equivalent at the beginning of the study.

In such a design, the major "rival hypothesis" concerns differences in the characteristics of the subjects in the four groups before the experimental intervention. For example, the patients on some wards may have had more extensive prior experience in self-medication, or their degree of psychiatric disturbance may have been lower. Osguthorpe and her associates recognized this potential problem and collected information about the subjects' medication knowledge (the dependent variable) both before the intervention (the alternative teaching strategies) and after its completion. The analyses took the preintervention test scores into account through the computation of *change scores*. That is, the investigators analyzed how much *improvement* in scores of the four groups had occurred following the intervention, rather than simply comparing the groups' final test scores. This type of analysis has the effect of removing any preintervention differences among the groups. The results of the study failed to support the hypothesis that the patients would be better informed using teaching methods other than the normal ward procedures.

Table 9-5. *Examples of Quasi-experimental and Pre-experimental Designs*

RESEARCH QUESTION	MANIPULATED VARIABLE	DESIGN	SUBJECTS
Is the use of a heart sound simulator effective in increasing the skills of critical-care nurses in recognition of heart sounds? (Harrell et al., 1990)	Exposure to an instructional module using a heart sound simulator	One group pretest-posttest design	40 critical-care registered nurses
What are the effects of participation in a special prenatal adolescent program on maternal and infant outcomes? (Slager-Earnest et al., 1987)	Participation in a special prenatal education program for young mothers versus non-participation in the program	Nonequivalent control group posttest only design	50 program participants 50 nonparticipants delivering at the same hospital
Does individualized or group instruction by nurses in a work setting have an effect on women's health knowledge, health beliefs, and the practice of breast self-exam? (Brailey, 1986)	Individual instruction versus group instruction versus no instruction	Nonequivalent control group pretest-posttest design	55 group instruction 50 individual instruction 49 no instruction
Does a special nursing protocol increase the rate of identification of battered women in an emergency department? (Tilden & Shepherd, 1987)	Use versus nonuse of a nursing interview protocol	Simple time series design	22 emergency room registered nurses
Is an individualized speech therapy program effective in increasing communication skills in aphasic and dysarthric patients? (Buckwalter et al., 1989)	Speech therapy versus withdrawal of speech therapy versus systematic attention without therapy	Time series with withdrawn and reinstituted treatment	36 brain-damaged patients with diagnoses of aphasia, dysarthria, or both
Does an intervention based on the nursing mutual participation model reduce the stress of parents with children in the pediatric intensive care unit (ICU)? (Curley, 1988)	Parents enrolled in a special nursing mutual participation model program versus parents receiving usual nursing care in the pediatric ICU	Time series with nonequivalent control group design	16 parents in the experimental intervention 17 parents in the comparison group

☰ SUMMARY

In this chapter we examined two important types of research that nurse researchers are increasingly using: (1) experiments and (2) quasi-experiments. *True experiments* are characterized by three fundamental properties. The first, *manipulation,* involves doing something to or acting on at least some of the subjects in a research study. The experimenter manipulates, or varies, the independent variable (often referred to as the *experimental treatment* or *intervention*) to see if the manipulation has an effect on the dependent variable or variables of interest. True experiments always require the second property, the utilization of a *control group,* whose performance on the dependent (or *outcome*) measures is used as a basis for assessing the performance of the experimental group on the same measures. The third requirement for an experiment is that subjects be assigned to control and experimental groups by a process known as *randomization.* The random assignment procedure can be accomplished by any method that allows every subject an equal chance of being included in any group. Such methods include flipping a coin, drawing names from a hat, and using a *table of random numbers.* Randomization does not guarantee that all groups will be equal, but this technique is the most reliable method for equating groups on all possible characteristics that could affect the outcome of the study.

The most basic experimental design is the *after-only* or *posttest-only design,* which involves collecting data from subjects after the experimental treatment has been introduced. When data are also collected before treatment (i.e., at *baseline*), the design is a *before–after* or *pretest–posttest design.* When an experimental design is used to test the efficacy of a clinical treatment in a large, heterogeneous population, the study is often referred to as a *clinical trial.* If pretest sensitization might obscure the effect of the treatment, a *Solomon four-group design* might be needed. When a researcher manipulates more than one variable at a time, the design is known as a *factorial experiment.* Such a design is efficient in that it permits two simultaneous experiments with one pool of subjects. Furthermore, with factorial designs we can test both *main effects* (effects resulting from the experimentally manipulated variables) and *interaction effects* (effects resulting from combining the treatments). In factorial designs, each independent variable is referred to as a *factor* and each factor consists of two or more *levels* of the treatment.

True experiments are considered by many as the ideal of science. We often want to know if our experimental treatment *causes* an observed outcome. Experiments come closer than any other type of research approach to meeting the criteria for inferring causal relationships. On the other hand, there are many situations in which an experimental design is impossible, owing to ethical or practical considerations. Experiments have also been criticized because of their artificiality.

Quasi-experiments involve manipulation but lack a comparison group or randomization. Quasi-experimental designs are designs in which efforts are made to introduce controls into the study to compensate in part for the absence of one or both of these important characteristics. In contrast, *pre-experimental designs* have no such safeguards and, therefore, are subject to ambiguity and multiple interpretations of results.

Several specific quasi-experimental designs were presented. The *nonequivalent control group design* involves the use of a control group (or *comparison group*) that is not designated by a randomization procedure. The problem with the use of such a comparison group is the possibility that the groups are initially different in ways that will affect the research outcomes, and so the collection of pretreatment data becomes an important means of assessing their initial equivalence. In studies in which there is no control group, a method for overcoming some of the difficulties in the interpretation of results is the collection of information over time before and after the treatment is instituted. Such a study is known as the *time series design.* An especially powerful design combines the features of the two most common quasi-experimental designs and is referred to as the *time series nonequivalent control group design*.

Despite some of the problems inherent in quasi-experimental designs, they may in some cases be more practical in the nursing field than the more rigorous experimental designs and, therefore, merit increased attention by nursing researchers. In evaluating the results of quasi-experiments, however, it is important to ask whether it is plausible that factors other than the experimental treatment caused or affected the obtained outcomes.

≡ STUDY SUGGESTIONS

1. A researcher is interested in studying the effect of sensitivity training for nurses on their behavior in crisis intervention situations. Describe how you would set up an experiment to investigate this problem.
2. Using the same situation described in study suggestion 1, describe two quasi- or pre-experimental designs that could be used to study the same problem. Discuss what the weaknesses of each would be.
3. Assume that you have ten individuals—Z, Y, X, W, V, U, T, S, R, and Q—who are going to participate in an experiment you are conducting. Using a table of random numbers, assign five individuals to Group I and five to Group II. Then randomly assign the groups to an experimental or control treatment.
4. Suppose that you were interested in testing the hypothesis that systematic relaxation procedures taught by nurses to presurgical patients would reduce stress. Describe what you might do to test this hypothesis using an experimental and quasi-experimental design. Compare the kinds of conclusions you could make with each approach.
5. In the section on randomization in this chapter, it was noted that the probability of obtaining deviant or nonequivalent groups through random assignment increases as the number of subjects in the experiment decreases. Why do you think this might be so?
6. In the hypothetical example of the hospital administration that wanted to study the effect of a new continuing education requirement on its nursing staff, pre-experimental and quasi-experimental designs were discussed. What might some of the problems be in trying to study this problem experimentally?
7. Using the notation presented in Figures 9-4 to 9-13, diagram a few of the research examples described in the text that are not already shown.

≡ SUGGESTED READINGS

METHODOLOGICAL REFERENCES

Battle, A.O. (1964). Quasi-experimental research designs in nursing. *Nursing Outlook, 12,* 30–32.

Brink, P.J., & Wood, M.J. (1989). *Advanced design in nursing research.* Newbury Park, CA: Sage.

Burns, N., & Grove, S.K. (1987). *The practice of nursing research: Conduct, critique, and utilization.* Philadelphia: W.B. Saunders. (Chapter 10).

Campbell, D.T., & Stanley, J.C. (1963). *Experimental and quasi-experimental designs for research.* Chicago: Rand McNally.

Christensen, L.M. (1988). *Experimental methodology.* Boston: Allyn and Bacon.

Clinton, J., Beck, R., Radjenovic, D., Taylor, L., Westlake, S., & Wilson, S.E. (1986). Time series designs in clinical nursing research. *Nursing Research, 35,* 188–191.

Cook, T.D., & Campbell, D.T. (1979). *Quasi-experimental design and analysis issues for field settings.* Chicago: Rand McNally.

Fetter, M.S., Feetham, S.L., D'Apolito, K., Chaze, B.A., Fink, A., Frink, B., Hougart, M., & Rushton, C. (1989). Randomized clinical trials: Issues for researchers. *Nursing Research, 38,* 117–120.

Harre, R. (1970). *The principles of scientific thinking.* Chicago: University of Chicago Press.

Kerlinger, F.N. (1973). *Foundations of behavioral research* (2nd ed.). New York: Holt, Rinehart & Winston. (Chapters 18 & 19).

Lazarsfeld, P. (1955). Foreword. In H. Hyman (Ed.), *Survey design and analysis.* New York: The Free Press.

Levine, E. (1960). Experimental designs in nursing research. *Nursing Research, 9,* 203–212.

Selltiz, C., Wrightsman, L.S., & Cook, S.W. (1976). *Research methods in social relations* (3rd ed.). New York: Holt, Rinehart & Winston. (Chapter 5).

Wilson, H.S. (1989). *Research in nursing* (2nd ed.). Menlo Park, CA: Addison-Wesley. (Chapter 6).

SUBSTANTIVE REFERENCES

Research Utilizing Experimental Designs

Anderson, C.J. (1981). Enhancing reciprocity between mother and neonate. *Nursing Research, 30,* 89–93.

Andrews, C.M., & Chrzanowski, M. (1990). Maternal position, labor, and comfort. *Applied Nursing Research, 3,* 7–13.

Beckie, T. (1989) A supportive-educative telephone program: Impact on knowledge and anxiety after coronary artery bypass graft surgery. *Heart and Lung, 18,* 46–55.

Cannon, K., Mitchell, K.A., & Fabian, T.C. (1985). Prospective randomized evaluation of two methods of drawing coagulation studies from heparinized arterial lines. *Heart and Lung, 14,* 392–395.

Damrosch, S.P., Gallo, B., Kulak, D., & Whitaker, C.M. (1987). Nurses' attributions about rape victims. *Research in Nursing and Health, 10,* 245–251.

Geden, E., Beck, N., Brouder, G., Glaister, J., & Pohlman, S. (1985). Self-report and psychophysiological effects of Lamaze preparation: An analogue of labor pain. *Research in Nursing and Health, 8,* 155–165.

Gill, N.E., Behnke, M., Conlon, M., McNeely, J.B., & Anderson, G.C. (1988). Effect of non-nutritive sucking on behavioral state in preterm infants before feeding. *Nursing Research, 37,* 347–350.

Greer, P.S. (1988). Head coverings for newborns under radiant warmers. *Journal of Obstetric, Gynecologic, and Neonatal Nursing, 17,* 265–271.

Guzzetta, C.E. (1989). Effects of relaxation and music therapy on patients in a coronary care unit with presumptive acute myocardial infarction. *Heart and Lung, 18,* 609–616.

Hargreaves, A., & Lander, J. (1989). Use of transcutaneous electrical nerve stimulation for postoperative pain. *Nursing Research, 38,* 159–161.

Heitkemper, M.M., Miller, J.C., & Shaver, J.F. (1989). The effect of restricted liquid feeding on gastrointestinal and adrenocortical variables in rats. *Western Journal of Nursing Research, 11,* 34–46.

Jacobs, M.K., McCance, K.L., & Stewart, M.L. (1986). Leg volume changes with EPIC and posturing in dependent pregnancy edema. *Nursing Research, 35,* 86–89.

Kurzuk-Howard, G., Simpson, L., & Palmieri, A. (1985). Decubitus ulcer care: A comparative study. *Western Journal of Nursing Research, 7,* 58–74.

Milde, F.K. (1988). The function of feedback in psychomotor skill learning. *Western Journal of Nursing Research, 10,* 425–434.

Miller, P., Sr., Wikoff, R., McMahon, M., Garrett, M.J., & Ringerl, K. (1988). Influence of a nursing intervention on regimen adherence and societal adjustments postmyocardial infarction. *Nursing Research, 37,* 297–302.

Sime, A.M., & Libera, M.B. (1985). Sensation information, self-instruction and responses to dental surgery. *Research in Nursing and Health, 8,* 41–47.

Research Utilizing Quasi-Experimental or Pre-Experimental Designs

Brailey, L.J. (1986). Effects of health teaching in the workplace on women's knowledge, beliefs, and practices regarding breast self-examination. *Research in Nursing and Health, 9,* 223–231.

Buckwalter, K.C., Cusack, D., Sidles, E., Wadle, K., & Beaver, M. (1989). Increasing communication ability in aphasic/dysarthric patients. *Western Journal of Nursing Research, 11,* 736–747.

Constantino, R.E. (1981). Bereavement crisis intervention for widows in grief and mourning. *Nursing Research, 30,* 351–353.

Curley, M.A. (1988). Effects of the nursing mutual participation model of care on parental stress in the pediatric intensive care unit. *Heart and Lung, 17,* 682–688.

Farr, L., Keene, A., Samson, D., & Michael, A. (1984). Alterations in circadian excretion of urinary variables and physiological indicators of stress following surgery. *Nursing Research, 33,* 140–146.

Harrell, J.S., Champagne, M.T., Jarr, S., & Miyana, M. (1990). Heart sound simulation: How useful for critical care nurses? *Heart and Lung, 19,* 197–202

Mills, M.E., Arnold, B., & Wood, C.M. (1983). Core-12: A controlled study of the impact of 12-hour scheduling. *Nursing Research, 32,* 356–361.

Mitchell, P.H., Ozuna, J., & Lipe, H.P. (1981). Moving the patient in bed: Effects on intracranial pressure. *Nursing Research, 30,* 212–218.

Munro, B.H., Creamer, A.M., Haggerty, M.R., & Cooper,

F.S. (1988). Effect of relaxation therapy on post-myocardial infarction patients' rehabilitation. *Nursing Research, 37,* 231–235.

Norris, S., Campbell, L.A., & Brenkert, S. (1982). Nursing procedures and alterations in transcutaneous oxygen tension in premature infants. *Nursing Research, 31,* 330–336.

Osguthorpe, N., Roper, J., & Saunders, J. (1983). The effect of teaching on medication knowledge. *Western Journal of Nursing Research, 5,* 205–215.

Parsons, L.C., & Wilson, M.M. (1984). Cerebrovascular status of severe closed head-injured patients following passive position changes. *Nursing Research, 33,* 260–264.

Parsons, L.C., Peard, A.L.S., & Page, M.C. (1985). The effect of hygiene interventions on the cerebrovascular status of severe closed head injured persons. *Research in Nursing and Health, 8,* 173–181.

Pender, N.J. (1985). Effects of progressive muscle relaxation training on anxiety and health locus of control among hypertensive adults. *Research in Nursing and Health, 8,* 67–72.

Santopietro, M.S. (1980). Effectiveness of a self-instructional module in human sexuality counseling. *Nursing Research, 29,* 14–19.

Slager-Earnest, S.E., Hoffman, S.J., & Beckan, C.J.A. (1987). Effects of a specialized prenatal adolescent program on maternal and infant outcomes. *Journal of Obstetric, Gynecologic, and Neonatal Nursing, 16,* 422–429.

Tilden, V.P., & Shepherd, P. (1987). Increasing the rate of identification of battered women in an emergency department. *Research in Nursing and Health, 10,* 209–215.

10
Non-experimental Research

When a researcher is in a position to introduce a "treatment," the effects of which he or she is interested in assessing, we say that the independent variable is being controlled or manipulated by the investigator. We noted in Chapter 9 that manipulation is a key element in true experiments, and in quasi- and pre-experimental designs as well. When experimentation or quasi-experimentation is possible, these approaches are generally the most highly effective methods for testing hypotheses concerning causal relationships among variables.

There are, nevertheless, a number of research problems that, for one or more reasons, do not lend themselves to an experimental or even quasi-experimental design. Let us suppose, for example, that we were interested in studying the effect of widowhood on physical and psychologic functioning. We could use as our dependent variables various physiologic and medical measures such as blood pressure, heart rate, and so on, as well as standard psychologic diagnostic tests, such as the Center for Epidemiological Studies Depression Scale. Our independent variable is widowhood versus nonwidowhood. Clearly, we would be unable to manipulate widowhood. Spouses become widows or widowers by a process that is neither random nor subject, ethically, to research control. Thus, we must proceed by taking two groups as they naturally occur (those who are widowed and those who are not) and comparing them in terms of psychologic and physical well-being.

There are essentially two broad classes of nonexperimental research. The first is *descriptive research*. Descriptive studies do not focus on relationships among variables. Their purpose is to observe, describe, and document aspects of a situation as it naturally occurs. Because the intent of such research is not to explain or to understand the underlying causes of the variables of interest, experimental designs are not required or even appropriate.

The second broad class of nonexperimental research, exemplified by the widowhood example, is *ex post facto research*. The literal translation of the Latin term *ex post facto* is "from after the fact." This expression is meant to indicate that the research in question has been conducted *after* the variations in the independent variable have occurred in the natural course of events. Ex post facto research attempts to understand relationships among phenomena as they naturally occur, without any researcher intervention.

Sometimes ex post facto research is referred to as correlational research.* The precise meaning of "correlational research" will become clearer when we have covered some statistical concepts. Basically, a *correlation* is an interrelationship or association between two variables— that is, a tendency for variation in one variable to be related to variation in another. For example, in human adults, height and weight tend to be correlated because there is a tendency for taller people to weigh more than shorter people.

Ex post facto/correlational studies often share a number of structural and design characteristics with experimental, quasi-experimental, and pre-experimental research. If we use the notation scheme outlined in Chapter 9 to symbolically represent the hypothetical widowhood study, we find that it bears a strong resemblance to the nonequivalent control group posttest-only design discussed in that chapter. Both designs are presented in Figure 10-1. As these diagrams show,

the pre-experimental design is distinguished from the ex post facto study only by the presence of an X, the manipulation of some experimental treatment by the researcher in the pre-experimental design.

The basic purpose of ex post facto research is essentially the same as experimental research: to determine the relationships among variables. The most important distinction between the two is the difficulty of inferring *causal* relationships in ex post facto studies because of the lack of manipulative control of the independent variables. In experiments, the investigator makes a prediction that a deliberate variation in X, the independent variable, will result in the occurrence of some event or behavior, Y (the dependent variable). For example, the researcher predicts that if some medication is administered, then patient improvement will ensue. The experimenter has direct control over the *"X"*: the experimental treatment can be administered to some and withheld from others, and subjects can be randomly assigned to an experimental group and a control group.

In ex post facto research, on the other hand, the investigator does not have control of the independent variable because it has already occurred. The examination of independent variable—the presumed causative factor—is done after the fact. As a result, attempts to draw any cause-and-effect conclusions are often problematic. Of course, even experimentation is insufficient to *prove* a causal relationship, but experimenters can place considerably more confidence in their inferences than can researchers using an ex post facto approach.

≡ *REASONS FOR CONDUCTING NONEXPERIMENTAL RESEARCH*

Many research studies involving human subjects, including the majority of nursing research investigations, are nonexperimental in nature. A brief look at the reasons that researchers conduct nonexperimental research should provide the reader with a better understanding of the value of such

* The use of the terms "ex post facto" and "correlational" is not entirely consistent in the literature on research methods. Some authors appear to use ex post facto to refer to all nonexperimental research that examines relationships among variables (Kerlinger, 1973); others use the term correlational for this purpose (Crano & Brewer, 1973). Still other researchers prefer to make a distinction between whether the intent of the study is causal and comparative (ex post facto) or merely descriptive of relationships (correlational) (Ary, Jacobs, & Razavich, 1979). In general, the terms will be used roughly equivalently in this chapter to designate studies of relationships among variables when the independent variable is not under the researcher's control.

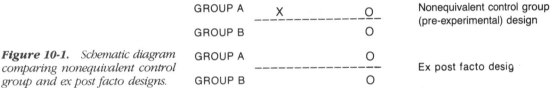

Figure 10-1. *Schematic diagram comparing nonequivalent control group and ex post facto designs.*

investigations—and the problems associated with them.

Independent Variable Inherently Not Manipulable

A vast number of characteristics are associated with individuals and institutions that are inherently not subject to experimental control. For instance, blood type, personality, medical diagnosis, and allergic reactions are examples of human characteristics that individuals bring with them to the research situation. Obviously, the effects of these characteristics on some phenomenon of interest cannot be studied experimentally. We simply cannot, for example, randomly confer upon incoming hospital patients various diagnoses to study the effect of the diagnosis on preoperative anxiety. Nevertheless, the relationship between these attribute variables, as they are sometimes called, and an entire range of dependent variables is quite often of considerable theoretical or practical interest. Does a person's cultural background affect his or her health beliefs? Does a patient's age affect the incidence of decubitus ulcer? What are the psychologic effects of multiple episodes of ventricular fibrillation? Such questions cannot be answered using experimental procedures.

Ethical Constraints on Manipulation

In nursing research, as in other fields in which human behavior is of primary interest, numerous variables could technically be manipulated but should not be manipulated for ethical reasons. If the nature of the independent variable is such that its manipulation could cause physical or mental harm to subjects, then that variable should not be controlled experimentally. For ex-

ample, if we were interested in studying the effect of prenatal care on infant mortality, it would be considered unethical to provide such care to one group of pregnant women but totally deprive a second group. What we would need to do is locate a naturally occurring group of mothers-to-be who have not received prenatal care. The birth outcomes of these women could then be compared with those of a group of women who had received appropriate care. The problem, however, is that the two groups of women are likely to differ in terms of a number of other characteristics such as age, education, nutrition, and health, any of which individually or in combination could have an impact on infant mortality, independent of the absence or presence of prenatal care. This is precisely why experimental designs are so strong in demonstrating cause-and-effect relationships.

Practical Constraints on Manipulation

There are many research situations in which it is simply not practical or even desirable to conduct a true experiment. Such constraints might involve insufficient time, lack of administrative approval, excessive inconvenience to patients or staff, or lack of adequate funds. For instance, let us suppose that we were interested in studying the effect of hospital noise levels on patient well-being and recovery. Certain areas of the hospital might be particularly noisy and other areas, much quieter. Say that we categorized all the rooms as either "above average" or "below average" in terms of noise intensity. Technically, it might be possible to randomly assign incoming patients to rooms, but this would typically be rather impractical. We must be content in this situation to perform an ex post facto study. We would collect information on patient well-being—number of hours slept, blood pressure, need for medications and so on—and compare groups exposed to the two different noise conditions on these various indices. Of course, we would want to control for a number of other variables that might confound our results. For example, we might want to restrict our study to patients with certain kinds of diagnoses, or to rooms of a particular type, such as semiprivate.

Research Perspective on Manipulation

Phenomenologically based studies seek to capture what people think, feel, and do in their naturalistic environments. Because of this goal, researchers conducting phenomenological or qualitative studies typically want as little disturbance as possible to the people or groups they are studying. Manipulation is neither attempted nor considered desirable; the emphasis is on the natural everyday world of humans. Thus, although phenomenological researchers sometimes focus on concepts that could be manipulated or could be affected by manipulation (e.g., dependency, coping, and decision making), they reject manipulation as a technique for studying certain problems.

☰ PURPOSES OF NONEXPERIMENTAL RESEARCH

Nonexperimental research is conducted for various reasons: to explain phenomena and test theoretical propositions, to predict the occurrence and magnitude of phenomena, and to describe various characteristics and conditions. This section examines nonexperimental research from the perspective of the purposes for which a study is undertaken.

Explanation, Causation, and Theory Testing

In many correlational or ex post facto studies, the researcher is interested in explaining phenomena and inferring causal relationships. For example, we might hypothesize that there is a correlation between the number of cigarettes smoked and the incidence of lung cancer, and empirical data would most likely corroborate this expectation. The inference we would like to make based on observed relationships is that cigarette smoking *causes* cancer. This kind of inference, however, is a fallacy that has been called *post hoc ergo propter* ("after this, therefore caused by this"). The fallacy lies in the assumption that one thing has caused another merely because it occurred chronologically before the other.

To illustrate here why such a cause-and-effect conclusion might not be warranted, let us assume (strictly for the sake of an example) that there is a preponderance of cigarette smokers in urban areas, but people living in rural areas are largely nonsmokers. Let us further assume that bronchogenic carcinoma is actually caused by the poor environmental conditions typically associated with cities and industrial areas. Therefore, we would be incorrect to conclude that cigarette smoking had caused lung cancer, despite the strong relationship that might be shown to exist between the two variables. This is because there is *also* a strong relationship between cigarette smoking and the "real" causative agent, living in a polluted environment. Of course, the cigarette smoking–lung cancer studies have in reality been replicated in so many different places with so many different groups of people that causal inferences are increasingly justified. This hypothetical example illustrates a famous research dictum: Correlation does not prove causation. That is, the mere existence of a relationship—even a strong one—between two variables is not enough to warrant the conclusion that one variable has caused the other.

Although correlational studies are inherently weaker than experimental studies in elucidating cause-and-effect relationships, different designs offer different degrees of supportive evidence. Below we consider some nonexperimental designs that have been used to examine causal relationships.

RETROSPECTIVE STUDIES

Retrospective studies are ex post facto investigations in which some phenomenon existing in the present is linked to other phenomena occurring in the past. That is, the investigator is interested in some presently occurring "effect" and attempts to shed light on previously occurring factors that have caused it. Many epidemiological studies are retrospective in nature, and this approach has been used by medical researchers for more than a century. Many of the early cigarette smoking–lung cancer studies were retrospective. In such studies, the researcher would begin with a sample of lung cancer victims and a sample of people without the disease. The researcher would then determine whether those in the cancer group were disproportionately likely to have been cigarette smokers.

In nursing research, as in medical research, retrospective studies are fairly common. Patient well-being, recovery, or satisfaction are phenomena that have been linked retrospectively to different nursing interventions or modes of treatment. Many studies in the field of nursing education have also been of this type.

In a sense, this kind of ex post facto study can be viewed as the converse of true experiments. In experiments, the researcher creates the "cause" by directly manipulating the independent variable and then observes the subsequent effect of the manipulation on some dependent variable. In contrast, in a retrospective study, the investigator begins with the "effect" and attempts to identify the previously occurring causative factors. Retrospective studies are considerably weaker than experiments in their ability to shed light on causal relationships. Findings from a single retrospective study are rarely convincing and, thus, often require confirmatory research efforts.

PROSPECTIVE STUDIES

A nonexperimental *prospective study* starts with an examination of presumed causes and then goes forward in time to the presumed effect. For example, a researcher might want to test the hypothesis that the incidence of rubella during pregnancy is related to malformations in the offspring. To test this hypothesis prospectively, the investigator would begin with a sample of pregnant women, including some of whom have contracted the disease during their pregnancy and others who have not. The subsequent occurrence of congenital anomalies would be observed. The researcher would then be in a position to test whether women who had contracted the disease during pregnancy were more likely to bear malformed babies than women who did not have rubella.

Prospective studies are often more costly than retrospective studies and perhaps are less common for this reason. Prospective research often requires large samples, particularly if the dependent variable of interest is rare, as in the example of malformed babies and maternal rubella. Another difficulty with prospective studies is that a substantial follow-up period may be necessary before the phenomenon or effect under investigation manifests itself, as is the case in prospective studies of cigarette smoking–lung cancer.

Despite these problems, prospective studies are considerably stronger than retrospective studies. For one thing, any ambiguity concerning the temporal sequence of phenomena usually is resolved in prospective research. In addition, samples are more likely to be representative, and investigators may be in a position to impose numerous controls to rule out competing explanations for observed effects. Finally, in prospective studies, the researcher can often obtain a "pretest" measure of the dependent variable. Despite these advantages, causal inferences cannot be made with the same degree of confidence in prospective correlational studies as in the case of experiments. Without the ability to manipulate the independent variable and randomly assign individuals to different conditions, there is no way to equate groups on all relevant factors. Because of this fact, alternative "causes' " or antecedents may compete with those that the researcher has hypothesized.

PATH ANALYTIC STUDIES

Path analysis is a technique that has been developed for elucidating hypothesized causal relationships among variables in a nonexperimental context. Using sophisticated statistical procedures, the researcher tests a hypothesized causal chain that is typically predicted on the basis of a theory or conceptual model. Path analytic procedures allow researchers to test whether nonexperimental data conform sufficiently to the model to justify causal inferences.

Figure 10-2 presents an illustration of a *path diagram.* This diagram summarizes the researcher's hypothesized casual linkages, which are indicated by the arrows. In this model, patients' compliance with a medical regimen is hypothesized to be a result of their capacity for self-care; this, in turn, is presumed to be affected by nursing actions, the severity of the patients' illnesses, and their self-esteem. In this model, capacity for self-care would be called a *mediating variable.* Nursing action is not hypothesized to

affect patient compliance directly. Rather, the effects of nursing action are believed to be mediated through effects on the patients' capacity for self-care.

To test a model such as that presented in Figure 10-2, the researcher would need to measure all of the variables in the model and then use appropriate statistical techniques. It is usually preferable to apply path analysis to data that have been collected prospectively. For instance, in the example used here, it would be more appropriate to collect information on the patients' self-esteem and the severity of their illnesses before measuring capacity for self-care and compliance. This is because relationships would be more difficult to tease out if all of the information were collected at a single point. If a relationship between capacity for self-care and self-esteem were found to exist at a single period of observation, for example, then it would be impossible to know whether the person's self-esteem had affected his or her capacity for self-care, or vice versa. Thus, although path analysis is a powerful tool for inferring causal relationships among variables collected nonexperimentally, it is less powerful than experimental designs because of potential problems of interpretation.

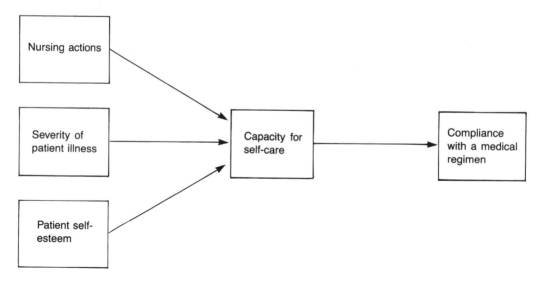

Figure 10-2. *Illustration of a path diagram.*

Prediction

Many situations exist in which it is useful to forecast how people will perform or behave. Predictive research is often used to facilitate decision making about individuals, such as in the selection of individuals for programs or special treatment. For example, let us suppose that a university nursing school has just begun a master's-level program in nursing research and that 30 students are admitted to the program during its first year of operation. These first 30 students have been selected from an applicant pool of approximately 100 individuals, and the principal criteria for selection were undergraduate grades and recommendations. However, numerous other pieces of information also are available about each new student, such as Graduate Record Examination (GRE) test scores, Miller Analogies test scores, rank in class, and so forth. Suppose that at the end of the first year we found that the 30 students varied considerably in their course performance. To reduce the probability of admitting students who will fare poorly in the new program, a study can be conducted to examine the relationship between various antecedent factors and the graduate grade point average of the first group of students. Findings, for example, might show that the scores on the quantitative section of the GRE test were more strongly related to performance in the new program than any other factor.

So far, the study has been completely retrospective. That is, the researcher identified preexisting characteristics of the students that were related to the dependent variable of interest, grade point average in the master's-level program. However, once this relationship is determined, it becomes possible to make some predictions about the kind of students who are likely to succeed in future years. Using sophisticated statistical procedures, prediction formulas can be developed that tell the program administrators how much weight should be given to different criteria in the selection of future students. The fundamental feature of prediction studies is the examination of relationships among variables in one group to make predictions about the behavior of another similar group.

Description

Scientists frequently focus on accurately describing natural phenomena and the relationships among them. In this section we discuss nonexperimental studies that are primarily descriptive in intent.

DESCRIPTIVE CORRELATIONAL STUDIES

Although there is considerable stress in scientific research on understanding what "causes" behaviors, conditions, and situations, researchers can often do little more than describe existing relationships without fully comprehending the complex causal pathways that exist. Thus, many of our research problems are often cast in noncausal terms. We ask, for example, whether men are less likely than women to achieve a bonding with their newborn infants, not whether or not a particular configuration of sex chromosomes has "caused" differences in parental attachment.

As in the case of other types of ex post facto research, the investigator engaged in a *descriptive correlational study* has no control over the independent variables. That is, there is no experimental manipulation or random assignment to groups. However, unlike other types of *ex post facto* studies—such as the cigarette smoking–lung cancer investigations—the aim of descriptive correlational research is to describe the relationship among variables rather than to infer cause-and-effect relationships.

Consider the following example. Suppose we have hypothesized that patients' adherence to prescribed hypertensive medication (as measured by changes in blood pressure readings) is related to their race/ethnicity. We may find, for example, that Hispanic patients have greater adherence to a medication regime than patients from other racial/ethnic backgrounds. Given the existence of this relationship, is it meaningful or reasonable to say that the person's ethnic background *caused* adherence? Clearly it is not. Yet the knowledge of a relationship is interesting and could lead to practical applications (such as an examination of the constraints to adherence among patients from other ethnic groups). In other words, descriptive correlational research is often quite useful in its own right and sometimes lays the groundwork for further, more rigorous research.

UNIVARIATE DESCRIPTIVE STUDIES

The purpose of descriptive studies is to obtain information about the current status of phenomena of interest. We use the term "univariate" here to distinguish descriptive correlational studies from those studies that intend simply to describe what exists in terms of frequency of occurrence (or its presence versus absence) rather than to describe the relationship between variables. For example, an investigator may wish to determine the health-care and nutritional practices of pregnant teenagers. Another investigator may wish to describe the coping strategies of patients diagnosed as having AIDS.

Univariate descriptive studies are not necessarily focused on only one variable. For example, a researcher might be interested in women's experience during menopause. The investigation might describe the frequency with which various symptoms are reported, the average age at menopause, the percentage of women seeking formal health care, and the percentage of women using medications to alleviate symptoms. There are multiple variables in this study, but the primary purpose is to describe the status of each and not to relate them to one another.

☰ STRENGTHS AND WEAKNESSES OF EX POST FACTO/ CORRELATIONAL RESEARCH

The quality of a study is not necessarily related to its approach: there are many excellent nonexperimental studies as well as seriously flawed experiments. Nevertheless, there is a continuum of design types in terms of capacity to reveal causal relationships. True experimental designs are at one end of that continuum, and retrospective correlational research is at the other, as shown in Figure 10-3. Descriptive studies are not included on this continuum because they are not intended to elucidate cause-and-effect relations.

Weaknesses of Ex Post Facto/ Correlational Research

Kerlinger (1973) has noted three major problems associated with ex post facto research: (1) the inability to actively manipulate the independent variable of interest, (2) the inability to randomly assign individuals to different treatments or groups, and (3) the possibility of faulty interpretation of study results.

In ex post facto studies, the researcher works with preexisting groups that were not formed by a random process but, rather, were formed by what might be termed a self-selecting process. Kerlinger (1973) has offered the following description of *self-selection*: "Self-selection occurs when the members of the groups being studied are in the groups, in part, because they differentially possess traits or characteristics extraneous to the research problem, characteristics

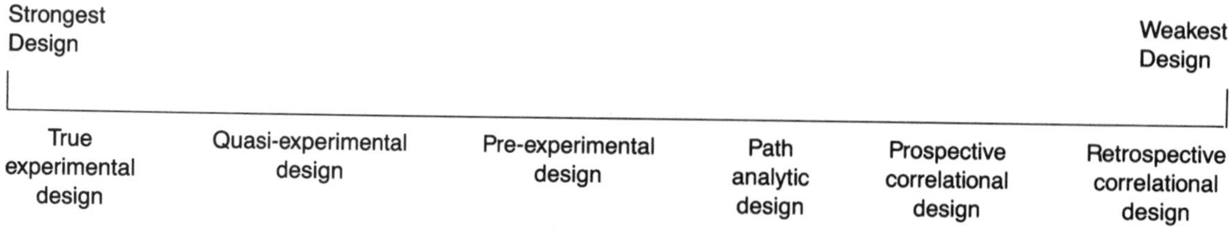

Strongest
Design

Weakest
Design

True experimental design	Quasi-experimental design	Pre-experimental design	Path analytic design	Prospective correlational design	Retrospective correlational design

Figure 10-3. *Continuum of research designs with respect to power to elucidate causal relationships.*

that possibly influence or are otherwise related to the variables of the research problem" (p. 381). As in the case of quasi-experimental or pre-experimental research, the researcher doing a correlational study cannot assume that the groups being studied were similar before the occurrence of the independent variable. Because of this fact, pre-existing differences may be a plausible alternative explanation for any observed differences on the dependent variable of interest.

To illustrate this problem, let us consider a hypothetical study in which the researcher is interested in examining the relationship between type of nursing program (the independent variable) and job satisfaction after graduation. If the investigator finds that diploma school graduates are more satisfied with their work than baccalaureate graduates one year after graduation, the conclusion that the diploma school program provides better preparation for actual work situations and, hence, leads to increased satisfaction may or may not be accurate. The students in the two programs undoubtedly differed to begin with in terms of a number of important characteristics such as personality, career goals, family economic circumstances, and so forth. That is, students self-selected themselves into one of the two programs; it may be the selection traits themselves that resulted in different job expectations and satisfactions.

A large part of the difficulty of interpreting correlational findings stems from the fact that, in the real world, behaviors, states, attitudes, and characteristics are interrelated (correlated) in complex ways. An example might help to make this clear. Let us suppose we were interested in studying the differences between the postoperative convalescent behavior of patients who had undergone surgery for two different medical problems—(1) hernia and (2) ulcers. Our independent variable in this hypothetical study is the type of medical problem. We might use one or more of the following as measures of the dependent variable (postoperative convalescent behavior): ratings of nurses on the degree of cooperativeness of the patient, number of times the patient calls the nurse for help, the patient's self-

ratings of distress, and the number of medications required to induce sleep or alleviate pain. Let us say that we find that the hernia patients receive a significantly lower rating by the nurses on degree of cooperation than the ulcer patients. We could interpret this finding to mean that particular medical problems and their accompanying surgical treatment produce different patterns of cooperative behavior in individuals. This relationship is diagrammed in Figure 10-4 (*A*). Note that, even with this interpretation, it is essentially impossible to separate the effects of the type of medical problem and type of surgical procedure, because one necessarily follows the other.

For the sake of this discussion, let us examine some alternative explanations for the findings. Perhaps there is a third variable that influences *both* the degree of convalescent cooperativeness and the type of medical ailment, such as the degree of physical activity to which an individual is accustomed. That is, it may be possible that hernia patients are usually engaged in a greater degree of physical activity than are ulcer patients, and this fact may be one of the causes of *both* the diagnosis and the inability to cope properly with the sedentary hospital routine. This set of relationships is diagrammed in Figure 10-4 (*B*).

A third possibility may be *reversed* causality, as shown in Figure 10-4 (*C*). Willingness to cooperate in general may be thought of as one aspect of a person's personality, and it is possible that the dynamics of a person's psychologic makeup results in the manifestation of different medical problems. In this interpretation, it is the person's disposition that causes the diagnosis and not vice versa.

Undoubtedly, the reader will be able to invent other alternatives. The point is that interpretations of *ex post facto* results should generally be considered tentative, particularly if the research has no theoretical basis.

Strengths of Ex Post Facto/ Correlational Research

In an earlier section of this chapter we discussed various constraints that limit the possi-

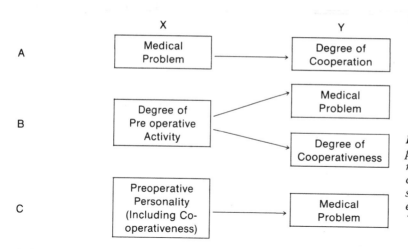

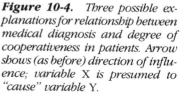

Figure 10-4. *Three possible explanations for relationship between medical diagnosis and degree of cooperativeness in patients. Arrow shows (as before) direction of influence; variable X is presumed to "cause" variable Y.*

bility of applying experimental designs to some research problems. Ex post facto and correlational research will continue to play a crucial role in nursing, medical, and social science research precisely because many of the interesting problems to be solved in those fields are not amenable to experimentation.

Despite our emphasis on causality in relationships, it has already been noted that in some kinds of research, such as predictive or descriptive research, a full understanding of causal networks may not be important. Furthermore, if the study is testing a hypothesis that has been deduced from an established theory, determining the direction of causation may be relatively straightforward, especially if powerful techniques such as path analysis have been used.

Correlational research is often an efficient and effective means of collecting a large amount of data about a problem area. For example, it would be possible to collect extensive information about the health histories and eating habits of a large number of individuals. Researchers could then examine which health problems are correlated with which diets. Thus, they could discover a large number of interrelationships in a relatively short amount of time. By contrast, an experimenter usually looks at only a few variables at a time. For example, one experiment might be devoted to manipulating foods high in cholesterol to observe the effects on certain medical symp-

toms, and another experiment could manipulate saccharin consumption, and so forth.

Finally, ex post facto research is often strong in realism and, therefore, has an intrinsic appeal for the solution of many practical problems. Unlike many experimental studies, ex post facto research is seldom criticized for its artificiality.

≡ RESEARCH EXAMPLES

We have used a number of hypothetical research problems to help explain many of the points made in this chapter. Table 10-1 presents a brief description of several actual nonexperimental studies that have been conducted by nurse researchers. Two nonexperimental studies are described in greater detail below.

A Two-Group Ex Post Facto Study

Tulman and Fawcett (1990), using the Roy Adaptation Model to guide them, compared employed and nonemployed mothers six months following childbirth in terms of demographic, health, psychosocial, and family variables. Data were collected from a sample of 92 women at multiple points following childbirth and, of these women, 53 (58 percent) were employed by six months postpartum. The data were collected by means of self-administered questionnaires. The questionnaires covered a broad range of variables, including demographics, functional status, social support, relations with husbands, and infant temperament.

The researchers found that, in comparing mothers who were employed at six months postpartum with those who were not, there were no differences in terms of such background characteristics as age, education, household income, and number of children. However, mothers who were employed at six months after delivery were more likely to report that they had fully regained their usual level of physical energy and that their infants were sleeping through the night. Employed women were also more likely than nonemployed women to report good relationships with their husbands. The two groups were comparable with respect to life satisfaction, satisfaction with the maternal role, confidence in mothering, social support, and functional status in nonoccupational areas (e.g., infant care responsibilities). The authors concluded that employed and nonemployed women are more alike than different during the first six months after delivery.

Table 10-1. *Examples of Nonexperimental Studies Conducted by Nurse Researchers*

PROBLEM STATEMENT	TYPE OF STUDY
What is the relationship between level of hope and type of coping styles on the one hand and level of grief resolution on the other among elderly widow(ers) after loss of a spouse? (Herth, 1990)	Descriptive correlational
What are the effects of fetal movement, ultrasound scans, and amniocentesis on maternal–fetal attachment and perception of fetal development in normal pregnancies? (Heidrich & Cranley, 1989)	Prospective
What is the effect of preexisting physical activity level on resting cardiovascular measures and the intensity of cardiovascular responses across the Valsalva maneuver in healthy adults? (Folta et al., 1989)	Retrospective
To what extent do nurses participate in the institutional ethics committees and in ethical decision making of hospitals, and what is their preparation for functioning in such roles? (Oddi & Cassidy, 1990)	Univariate descriptive
What are the effects of stress on family functioning among high-risk and low-risk parents eight months following the birth of a child? (Mercer & Ferketich, 1990)	Path analytic
Does the health behavior of the elderly vary as a function of sex, age, socioeconomic status, and marital status? Are those elderly people who engage in more health-promoting behavior healthier? (Brown & McCreedy, 1986)	Descriptive correlational; retrospective
To what extent do individual and situational factors affect coping and psychosocial health dysfunction among widows and widowers? (Gass & Chang, 1989)	Path analytic
What are the factors that best predict successful performance on the NCLEX-RN examination? (Jenks et al., 1989)	Prediction
What are the visiting and telephoning patterns of families of very low birthweight infants during their initial hospitalization? What factors are related to visiting and telephoning? (Brown et al., 1989)	Descriptive; descriptive correlational

This study was clearly nonexperimental. The researchers had no control over whether the women returned to work or not six months after childbirth. This example illustrates the use of an ex post facto design in a situation in which it would be feasible technically to manipulate the independent variable (employment status), although it would be highly unethical to do so. This study also illustrates some of the interpretive difficulties that emerge in an ex post facto study. For example, the finding that employed mothers were more likely than nonemployed mothers to report that they had fully regained their usual level of energy could mean that mothers are most likely to return to work once they feel physically ready for the demands of the workplace. Alternatively, it could be that getting back to work in and of itself had an energizing effect on the women. As a third possibility, it could also be that women who were predisposed to return to work quickly were especially likely to think positively or to be stoical. Thus, ex post facto research permits numerous rival hypotheses.

A Descriptive Correlational Study

McKeever and Galloway (1984) were interested in the effects of nongynecologic surgery on menstrual cycle alterations among adolescent and adult surgical patients. Portions of the study were purely descriptive, in keeping with the fact that little information was available concerning the incidence of menstrual cycle alterations following surgery. For example, the investigators wanted to answer the basic question: Is the menstrual cycle length affected by surgery performed under general anesthesia? In addition, they sought information about how a number of variables were interrelated. For example, one of the research questions was: Is there is a relationship between the menstrual cycle phase at the time of surgery and the onset of the first postoperative menses? They also examined whether the patients' perceptions of stress during hospitalization were related to postoperative menstrual cycle alterations.

Data for this investigation were obtained from a sample of 77 women aged 12 to 45, all of whom reported having had regular menstrual cycles before hospitalization. The subjects were interviewed within 72 hours of surgery and again six weeks later. The results revealed that the majority of women in the sample experienced a postoperative menstrual cycle length alteration, although the alteration was found to be unrelated to menstrual phase at the time of surgery. The women who experienced no alterations were those who encountered relatively low levels of both physiologic and psychologic stress. High stress was especially likely to be associated with an early onset of menses.

This study is clearly nonexperimental in nature. The investigators did not manipulate any variables. Unlike the preceding example, this research studied variables that are inherently non-manipulable. That is, the investigators could not manipulate the phase of the patients' menstrual cycle at the time of surgery nor their perceived level of stress during hospitalization. The investigators acknowledged that the results of their study were open to various interpretations and concluded that the "effects of environmental, social, and psychological stressors on the menstrual cycle should be explored further" (p. 45).

≡ SUMMARY

Nonexperimental research includes two broad categories: (1) descriptive research and (2) ex post facto/correlational research. *Descriptive research* is designed to summarize the status of phenomena of interest as they currently exist. *Ex post facto* or *correlational studies* are research investigations designed to examine the relationships among variables. Unlike experimental or quasi-experimental studies, however, ex post facto research lacks active manipulation of the independent variable. Because the investigation of the independent variable is done after the fact—that is, after it has occurred in the natural course of events—it becomes difficult to draw cause-and-effect conclusions. It is for this reason that, methodologically speaking, experimental studies are considered more rigorous.

There are basically three types of constraints that preclude experimentation and, therefore, make a nonexperimental approach useful or necessary. First, a number of independent variables, such as height, sex, and race, are human characteristics that are not amenable to control and randomization. Second, other independent variables are technically manipulable but are ethically inappropriate for experimental purposes with human subjects, as in the case of smoking versus not smoking cigarettes. Third, it may often be impractical or impossible to manipulate variables owing to insufficient time, inconvenience, administrative barriers, or prior manifestation of the phenomena of interest. In addition to these constraints, researchers sometimes deliberately choose not to manipulate variables to get a more realistic understanding of phenomena as they operate in naturalistic settings.

A number of special types of nonexperimental studies were briefly described in this chapter. Some nonexperimental studies attempt to elucidate causal relationships. *Retrospective studies* are investigations in which the researcher observes the manifestation of some phenomenon (the dependent variable) and tries to retrospectively identify its antecedents or causes (the independent variable). *Prospective studies* start with an observation of presumed causes and then go forward in time to observe the consequences. Prospective research is typically initiated after evidence of important relationships are suggested by retrospective investigations. *Path analytic studies* use sophisticated statistical procedures to test causal relationships predicted on the basis of a theory or conceptual model.

Prediction studies use retrospective information about the relationships among variables in one group to make a forecast about the outcomes of another similar group. *Descriptive correlational studies* are less concerned with determining cause-and-effect relationships than with a description of how one phenomenon is related to another. *Univariate descriptive research* provides information on the occurrence, frequency of oc-currence, or average value of the variables of interest without examining how variables are interrelated.

The primary weakness of ex post facto and correlational research is that the researcher lacks experimental control, both in terms of inability to manipulate the independent variable and inability to randomly assign subjects to treatment groups. The problem of *self-selection* into groups is associated with the inability to randomize. Because of this lack of control, ex post facto and correlational research are more likely to run the risk of erroneous interpretation of results than experimental research.

On the other hand, because experimentation is often unfeasible or impractical in many research situations, ex post facto and correlational studies are considered important in nursing research. Correlational research is generally an efficient and useful method of collecting a large amount of data in a relatively short period. Finally, ex post facto studies are typically strong in terms of their realism.

≡ *STUDY SUGGESTIONS*

1. A nurse researcher is interested in studying the success of several different approaches to feeding patients with dysphagia. Can the researcher use an ex post facto design to examine this problem? Why or why not? Could an experimental or quasi-experimental approach be used? How?

2. A nurse researcher is planning to investigate the relationship between the social class of hospitalized children and the frequency and content of children-initiated communications with the nursing staff. Which is the independent variable and which is the dependent variable? Would you classify this research as basically experimental or correlational, or could both approaches be used?

3. In the example in the chapter involving hernia and ulcer patients, three interpretations of the results were advanced. Describe one or two other possibilities.

4. Classify the following list of potential independent variables in terms of whether it would be impossible, unethical, or impractical to manipulate the variable and, hence, to conduct an experiment: psychiatric disorder, method of contraception, individual's weight, preoperative anxiety in patients, body temperature, method of asthma therapy, white blood cell count, heroin addiction, membership in a professional nursing association, marital status.

5. Design a hypothetical descriptive study in some setting of interest. What kind of variables would you be interested in examining?

6. Read one of the studies listed under "Substantive References." Identify the independent and dependent variables. Could the study have used an experimental or quasi-experimental design? Why or why not? Diagram (if appropriate) the directionality of the cause/effect relationship as shown in Figure 10-4. Can you offer an alternative explanation?

7. In the section on prospective studies, an example relating to rubella and congenital anomalies was cited. How could such a problem be studied retrospectively? Would an experimental approach with humans be possible? Why or why not?

☰ SUGGESTED READINGS

METHODOLOGICAL REFERENCES

Ary, D., Jacobs, L.C., & Razavich, A. (1979). *Introduction to research in education* (2nd ed.). New York: Holt, Rinehart & Winston. (Chapters 3 & 4).

Brink, P.J., & Wood, M.J. (1989). *Advanced design in nursing research*. Newbury Park, CA: Sage.

Burdette, W.J., & Gehan, E.A. (1970). *Planning and analysis of clinical studies*. Springfield, IL: Charles C Thomas. (Chapters 3 & 4).

Burns, N., & Grove, S.K. (1987). *The practice of nursing research: Conduct, critique, and utilization*. Philadelphia: W.B. Saunders. (Chapter 10).

Crano, W.D., & Brewer, M.B. (1973). *Principles of research in social psychology*. New York: McGraw-Hill. (Chapter 5).

Kerlinger, F. (1973). *Foundations of behavioral research* (2nd ed.). New York: Holt, Rinehart & Winston. (Chapter 22).

Spector, P.E. (1981). *Research designs*. Beverly Hills: Sage.

Waltz, C., & Bausell, R.B. (1981). *Nursing research: Design, statistics, and computer analysis*. Philadelphia: F.A. Davis.

Woods, N.F., & Catanzaro, M. (1988). *Nursing research: Theory and practice*. St. Louis:C.V. Mosby. (Chapters 9 & 10).

SUBSTANTIVE REFERENCES

Aaronson, L.S., & MacNee, C.L. (1989). The relationship between weight gain and nutrition in pregnancy. *Nursing Research, 38,* 223–227.

Barkauskas, V.H., Chen, S.C., & Chen, E.H. (1985). Health problems encountered by nurse practitioners and physicians in family practice clinics. *Western Journal of Nursing Research, 7,* 101–115.

Blackburn, S., & Lowen, L. (1986). Impact of an infant's premature birth on the grandparents and parents. *Journal of Obstetric, Gynecologic, and Neonatal Nursing, 15,* 173–178.

Brown, J.S., & McCreedy, M. (1986). The hale elderly: Health behavior and its correlates. *Research in Nursing and Health, 9,* 317–329.

Brown, L.P., York, R., Jacobsen, B., Gennaro, S., & Brooten, D. (1989). Very low birth-weight infants: Parental visiting and telephoning during initial infant hospitalization. *Nursing Research, 38,* 233–236.

Campbell, J.C. (1989). A test of two explanatory models of women's responses to battering. *Nursing Research, 38,* 18–24.

Dawson, C. (1985). Hypertension, perceived clinician empathy, and patient self-disclosure. *Research in Nursing and Health, 8,* 191–198.

Folta, A., Metzher, B.L., & Therrien, B. (1989). Preexisting physical activity level and cardiovascular responses across the Valsalva maneuver. *Nursing Research, 38,* 139–143.

Gass, K.A., & Chang, A.S. (1989). Appraisals of bereavement, coping, resources, and psychosocial health dysfunction in widows and widowers. *Nursing Research, 38,* 31–36.

Heidrich, S.M., & Cranley, M.S. (1989). Effect of fetal movement, ultrasound scans, and amniocentesis on maternal–fetal attachment. *Nursing Research, 38,* 81–84.

Herth, K. (1990). Relationship of hope, coping styles, concurrent losses, and setting to grief resolution in the elderly widow(er). *Research in Nursing and Health, 13,* 109–117.

Jackson, B.B. (1990). Social support and life satisfaction of black climacteric women. *Western Journal of Nursing Research, 12,* 9–23.

Jenks, J., Selekman, J., Bross, T., & Paquet, M. (1989). Success in NCLEX-RN: Identifying predictors and optimal timing for intervention. *Journal of Nursing Education, 28,* 112–118.

McKeever, P., & Galloway, S.C. (1984). Effects of non-gynecological surgery on the menstrual cycle. *Nursing Research, 33,* 42–46.

Mercer, R.T., & Ferketich, S.L. (1990). Predictors of family functioning eight months following birth. *Nursing Research, 39,* 76–82.

Metheny, N.A., Spies, M., & Eisenberg, P. (1986). Frequency of nasoenteral tube displacement and associated risk factors. *Research in Nursing and Health, 9,* 241–247.

Nelson, B.J., & Blasdell, A.L. (1988). Comparing quality on eight- and twelve-hour shifts. *Nursing Management, 19,* 64A–64H.

Norbeck, J.S., & Anderson, N.J. (1989). Psychosocial predictors of pregnancy outcomes in low-income black, Hispanic, and white women. *Nursing Research, 38,* 204–209.

Nuttall, P. (1988). Maternal responses to home apnea monitoring of infants. *Nursing Research, 37,* 354–357.

Oddi, L.F., & Cassidy, V.R. (1990). Participation and perception of nurse members in the hospital ethics committee. *Western Journal of Nursing Research, 12,* 307–317.

Packard, J.S., & Motowidlo, S.J. (1987). Subjective stress, job satisfaction, and job performance of hospital nurses. *Research in Nursing and Health, 10,* 253–261.

Saltzer, E.B., & Golden, M.P. (1985). Obesity in lower and middle socioeconomic status mothers and their children. *Research in Nursing and Health, 8,* 147–153.

Scalzi, C.C. (1990). Stress in top-level nurse executives. *Western Journal of Nursing Research, 12,* 85–94.

Shannahan, M.D., & Cottrell, B.H. (1985). Effect of the birth chair on duration of second stage labor, fetal outcome and maternal blood loss. *Nursing Research, 34,* 89–92.

Tulman, L., & Fawcett, J. (1990). Maternal employment following childbirth. *Research in Nursing and Health, 13,* 181–188.

11
Additional Types of Research

In Chapters 9 and 10 we explored research that differed in terms of one dimension: the tightness of the controls introduced by the investigator for the purpose of inferring cause-and-effect relationships. All research studies can be categorized as either experimental, quasi- or pre-experimental, or nonexperimental in design.

The discussion of experimental versus nonexperimental research, although useful in introducing some concepts of research design, nevertheless fails to provide the beginning researcher with a sense of the full range of purposes of nursing research. This chapter is devoted to examining additional types of research not already discussed in previous chapters: survey research, field studies, evaluation research, needs assessments, historical research, case studies, secondary analysis, meta-analysis, and methodological research. These nine types of research are not necessarily linked to a specific type of research design, as shown in Figure 11-1.

≡ *SURVEY RESEARCH*

A *survey* is designed to obtain information from populations regarding the prevalence, distribution, and interrelations of variables within those populations. The decennial census of the U.S. population is one example of a survey. Political opinion polls, such as those conducted by Gallup or Harris, are other examples. Although the distinction between a population and a sample was pointed out in Chapter 4, it is useful to repeat it here. *Population* refers to the entire set of individuals (or objects) having a common characteristic. For example, all registered nurses (RNs) in the United States constitute one population and all parents of physically handicapped children con-

	Experimental	Quasi-Experimental	Correlational/ Ex Post Facto	Descriptive
Survey Research			X	X
Field Study			X	X
Evaluation Research	X	X	X	X
Needs Assessments			X	X
Historical			X	X
Case Study		X	X	X
Secondary Analysis			X	X
Methodological	X	X	X	X
Meta-Analysis			X	X

Figure 11-1. *Possible designs for various types of research.*

stitute another. Any subset from a population is called a *sample.* When surveys use samples of individuals as subjects, as they usually do, they are often referred to as *sample surveys* (as opposed to a *census,* which covers the entire population).

The term *survey* can be used to designate any research activity in which the investigator gathers data from a portion of a population for the purpose of examining the characteristics, opinions, or intentions of that population. For example, a researcher could do a survey of blood types by analyzing blood samples from a population of Red Cross donors. However, in practice, surveys generally refer to studies in which information is obtained from a sample of individuals by means of self-report—that is, the subjects respond to a series of questions posed by the investigator.

The Content of Survey Research

The content of a self-report survey is essentially limited only by the extent to which respondents are willing to report on the topic. Any information that can reliably be obtained by directly asking a person for that information is acceptable for inclusion in a survey.

Often, a survey focuses on what people do: how or what they eat, how they care for their health needs, their compliance in taking medications, what kinds of family-planning behaviors they engage in, what their sleeping patterns are, and so forth. In some instances, particularly in political surveys, the emphasis is on what people

plan to do—how they plan to vote, for example. Surveys also collect information on people's knowledge, opinions, attitudes, and values. For example, we might be interested in learning about the public's knowledge of and attitude toward health maintenance organizations. Another example would be a survey of nurses' opinions about proposed legislation to expand the activities of nurse practitioners.

Almost invariably, survey researchers ask respondents for information about their personal background or situation. Most surveys secure data on many of the following characteristics: age, sex, race/ethnicity, marital status, education, religion, employment status, occupation, income, father's and mother's education, race, and family size. Demographic characteristics such as these are rarely the focus of any survey except in the case of a national census. There are, however, two important reasons for collecting background data. First, personal characteristics such as age, education, and sex have been shown repeatedly to be related to a person's behavior and attitudes. These variables, in other words, often play a valuable explanatory role. The second reason for collecting this information is to enable the researcher to compare characteristics of the sample with those of the population. If it is known, for instance, that the population under examination comprises approximately 50% men and 50% women, one might have reason to question the validity of conclusions based on the survey of a sample in which 85% of the respondents were women.

Types of Survey Techniques

Survey data can be collected in a number of ways. The three most common methods are (1) personal interviews, (2) telephone interviews, and (3) mailed questionnaires.

The most powerful method of securing survey information is through *personal interviews,* the method in which interviewers meet with individuals face-to-face and secure information from them. In most cases, the interviewer will use a carefully developed set of questions, referred to as an *interview schedule.* The time needed for a personal interview varies considerably from study to study and from respondent to respondent. Some interviews may be completed in a matter of minutes; others may take literally hours to complete. Generally, personal interviews are rather costly. They require considerable planning and interviewer training to be successful; they also tend to involve a lot of personnel time. Nevertheless, personal interviews are regarded as the most useful method of collecting survey data because of the depth and quality of the information they yield. Furthermore, personal interviews usually result in a high number of "returns," that is, relatively few people refuse to be interviewed in person.

Telephone interviews are a less costly, but often less effective, method of gathering survey information. Whenever detailed information is needed from respondents, a personal interview is usually preferable. When the interviewer is unknown, respondents may be uncooperative and unresponsive in a telephone situation. Telephone interviews inherently lack the ability to build rapport, which is a feature of face-to-face interviews. However, telephoning can be a convenient method of collecting a lot of information quickly if the interview is short, specific, and not too personal, or if the researcher has had prior personal contact with the subjects. Among nurse researchers, telephone surveys are relatively rare.

Questionnaires differ from interviews primarily in that they are self-administered. That is, the respondent reads the questions on the schedule and gives an answer in writing. A person associated with the survey may or may not be present at the time the questionnaire is completed to answer questions that arise. Because of this fact, and because respondents differ considerably in their reading levels and in their ability to communicate in writing, questionnaires are *not* merely a printed form of an interview schedule. Great care must be taken in the development of a questionnaire to word questions clearly, simply, and unambiguously. The most common way of distributing questionnaires is through the mail. Compared with personal interviews, the cost of a mailed questionnaire is quite low, especially if the population is spread over a wide geographical area.

Advantages and Disadvantages of Surveys

The greatest advantage of survey research is its flexibility and broadness of scope. It can be applied to many populations, it can focus on a wide range of topics, and its information can be used for many purposes. Good surveys can be much more costly than experiments, but when one considers the amount of information obtained in the course of normal surveys, they are not uneconomical.

However, a number of limitations of survey research should be considered. First, the information obtained in most surveys tends to be relatively superficial. Interviews and questionnaires rarely probe deeply into such complexities as contradictions of human behavior and feelings. Survey research is better suited to extensive rather than intensive analysis. A second drawback of survey research is one we mentioned previously in connection with ex post facto research: survey data do not permit the researcher to have much confidence in inferring cause-and-effect relationships. Survey researchers have no control over independent variables (that is, they do not manipulate any variables). Another difficulty with survey research is that it tends to be demanding of personnel time and other resources. In a large survey, literally dozens of workers may be required to administer the interviews. Although smaller survey studies can often be successfully completed by a small group of researchers, even localized surveys generally require a considerable investment of time and energy and rarely result in any findings before months of effort.

Survey Research Examples

Table 11-1 presents a brief description of several surveys that have been undertaken by nurse researchers. A more complete description of a nursing research survey is presented below.

> Wiley and her colleagues (1990) conducted a survey to determine nurses' concerns, opinions, and precautions related to caring for patients infected with the human immunodeficiency virus (HIV). The survey involved the mailing of a questionnaire and a self-addressed return envelope to approximately 600 nurses who worked at a medical center in a large midwestern city. The sample included all staff nurses employed in the ambulatory/home health care unit of the hospital, and all staff nurses in seven inpatient critical care units (e.g., emergency room, labor and deliv-

> ery). Of the 600 nurses who were invited to participate in the survey, a total of 323 (54%) completed and returned a questionnaire.

> The questionnaire, called the HIV-Impact Questionnaire, consisted primarily of 15 statements concerning HIV with which the nurses were asked to indicate levels of agreement or disagreement. The statements focused on three main topics: concerns about acquiring a work-related HIV infection; opinions about HIV-related agency policies; and use of HIV-infection control precautions.

> Twenty percent of the nurses in the survey reported HIV exposure and 24 percent reported no exposure; the remaining 56 percent of the nurses did not know if they had been exposed. HIV-exposed nurses were more likely than others to report worrying about becoming infected and considering a change in specialty or profession because of associated risks. Over one-half of the sample said that if the agency gave them the option, they would refuse assignment to HIV-infected patients. The researchers concluded that HIV-infected nurses need support in dealing with their concerns and need more information about HIV-infection control.

Table 11-1. *Examples of Nursing Research Surveys*

PROBLEM STATEMENT	TYPE	SAMPLE
What are the perceptions and attitudes of nurses toward nursing impairment? (Hendrix et al., 1987)	Mailed questionnaire	1,047 RNs
What is the relationship between consumer characteristics and their intention to use family nurse practitioner services? (Smith & Shamansky, 1983)	Telephone interview	239 households in Seattle
What are the factors associated with lower back pain in nurses? (Mandel & Lohman, 1987)	Mailed questionnaire	428 RNs
Do individuals believe that if they follow recommendations for coronary heart disease risk factor reduction their chances of developing heart disease will be decreased? (Lile, 1990)	Distributed questionnaires	317 adults aged 20–60
What are pregnant women's reasons for delaying prenatal care? (Young et al., 1989)	Personal interviews	201 pregnant women
What is the impact of shared values on staff nurses' job satisfaction and perceived productivity? (Kramer & Hafner, 1989)	Group-administered questionnaire	2,297 staff nurses

Through the use of a survey, the researchers were able to collect data from a large sample of nurses. They chose to use a mailed questionnaire as a method of data collection. This method, while economical, resulted in only a moderate rate of response. As acknowledged by the researchers themselves, it is possible that HIV-exposed nurses were more likely than others to respond to the questionnaire, given their greater interest in a survey of this type. This, in turn, would bias the results, since HIV-exposed nurses had different opinions than did non-exposed nurses. Nevertheless, the survey yielded information that has considerable relevance for nurses and nursing administrators, and merits replication.

≡ *FIELD STUDIES*

Qualitative research that aims at describing and exploring phenomena in naturalistic settings is frequently referred to as *field research*. Field studies are investigations that are done "in the field," in such social settings as hospitals, clinics, intensive care units, nursing homes, housing projects, and so on. The purpose of field studies is to examine in an in-depth fashion the practices, behaviors, beliefs, and attitudes of individuals or groups as they normally function in real life. Unlike surveys, field studies are often intensive rather than extensive, and data are collected in a variety of ways. In field studies, the researcher, by definition, engages in field work (i.e., goes out to the setting where the subjects normally operate). The data that are collected are usually narrative materials, based on researcher observation, conversations with subjects, or available documents. The aim of the field researcher is to "get close" to the people under study to really understand a problem or situation from their perspective.

Anthropologists have engaged in field research for decades in their efforts to understand the functioning of human cultures. Nurse researchers, because of their interest in nurse–patient–environment interactions, are becoming increasingly interested in field research. Examples of the kinds of nursing problems that could

fruitfully be addressed through field research include the following: What are the health-care needs of the homeless, and what are the barriers to providing that care? What environmental conditions and stresses lead to dysfunctional parenting and child abuse? What types of interpersonal style characterize hospitalized psychiatric patients?

Characteristics of Field Research

In traditional scientific research, a heavy emphasis is placed on control and objectivity. In field research, the researcher continually uses subjective judgments about whom to interview, what to observe, what questions to ask, and so on. In field research, the main instrument of data collection *is* the researcher, rather than technical apparatus or formal written tools.

Typically, data collection and analysis are ongoing, simultaneous activities in the field. The analysis of information often leads the investigator to pursue new avenues of inquiry. In traditional approaches, data to be collected are prespecified and generally remain unanalyzed until all the data are "in."

Field research is typically less linear than other types of research. That is, the steps do not follow a linear progression such as that suggested in Chapter 4. The field researcher may begin with only a general problem area or hypothesis to be explored, or hypotheses may be generated in the course of data collection and analysis and pursued more rigorously in subsequent data collection. Field researchers try to remain open and flexible about the research process in the hope that such flexibility will allow them to pursue the realities of the subjects' experience as that experience is lived.

Conducting Field Research

Wilson (1989) has identified the following five stages that are typically undertaken in field research:

Stage I. Identifying the setting in which the field-work will take place and assessing the appropriateness of the setting for the problem of interest.

Stage II. Gaining access to the people or groups to be studied, including the development of strategies to use in approaching "gatekeepers."

Stage III. Assuming an appropriate role (appropriate in terms of research aims or the demands and constraints of those under study) in the social setting, on a continuum ranging from full participant in the setting to complete observer.

Stage IV. Collecting, recording, analyzing, and interpreting data.

Stage V. Fulfilling commitments made to gain access to the social setting, and leaving the field.

Appraisal of Field Research

Field studies are strong on realism because they are done in natural settings without structure or controls imposed by the researcher. Because of the in-depth and flexible nature of field studies, they often provide a depth of understanding of social phenomena that is unattainable with more traditional methods of scientific research. For example, Norris' (1975) in-depth study of restlessness led to a careful delineation of the meaning of this phenomenon and a description of its precursors.

Some of the very elements that make field research strong are potential problem areas. During data collection and analysis, the researcher is so thoroughly immersed in the phenomenon that the risk of bias becomes great. Perhaps the most problematic aspect of field research, however, is the difficulty with which investigators describe how they have arrived at their conclusions. Field research can almost never be replicated because the methods evolve *in situ*. It is often difficult to evaluate whether two independent field researchers would come to different conclusions based on the same investigation. Because of these problems, field research has sometimes been characterized by hard-line scientists as "soft" and "fuzzy."

Examples of Field Studies

Nurse researchers are increasingly going "into the field" to gather rich, qualitative data on problems of importance to nursing. Table 11-2 presents a summary of several field studies. A more detailed description of a field study is provided below.

Madeleine Leininger has been a leader in an area she calls *ethnonursing research,* which she defines as "the study and analysis of the local or indigenous people's viewpoints, beliefs, and practices about nursing care behavior and processes of designated cultures" (Leininger, 1985, p. 38). One of the many field studies she has conducted focused on black and white residents of a rural community in central Alabama (Leininger, 1985, pp. 195–216). The purpose of the research was to systematically study the care and health values, beliefs, attitudes, and general "lifeways" of these two cultural groups. Among the many research questions addressed by her research were the following: "What is the general lifeway of the Black and White villagers, especially related to care and health cultural expressions?" and "What are the perceived differences and similarities between the rural folk and the urban professional health care practices?" (p. 196).

To address these research questions, Leininger spent ten months in the field, intensively studying a community of under 3000 people that she called Friendly Village and, for the purposes of "reflective comparison," a similar community called Pecan Village. During the ten months of her fieldwork, Leininger observed the living habits and customs of the residents of these communities, participated in some of their lifeways, and interviewed approximately 90 Friendly Villagers. Sixty of them were selected for in-depth observation and interviewing.

Through such intensive study, the investigator was able to gain rich information about how people in this culture felt about health and health care, and about how those beliefs influenced their health behavior. Only a few examples of the kinds of in-depth insights she derived from her research can be presented here. For example, a dominant theme that emerged in connection with the meaning of health to the villagers was that "health means being able to do your work in the home, church, and community" (p. 204). Leininger also learned the strength of the villagers' perceived linkage between health and religion. From the villagers' viewpoint, it made no sense to speak of health without considering spiritual health as a total process of living; health in that community was associated with living properly by the Bible and doing what God teaches. A full understanding of such beliefs would clearly be important to the provision of culturally acceptable health care in such communities.

≡ *EVALUATION RESEARCH*

Evaluative research is an "applied" form of research. Basically, *evaluation research* involves finding out how well a program, practice, procedure, or policy* is working. Its goal is to assess or evaluate the success of a program. In other words, evaluative research deals with the question of how well the program is meeting its objectives. In nursing practice, nursing administration, and nursing education, there is obviously a need to sit back and pose such questions as, How are we doing? Are we accomplishing our goals? For example, a clinical nurse may want to evaluate the effectiveness of structured, as opposed to casual, observations of patients in the development of nursing-care plans. A nursing administrator may want to assess the success of certain hospital policies and practices with respect to nurses' performance and job satisfaction. A nursing educator may want information concerning the effectiveness of an autotutorial approach in teaching nurs-

* For the most part, we will use the term "program" throughout our discussion, but the reader should be aware that this term is meant to include practices, procedures, and policies as well.

Table 11-2. *Examples of Nursing Research Field Studies*

PROBLEM STATEMENT	FIELD SETTING
What is the interactive process by which adults learn about and manage contraceptive practices? (Swanson, 1988)	Community-based sites offering family planning and reproductive health services in California
What patterns of behaviors in the everyday life of nurses as women interface with their interactions with physicians as men, and what patterns of gender role behavior do nurses exhibit in their professional role? (Katzman & Roberts, 1988)	A nonprofit hospital in the northeastern United States
What are the folk medicine practices and the health-care practices of Hmong refugees in the United States? (Cheon-Klessig et al., 1988)	A Hmong community in the United States
What are the childbearing beliefs and knowledge of conception and fetal development among Cambodian refugee women? (Kulig, 1990)	A Cambodian community in a city in the western provinces of Canada
What are the sources of job stress among psychiatric technicians who care for the mentally retarded in a state institution, and how are social resources used to reduce job stress? (Browner, 1987)	A state residential facility that provides care for the severely and profoundly mentally retarded

ing students how to administer subcutaneous injections.

In evaluations, the research objective is utilitarian. The purpose of the evaluation is to answer the practical questions of people who must make decisions: Should the program be continued? Do current practices need to be modified or should they be abandoned altogether? Should the new intervention be replicated in other settings? Do the costs of implementing the program outweigh the benefits? When programs are found to be only partially effective, evaluation research can often provide directions for making improvements.

Evaluation research has an important role to play both in localized settings and in programs at the national level. Evaluations are often the cornerstone of an area of research known as *policy research;* nurses have become increasingly aware of the potential contribution their research can make to the formulation of national and local health policies and thus are undertaking evaluations that have implications for such policies.

Evaluation Research Models

There are various schools of thought concerning the conduct of evaluation research. In this section we will examine briefly two that are, in a sense, at opposite ends of the spectrum. Other evaluation models fall between these extremes; the reader interested in pursuing evaluation research might want to consult the references at the end of this chapter.

The traditional strategy for the conduct of evaluation research consists of four broad phases: (1) determining the objectives of the program, (2) developing a means of measuring the attainment of those objectives, (3) collecting the data, and (4) interpreting the data *vis-à-vis* the objectives. These steps sound rather straightforward—much like the steps in most research studies. Often, the most difficult task is to spell out in detail the goals of a program or practice. Typically, there are numerous objectives of a program, and these objectives may be vague. For example, the principal goal of many nursing practices is the improve-

ment of patient care. This aim, though laudable, is so vague as to be almost meaningless in terms of evaluating its realization. What exactly do we *mean* by improving patient care? How will we know if we have succeeded?

The term behavioral objective, frequently referred to in evaluation research literature, is a concept that has evolved as a means of coping with the broadness and fuzziness of program goals. A *behavioral objective* is the intended outcome of a program stated in terms of the behavior of the individuals at whom the program is aimed. Thus, the goal of "improved patient care" might in one instance translate as "the patient will learn how to cough productively following surgery" or in another as "the patient will walk the length of the corridor within five days after surgery." Note that behavioral objectives always focus on the behavior of the *beneficiaries,* rather than the *agents,* of the program. In the previous examples, the objectives were worded to reflect the intended behavioral outcome of the *patient*—not the behavior of the nurse. It would be inappropriate, for example, to use the objective "the nurse will teach patients to measure their heart rate by counting their radial pulse for a full minute."

The emphasis on behavioral objectives can be taken to extremes. There are many times when our interest centers on psychologic dimensions such as morale or an emotion (e.g., anxiety) that do not always manifest themselves in behavioral terms. However, the evaluator who tries to formulate program goals in terms of behavioral objectives will almost always find that the goals are less vague and diffuse than they might otherwise have been.

Once the program goals have been delineated, the evaluation using a traditional approach can be designed much like other research studies. An evaluation can use either an experimental design (with subjects randomly assigned to either the program being evaluated or to a control group), a quasi-experimental design, or a nonexperimental design. The final step in the classical evaluation model is to analyze the data in such a way that some decisions can be made about the program or practice under consideration, or some action can be taken to make the program more effective.

The traditional model of evaluation has sometimes been criticized by a number of writers for a certain narrowness of conceptualization. One alternative evaluation model is the so-called *goal-free approach*. Proponents of this model argue that programs may have a number of consequences besides accomplishing the official objectives of the program and that the classical model is handicapped by its inability to investigate these other effects. According to advocates of goal-free evaluation, the mere knowledge of the program objectives has the potential of biasing the evaluator by suggesting the areas of the program that should be researched.

Thus, goal-free evaluation represents an attempt to evaluate the outcomes of a program in the absence of information about *intended* outcomes. The job of the evaluator—a demanding one—is basically that of describing the repercussions of a program or practice on various components of the overall system. A goal-free evaluation of a procedure to reduce preoperative anxiety, for example, might assess the impact of the procedure not only on patients but also on other individuals such as staff, administrators, and visitors of the patients *and* on other procedures, policies, or costs. The goal-free evaluation model is, in many respects, congruent with the medical model of patient evaluation, with its concern for monitoring possible side effects of a treatment.

The goal-free model might often be a profitable approach, and certainly leaves more room for creativity on the part of the evaluator. In many cases, however, the model may not be practical because there are seldom unlimited resources (personnel, time, or money) for the conduct of an evaluation. Decision makers may need to know, quite simply, whether objectives are being met so that immediate decisions can be made. In the final analysis, the choice of a model will depend, to a large extent, on the informational needs of the decision maker and on the position of the evaluator within the organization.

Types of Evaluations

Evaluations are undertaken to answer a variety of questions about a program or policy. This section briefly describes evaluations designed to address different types of questions. In evaluations of large-scale interventions (sometimes called *demonstrations*), the evaluator might well undertake all of the evaluation activities discussed here.

PROCESS OR IMPLEMENTATION ANALYSES

A *process* or *implementation analysis* is undertaken when there is a need for descriptive information about the process by which a program or procedure gets implemented and how it functions in actual operation. A process analysis is typically designed to address such questions as the following:

Does the program function in the real world the way its designers intended it? What appear to be the strongest and weakest aspects of the program? What exactly *is* the treatment, and how does it differ (if at all) from traditional practices?

What was the process by which the program was shaped and became fully operational?

What, if any, were the barriers to successfully implementing the program? How have the staff dealt with these barriers? What factors facilitated the implementation process?

What were the characteristics of the participants, the staff, and the setting of the program? Did the program serve the clients for whom the program was designed?

How do staff and clients like the program? Have there been any problems in recruiting people to participate in the program? Have there been any problems with staff turnover?

Have staff been adequately trained to implement the program? If staff turnover has occurred, has training for replacement staff been adequate?

Can the program be readily replicated in a new setting, or was its implementation affected by something unique in the setting in which it first operated?

A process analysis might be undertaken with the aim of improving a new or ongoing program; in such a situation, the evaluation may be referred to as a *formative evaluation*. In other situations, the purpose of the process analysis might be primarily to carefully describe a program so that it can be replicated by others. In either case, a process analysis typically involves an in-depth examination of the operation of a program, often involving the collection of both qualitative and quantitative data. The information is typically gathered through interviews with staff and clients, through observation of the program in operation, and through an analysis of records relating to the program. Thus, process analyses are typically broad-based examinations designed to answer questions about the functioning of a program.

OUTCOME AND IMPACT ANALYSES

Evaluations typically focus on whether a program or policy *works*—that is, whether it is effective in meeting its objectives. Evaluations that assess the worth of a program are sometimes referred to as *summative evaluations*. The intent of such evaluations is to help people decide whether the program should be discarded, replaced, modified, continued, or replicated.

Researchers who specialize in evaluation research sometimes distinguish between an outcome analysis and an impact analysis. An *outcome analysis* tends to be fairly descriptive and does not utilize a rigorous design. Such an analysis simply documents the extent to which the goals of the program are attained—that is, the extent to which positive outcomes occur. For example, a program might be designed in a poor rural community to encourage women to obtain prenatal care. An outcome analysis might document the percentage of women delivering babies in the community who had obtained such care, the percentage of low-birthweight infants, the incidence of neonatal mortality, and so on. These outcomes might be compared with rates in a period before

the implementation of the special program, as a means for putting the outcomes in a broader context.

An *impact analysis*, by contrast, attempts to carefully identify the *net impacts* of an intervention—that is, the impacts that can be attributed exclusively to the intervention rather than to other factors. Impact analyses almost always utilize an experimental or quasi-experimental design, because the aim of such evaluations is to attribute a causal influence to the special intervention. In the example above, let us suppose that the program to encourage prenatal care involved having nurses make home visits to women in the community to explain the benefits of early care during pregnancy. If the visits could be made to pregnant women on a random basis, the labor and delivery outcomes of the group of women receiving the home visits and those not receiving them could be compared to determine the net impacts of the intervention. Impact analyses clearly provide more conclusive evidence than outcome analyses about the effectiveness of a program.

COST–BENEFIT ANALYSES

New programs or policies are often expensive to implement. Therefore, evaluations sometimes include a *cost–benefit analysis* to determine whether the benefits of the program outweigh the costs, in terms of monetary value. Cost–benefit analyses are typically done in connection with impact analyses—that is, when there is solid evidence regarding the net impacts of an intervention.

In some cases, a cost–benefit analysis cannot meaningfully be conducted because it is impossible to put a dollar value on the outcome. For example, if the program to encourage prenatal care resulted in a lowering of neonatal mortality by 2%, such an outcome would not lend itself to a cost–benefit analysis because the costs of an infant's death are not primarily financial. On the other hand, if the intervention lowered the rate of low birthweight infants, a cost–benefit analysis could be readily conducted. In such a situation, the evaluator would need to compare the total cost of operating the home visitation program against the total cost required to treat the low birthweight infants (i.e., to treat the number of low-birthweight infants in the control group in excess of those that occurred in the experimental group). The question is whether the cost of the preventive intervention is offset by eventual savings in treatment costs. When cost–benefit analyses can be performed, decision makers often have a solid basis for deciding on whether a program should be continued and expanded.

Obstacles and Problems in Evaluation Research

All research projects encounter difficulties that are usually unanticipated. Evaluation researchers often come up against several obstacles that can be foreseen because they emerge so frequently. In this section we will briefly review several of the most recurrent problem areas in the hope that advanced planning may help to alleviate the difficulties.

Evaluation research can be threatening to individuals. Even when the focus of an evaluation is on a nontangible entity, such as a program, procedure, policy, or the like, it is *people* who developed the entity and are implementing it. People tend to think that they, or their work, are being evaluated and may in some cases feel that their job or reputation is at stake. Evaluation researchers, thus, need to have more than methodological skills: they need to be diplomats, adept in interpersonal dealings with people. If the people operating a program are defensive and noncooperative, the evaluation could be unproductive.

Even when program staff are not on the defensive, they can be reluctant to cooperate for other reasons. If they are convinced about the merit of the program or policy that is being evaluated, they may not see the need for more objective information. They may believe that their time is better spent in providing services to people than in helping a researcher evaluate the adequacy of their services.

Yet another difficulty that many evaluation researchers encounter is the problem of ascertaining the goals of the program. In the classical approach to evaluating a program, the evaluator must have a clear idea of what the program is attempting to accomplish. When a program or practice has a simple goal, the evaluator need only develop some method of measuring its attainment. More often, however, the objectives of a program are multiple and diffuse; in many cases, the goals refer to behaviors or conditions in the distant future.

This list of barriers or obstacles to conducting effective evaluation is not intended to discourage researchers but rather to alert people about to embark on such endeavors to the more frequent evaluation problems. Difficulties arise in all research projects—permissions can be delayed, telephones malfunction, research personnel become ill, and so forth. In evaluation research, however, the researcher must often contend with a characteristic set of problems that are organizational, interpersonal, or political in nature. The wise person will enter an evaluation project with eyes wide open, aware of the obstacles that may arise, yet sensitive to the genuine contribution that evaluations can make to program functioning and to the improvement of health care and the development of health-care policy.

Example of Evaluation Research

Many of the studies undertaken by nurse researchers could be considered evaluations; most of the published evaluations are ones that would be considered summative in nature. Table 11-3 presents several evaluation studies that have been conducted by nurse researchers. Below we describe an evaluation study in greater detail.

> Mills and her colleagues (1985) evaluated the effectiveness of an inpatient cardiac education program. The group education program was implemented because of the large number of patients being treated at the hospital (the Little Rock Veterans Administration Medical Center) with a diagnosis of ischemic heart disease. The patient education program consisted of

five 1-hour classes. The objectives of the program were to increase patients' knowledge in specific areas and to increase postdischarge compliance with a prescribed treatment plan. A number of behavioral objectives were developed. For example, one of the objectives for the first of the five classes was as follows: The patient will be able to describe what happens to the heart muscle when a person has a heart attack.

A total of 277 patients participated in the study. A 23-item multiple-choice test of knowledge was administered to subjects before the treatment (the five classes) and then upon completion of the course. Four weeks after discharge from the program, participants were again contacted and asked to complete a behavior assessment (compliance) questionnaire. The results revealed that there were significant gains in knowledge, as measured by the test, after the patients completed the education program.

The design for this portion of the study can best be described as pre-experimental, because there was no control group of subjects who were *not* exposed to the intervention. However, the investigators did incorporate a design element that gives us greater confidence that the increase of knowledge did not merely reflect the patients' familiarity with the test. Some subjects were randomly assigned to a group that did not receive an initial test of knowledge. There were no differences between the two groups in terms of their posttreatment test scores, so it seems reasonable to conclude that the knowledge gain reflects a program impact rather than experience with the test.

A further analysis indicated that the greater the number of classes a patient attended and the higher the posttest knowledge scores, the higher the compliance with the prescribed treatment plan. Unfortunately, these findings do not allow us to conclude that compliance can be increased by increasing a patient's exposure to an educational program. More highly motivated patients were probably more likely to attend more classes; therefore, it is plausible that self-selection factors

Table 11-3. *Examples of Nursing Research Evaluations*

PROBLEM STATEMENT	TYPE
Is the aerobic capacity of overweight, middle-aged women positively affected by participation in a 16-week intensity controlled dance-exercise program? (Gillett & Eisenman, 1987)	Impact analysis
What is the process of home care for the child dying of cancer as it involves the family, nurse, and physician? (Martinson et al., 1986)	Process analysis
Is a home training program to teach circumvaginal muscle (CVM) exercise effective in increasing the pressure developed by the CVM? (Dougherty et al., 1989)	Impact analysis
What are the patient recollections of the critical-care experience in a special critical-care nurses demonstration project? (Simpson et al., 1989). How was the project characterized in terms of nurse–physician collaboration, administration of nursing services, work and information flow, and staff morale? (Mitchell et al., 1989)	Process analysis
What are the outcomes of a special critical-care nurses' demonstration project in terms of mortality ratios, rate of complications, and fiscal costs? (Mitchell et al., 1989)	Outcome analysis, cost-benefit analysis
What is the impact of a comprehensive discharge planning protocol implemented by a gerontological nurse specialist in terms of post-discharge outcomes? (Naylor, 1990)	Impact analysis

influenced the relationship between class attendance and compliance scores.

☰ NEEDS ASSESSMENTS

Like evaluation research, a needs assessment represents an effort to provide a decision maker or policy maker with information for action. As the name implies, a *needs assessment* is a study in which a researcher collects data for estimating the needs of a group, community, or organization. A needs assessment provides informational input in a planning process.

A needs assessment generally is undertaken by agencies or groups that have a service component. Nursing educators may wish to assess the needs of their clients (students); hospital staff members may wish to learn the needs of those they serve (patients); a mental health outreach clinic may wish to gather information on the needs of some target population (e.g., adolescents in the community). Because resources are seldom limitless, information that can help in establishing priorities is almost always valuable. Needs assessments are useful in this capacity not only when a program or policy becomes established but also after the program is in operation. Organizations and communities are dynamic entities whose needs are almost always in transition. A program whose objectives are structured to meet the needs of the group at one point may find that it becomes ineffective because the objectives are no longer meaningful. Thus, although an evaluation might seek to ascertain if a program is attaining its objectives, the aim of needs assessments is to determine if the objectives of a program are meeting the needs of the individuals who are supposed to benefit from it.

Needs Assessment Approaches

The methods of a needs assessment may vary considerably in complexity, cost, and length of time required to perform the study. The various approaches noted here are not necessarily mutually exclusive. Several methods often are used quite profitably to supplement one another in a single study. The *key informant approach,* as the name implies, collects information concerning the needs of a group from key individuals who are presumed to be in a position to know those needs. These key informants could be community leaders, prominent health-care workers, agency directors, or other knowledgeable individuals. Questionnaires or interviews are generally used to collect the data.

Another method is the *survey approach* in which data are collected from a sample from the target group whose needs are being assessed. In a survey, there would be no attempt to question only people who are in positions of authority or who are knowledgeable. Any member of the group or community could be asked to give his or her viewpoint.

Another alternative is to use an *indicators approach,* which relies on inferences made from statistics available in existing reports or records. For example, a nurse-managed clinic that is interested in analyzing the needs of its clients could examine over a 5-year period the number of appointments that were kept, the employment rate of its clients, the changes in risk appraisal status, methods of payment, and so forth. The indicators approach is very flexible and may also be quite economical because the data are generally available but need organization and interpretation.

The final phase of a needs assessment almost always involves the development of recommendations. These recommendations for action typically involve the delineation of priorities as revealed by the findings, but the suggestions are rarely entirely objective. The role of the researcher conducting a needs assessment is often that of making judgments about priorities in light of considerations such as costs and feasibility and in advising on means by which the most highly prioritized needs can be serviced.

Example of a Needs Assessment

Derdiarian (1986) studied the informational needs of men and women who had received their first cancer diagnosis within the previous three weeks. Prior research had suggested that cancer patients lack information about their disease and its implications, and that the lack of knowledge interferes with their adjustment.

Data for the study were gathered through interviews with a sample of 60 patients recently diagnosed as having cancer. The sample included men and women aged 18 to 70 in different stages of cancer. The interview schedule, referred to as the Derdiarian Informational Needs Assessment, incorporated questions that were based primarily on a theory of stress and coping. The results indicated that all of the patients' major informational needs could be classified in four major categories: disease-related, personal, family-related, and social relationships. The results indicated that the highest need was for disease-related information—about treatments and about prognosis. In the personal category, the patients indicated the highest need for information about implications of the disease for physical well-being. Further analyses revealed that there was relatively little variation in the patients' informational needs according to their age, gender, or stage of cancer.

The researcher wanted to better understand the informational needs of cancer patients from their own perspective, rather than from the perspective of health care workers. She used a survey to gather data from members of the target population (recently informed cancer patients), using personal interviews as her data collection approach. On the basis of her assessment of patient needs, the researcher concluded that her findings had implications for teaching and counseling cancer patients when they are first informed of their illness.

≡ *HISTORICAL RESEARCH*

Historical research is the systematic collection and critical evaluation of data relating to past occurrences. Generally, historical research is undertaken to test hypotheses or to answer questions concerning causes, effects, or trends relating to past events that may shed light on present behaviors or practices. An understanding of contemporary nursing theories, practices, or issues can often be enhanced by an investigation of a specified segment of the past. Particularly in this time when nurses are working to define and extend their professional roles, a knowledge of the roots of nursing has the capacity to put nursing theories and procedures into an appropriate context. For example, the struggles experienced by several states in enacting new laws that recognize nurses as independent practitioners had their roots in the "handmaiden to the physician" attitude so long accepted by physicians, nurses, and society at large.

The steps involved in performing historical research are quite similar to those for other types of research: the historical researcher defines a problem area, develops hypotheses or specific questions, collects data according to a systematic framework, analyzes the data, and interprets the findings. Historical research differs from other types of research, however, in two important respects. First, considerable effort is usually required to identify data sources on events, situations, and human behavior occurring in the past. Second, because the researcher has no control over the quality of data available, another research task involves the critical evaluation of gathered information.

Historical research is inherently nonexperimental. The researcher can neither manipulate nor control the variables, nor is there any possibility of random assignment. In fact, the historical researcher must cope with a number of handicaps. In ex post facto or survey research, the investigator may not be able to manipulate variables but usually there are opportunities to construct or select the data collection instrument. Historical researchers, however, have no control over the documents, records, or artifacts available for study. The historical researcher is at a similar disadvantage with regard to sampling. Only surviving records can be consulted, and these records may contain a number of biases.

Formulation of the Problem and Hypotheses

Like other forms of research, it is important for the historical researcher to formulate a feasible, well-articulated problem area to explore. It is easy for a historical problem to become unmanageable because there is less closure than in a study that creates new data. That is, the researcher may lack a definitive end point at which the data can be said to have been collected. On the other hand, a unique problem in historical research is that a sufficient quantity of data (of adequate quality) may be unavailable. Thus, the historical researcher should be familiar enough with the problem area to choose a well-defined topic that can be studied in depth and for which there are at least enough data to permit a test of some hypotheses or provide answers to specific questions.

The student should be careful not to confuse historical research with a review of the literature, although a literature review will undoubtedly be an early step in the research process. The purpose of historical research should be to explain the present or to anticipate future events; it is not merely to find out what is already known about an issue and to paraphrase it. Like other types of research, historical inquiry has as its goal the discovery of new knowledge.

One important difference between historical research and a literature review is that a historical researcher is often guided in the collection of information by the formulation of specific hypotheses or questions. The hypotheses represent attempts at explaining and interpreting the conditions, events, or phenomena under investigation. Hypotheses in historical research are not usually tested in a statistical sense. They are, generally, broadly stated conjectures about relationships among historical events, trends, and phenomena. For example, it might be hypothesized that a relationship exists between the presence or absence of war on the one hand and the amount of scientific nursing knowledge generated on the other. This hypothesis could be tested by analyzing research trends in nursing during the twentieth century.

Collection of Historical Data

Data for historical research are usually in the form of written records of the past: periodicals, diaries, books, letters, newspapers, minutes of meetings, legal documents, and so forth. However, a number of nonwritten materials may also be of interest. For example, physical remains and objects are potential sources of information. Visual materials such as photographs, films, and drawings are forms of data, as are audio materials such as records, tapes, and so forth. It is evident that many of these materials may be difficult to obtain and even written materials will not always be conveniently indexed by subject, author, or title. The identification of appropriate historical materials may require a considerable amount of time, effort, and detective work. Fortunately, there exist several archives of historical nursing documents, such as the collections at several universities (e.g., Boston University, Columbia University, Radcliffe College, and Johns Hopkins University) as well as collections at the National Library of Medicine, the Nursing Museum in Philadelphia, the American Journal of Nursing Company, and the National League for Nursing. Fairman (1987) identified additional sources for those interested in nursing history.

If the event or phenomenon of interest occurred recently, then it may be possible to identify living people who participated in or witnessed the event or who personally knew a historical figure. When this is the case, interviews with such people contribute another form of data.

Historical materials generally are classified as either primary or secondary sources. A *primary source* is first-hand information, such as original documents, relics, or artifacts. Examples are Louisa May Alcott's book *Hospital Sketches,* minutes of early American Nurses Association meetings, hospital records, and so forth. Primary sources represent the most direct link with historical events or situations: only the narrator (in the case of written materials) intrudes between original events and the historical researcher.

Secondary sources are second- or third-hand accounts of historical events or experiences. For example, textbooks, encyclopedias, or other reference books are generally secondary sources. Secondary sources, in other words, are discussions of events written by individuals who are summarizing or interpreting primary source materials. Primary sources should be used whenever possible in historical research. The further removed from the historical event the information is, the less reliable, objective, and comprehensive the data are likely to be. Of course, primary sources generally are more difficult to locate and use, but historical research that relies exclusively or heavily on secondary materials is bound to have numerous limitations.

Evaluation of Historical Data

Historical evidence usually is subjected to two types of evaluation, which historians refer to as external and internal criticism. *External criticism* is concerned basically with the authenticity and genuineness of the data. For example, a nursing historian might have a diary presumed to be written by Dorothea Dix. External criticism would involve asking such questions as, Is this the handwriting of Ms. Dix? Is the paper on which the diary is written of the right age? Are the writing style and ideas expressed consistent with her other writings?

There are various scientific techniques available to determine the age of materials, such as x-ray and radioactive procedures. However, other flaws may be less easy to detect. For example, there is the possibility that material of interest may have been written by a ghost writer—that is, by someone other than the person in whom we are really interested. There is also the potential problem of mechanical errors associated with transcriptions, translations, or typed versions of historical materials. Furthermore, even if a document or object is original, it is possible that alterations were made at a later point. There may be no way to prove the authenticity of historical ma-

terials. If the researcher finds any reason to question the genuineness of the documents or objects, however, great caution should be exercised in their use.

Internal criticism of historical data refers to the evaluation of the worth of the evidence. The focus of internal criticism is not so much on the physical aspects of the materials but rather on their content. An important issue here is the accuracy or truth of the data. For example, the historical researcher must question whether a writer's representations of historical events are unbiased. It may also be appropriate to ask if the author of a document was in a position to make a valid report of an event or occurrence, or whether the writer was competent as a recorder of fact. Evidence bearing on the accuracy of historical data might include one of the following: comparisons with other people's accounts of the same event to determine the degree of agreement; knowledge of the time at which the document was produced (reports of events or situations tend to be more accurate if they are written immediately following the event, such as in diaries or minutes of a meeting); knowledge of the point of view or biases of the writer; and knowledge of the degree of competence of the writer to record events authoritatively and accurately.

Data Synthesis and Analysis

After evaluating the authenticity and accuracy of historical data, the researcher must begin to pull the materials together, to analyze them, and to test the research hypotheses. Data that have passed the tests of internal and external criticism are not uniformly useful: the relative value of the various sources must be weighed. The historical researcher must be extremely careful at this point because the analysis of historical information involves logical processes rather than statistical ones and, therefore, the possibility of subjectivity arises. That is to say, the researcher must take care not to disregard evidence that either contradicts or fails to support the hypotheses. In essence, the final steps of historical research involve a considerable amount of decision making. The entire mass of evidence must be organized and weighed, and problems about inconsistencies must be resolved. Judgments have to be made, but they should be made in as objective a manner as possible.

Once the data have been organized, analyzed, and synthesized, conclusions and interpretations need to be formulated. The historical researcher, to a greater degree than other researchers, must be cautious in generalizing the results of the research because events can never be duplicated exactly.

Example of Historical Research

Table 11-4 summarizes several published historical studies conducted by nurse researchers. A more detailed example is described below.

Hardy (1988) conducted a historical study that focused on the American Nurses' Association (ANA) policies with respect to federal funding for nursing education between 1952 and 1972. Data concerning forces internal to the ANA, interorganizational health care relationships, the political climate in the federal government, and trends in higher education were gathered from nursing and government sources. The data were grouped into three sequential periods: 1952 to 1959, 1959 to 1969, and 1969 to 1972. A major purpose of the study was to use the information concerning the three periods as a basis for developing policy implications.

The primary sources used for collecting data included minutes of ANA and other nursing committees, reports of nursing committees, letters between ANA nursing leaders and congressional personnel, memoes from ANA leadership to state level nursing leaders, and congressional records and statutes. Secondary sources included material from nursing texts, journal articles, and pamphlets from nursing organizations.

Hardy's historical analysis led to some interesting conclusions. The analysis and synthesis of her rich array of data revealed that the ANA policy for federal funding was influenced to a large ex-

Table 11-4. *Examples of Historical Nursing Studies*

PROBLEM STATEMENT	SOURCE
What is the historical meaning of the concept of "caring" for nursing, and what is the relationship between nursing, womanhood, and the concept of caring over the course of the past century?	Reverby, 1987
How have nurses historically used the political system to shape health policies affecting patient welfare and nurses' working conditions?	Rogge, 1987
What are some of the conflicts of loyalties that nurses have historically faced, and how have these conflicted loyalties hindered the attainment of their own goals?	Baer, 1989
How have solutions to past nursing shortages contributed to current nursing shortages?	King, 1989
What common themes are revealed in letters written by nurses caring for service personnel during World War I?	Baer, 1987

tent by forces within nursing, the political climate in Washington, and societal trends in higher education. For example, the policy developed during the 1952 to 1959 period endorsed federal funding for all types of nursing education. Between 1959 to 1969, the policy supported collegiate education. The policies reverted to more broad-based nursing educational funding during 1969 to 1972. Hardy noted that the strong collaborative efforts developed among nursing organizations may have contributed to the continued federal funding support that nursing education currently receives.

☰ *CASE STUDIES*

Case studies are in-depth investigations of an individual, group, institution, or other social unit. The researcher conducting a case study attempts to analyze and understand the variables that are important to the history, development, or care of the subject or the subject's problems. As befits an intensive analysis, the focus of case studies is typically on determining the dynamics of *why* the subject of the investigation thinks, behaves, or develops in a particular manner, rather than *what* his or her status, progress, actions, or thoughts are. It is not unusual for probing research of this type to require a rather detailed study over a considerable period. Data are often collected that relate not only to the subject's present state but also to past experiences and situational and environmental factors relevant to the problem being examined.

The Functions of Case Studies

Case studies are a useful way to explore phenomena that have not been rigorously researched. For example, as new reproductive technologies have emerged (such as *in vitro* fertilization), several case studies have reported on the experiences of the couple undergoing treatment, laying the groundwork for more extensive research.

The information obtained in case studies can be extremely useful in the production of hypotheses to be tested more rigorously in subsequent research. Indeed, many writers consider this the most obvious and direct scientific function of case materials. For example, Freud's case studies of clients with personality disorders and problems led him to formulate an elaborate theoretical system. Although Freud did not test the hypotheses implied by his theories, some of the relationships suggested by his work have been studied more systematically by subsequent investigators. The intensive probing that characterizes case studies often leads to insights concerning previously unsuspected relationships. Furthermore, in-depth case studies may serve the very important role of clarifying concepts and variables or of elucidating ways to measure them.

Case studies sometimes are used in conjunction with large-scale research projects to serve in an illustrative capacity. Research reports that are filled with extensive statistical information often fail to convey some of the richness of the real-life subject matter. Qualitative case materials presented in such a context can be extremely effective in elucidating certain points or in imparting a more realistic impression to data that might otherwise appear far removed from practical concerns.

It is often risky to make predictions or generalizations to a broader population based on case study data. However, it may be perfectly reasonable to predict the future behavior of an individual who is the subject of the case study based on events or relationships experienced by the person in the past.

Case Study Methods

Unlike many of the types of research we have discussed in earlier chapters, there is no clear-cut, specified technique associated with case studies. The first step, as one might expect, is to delineate the problem area to be studied. This is seldom difficult in case studies because the majority of such studies seem to arise from attempts to solve a specific practical problem, as often happens in nursing and other clinical situations. Once the problem area and the case or cases to be studied have been identified, the researcher must develop a research design and a data collection plan.

Most case studies are nonexperimental; in such studies, the researcher obtains a wealth of descriptive information and may examine relationships among different variables, or may examine trends over time. Some case studies, however, involve the administration of a treatment and an analysis of ensuing consequences on the individual. Such studies are sometimes referred to as *single-subject experiments*. Time series designs are often especially appropriate in such situations. For example, suppose we were interested in examining the effect of a therapeutic approach on the behavior of an autistic child. We would begin by isolating one or more specific behaviors as a measure of the child's status, as for example, the child's ability to play quietly without becoming violent or the child's willingness to take medications. Before instituting any treatment (therapy), we would record the child's baseline behavior on the criterion measures for a short time. Once therapy begins, we would carefully monitor and record criterion measures either until the desired behavior patterns were obtained or for a specified time. Because other events or circumstances in the child's life could be responsible for improved behavior, the design would be strengthened by having a *reversal phase,* that is, a period in which the treatment is withheld. If there is subsequent deterioration in the subject's behavior pattern, we would have more confidence that it is the treatment, rather than extraneous factors, that is producing the desired effect.

Finally, as a further check, the treatment could be reinstituted, and further measurements of the criterion variable made. Figure 11-2 presents some hypothetical data for the example of the autistic child's play behavior using such a design, which is the design that was diagrammed in Chapter 9 as Figure 9-13. These data provide rather clear-cut evidence of the treatment's efficacy; in reality, the data would typically be less conclusive.

There is considerable freedom in selecting or devising a way to gather data for case studies. Virtually all the data-collecting methods available in research are amenable to use in a case study: questionnaires and interviews, observation schemes, rating devices, physiologic measures, personal documents such as diaries or letters, statistical records, and so forth. The researcher

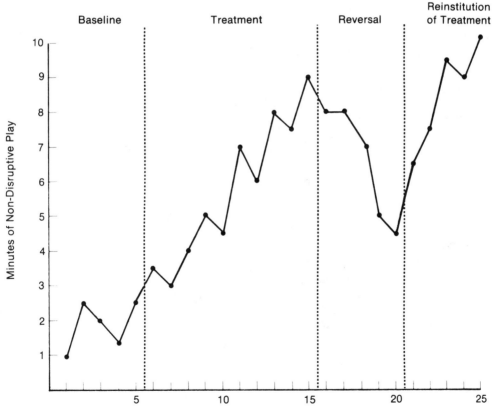

Figure 11-2. *Hypothetical example of an autistic child's play behavior.*

may select one of these techniques or may combine several. Case studies frequently involve the collection of both qualitative and quantitative data.

Finally, the data collected must be analyzed and interpreted. Because the investigator becomes well acquainted with the subject, and because there are typically no controls or comparisons to put the data into broader perspective, there may be a risk of subjectivity or bias in performing case studies. It is wise to be conservative in interpreting case study data.

Strengths and Weaknesses of Case Studies

Unquestionably the greatest advantage of case studies is the depth that is possible when a limited number of individuals, institutions, or groups is being investigated. A common complaint leveled at other types of research is that the data tend to be rather superficial. Case studies provide the researcher with the opportunity of having an intimate knowledge of the subject's condition, thoughts, feelings, actions (past and present), intentions, and environment.

On the other hand, this same strength is a potential weakness, because the familiarity of the researcher with the subject may make objectivity more difficult. Objectivity may be particularly problematic if the data are collected by observational techniques for which the researcher is the main (or only) observer.

Perhaps the most serious disadvantage of the case study method is its lack of generalizability. That is, if the researcher reveals the existence of important relationships, it is generally difficult to argue that the same relationships would manifest themselves in other subjects.

Example of a Case Study

Baltes and Zerbe (1976) conducted a case study of an elderly woman living in a nursing home who, although physically able, was not feeding herself. The researchers hypothesized that a change in environmental conditions would result in a change in the subject's self-feeding behaviors.

The investigators observed and recorded the subject's eating behavior during breakfast, dinner, and supper for one week before beginning any treatment. The treatment consisted of prompting the subject to feed herself by giving verbal instructions, placing the spoon in the subject's hand, and progressively raising it to her mouth. As soon as the subject responded to any stage of the treatment, reinforcement of the positive self-feeding behavior occurred by providing flowers, music, and liquids. Non−self-feeding behaviors of the subject resulted in removing the flowers, stopping the music, and turning the investigator's back to the subject. As soon as the subject began to feed herself, the positive reinforcers returned.

The results of the study supported the hypothesis that changes in environmental conditions resulted in a change in the subject's self-feeding behavior. The presence of flowers, music, and social interaction enhanced self-feeding. Return to the environmental conditions existing before the study produced a decline in self-feeding behavior.

This case study involved the administration of a treatment. Baseline data were collected before instituting the treatment. Once the subject began to feed herself in a consistent fashion, the treatment was withheld, i.e., the reversal phase was implemented. As the subject's self-feeding behavior declined during the reversal phase, the investigators gained more confidence that the change in self-feeding behavior resulted from the treatment. The treatment was not reinstituted in this study because the subject died.

≡ SECONDARY ANALYSIS

The types of research reviewed thus far have an important characteristic in common—the investigator must collect or organize new data. This section deals with research projects that use previously gathered data.

The amount of research conducted every

year in such fields as nursing, medicine, public health, nutrition, the life sciences, and the social sciences is overwhelming. In a typical research project, more data are collected than the investigator actually analyzes. Even when the initial researcher does utilize all of the data, he or she does not typically exhaust the possibilities of examining the relationships among the variables. This is particularly true of large-scale data sets, such as the ones collected by the National Center for Health Statistics (NCHS) and the Center for Epidemiologic Studies, but may be true of smaller research projects as well. It is, therefore, becoming increasingly common for researchers to use available data to test their research hypotheses. This type of research activity, referred to as *secondary analysis,* is extremely valuable because it is efficient and economical.

Secondary Analysis Approaches

Let us explore some of the possibilities of secondary analysis by considering a hypothetical example. Suppose that an investigator were interested in exploring staff attitudes toward mental illness and modes of patient treatment in psychiatric hospitals and the relationship between these attitudes and a variety of patient outcomes (e.g., number of patients released on trial visits, number of hours of restraint or seclusion, number of unauthorized absences of the patients, and so forth). Let us assume that the researcher has collected the attitudinal information from several hundred staff members in five hospitals by means of a questionnaire, which also included a number of background information questions about each staff person, such as position, number of years of experience, age, education, sex, and so forth. The original research study, however, does not make use of this background information (except to describe the sample), because the focus of the investigation is on hospital units, not on individual staff members. Thus, the original investigator may find that in hospital units where the staff as a whole tended to view patients unfavorably and tended to interpret hospital rules in an authoritarian manner, there also tended to be fewer patients released on trial visits, a greater number of patient elopements, and a higher number of hours during which patients were secluded or restrained. At this point, the researcher has tested the hypotheses that guided the initial study yet has left unanalyzed a considerable amount of data.

At some subsequent point, a nurse researcher might hypothesize that an authoritarian attitude toward mentally ill patients among the nursing staff is related to the nurse's age, educational background, status in the nursing hierarchy, and other background characteristics. The information collected in the original study could provide the nurse researcher with an excellent opportunity for testing the new hypotheses. In such a situation, the unit of analysis would be individual staff members and would be restricted only to nursing personnel. This secondary analysis would ignore the data relating to patient outcomes, because they are irrelevant to the hypotheses of the new investigation.

This example illustrates a number of avenues for secondary analyses. First, variables that are unanalyzed in an initial investigation are prime targets for further research. Furthermore, different relationships among variables can be explored in later uses of the data. In our example, the attitudinal variables that were the independent variables in the primary analysis became the dependent variables in the secondary analysis. That is, the initial analysis used the staff attitudes to "explain" patient outcomes; the secondary analysis used background characteristics to "explain" nursing staff attitudes.

The example shows two other approaches adopted in secondary analyses. Whereas the initial researcher utilized data from all subjects, the investigator in the later project was interested in only a subsample, the nursing personnel. It is frequently the case that secondary analysis concentrates on a particular subgroup rather than on the entire sample. A study that examined nursing students' withdrawal from a nursing program might generate data useful for further research on the needs and problems of minority nursing dropouts. An investigation of health habits and health-related behaviors in urban areas could produce information of interest to a researcher concerned with pica practice among urban children.

Another possibility for secondary analysis illustrated by our example is a change in the unit of analysis. In this example, the original research was concerned with aggregate data, that is, with the data from several individuals collapsed (averaged) within a bigger unit—the hospital ward. The researcher could have used an even larger unit—the hospital as a whole. The secondary analysis used the most basic element (individual responses) as the unit of analysis.

Secondary analysis can be particularly powerful if it is possible to obtain two or more data sets with comparable variables. If similar relationships between variables are revealed in different samples or populations, then the researcher can be much more confident that the results are generalizable to other groups. Secondary analyses of data sets that complement each other in this way can be particularly valuable in formulating general propositions or theories.

Sources of Data for Secondary Analysis

A major source of secondary data of interest to nurse researchers is the various surveys sponsored by NCHS. For example, NCHS periodically conducts such national surveys as the National Health Interview Survey (NHIS) and the Health Promotion and Disease Prevention (HPDP) Survey, both of which gather health-related information from thousands of individuals all over the United States. Box 11-1 presents a description of one survey conducted by NCHS, to give readers a sense of the kind of data sets that are available for secondary analysis.

In recent years, a number of groups such as university institutes and federal agencies have been attempting to organize data and make them available to researchers for secondary analysis. The policies regulating the public use of data vary from one organization to another, but it is not unusual for data to be provided to an interested researcher at about the cost for duplication plus handling. Thus, in some cases in which the gathering of the data involved an expenditure of hundreds of thousands of dollars, reproduced materials may be supplied for less than 1% of the initial costs.

Secondary analysis of large-scale data sets is becoming increasingly feasible because of the development of data libraries, such as the International Data Library and Reference Service at the University of California (Berkeley) or the Roper Public Opinion Research Center at Williams College (Williamstown, Massachusetts). In addition, a number of groups, in some cases funded by the National Science Foundation, are attempting to inventory and catalog the data libraries, such as the Council of Social Science Data Archives in New York City. The federal government sometimes sponsors the establishment of data archives on health-related topics. For example, the U.S. Office of Population Affairs sponsors the Data Archive on Adolescent Pregnancy Prevention. Many universities and research institutes within universities maintain "libraries" of data sets from large national surveys.

Small-scale, localized studies are unlikely to be included in data libraries. Nevertheless, the research community often cooperates in supplying data for secondary analysis to other researchers. An investigator may learn of existing data that are suitable for his or her research needs from colleagues, or in a journal article, report, or a presentation at a professional conference. In such an event, it may well be worth exploring the possibility of borrowing the data or of engaging in a collaborative research activity.

Strengths and Weaknesses of Secondary Analysis

The use of available data makes it possible for the researcher to bypass time-consuming and costly steps in the research process. Investigators engaged in a secondary analysis can typically proceed directly from the formulation of research hypotheses to a testing of those hypotheses. There is no need to obtain a sample, design an instrument, or gather the data. Thus, the greatest advantage of secondary analysis is its expediency.

On the other hand, there are numerous disadvantages in working with existing data. If an investigator does not play a role in collecting the data, the chances are pretty good that the data set will be deficient or problematic in one or more ways, such as in the sample used, the variables measured, and so forth. The researcher may continuously face "if only" problems: if only they had asked a question about _____, or if only they had included _____ in their sample. Furthermore, one always takes a risk of obtaining data that are inaccurate or erroneous. Errors can enter into the research endeavor at a number of phases: the interviewers may have been inexperienced, clerical errors can be made, questionnaires can be lost, and so forth. This is not to say that errors do not arise in one's own project, but at least with self-collected data the problem areas are more likely to be known. It is usually easier, in any event, to work with one's own mistakes than with someone else's. Finally, it may be difficult, if not impossible, to find data relevant to a research area of interest.

Examples of Secondary Analysis

As nurse researchers have become increasingly skilled in analyzing large data sets with sophisticated statistical procedures, they have also turned increasingly to undertaking secondary analyses. Table 11-5 presents a few examples, and one detailed example is discussed below.

For more than a decade, the U.S. Department of Education has sponsored large-scale surveys of high school students for the purpose of understanding how educational variables later affect the life outcomes of students. The first of these surveys involved some 19,000 male and female seniors selected from a national sample of high schools in 1971–1972. The study, referred to as the National Longitudinal Study of the Class of 1972, or NLS-72, has subsequently obtained follow-up data from the same students in 1973, 1974, 1976, 1979, and 1986.

Dunkelberger and Aadland (1984)

BOX 11-1 DESCRIPTION OF A SURVEY CONDUCTED BY THE NATIONAL CENTER FOR HEALTH STATISTICS AND AVAILABLE FOR SECONDARY ANALYSIS

Name:	1988 National Health Interview Survey (NHIS), Child Health Supplement
Purpose:	To provide detailed information on the physical and mental health, school performance and behavior of children in the United States
Design:	Data were collected from a national sample of households as part of the NHIS. The Child Health Supplement involved the collection of information for one child aged 0 to 17 years in each family having such a child. In families with more than one eligible child, one was selected at random. A knowledgeable adult member of the household (usually the biologic mother) served as a proxy respondent for each selected child.
Sample:	A nationally representative sample of approximately 20,000 children
Content:	The 1988 Child Health Supplement covers the following topics: child care arrangements (for children under age 6 years); residential mobility; circumstances surrounding birth; accidental injuries; chronic medical conditions and their effects; smoking in household (current and during pregnancy); preventive health care and habits; behavior in school; need for use of psychologic counseling; behavior problems; sleep habits; and background characteristics of the family.

made use of this publicly available data set, using data collected through 1979, to examine patterns of attainment of nursing careers. From the thousands of participants in the NLS survey, the investigators selected three sub-groups for secondary analysis: (1) those who expected to become nurses while they were in high school and went on to do so, (2) those who expected to become nurses while in high school but failed to do so, and (3) those who did not expect a nursing career but went on to become nurses. A total of 768 subjects in the NLS sample fell into one of these categories.

The investigator's analyses revealed that only 34% of those who planned to become nurses actually did so. Background variables were found to be related to nonattainment of a nursing career goal. Those who failed to become nurses despite their early interest were more often from low socioeconomic backgrounds and were more often nonwhite than those in the other two groups. However, among the subjects who did ultimately become nurses, few characteristics distinguished those who had articulated their goals in high school from those who had not.

This study capitalized on available data to answer questions about patterns of pursuing a nursing career. Such data, involving a survey of a national sample of students over a 7-year period, would have been prohibitively expensive if the investigators had had to collect the information themselves.

≡ META-ANALYSIS

Chapter 6 described the function of a literature review as a preliminary step in a research project. However, there is growing recognition of the fact that the careful integration of knowledge on a topic in itself constitutes an important scholarly endeavor that can contribute new knowledge.

The procedure known as *meta-analysis* represents an application of statistical procedures to findings from research reports. In essence, meta-analysis regards the findings from one study as a single piece of "data." The findings from multiple studies on the same topic can, therefore, be combined to yield a data set that can be analyzed in a manner similar to that obtained from individual subjects.

Meta-analysis Procedures

The earliest form of nonnarrative research integration used what has been referred to as the *voting method*. This procedure involves tallying the outcomes of previous studies to determine

Table 11-5. *Examples of Secondary Analyses by Nurse Researchers*

PROBLEM STATEMENT	DATA SET USED
What are the personal and social factors that predict a positive life outlook of older single women? (Hoeffer, 1987)	1975 National Survey of the Aged
Does the labor force participation among RNs differ from that of women in comparable occupations? (Greenleaf, 1983)	Pooled national surveys, 1972–1980, General Social Surveys
What factors are related to job satisfaction among recent graduates of nursing programs? (Munro, 1983)	The National Longitudinal Survey of the High School Class of 1972
What is the risk of disabling back disorders among nursing personnel in comparison with that of employees in other occupations? (Jensen, 1987)	Bureau of Labor Statistics Supplementary Data System

what outcome has received the greatest empirical support. For example, suppose we were reviewing studies that investigated whether exposing low-birthweight infants to auditory stimulation resulted in improved behavioral development compared with infants with no special treatment. There are three possible outcomes: (1) a gain for infants exposed to auditory stimulation, (2) a gain for those not exposed, and (3) no group difference. An analysis using the voting method would involve counting which of these three outcomes was obtained most frequently in studies performed to date.

The voting method has since been superseded by methods of considerable sophistication and complexity. Because beginning researchers may have no statistical background, a discussion of actual statistical procedures cannot be included here. Suffice it to say that these methods, described in detail by Glass, McGaw, and Smith (1981), generally involve the calculation of an index known as the *effect size,* which quantifies how different two groups are with respect to the dependent variable. The effect size statistic is computed in such a way that it is independent of the method of measuring the dependent variable. For example, Falbo and Polit (1985) compared the effect of being raised with and without siblings on a child's development. In studying the intellectual development of only children and siblings, the results of studies using a variety of measures of intellectual ability (Scholastic Aptitude Test scores, Wechsler IQ scores, Raven Progressive Matrices scores, and so on) were combined.

Because the effect-size statistic is a numerical value, it is possible to perform analyses focusing on the relationship between the effect size and other variables. In other words, it is possible to test hypotheses concerning variations in the effect size. For example, Falbo and Polit (1985) found that, across numerous studies, only children scored higher on tests of ability than children raised with siblings. However, the difference was especially pronounced among younger children and diminished in magnitude with older subjects. Thus, meta-analysis permitted an exam-

ination of the relationship between age and only child/nononly child differences in ability.

Advantages and Disadvantages of Meta-analysis

Traditional narrative reviews of the literature are handicapped by several factors uncharacteristic of meta-analysis. The first is that if the number of studies on a specific topic is large and if the results are inconsistent, then it is difficult to draw conclusions. The second is that narrative reviews are often subject to potential biases. The researcher may unwittingly give more weight to findings that are congruent with his or her own viewpoints. Third, in narrative reviews it is seldom possible to examine relationships between the findings and other study variables. Thus, meta-analytic procedures provide a convenient and objective method of integrating a large body of findings and of observing patterns and relationships that might otherwise have gone undetected. Furthermore, meta-analysis provides information about the magnitude of differences and relationships. Meta-analysis can thus serve as an important scholarly tool in theory development and in pointing the way for new areas of research.

Meta-analysis has also been criticized on a number of grounds. One issue has been called the "fruit problem"—that is, the possibility of combining studies that conceptually do not belong with each other (apples and oranges). Another issue is that there is generally a bias in the studies appearing in published sources. Studies in which no differences or no relationships have been found are less likely to be published and, therefore, less likely to be included in the meta-analysis. Narrative literature reviews are subject to the same two problems, but these problems may take on added significance in a meta-analysis because the quantitative results make the conclusions seem more concrete and absolute. Another problem is that a research report could provide general information about the study's findings but might not include sufficient quantitative information for computing an effect size. Despite these potential problems, careful and thorough meta-analyses represent an important advancement to the scientific community.

Example of a Meta-analysis

Devine and Cook (1983) performed a meta-analysis of 49 studies that investigated the effect of psychoeducational interventions on patients' length of postsurgical hospital stay. Their research examined whether interventions such as teaching skills to reduce pain, providing psychologic support, and providing information about the surgical procedures were associated with reductions in hospital stay. Their analyses also involved the testing of several hypotheses. For example, because the average hospital stay has declined over time, the question of whether the effects (if any) of interventions have remained stable over time or were subject to "floor effects" (i.e., perhaps the lower limit of length of patient stay has been reached, regardless of psychoeducational interventions) was raised.

Devine and Cook did a thorough review of both published and unpublished sources. Their analysis revealed that across the 49 studies, interventions reduced hospital stay by about 1.25 days on average. They found that this reduction did not depend on whether the study was published or unpublished or on whether the discharging physician was aware of the patients' experimental condition. They also found that the beneficial effects of the psychoeducational intervention became smaller over time.

This research provided not only a summary of the effectiveness of the interventions but also an estimate of the magnitude of the effect. Furthermore, Devine and Cook were able to address several questions about variations in the effect over time and across studies with different methods. Their review provided considerably more information than could have been obtained with more traditional methods of review.

≡ *METHODOLOGICAL RESEARCH*

We conclude this chapter with a brief discussion of research whose central aim is to make a contribution to the methods used in performing research. *Methodological research* refers to controlled investigations of the ways of obtaining, organizing, and analyzing data. Methodological studies address the development, validation, and evaluation of research tools or techniques. Nurse researchers in recent years have become increasingly interested in methodological research. This is not surprising in light of growing demands for sound and reliable measures and for sophisticated procedures for obtaining and analyzing data.

The methodological researcher may, to take an example, concentrate on the development of an instrument that accurately measures patients' satisfaction with nursing care. The researcher in such a case is not interested in the level of patient satisfaction nor in how such satisfaction relates to characteristics of the nurses, the hospital, or the patients. The goal of the researcher is to develop an effective, serviceable, and trustworthy instrument that can be used by other researchers, and to evaluate his or her success in accomplishing this goal.

Another example of methodological research would be a study that investigated procedures for enhancing the rate of response to mailed questionnaires. The investigator might use a true experimental design in which subjects might be randomly assigned to one of three types of cover letters accompanying the questionnaire: (1) a simple cover letter requesting cooperation, written by the investigator; (2) a cover letter written on the official stationery of some important and prominent person, such as the head of a state licensing board for nurses; and (3) a cover letter that promised the prospective participant a reward (monetary or otherwise) for cooperating in the study.

Methodological research may seem less exciting and less rewarding than substantive research, but it is virtually impossible to conduct outstanding and meaningful research on a substantive topic with inadequate research tools. Studies of a methodological nature are indispensable in any scientific discipline, and perhaps especially so when a field is relatively new and deals with highly complex, intangible phenomena such as human behavior or welfare, as is the case in nursing research.

Examples of Methodological Research

In 1981, an entire issue of the journal *Nursing Research* was devoted to methodological research—specifically, to studies designed to develop, improve, or evaluate measuring tools for nursing research. For example, Mishel (1981) discussed the development of a conceptual model for understanding the role of "uncertainty in illness" as an important determinant of patients' experiences in illness, treatment, and hospitalization. Based on the model, a 30-item test was developed: the Mishel Uncertainty in Illness Scale (MUIS). The article described the procedures that the author used in three separate validation studies to evaluate the utility of the new instrument. The author concluded that "the MUIS appears to be a useful instrument for investigating the role of uncertainty in illness and recovery" (p. 263).

Another example from the same issue of *Nursing Research* is the study of Brandt and Weinert (1981), who described the development of the Personal Resource Questionnaire (PRQ), a 25-item instrument designed to measure the availability and intensity of a person's social supports. The focus of the report was methodological considerations; that is, the authors described the steps that were taken to develop, refine, and evaluate the worth of the PRQ.

Careful methodological research has as its ultimate goal the improvement of the quality of research with a more substantive focus. The two instruments just described have subsequently been subjected to further methodological assessments and used in many other research studies. For example, Brandt (1984) used the PRQ to examine whether mothers of children with a developmental delay varied their discipline in relation to the amount of social support available to them; Aaronson (1989) used the PRQ in a study of the effects of social support on health behavior during pregnancy; and Yarcheski and Mahon (1989) used this instrument to test a causal model of positive health practices among adolescents. With regard to the MUIS, Mishel and Braden (1988) used the scale to explore factors related to reductions in uncertainty in illness among women with gynecologic cancer; Webster and Christman (1988) examined the relationship between uncertainty in illness and the use of various coping strategies among patients with myocardial infarction; and Yarcheski (1988) used the MUIS with a sample of chronically ill adolescents and their parents to examine the relationship between uncertainty in illness and future time perspective. Davis (1990) used both the MUIS and the PRQ in her study of illness uncertainty, social support, and stress among patients recovering from a major health crisis and their family care givers.

☰ SUMMARY

Survey research is the branch of research that examines the characteristics, behaviors, attitudes, and intentions of a group of people by asking individuals belonging to that group (typically only a subset) to answer a series of questions. Survey research is an extremely flexible research approach and, therefore, is quite diversified with respect to populations studied, scope, content, and purpose. The most powerful method of collecting survey information is the *personal interview* in which interviewers meet with participants in a face-to-face situation and question them directly. This method has the advantage of encouraging cooperation, which results in higher response rates and a better quality of data. *Tele-*

phone interviews have grown in popularity in recent years but, although this approach is convenient and economical, it is not recommended when the interview is long or detailed or when the questions are sensitive or highly personal. *Questionnaires* are self-administered; that is, questions are read by the respondent, who then gives a written response. Questionnaires are often distributed through the mail, but because of the generally low response rates of mailed surveys, some type of personal contact generally is recommended.

Field studies are in-depth studies of people or groups conducted in naturalistic settings—that is, in the "field." The aim of the researcher is to "get close" to some phenomenon as it evolves in real life (i.e., to obtain first-hand information about how people think, act, and feel relative to the phenomenon of interest). Field research generally involves the simultaneous collection and analysis of narrative, qualitative materials that may be collected through in-depth interviews, through observations of naturally occurring events and behavior, and through an examination of available documents. One of the most difficult aspects of field studies often is gaining entry into the group being studied.

Evaluation research is the process of collecting and analyzing information relating to the functioning of a program, policy, or procedure to assist decision makers in choosing a course of action. Various evaluation models have been developed. The *classical approach* evaluates the congruence between the goals of the program and actual outcomes. Goals are typically phrased in the form of *behavioral objectives,* which delineate the intended outcomes of a program in terms of the behaviors of the program's beneficiaries. The *goal-free approach* attempts to understand all of the effects of a program, whether or not they were intended. Evaluations are typically undertaken to answer a variety of questions. *Process* or *implementation analyses* are undertaken to describe the process by which a program gets implemented and how it is functioning in practice. When such analyses are undertaken with the

intent of improving the program, they are sometimes referred to as *formative evaluations.* Evaluations that test the effectiveness of a program are sometimes called *summative evaluations.* Such evaluations may take the form of *outcome analyses,* which basically describe the status of some condition following the introduction of some intervention, or *impact analyses,* which typically use rigorous designs to test whether the intervention caused any *net impacts. Cost–benefit analyses* attempt to answer the question of whether the monetary costs of a program are outweighed by the monetary benefits.

Needs assessments are another type of applied research aimed at providing useful information for planners and decision makers. A needs assessment is an investigation of the needs of a group, community, or organization for certain types of services or policies. Because organizations and groups are almost constantly in transition and because their needs may change through time, needs assessments can serve a useful purpose both before *and* after a service program is in operation. Several techniques or approaches are used in the conduct of needs assessments, notably the *key informant, survey,* or *indicator* approaches.

Historical research is the systematic attempt to establish facts and relationships concerning past events. The historical researcher utilizes the scientific method insofar as possible to answer questions or test hypotheses by objectively evaluating and interpreting available historical evidence. Historiographers are at a disadvantage from a research point of view in that they can neither manipulate nor randomize anything, nor have they much control over the quality and quantity of their data. The data are usually in the form of written records from the past (such as letters, diaries, or legal documents), but physical artifacts and audio or visual materials represent another potential source of information. Historical data are normally subjected to two forms of evaluation: (1) *external criticism,* which is concerned with the authenticity of the source, and (2) *internal criticism,* which assesses the worth of the evidence.

Case studies are intensive investigations of a single entity or a small number of entities. Typically, that entity is a human, but groups, organizations, families, or communities may sometimes be the focus of concern. In a case study, the investigator examines the individual in-depth by probing into the history or development of the subject with respect to the characteristics or behaviors of interest. Case studies can be quite valuable in the production of hypotheses or the demonstration of some clinical approach that could be subjected to more rigorous testing. When an intervention is being demonstrated or assessed, it may be possible to conduct a *single subject experiment*. Such studies generally involve collecting data over an extended period using a time series design. The case study offers the potential of great depth but runs the risk of subjectivity and severely limited generalizability.

Secondary analysis refers to research projects in which the investigator analyzes previously collected data. Research studies typically produce more data than can be analyzed at one time, and, hence, existing data sets offer an economical and efficient means of testing hypotheses. Four possible approaches to secondary analysis were explored. The secondary investigator may (1) examine unanalyzed variables, (2) test unexplored relationships, (3) focus on a particular subsample, or (4) change the *unit of analysis*. The use of existing data offers the potential of saving time and resources, but the secondary analyst pays for this efficiency by the inability to gather *exactly* the kinds of data that he or she needs and by the possibility of working with inaccurate or problematic data sets.

Meta-analysis is a method of integrating the findings of prior research using statistical procedures. Meta-analyses typically involve the calculation of an *effect size* that quantifies relationships and differences between groups. Effect sizes from numerous studies can then be averaged to provide a numerical estimate of the magnitude of relationships; effect size variations can also be studied in relation to sample characteristics and study approaches. Although meta-analytic procedures are subject to some constraints and problems, they represent an important avenue of integration and theory development.

In *methodological research,* the investigator is concerned with the development, validation, and assessment of methodological tools or strategies. The researcher conducting a methodological study focuses primarily on increasing knowledge with respect to the methods used in performing scientific research rather than contributing to some substantive area. In nursing research, methodological studies are playing an increasingly important role in refining and improving the techniques for analyzing nursing problems, particularly in the development of useful measuring tools.

≡ STUDY SUGGESTIONS

1. Read one of the studies listed under "Substantive References: Survey Research." Ascertain the type of questions (background information, behavioral data, attitudes, and so forth) asked in the survey.

2. Suppose you were interested in studying the attitude of nurses toward caring for patients with AIDS. Would you use a personal interview, telephone interview, or questionnaire to collect your data? Why?

3. An investigator is interested in doing a field study focusing on efforts of drug addicts to shake their addiction. Where might such a field study take place? How might the researcher gain entry into an appropriate setting?

4. A psychiatric nurse therapist working with emotionally disturbed children is interested in evaluating a program of play therapy. Explain how you might proceed if you were to use
   a. the classical evaluation model
   b. a goal-free approach
   Which approach do you think would be more useful, and why?

5. For each of the following practices or procedures derive one or more hypothetical objectives and state them as *behavioral* objectives:
   a. a crisis intervention program for drug abusers
   b. procedures to educate primaparas with respect to breast-feeding of their infants
   c. a program to interest nursing students in working with elderly people
   d. an instructional unit to teach student nurses how to administer subcutaneous injections
6. Explain how you would use the key informant, survey, and indicator approaches to assess the need to teach Spanish to nurses in a given community.
7. Identify a problem for study using the historical research approach. Formulate hypotheses. What might serve as primary sources for the data? How would you check the data for internal criticism?
8. Read one of the reports listed under "Substantive References: Secondary Analysis." Develop some hypotheses that could be tested using the same data set.
9. Read one of the reports listed under "Substantive References: Meta-analysis." Identify the conclusions reached by the researchers that would have been impossible in a narrative literature review.

≡ SUGGESTED READINGS

METHODOLOGICAL REFERENCES

Backstrom, C.H., & Hursh, G.D. (1981). *Survey research* (2nd ed.). Evanston, IL: Northwestern University Press.

Barlow, D.H., & Hersen, M. (1973). Single-case experimental designs. *Archives of General Psychiatry, 29,* 319–325.

Boruck, R.F. (1978). *Secondary analysis.* San Francisco: Jossey-Bass.

Christy, T.E. (1975). The methodology of historical research. *Nursing Research, 24,* 189–192.

Dillman, D. (1978). *Mail and telephone surveys: The Total Design Method.* New York: John Wiley and Sons.

Fairman, J.A. (1987). Sources and references for research in nursing history. *Nursing Research, 36,* 56–59.

Foreman, P.B. (1971). The theory of case studies. In B.J. Franklin & H.W. Osborne (Eds.), *Research methods: Issues and insights* (pp. 187–205). Belmont, CA: Wadsworth.

Fowler, F.J. (1984). *Survey research methods.* Beverly Hills, CA: Sage.

Glass, G.V., McGaw, B., & Smith, M.L. (1981). *Meta-analysis of social research.* Beverly Hills: Sage.

Guba, E.G., & Lincoln, Y.S. (1981). *Effective evaluation: Improving the usefulness of evaluation results through responsive and naturalistic approaches.* San Francisco: Jossey-Bass.

Hedges, L.V., & Olkin, I. (1985). *Statistical methods for meta-analysis.* Orlando, FL: Academic Press.

Holm, K. (1983). Single subject research. *Nursing Research, 32,* 253–255.

Hulley, S.B., & Cummings, S.R. (1988). *Designing clinical research: An epidemiological approach.* Baltimore: Williams and Wilkins. (Chapter 6).

Hyman, H.H. (1972). *Secondary analysis of sample survey: Principles, procedures and potentialities.* New York: John Wiley and Sons.

Kiecolt, K.J., & Nathan, L.E. (1985). *Secondary analysis of survey data.* Beverly Hills, CA: Sage.

Leininger, M. (Ed.) (1985). *Qualitative research methods in nursing.* New York: Grune & Stratton.

Lynn, M.R. (1989). Meta-analysis: Appropriate tool for the integration of nursing research? *Nursing Research, 38,* 302–305.

McCain, N.L., Smith, M.C., & Abraham, I.L. (1986). Meta-analysis of nursing interventions. *Western Journal of Nursing Research, 8,* 155–167.

McKillip, J. (1986). *Need analysis: Tools for the human services and education.* Beverly Hills, CA: Sage.

Meier, P., & Pugh, E.J. (1986). The case study: A viable approach to clinical research. *Research in Nursing and Health, 9,* 195–202.

Notter, L.E. (1972). The case for historical research in nursing. *Nursing Research, 21,* 483.

Rosenthal, R. (1984). *Meta-analytic procedures for social research.* Beverly Hills, CA: Sage.

Rossi, P.H. (1984). *Handbook of survey research.* New York: Academic Press.

Rossi, P.H., & Freeman, H.E. (1979). *Evaluation: A systematic approach.* Beverly Hills: Sage.

Schatzman, L., & Strauss, A. (1982). *Field research: Strategies for a natural sociology* (2nd ed.). Englewood Cliffs, NJ: Prentice-Hall.

Schulberg, H.C., & Baker, F. (1979). *Program evaluation in the health fields* (Vol. 2). New York: Human Sciences Press.

Shields, M. (1974). An evaluation model for service programs. *Nursing Outlook, 22,* 448–451.

Sorenson, E.S. (1988). Historiography: Archives as sources of treasure in historical research. *Western Journal of Nursing Research, 10,* 666–670.

Stewart, D.W. (1984). *Secondary research: Information services and methods.* Beverly Hills, CA: Sage.

Warheit, G.J., Bell, R.A., & Schwab, J.J. (1975). *Planning for change: Needs assessment approaches.* Washington, DC: National Institute of Mental Health.

Wilson, H.S. (1989). *Research in nursing* (2nd ed.). Menlo Park, CA: Addison-Wesley. (Chapter 12).

Yin, R.K. (1984). *Case study research.* Beverly Hills, CA: Sage.

SUBSTANTIVE REFERENCES

Survey Research

Damrosch, S.P., & Strasser, J.A. (1988). A survey of doctorally prepared academic nurses on qualitative and quantitative research issues. *Nursing Research, 37,* 176–180.

Deets, C., & Froebe, D.J. (1984). Incentives for nurse employment. *Nursing Research, 33,* 242–246.

Hendrix, M.J., Sabritt, D., McDaniel, A., & Field, B. (1987). Perceptions and attitudes toward nursing impairment. *Research in Nursing and Health, 10,* 323–333.

Kramer, M., & Hafner, L.P. (1989). Shared values: Impact on staff nurse job satisfaction and perceived productivity. *Nursing Research, 38,* 172–177.

Lile, J.L. (1990). Beliefs about coronary heart disease among selected southwestern residents. *Applied Nursing Research, 3,* 71–72.

Lusk, S.L., Disch, J.M., & Barkauskas, V.H. (1988). Interest of major corporations in expanded practice of occupational health nurses. *Research in Nursing and Health, 11,* 151–152.

Mandel, J.H., & Lohman, W. (1987). Low back pain in nurses. *Research in Nursing and Health, 10,* 165–170.

Moore, M.N. (1989). Tenure and the university reward structure. *Nursing Research, 38,* 111–116.

Shamansky, S.L., Schilling, L., & Holbrook. T.L. (1985).

Determining the market for nurse practitioner services. *Nursing Research, 34,* 242–247.

Smith, D.W., & Shamansky, S.L. (1983). Determining the market for family nurse practitioner services: The Seattle experience. *Nursing Research, 32,* 301–305.

Wiley, K., Heath, L., Acklin, M., Earl, A., & Barnard, B. (1990). Care of HIV-infected patients: Nurses' concerns, opinions, and precautions. *Applied Nursing Research, 3,* 27–33.

Young, C., McMahon, J.E., Bowman, V., & Thompson, D. (1989). Maternal reasons for delayed prenatal care. *Nursing Research, 38,* 242–243.

Field Studies

Alade, M.O. (1989). Teenage pregnancy in Ile-Ife, Western Nigeria. *Western Journal of Nursing Research, 11,* 609–613.

Barbee, E.L. Tensions in the brokerage role: Nurses in Botswana. *Western Journal of Nursing Research, 9,* 244–256.

Browner, C.H. (1987). Job stress and health: The role of social support at work. *Research in Nursing and Health, 10,* 93–100.

Cheon-Klessig, Y., Camilleri, D.D., McElmurry, B.J., & Ohlson, V.M. (1988). Folk medicine in the health practice of Hmong refugees. *Western Journal of Nursing Research, 10,* 647–660.

Dougherty, M.C., Courage, M.M., & Schilling, L.S. (1985). Ethnographic nursing research in a black community. In M.M. Leininger (Ed.), *Qualitative research methods in nursing.* New York: Grune & Stratton.

Katzman, E.M., & Roberts, J.I. (1988). Nurse–physician conflicts as barriers to the enactment of nursing roles. *Western Journal of Nursing Research, 10,* 576–590.

Kulig, J.C. (1990). Childbearing beliefs among Cambodian refugee women. *Western Journal of Nursing Research, 12,* 108–118.

Leininger, M.M. (1985). Southern rural black and white American lifeways with a focus on care and health phenomena. In M.M. Leininger (Ed.), *Qualitative research methods in nursing.* New York: Grune & Stratton.

Norris, C.M. (1975). Restlessness: A nursing phenomenon in search of a meaning. *Nursing Outlook, 23,* 103–107.

Swanson, J.M. (1988). The process of finding contraceptive options. *Western Journal of Nursing Research, 10,* 492–503.

Wing, D.M. (1990). A cross-cultural field study of nurses and political strategies. *Western Journal of Nursing Research, 12,* 373–385.

Evaluations and Needs Assessments

Derdiarian, A.K. (1986). Informational needs of recently diagnosed cancer patients. *Nursing Research, 35,* 276–281.

Dougherty, M., Bishop, K., Mooney, R., & Gimotty, P. (1989). The effect of circumvaginal (CVM) exercise. *Nursing Research, 38,* 331–335.

Frank, P. (1979). A survey of health needs of older adults in North West Johnson County, Iowa. *Nursing Research, 28,* 360–368.

Gillett, P.A., & Eisenman, P.A. (1987). The effect of intensity controlled aerobic dance exercise on aerobic capacity of middle-aged, overweight women. *Research in Nursing and Health, 10,* 383–390.

Golas, G.A., & Parks, P. (1986). Effect of early postpartum teaching on primiparas' knowledge of infant behavior and degree of confidence. *Research in Nursing and Health, 9,* 209–214.

Hain, M.J., & Chen, S.C. (1976). Health needs of the elderly. *Nursing Research, 25,* 433–439.

Kasper, J.W., & Nyamathi, A.M. (1988). Parents of children in the pediatric intensive care unit: What are their needs? *Heart and Lung, 17,* 574–581.

Martinson, I.M., Moldow, D.G., Armstrong, G.D., Henry, W.F., Nesbit, M.E., & Kersey, J.H. (1986). Home care for children dying of cancer. *Research in Nursing and Health, 9,* 11–16.

Mills, G., Barnes, R., Rodell, D., & Terry, L. (1985). An evaluation of an inpatient cardiac patient/family education program. *Heart and Lung, 14,* 400–406.

Mitchell, P.H., Armstrong, S., Simpson, T.F., & Lentz, M. (1989). American Association of Critical-Care Nurses Demonstration Project: Profile of excellence in critical care nursing. *Heart and Lung, 18,* 219–237.

Moss, J.R., & Craft, M.J. (1989). Visual estimation accuracy. *Western Journal of Nursing Research, 11,* 352–360.

Naylor, M.D. (1990). Comprehensive discharge planning for hospitalized elderly. *Nursing Research, 39,* 156–161.

Norris, L., & Grove, S. (1986). Investigation of selected psychsocial needs of family members of critically ill adult patients. *Heart and Lung, 15,* 194–199.

Simpson, T.F., Armstrong, S., & Mitchell, P. (1989). American Association of Critical-Care Nurses Demonstration Project: Patients' recollections of critical care. *Heart and Lung, 18,* 325–332.

Wooldridge, J.B., & Jackson, J.G. (1988). Evaluation of bruises and areas of induration after two techniques of subcutaneous heparin injection. *Heart and Lung, 17,* 476–482.

Historical Research

Baer, E.D. (1985). Nursing's divided house—An historical view. *Nursing Research, 34,* 32–38.

Baer, E.D. (1987). Letters to Miss Sanborn: St. Vincent Hospital nurses' accounts of World War I. *Journal of Nursing History, 2,* 17–32.

Baer, E.D. (1989). Nursing's divided loyalties: An historical case study. *Nursing Research, 38,* 166–171.

Buhler-Wilkerson, K. (1985). Public health nursing: In sickness or in health? *American Journal of Public Health, 75,* 1155–1161.

Church, O.M. (1985). Emergence of training programs for asylum nursing at the turn of the century. *Advances in Nursing Science, 7,* 35–46.

Hardy, M.A. (1988). Political savvy or lost opportunity? Evolution of the American Nurses' Association policy for nursing education funding, 1952–1972. *Journal of Professional Nursing, 4,* 205–217.

King, M.G. (1989). Nursing shortage, circa 1915. *Image: Journal of Nursing Scholarship, 21,* 124–127.

Norman, E.M. (1989). The wartime experience of military nurses in Vietnam, 1965–1973. *Western Journal of Nursing Research, 11,* 219–233.

Reverby, S. (1987). A caring dilemma: Womanhood and nursing in historical perspective. *Nursing Research, 36,* 5–11.

Rogge, M.M. (1987). Nursing and politics: A forgotten legacy. *Nursing Research, 36,* 26–30.

Silverstein, N.G. (1985). Lillian Wald at Henry Street, 1893–1895. *Advances in Nursing Science, 7,* 1–12.

Wheeler, C.E. (1985). *The American Journal of Nursing* and the socialization of a profession, 1900–1920. *Advances in Nursing Science, 7,* 20–34.

Case Studies

Anderson, J.M. (1985). Perspectives on the health of immigrant women: A feminist analysis. *Advances in Nursing Science, 8,* 61–76.

Baltes, M.M., & Zerbe, M.B. (1976). Reestablishing self-feeding in a nursing home resident. *Nursing Research, 25,* 24–26.

Peterson, B.H. (1985). A qualitative clinical account and analysis of a care situation. In M.M. Leininger

(Ed.). *Qualitative research methods in nursing.* New York: Grune & Stratton.

Wilson, H.S. (1982). *Deinstitutionalized residential care for the mentally disordered: The Soteria House approach.* New York: Grune & Stratton.

Secondary Analysis

Cohen, M.Z., & Loomis, M.E. (1985). Linguistic analysis of questionnaire responses: Methods of coping with work stress. *Western Journal of Nursing Research, 7,* 357–366.

Dunkelberger, J.E., & Aadland, S.C. (1984). Expectation and attainment of nursing careers. *Nursing Research, 33,* 235–240.

Greenleaf, N.P. (1983). Labor force participation among registered nurses and women in comparable occupations. *Nursing Research, 32,* 306–322.

Hoeffer, B. (1987). Predictors of life outlook of older single women. *Research in Nursing and Health, 10,* 111–117.

Jensen, R.C. (1987). Disabling back injuries among nursing personnel. *Research in Nursing and Health, 10,* 29–38.

Johansen, S., Bowles, S., & Haney, G. (1988). A model for forecasting intermittent skilled home nursing needs. *Research in Nursing and Health, 11,* 375–382.

Munro, B.H. (1983). Job satisfaction among recent graduates of schools of nursing. *Nursing Research, 32,* 350–361.

Munro, B.H. (1980). Dropouts from nursing education: Path analysis of a national sample. *Nursing Research, 29,* 371–377.

Meta-analysis

Broome, M.E., Lillis, P.P., & Smith, M.C. (1989). Pain interventions with children: A meta-analysis of research. *Nursing Research, 38,* 154–158.

Brown, S.A. (1988). Effects of educational interventions in diabetes care: A meta-analysis of findings. *Nursing Research, 37,* 223–230.

Burckhardt, C.S. (1987). The effect of therapy on the mental health of the elderly. *Research in Nursing and Health, 10,* 277–285.

Devine, E.C., & Cook, T.D. (1983). A meta-analytic analysis of effects of psychoeducational interventions on length of post-surgical hospital stay. *Nursing Research, 32,* 267–274.

Falbo, T., & Polit, D. (1985). A meta-analysis of the only child literature. *Pediatric Nursing, 11,* 356–360.

Heater, B.S., Becker, A.M., & Olson, R.K. (1988). Nursing interventions and patient outcomes: A meta-analysis of studies. *Nursing Research, 37,* 303–307.

Hyman, R.B., Feldman, H.R., Harris, R.B., Levin, R.F., & Malloy, G.B. (1989). The effects of relaxation training on clinical symptoms: A meta-analysis. *Nursing Research, 38,* 216–220.

Johnson, J.H. (1988). Differences in the performance of baccalaureate, associate degree, and diploma nurses: A meta-analysis. *Research in Nursing and Health, 11,* 183–197.

McCain, N.L., & Lynn, M.R. (1990). Meta-analysis of a narrative review: Studies evaluating patient teaching. *Western Journal of Nursing Research, 12,* 347–358.

Schwartz, R., Moody, L., Yarandi, H., & Anderson, G.C. (1987). A meta-analysis of critical outcome variables in nonnutritive sucking in preterm infants. *Nursing Research, 36,* 292–295.

Wilkie, D.J., Saverda, M.C., Holzemer, W.L., Tesler, M.D., & Paul, S.M. (1990). Use of the McGill Pain Questionnaire to measure pain: A meta-analysis. *Nursing Research, 39,* 36–41.

Methodological Research

Blank, D.M. (1985). Development of the infant tenderness scale. *Nursing Research, 34,* 211–216.

Brandt, P.A., & Weinert, C. (1981). The PRQ—A social support measure. *Nursing Research, 30,* 277–280.

Brown, M.S., & Kodadek, S.M. (1987). The use of lie scales in psychometric measures of children. *Research in Nursing and Health, 10,* 87–92.

Cox, C.L. (1985). The Health Self-Determination Index. *Nursing Research, 34,* 177–183.

Fenton, M.V. (1987). Development of the Scale of Humanistic Nursing Behaviors. *Nursing Research, 36,* 82–87.

Hester, N.O. (1984). Child's health self-concept scale: Its development and psychometric properties. *Advances in Nursing Science, 7,* 45–55.

Miller, J.F., & Powers, M.J. (1988). Development of an instrument to measure hope. *Nursing Research, 37,* 6–10.

Mishel, M.H. (1981). The measurement of uncertainty in illness. *Nursing Research, 30,* 258–263.

Quinless, F.W., & Nelson, M.M. (1988). Development of a measure of learned helplessness. *Nursing Research, 37,* 11–15.

Thomas, S.D., Hathaway, D.K., & Arheart, K.L. (1990). Development of the General Health Motivation

Scale. *Western Journal of Nursing Research, 12,* 318–335.

Woods, N.F., Most, A., & Dery, G.K. (1982). Estimating premenstrual distress: A comparison of two methods. *Research in Nursing and Health, 5,* 81–92.

OTHER REFERENCES CITED IN CHAPTER 11

Aaronson, L.S. (1989). Perceived and received support: Effects on health behavior during pregnancy. *Nursing Research, 38,* 4–9.

Brandt, P.A. (1984). Stress-buffering effects of social support on maternal discipline. *Nursing Research, 33,* 229–234.

Davis, L.L. (1990). Illness uncertainty, social support, and stress in recovering individuals and family care givers. *Applied Nursing Research, 3,* 69–71.

Mishel, M.H., & Braden, C.J. (1988). Finding meaning: Antecedents of uncertainty in illness. *Nursing Research, 37,* 98–103.

Webster, K.K., & Christman, N.J. (1988). Perceived uncertainty and coping post myocardial infarction. *Western Journal of Nursing Research, 10,* 384–400.

Wilson-Barnett, J., & Osborne, J. (1983). Studies evaluating patient teaching: Implications for practice. *International Journal of Nursing Studies, 20,* 33–44.

Yarcheski, A. (1988). Uncertainty in illness and the future. *Western Journal of Nursing Research, 10,* 401–413.

Yarcheski, A., & Mahon, N.E. (1989). A causal model of positive health practices: The relationship between approach and replication. *Nursing Research, 38,* 88–93.

12
Principles of Research Design

Chapters 9 through 11 introduced the reader to a wide variety of research approaches, but paid relatively little attention to a consideration of how the investigator would go about designing the study. Because many of the issues relating to research design are common to several types of research, it was considered preferable to deal with these issues in a single chapter. The principal aim of this chapter is to introduce design techniques that strengthen the quality of many types of research studies or enhance the interpretability of their findings.

≡ *PURPOSES AND DIMENSIONS OF RESEARCH DESIGN*

Research design refers to the researcher's overall plan for obtaining answers to the research questions and testing the research hypotheses. The research design spells out the strategies that the researcher adopts to develop information that is accurate, objective, and meaningful. Typically, the research design delineates the following aspects of the study:

Will there be an intervention? In some cases, nurse researchers want to test the effects of some specific intervention (e.g., a program to promote breast self-examination), but in others, they want to observe phenomena as they naturally occur. This dimension refers to the distinction between experimental versus nonexperimental designs, a topic discussed at length in Chapters 9 and 10. When there is an experimental intervention, the specification of the design should spell out the full nature of that intervention.

What type of comparisons will be made? Generally, researchers need to develop some type of comparison within their studies so that their results will be interpretable. Sometimes the comparison involves examining differences between two or more groups. For example, suppose a researcher wanted to study the emotional consequences of having an abortion. To do this, the researcher might compare the emotional status of women who had an abortion with women from the same health clinic who delivered a baby but whose pregnancy had not been wanted. If the researcher had not used a comparison group, it would have been difficult to know whether the emotional status of the abortion group members was distinctive. Sometimes researchers use a "before" and "after" comparison (e.g., comparing patients' stress preoperatively and postoperatively) and sometimes they use several comparisons to more fully understand the phenomena of interest.

What procedures will be used to control extraneous variables? As noted in Chapter 4, the complexity of relationships among human characteristics makes it difficult to unambiguously answer research questions unless efforts are made to isolate the independent and dependent variables and control other factors extraneous to the research question. Thus, one important feature of the research design is the specification of steps that will be taken to control extraneous variables. This chapter discusses techniques for achieving control in research studies.

When and how many times will data be collected from research subjects? In most studies, data are collected from subjects at a single point in time. For example, patients might be asked to complete a questionnaire about their nutritional practices. However, some designs call for multiple contacts with subjects, either to determine how things have changed over time, to determine the stability of some phenomenon, or to develop some sense of a "baseline" against which the effect of some treatment can be compared. The research design also designates *when,* relative to other events, the data

will be collected (e.g., one day postoperatively, in the thirtieth week of gestation, and so forth).

In what setting will the study take place? Sometimes studies take place in naturalistic environments, such as in clinics, people's homes, and so on. Other studies are conducted in highly controlled "laboratory" * settings. Most nursing research occurs in fairly naturalistic environments, but studies in laboratory-type settings have also been conducted.

The research design incorporates some of the most important methodological decisions that the researcher makes in conducting a research study. Other aspects of the study—the data collection plan, the sampling plan, and the analysis plan—also involve important decisions, but the research design stipulates the fundamental form that the research will take. For this reason, it is important to have a good understanding of design options when embarking on a research project.

≡ TECHNIQUES OF RESEARCH CONTROL

A major purpose of research design for most research questions is to maximize the amount of control that an investigator has over the research situation and variables. As discussed in Chapter 4, the researcher needs to control extraneous variables to determine the true nature of the relationship between the independent and dependent variables under investigation. *Extraneous variables* are variables that have an irrelevant association with the dependent variable and that can confound the testing of the research hypothesis. There are two basic types of extraneous variables: (1) those that are intrinsic to the subjects of the

---

* The term "laboratory" typically connotes a setting in which scientific equipment is installed. Here, the term is used in a general sense to refer to a physical location apart from the routine of daily living, which is used by the researcher as the site for the collection of data and where subjects report to participate in the research project.

study and (2) those that are external factors stemming from the research situation.(Many of the control techniques outlined in this chapter are not normally invoked in field studies or studies within the phenomenological tradition, in which the aim is for the research setting to be as natural as possible.)

Controlling External Factors

In scientific research, the researcher usually takes steps to minimize situational contaminants. The researcher should generally seek to make the conditions under which the data are collected as similar as possible for every participant in the study. The control that a researcher imposes on a study by attempting to maintain constancy in the research conditions probably represents one of the earliest forms of scientific control.

The environment has been found to exert a powerful influence on people's emotions and behavior. In designing research, therefore, the investigator needs to pay attention to the environmental context within which the study is to be conducted. Control over the environment is most easily achieved in laboratory experiments in which all subjects are brought into an environment that the experimenter is in a position to arrange. Researchers have much less freedom in controlling the environment in studies that occur in natural settings. This does not mean that the researcher should abandon all efforts to make the environments as similar as possible. For example, in conducting a survey in which the information is to be gathered by means of an interview, the researcher should attempt to conduct all interviews in basically the same kind of environment. That is, it would not be desirable to interview some of the respondents in their own homes, some in their place of work, some in the researcher's office, and so forth. In each of these settings, the participant normally assumes different roles (e.g., wife, husband, parent; employee; and client or patient) and responses to questions may be influenced to some degree by the role in which the respondent is operating.

One of the advantages of conducting a study in an artificial setting such as a laboratory is that the researcher has greater confidence of having control over the independent and extraneous variables. In real-life settings, even when there are randomly assigned groups, the differentiation between groups may be difficult to control. Let us look at another example to see why this is so. Suppose we are planning to teach nursing students a unit on dyspnea, and we have used a lecture-type approach in the past. If we are interested in trying an individualized, autotutorial approach to cover the same material and want to evaluate the effectiveness of this method before adopting it for all students, we might randomly assign students to one of the two methods. Scores on a test covering the content of the unit could be used as the dependent or criterion variable. But now, suppose the students in the two groups talk to one another about their learning experiences. Some of the lecture-group students might go through parts of the programmed text. Perhaps some of the students in the autotutorial group will sit in on some of the lectures. In short, field experiments are often subject to the problem of *contamination of treatments.* In the same study, it would also be difficult to control other variables, such as the time or place in which the learning occurs for the individualized group.

Another external factor that should be controlled is the time factor. Depending on the topic of the study, the dependent variable may be influenced by the time of day or time of year in which the data are collected, or both. It would, in such cases, be desirable for the researcher to strive for constancy of times across subjects. If an investigator were studying fatigue or perceptions of physical well-being, it would probably matter a great deal whether the data were gathered in the morning, afternoon, or evening, or in the summer as opposed to the winter. Although time constancy is not always critical, it is often relatively easy for the researcher to control and should, therefore, be sought whenever possible.

Another aspect of maintaining constancy of conditions concerns constancy in the communications to the subjects and in the treatment itself in the case of experiments or quasi-experiments. In most research efforts, the researcher informs participants about the purpose of the study, what use will be made of the data, under whose auspices the study is being conducted, and so forth. This information generally should be prepared ahead of time, and the same message should be delivered to all subjects. In most research situations, there should be as little ad libbing as possible.

In studies involving the implementation of a treatment, care should be taken to adhere to the specifications (often referred to as *research protocols*) for that treatment. For example, in experiments to test the effectiveness of a new drug to cure a medical problem, the researcher would have to take great care to ensure that the subjects in the experimental group received the same chemical substance and the same dosage, that the substance was administered in the same way, and so forth. Some treatments are much "fuzzier" than in the case of administering a drug, as is the case for most nursing interventions. In such a situation, the investigator should spell out in detail the exact behaviors required of the personnel responsible for delivering or administering the treatment.

One of the features that distinguishes non-experimental research from experimental and quasi-experimental studies is that if the researcher has not manipulated the independent variable, then there is no means of ensuring constancy of conditions. Let us take as an example an ex post facto study that attempts to determine if there is a relationship between a person's knowledge of nutrition and his or her own eating habits. Suppose the investigator finds no relationship between nutritional knowledge and eating patterns. That is, the investigator finds that people who are well-informed about nutrition are just as likely as uninformed people to maintain inadequate diets. In this case, however, the researcher has had no control over the source of a person's nutritional knowledge (the independent variable). This knowledge was measured after the fact (*post facto*), and the conditions under which the information was obtained cannot be assumed to be constant or even similar. The researcher may conclude from the study that it is useless to teach nutrition to people because knowledge has no impact on their eating behavior. It may be, however, that different methods of providing nutritional information vary in their ability to motivate people to alter their nutritional habits. Thus, the ability of the investigator to control or manipulate the independent variable of interest may be extremely important in understanding the relationships between variables, or the absence of relationships.

Controlling Intrinsic Factors

Characteristics of the participants in a scientific study almost always need to be controlled for the findings to be interpretable. The control of intrinsic extraneous variables is especially important when the dependent variable is psychosocial rather than biophysiologic in nature. That is because psychosocial variables (e.g., stress) are more susceptible than physiologic ones (e.g., body temperature and heart rate) to the influence of individual characteristics (e.g., sex, social class, and marital status). This section describes six specific ways of controlling extraneous variables associated with subject characteristics.

RANDOMIZATION

We have already discussed the most effective method of controlling individual extraneous variables—randomization. The primary function of *randomization* is to secure comparable groups, that is, to equalize the groups with respect to the extraneous variables. A distinct advantage of random assignment, compared with other methods of controlling extraneous variables, is that randomization controls *all* possible sources of extraneous variation, without any conscious decision on the researcher's part about which variables need to be controlled.

Suppose, for example, that we were interested in assessing the effect of a physical training program on cardiovascular functioning among nursing home residents. Characteristics such as the individuals' age, sex, prior occupation, history of smoking, and length of stay in the nursing home could all affect the patients' cardiovascular system, independently of the physical training program. The effects of these other variables are extraneous to the research problem and should be controlled. Through randomization, we could expect that an experimental group (receiving the physical training program) and control group (not receiving the program) would be comparable in terms of these as well as any other factors that influence cardiovascular functioning.

HOMOGENEITY

When randomization is not feasible, there are alternative methods of controlling intrinsic subject characteristics that could contaminate the relationships under investigation. A second method is to use only subjects who are homogeneous with respect to those variables that are considered extraneous. The extraneous variables, in this case, are not allowed to vary. In the example of the physical training program, if sex were considered to be an important confounding variable, the researcher might wish to use only men (or only women) as subjects. Similarly, if the re-

searcher were concerned about the effects of the subjects' age on cardiovascular functioning, participation in the study could be limited to those within a specified age range. This method of utilizing a homogeneous subject pool is fairly easy and offers considerable control. However, the limitation of this approach lies in the fact that the research findings can only be generalized to the type of subjects who participated in the study. If the physical training program were found to have beneficial effects on the cardiovascular status of a sample of men aged 65 to 75, its usefulness for improving the cardiovascular status of women in their eighties would be strictly a matter of conjecture.

BLOCKING

A third approach to controlling extraneous variables is to include them in the design of a study as independent variables. To pursue our example of the physical training program, if sex were thought to be a confounding variable, it could be built into the study design (Fig. 12-1). This procedure would allow us to make an assessment of the impact of our training program on the cardiovascular functioning of both elderly men and women. Furthermore, although the reason for this may be unclear until the reader is familiar with inferential statistics, this ap-

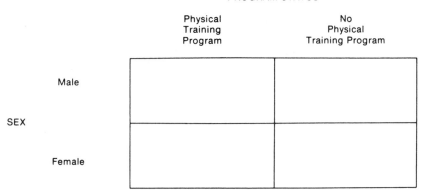

Figure 12-1. *Schematic diagram of a randomized block design.*

proach has the advantage of adding greater precision and enhancing the likelihood of detecting differences between our experimental and control groups.

Let us consider this third approach in greater detail. We will refer to the design shown in Figure 12-1 as a *randomized block design.** The variable sex, which cannot be manipulated by the researcher, is known as a *blocking variable*. In an experiment to test the effectiveness of the physical training program, the experimenter obviously could not randomly assign subjects to one of four cells: the sex of the subjects is a "given." However, the experimenter can and should randomly assign males and females separately to the experimental and control conditions. Let us say that there are 40 males and 40 females available for the study. The researcher *should not* take the 80 subjects and assign half to the physical training program group and the other half to the "no program" group. Rather, the randomization procedure should be performed separately for the two sexes, thereby guaranteeing 20 subjects in each cell of the four-cell design.

The design can be extended to include more than one blocking variable, as shown in Figure 12-2. In this design, the age of the subject has been included to control for this second extraneous variable. Once again, the experimenter should randomly assign subjects from each block to either the experimental or control conditions. In other words, half of the men aged 66 to 70 would randomly be assigned to the program, as would half of the men aged 71 to 75, and so forth. Although in theory the number of blocks that could be added is unlimited, practical concerns usually dictate a relatively small number of blocks

(and, hence, a small number of extraneous variables that can be controlled). Expansion of the design usually requires that a larger subject pool be used. As a general rule of thumb, a minimum of 20 to 30 subjects per cell is often recommended. This means that, whereas a minimum of 80 subjects would be needed for the design in Figure 12-1, 240 subjects would be needed for the design in Figure 12-2. This suggests that, if a decision is made to introduce extraneous variables into the design of a study, great care should be taken to choose the most relevant subject characteristics as the blocking variables.

Strictly speaking, the type of design we have discussed is appropriate only in experimental studies, but, in reality, it is used quite commonly in quasi-experimental and ex post facto studies as well. If an investigator were studying the effects of a physical training program on cardiovascular functioning after the fact (i.e., subjects self-selected themselves into one of the two groups and the researcher had no control over who was included in each group), he or she might want to set up the analysis in such a way that differential effects for men and women would be analyzed. The design structure would look the same as the one presented in Figure 12-1, although the implications and conclusions that could be drawn from the results would be quite different than if the researcher had been in control of the manipulation and randomization procedures.

MATCHING

A fourth method of dealing with extraneous variables is known as matching. *Matching* involves using knowledge of subject characteristics to form comparison groups. If a matching procedure were to be adopted for our physical training program example, and age and sex were the extraneous variables of interest, we would need to match each subject in the experimental group with one in the control group with respect to age and sex. If the subjects could be assigned on a random basis, we would actually have a special

---

* The terminology for this design varies from text to text. Some authors (e.g., Kerlinger, 1973) refer to this as a factorial design; others call it a levels-by-treatment design. We have chosen not to use the term "factorial" because sex is not under experimental control and, hence, complete randomization is impossible. (See Dayton, 1970, for this use of randomized block design.)

PROGRAM STATUS

SEX	AGE GROUP	Physical Training Program	No Physical Training Program
	66–70		
Male	71–75		
	76–80		
	66–70		
Female	71–75		
	76–80		

Figure 12-2. *Schematic diagram of a randomized block design.*

type of randomized block design with one subject per cell.*

However, matching is usually a *post hoc* attempt to approximate this experimental blocking design. That is, the researcher may begin with 20 subjects who participate in the training program and then create a control group by matching, one by one, individuals from the general population in terms of age and sex of the experimental subjects. Studies using such a pair-matching procedure to equate two (or more) groups are sometimes referred to as *case-control studies*. This design is very common in epidemiological research.

Despite the intuitive appeal of such a design, there are reasons why matching should be avoided if possible. First, to match effectively, the researcher must know in advance what the relevant extraneous variables are. Second, after two or three variables, it often becomes impossible to match adequately. Let us say that we are interested in controlling for the age, sex, race, and length of nursing home stay of the subjects. Thus, if subject 1 in the physical training program were a black woman, aged 80, whose length of stay is five years, the researcher would need to seek another woman with these same or similar characteristics as a comparison group counterpart. With more than three variables, the matching procedure becomes extremely cumbersome, if not impossible. For these reasons, matching as a technique for controlling extraneous variables should, in general, be used only when other, more powerful procedures are not feasible, as might be the case for some ex post facto studies.

* In this special case, the requirement of 20 to 30 cases per cell is irrelevant because no attempt is made to assess the effects of the extraneous variables on the dependent variable. Matching merely attempts to produce equivalent groups for comparison purposes. The requirement of 20 to 30 cases per cell stems from the fact that an estimate of an effect of a treatment is unstable (can fluctuate markedly from one individual to the next) when the number of cases is small. However, if the researcher is not interested in how, for example, the physical training program affects males versus females, but is interested in securing equivalent groups, matching on a one-to-one basis and then randomly assigning subjects to conditions is acceptable.

Sometimes, as an alternative to pair-matching (in which subjects are matched on a one-to-one basis for every matching variable), researchers choose to have a *balanced design* with regard to key extraneous variables. In such situations, the researcher attempts only to ensure that the composition of the groups being compared have proportional representation with regard to variables believed to be correlated with the dependent variable. For example, if gender and race were the two extraneous variables of interest in our example of the physical training program, the researcher adopting a balanced design would strive to ensure that the same percentage of men and women (and the same percentage of white and black subjects) were in the group participating in the physical training program as in a comparison group of nonparticipants. Such an approach is much less cumbersome than pair-matching, but also has similar limitations. Nevertheless, both pair-matching and balancing are generally preferable to failing to control for intrinsic subject characteristics at all.

ANALYSIS OF COVARIANCE

A fifth method of controlling unwanted variables is through statistical procedures. It is recognized that, at this point, many readers may be unfamiliar with basic statistical procedures, let alone the sophisticated techniques referred to here. Therefore, a detailed description of a powerful statistical control mechanism, known as analysis of covariance, will not be attempted. The interested reader with a background in statistics should consult Chapter 22 or a textbook on advanced statistics for fuller coverage of this topic. However, because the possibility of statistical control may mystify readers, we will explain the underlying principle with a simple illustration.

Returning to the physical training program example, suppose we have a group that is undergoing a physical training program and another group that is not. The groups represent intact groups (e.g., residents of two different nursing homes, only one of which is offering the physical training program), and therefore randomization is impossible. As our measures of cardiovascular functioning, suppose we use maximal oxygen consumption and resting heart rate. As with most things in life, there undoubtedly will be individual differences on these two measures. The research question is, "Can some of the individual differences be attributed to a person's participation in the physical training program?" Unfortunately, the individual differences in cardiovascular functioning are also related to other, extraneous characteristics of the subjects, such as age. The large circles in Figure 12-3 may be taken to represent the total variability (extent of individual differences) for both groups on, say, resting heart rate. A certain amount of that total variability can be explained simply by virtue of the subject's age, which is schematized in the figure as the small circle on the left in Figure 12-3 (A). Another part of the variability can be explained by the subject's participation or nonparticipation in the physical training program, represented as the small circle on the right in (A). In (A), the fact that the two small circles (age and participation in program) overlap indicates that there is a relationship between those two variables. In other

words, subjects in the group receiving the physical training program are, on average, either older or younger than members of the comparison group. Therefore, age should be controlled. Otherwise, it will be impossible to determine whether differences in resting heart rate should be attributed to age differences or differences in program participation.

Analysis of covariance can accomplish this control function by statistically removing the effect of the extraneous variable on the dependent variable. In the illustration, that portion of heart rate variability that is attributable to age could be removed through the analysis of covariance technique. This is designated in Figure 12-3 (A) by the darkened area in the large circle; (B) illustrates that the final analysis would examine the effect of program participation on heart rate after removing the effect of age. With the variability of heart rate resulting from age controlled, we can have a much more precise estimate of the effect of the training program on heart rate. Note that even after removing the variability resulting from age, there is still individual variability not associated with the program treatment—the bottom half of

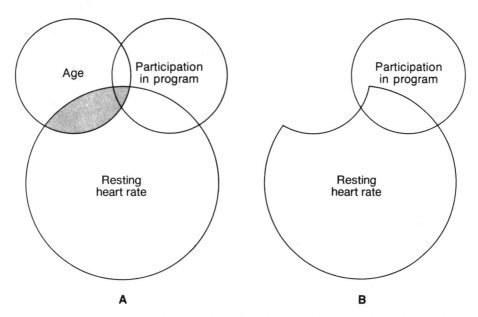

Figure 12-3. *Schematic diagram illustrating the principle of analysis of covariance.*

the large circle in (B). This means that the precision of the study can probably be further enhanced by controlling additional extraneous variables, such as sex, type of previous occupation, and so forth. The analysis of covariance procedure can accommodate multiple extraneous variables. When pretest measures of the dependent variables have been obtained, these are often controlled statistically through analysis of covariance.

REPEATED MEASURES

The sixth technique uses the subjects themselves as their own controls. In some experiments, one group of subjects can be exposed to more than one condition or treatment. This type of design, known as a *repeated measures design,* has the advantage of ensuring the highest possible degree of equivalence between subjects exposed to different conditions. Suppose that we were interested in studying the relationship between the content of a patient's talk and nurses' listening behavior. We might set up a laboratory experiment rather than a field experiment to control for a host of confounding environmental or situational factors. Let us say that a simulated hospital room is created, and a confederate of the researcher poses as a hospital patient. Our subjects (nurses) enter the room with instructions to perform certain nursing routines. Now suppose that the three types of verbal content we are interested in are conversation relating to (1) physical pain, (2) emotional pain such as fear and loneliness, and (3) general talk about the weather and so forth. The confederate patient would learn three "scripts" relating to these areas; we could then assess the nurses' listening behavior by having them later answer questions about what the patient said. How could we proceed to conduct this study? We *could* start with 30 nurses and then randomly assign ten to each of the three conditions. Then each group would only be exposed to one of the three scripts. In such a study, two important extraneous variables might be the nurses' specialty area and their number of years of experience. The randomization procedure would probably control for such differences, but with only ten subjects per condition, it might be possible by chance alone to get a group that overrepresents nurses with, say, a psychiatric specialty. An alternative would be to use a repeated measures design wherein all 30 nurses are exposed to all three scripts. This would clearly guarantee equivalence across conditions, thereby controlling extraneous variables. Furthermore, repeated measures provide the researcher with more data: in the example, we would have 90 pieces of information (30 subjects × three conditions).

Repeated measures designs often are inappropriate because of the problem of carry-over effects. When subjects are exposed to two different treatments or conditions, they may be influenced in the second condition by their experience in the first condition. Because the two (or more) treatments are not applied simultaneously, the order of the treatment may be important in affecting the subject's performance. The procedure of *counterbalancing* is frequently used in conjunction with repeated measures designs to minimize the impact of ordering effects. In our example of nurses' listening behavior, the order of presentation of the three scripts would be systematically varied so that the attention paid to a given conversation would not depend on whether it was heard first, second, or third. Table 12-1 illustrates a counterbalanced order of presentation for the first 12 subjects in our hypothetical experiment. In sum, repeated measures can be a useful and efficient design for eliminating extraneous variables, but when carry-over effects from one condition to another are anticipated, as might be the case in many medical or nursing interventions, the researcher will need to seek other designs.

Evaluation of Control Methods

Overall, the random assignment of subjects to groups is the most effective approach of managing extraneous variables, because randomization tends to produce a "canceling out" of individual variation on all possible extraneous variables. Repeated measures designs, although also useful

Table 12-1. *Counterbalanced Order of Presentation of Patient Scripts*

SUBJECT	FIRST	SECOND	THIRD
1	A	B	C
2	B	C	A
3	C	A	B
4	A	C	B
5	C	B	A
6	B	A	C
7	A	B	C
8	B	C	A
9	C	A	B
10	A	C	B
11	C	B	A
12	B	A	C

A, Script dealing with physical pain.

B, Script dealing with emotional pain.

C, Script dealing with "small talk."

the control procedures is generally preferable to the absence of attempts to control intrinsic extraneous variables.

All six of the control techniques discussed in this section have been profitably used by nurse researchers. Table 12-2 presents some research examples of the use of these procedures.

≡ INTERNAL AND EXTERNAL VALIDITY

One method of evaluating the adequacy of a research design is to assess its internal and external validity. *Internal validity* is attained in a study when the findings can be shown to result only from the effect of the independent variable of interest and cannot be interpreted as reflecting the effects of extraneous variables. *External validity* is attained when the results can confidently be generalized to situations outside of the specific research setting.

Internal Validity

The control mechanisms reviewed in the previous section are all strategies for improving the internal validity of research studies. If the researcher is not careful in managing extraneous variables and in other ways controlling the design of the study, there may be reason to challenge the conclusion that the subjects' performance on the dependent measure resulted from the effect of the independent variable.

True experiments possess a high degree of internal validity because the use of control procedures (manipulation and randomization) enables the researcher to rule out most alternative explanations for the results. With quasi-experimental, pre-experimental, or ex post facto designs, the investigator must always contend with competing explanations for the obtained results. These competing explanations, referred to as *threats to internal validity,* have been grouped into several classes, a few of which are examined here.

in controlling all possible sources of extraneous variation, cannot be applied to many nursing research problems. The remaining alternatives to randomization—homogeneity, blocking, matching, and analysis of covariance—have one disadvantage in common: the researcher must know or predict in advance the relevant extraneous variables. To select homogeneous samples, develop a blocking design, match, or perform an analysis of covariance, the researcher must make a decision about what variable or variables need to be measured and controlled. This constraint may pose severe limitations on the degree of control that is possible, particularly because the researcher can seldom deal explicitly with more than two or three extraneous variables at a time.

Although we have repeatedly hailed randomization as the ideal mechanism for controlling extraneous subject characteristics, it is clear that randomization is not always possible. For example, if the independent variable cannot be manipulated, then other techniques must be used. In ex post facto and quasi-experimental studies, the control options available to researchers include homogeneity, blocking, matching, and analysis of covariance. The use of any of

HISTORY

The threat of *history* refers to the occurrence of external events, which happen at about the same time as the introduction of the independent variable, that can affect the dependent variables. For example, suppose we were studying the effectiveness of a county-wide nurse outreach program designed to encourage pregnant women in rural areas to improve their health-related practices before delivery (e.g., better nutritional practices, cessation of smoking and drinking, and earlier prenatal care). The program might be evaluated by comparing the average birthweight of infants in the 12 months before the outreach program with the average birthweight of those born in the 12 months after the program was introduced. However, suppose that one month after the new program was launched, a highly publicized docudrama regarding the inadequacies of prenatal care for poor women was aired on national television. Our dependent variable in this case, infants' birthweight, might now be affected by both the intervention and the messages in the docudrama, and it becomes impossible for us to "unconfound" the two effects. In a true experiment, history generally is not a threat to the internal validity of a study because we can often assume that external events are as likely to affect the experimental as the control group.

Table 12-2. *Examples of Studies Controlling for Extraneous Variables by Various Methods*

RESEARCH QUESTION	METHOD OF CONTROL	EXTRANEOUS VARIABLES CONTROLLED
Does shoulder exercise therapy affect range of motion during early convalescence after coronary artery bypass surgery? (Shaw et al., 1989)	Randomization	All
Are there differences in resting systolic blood pressure and in systolic blood pressure across the Valsalva maneuver as a function of ethnic group? (Lu et al., 1990)	Homogeneity	Age; history of cerebrovascular, cardiovascular, and respiratory disease; hypertension; weight
What are the effects of choice and predictability information regarding barium enema on patients' distress, compliance, and satisfaction? (Wallston et al., 1987)	Blocking	Desire for control, prior experience with barium enema
	Analysis of covariance	Education
	Randomization	All others
Do the parents of children who are sexually abused in day care demonstrate greater psychologic distress than parents of nonabused children? (Kelley, 1990)	Matching	Age, gender, social class, length of attendance in day care
Do women who choose alternative delivery experiences differ from women who choose conventional birth experiences in terms of anxiety, hostility, or depression? (Littlefield et al., 1990)	Analysis of covariance	Maternal age
Do Type A and Type B cardiac patients differ in their blood pressure and heart rate responses during routine verbalization? (Thomas & Friedman, 1990)	Repeated measures	All

When this is the case, any differences in the groups that emerge at the end of the study represent effects over and above those created by external factors.

SELECTION

The term *selection* encompasses biases resulting from pretreatment differences between groups. When individuals are not assigned randomly to groups, we must always be aware of the possibility that the groups are nonequivalent. They may differ, in fact, in ways that are quite subtle and difficult to detect. If the groups are nonequivalent, the researcher is faced with the possibility that any group differences on the dependent variable are the result of initial differences rather than the effect of the independent variable. For example, if a researcher found that women with a fertility problem were more likely to be depressed than women who were mothers, it would be impossible to conclude that the two groups differed in terms of depression *because* of their differences in reproductive statuses; the women in the two groups might have been different in terms of psychologic adjustment to begin with. The problem of selection is clearly reduced when the researcher can collect data regarding the characteristics of the subjects before the occurrence of the independent variable, but this is often difficult to accomplish. In the outreach program example, the best design would involve the collection of information on the subjects' level of depression even before the women's attempts to become pregnant. Selection bias is one of the most problematic and frequently encountered threats to the internal validity of studies not using an experimental design.

Selection biases also often interact with other biases to compound the threat to the internal validity of the study. For example, if the comparison group is different from the experimental group or main group of interest, then the characteristics of the members of the comparison group could lead them to have different intervening experiences, thereby introducing both history and selection biases into the design.

MATURATION

In a research context, *maturation* refers to processes occurring within the subjects during the course of the study as a result of time rather than as a result of a treatment or independent variable. Examples of such processes include physical growth, emotional maturity, fatigue, and the like. For example, if we wanted to evaluate the effects of a special sensorimotor development program for developmentally retarded children, we would have to consider that progress does occur in these children even without special assistance. A design such as a one group pretest–posttest design (see Fig. 9-7 in Chapter 9), for example, would be highly susceptible to this threat to internal validity.

Maturation would be a relevant consideration in many areas of nursing research. Remember that "maturation" here does not refer to aging or developmental changes exclusively but, rather, to any kind of change that occurs with the individual as a function of time. Thus, wound-healing, postoperative recovery, and many other bodily changes that can occur with little or no nursing or medical intervention must be considered as an explanation for outcomes to subjects that rivals an explanation based on the effects of a treatment.

TESTING AND INSTRUMENTATION

The effects of taking a pretest on the scores of a posttest are known as *testing* effects. It has been documented in numerous studies, particularly in those dealing with opinions and attitudes, that the mere act of collecting information from people changes them. Let us say that we administer to a group of nursing students a questionnaire dealing with their attitudes toward euthanasia. We then proceed to acquaint the students with various arguments that have been made for and against euthanasia, outcomes of court cases, and the like. At the end of instruction, we give them the same attitude measure as before and observe whether their attitudes have changed as a function of the instruction. The problem here is that the first administration of the questionnaire might sensitize the students to issues that they had not contemplated before. The sensitization may, in fact, result in attitude changes whether or not instruction follows. If a comparison group is not used in the study, it becomes impossible to segregate the effects of the instruction from the effects of having taken the pretest (as well as from the effects of history, maturation, and so forth). In true experiments, testing may not be a problem because its effects would be expected to be approximately equal in all groups, but the Solomon four-group design (discussed in Chapter 9) could be used if the researcher wanted to segregate the effects of the intervention from those of the pretest. Sensitization, or testing, problems are typically much more likely to occur when we are exposing the subjects to controversial or novel material in the pretest.

Another threat that is related to the researcher's measurements is referred to as the threat of *instrumentation*. This bias reflects changes in the researcher's measuring instruments between an initial point of data collection and a subsequent point. For example, if the researcher uses one measure of stress at baseline, and a different measure at follow-up, then any changes might reflect changes in the measuring tool rather than the effects of the independent variable. Instrumentation effects could occur even if the same measure is used if the measuring tool yields more accurate measures on the second administration (e.g., if the people collecting the data are more experienced) or less accurate measures (e.g., if the people collecting the data become bored or fatigued).

MORTALITY

Mortality refers to the differential loss of subjects from comparison groups. The loss of subjects during the course of a study, often referred to as *attrition,* may differ from one group to another because of *a priori* differences in interest, motivation, and the like. For example, suppose we used a nonequivalent control group design to assess the morale of the nursing personnel from two different hospitals, one of which was

initiating the problem-oriented method of charting. The dependent variable, nursing staff satisfaction, is measured in both hospitals before and after the intervention. Comparison group members, who may have no particular commitment to the study, may decline to complete a posttest questionnaire because of lack of incentive. Those who do fill it out may be unrepresentative of the group as a whole—they may be those who are most enthusiastic about their work environment, for example. If this were the case, it might appear that the morale of the nurses in the comparison hospital had improved over time, but this improvement might only be an artifact of the "mortality" of a biased segment of this group. In clinical nursing studies, the problem of attrition may be especially acute because of patient discharge and death.

INTERNAL VALIDITY AND RESEARCH DESIGN

Quasi-experimental and ex post facto studies are especially susceptible to threats to internal validity. The threats just described (as well as others, which are less frequently of concern to nurse researchers) represent alternative explanations that compete with the independent variable as a cause of the dependent variable. The aim of a good research design is to rule out these competing explanations.

A good experimental design will normally control for these factors, but it must not be assumed that in a true experiment the researcher need not worry about them. For example, if constancy of conditions is not maintained for experimental and control groups, then history might be a rival explanation for any group differences. Mortality is, in particular, a salient threat in true experiments. Because the experimenter does things differently with the experimental and control groups, subjects in the groups may drop out of the study differentially. This is particularly apt to happen if the experimental treatment is painful, inconvenient, or time consuming, or if the control condition is boring or considered a nuisance. When this happens, the subjects remaining in the study may differ from those who left in important ways, thereby nullifying the initial equivalence of the groups.

External Validity

External validity refers to the generalizability of the research findings to other settings or samples. Research is almost never conducted with the intention of discovering relationships among variables for one group of people at one point in time. The aim of research is typically to reveal enduring relationships, the understanding of which can be used to improve the human condition. If a nursing intervention under investigation is found to be successful, others will want to adopt the procedure. Therefore, an important question is whether the intervention will "work" in another setting and with different patients. Researchers should routinely ask themselves: To what populations, environments, and conditions can the results of the study be applied?

Strictly speaking, the findings of a study can only be generalized to the population of subjects from which a study sample has been randomly selected. If an investigator were studying the effects of a newly developed therapeutic treatment for heroin addicts, then the researcher might begin with a population of addicts in a particular clinic or drug treatment center. From this population, a random sample of drug users could be selected for participation in the study. Individuals from the sample would then be randomly assigned to one of two or more conditions assuming that an experiment were possible. If the results revealed that the new therapeutic treatment was highly effective in reducing recidivism among the sample of addicts, can it be concluded that all addicts in the United States would benefit from the treatment? Unfortunately, no. The population of heroin addicts undergoing treatment in one particular facility may not be representative of all addicts. For example, the facility in question may attract drug users from certain ethnic, socioeconomic, or age groups. Perhaps the new treatment is only effective with individuals from such groups.

Of relevance here is Kempthorne's (1961) distinction between accessible populations and target populations. The *accessible population* is the population of subjects available for a particular study. In our drug treatment example, all the heroin addicts in treatment at a particular treatment center would constitute the accessible population. When random procedures have been used to select a sample from an accessible population, there is no difficulty in generalizing the results to that group.

The *target population* is the total group of subjects about whom the investigator is interested and to whom the results could reasonably be generalized. This second type of generalization is considerably more risky than the first and cannot be done with as much confidence as in the case of generalizations to the accessible population. The adequacy and utility of this type of inference hinges very strongly on the similarity of the characteristics of the two populations. Thus, the researcher must be aware of the characteristics of the accessible population and, in turn, define the target population to be like the accessible population. In the drug treatment example, the accessible population might predominantly comprise voluntarily admitted white males in their twenties living in New York City. Although we might ideally like to generalize our results to all drug addicts, we would be on much safer ground if we defined our target population as young, urban, white men who present themselves for treatment.

In addition to characteristics of the sample that limit the generalizability of research findings, there are various characteristics of the environment or research situation that affect the study's representativeness and, hence, its external validity. These characteristics should be considered in developing a research design and in interpreting results once the data have been collected. Among the most noteworthy threats to the external validity of studies are the following five effects:

1. *The Hawthorne effect.* Subjects in an investigation may behave in a particular manner largely because they are aware of their participation in a study. If a certain type of behavior

or performance is elicited only in a research context, then the results cannot be generalized to more natural settings. This threat to external validity was discussed at greater length in Chapter 9.

2. *Novelty effects.* When a treatment is new, subjects and research agents alike might alter their behavior in a variety of ways. People may be either enthusiastic or skeptical about new methods of doing things. The results may reflect these reactions to the novelty; once the treatment is more familiar, the same results may fail to appear.

3. *Interaction of history and treatment effect.* The results may reflect the impact of the treatment *and* some other events external to the study. When the treatment is implemented again in the absence of the other events, different results may be obtained. For example, if a dietary intervention for people with high cholesterol levels was being evaluated shortly after extensive media coverage of research demonstrating a link between consumption of oat bran and reduction in cholesterol levels, it would be difficult to know whether any observed effects would be observed again if the intervention were implemented several months later with a new group of people.

4. *Experimenter effects.* The performance of the subjects may be affected by characteristics of the researchers. The investigators often have an emotional or intellectual investment in demonstrating that their hypotheses are correct and may unconsciously communicate their expectations to the subjects or they may be somewhat biased in their observations. If this is the case, any observed relationships in the original study might be difficult to replicate in a more neutral situation.

5. *Measurement effects.* In research studies, the investigators collect a considerable amount of data, such as pretest information, background data, and so forth. The results may not apply to another group of people who are not also exposed to the same data-collection procedures.

In conclusion, the researcher should strive to design studies that are strong with respect to both internal and external validity. In some instances, however, the requirements for ensuring one type of validity may interfere with the possibility of achieving the second. That is, if the researcher exerts a high degree of control over a study in an effort to maximize internal validity, the setting may become highly artificial and pose a threat to the generalizability of the findings to more naturalistic environments. Thus, it is often necessary to reach a compromise by introducing sufficient controls while maintaining some semblance of realism. In this regard, the concept of replication, or the repeating of a study in a new setting with new subjects, is an extremely important one. Much greater confidence can be placed in the findings of a study if it can be demonstrated that the results can be replicated in other settings and with new subjects.

☰ CHARACTERISTICS OF GOOD DESIGN

The criteria of internal and external validity represent one frame of reference for evaluating the quality of research designs. In this section we briefly examine the characteristics of good design from a somewhat less technical point of view.

Appropriateness for Research Question

The requirement that the research design should be appropriate for the questions being asked seems so obvious that it may be overlooked. Generally, a given research problem can be handled adequately with a number of different designs, so that the researcher typically has some flexibility in selecting a design. Yet many designs will be completely unsuitable for dealing with the research problem. For example, if a researcher were interested in comparing the effects of two drugs on sleep promotion, it is unlikely that a repeated measures design would be appropriate, given the interactive nature of many drugs. As another example, a loosely structured research design such as those often used in field studies might be inappropriate to address the question of whether nonnutritive sucking opportunities among premature infants facilitate early oral feedings. On the other hand, a tightly controlled study may unnecessarily restrict the researcher interested in understanding the processes by which nurses make diagnoses. This chapter has emphasized techniques of control normally associated with highly structured, scientific research, but there are many research questions of interest to nurses for which such designs may be unsuitable.

Lack of Bias

A second characteristic of good research design in traditional scientific studies is that it results in data that are not biased. Bias can operate in a variety of ways, some of which are very subtle. The most pervasive source of bias is in the allocation of subjects to groups. When groups are formed on a nonrandom basis, the risk of selection bias is always present. The investigator is not necessarily responsible for the bias, however; in ex post facto studies in which subjects "self-select" themselves into groups, the biases might be quite beyond the researcher's control.

In studies in which the data are collected by means of observation, the researcher's preconceptions might unconsciously bias the objective collection of data. In such a case, the researcher should take a number of steps to minimize this risk. Whenever possible, double-blind procedures are highly recommended. The double-blind technique removes observer biases by virtue of the fact that neither the subject nor the observer (or person collecting the data) knows in which group a given subject is. When this approach is not feasible, it is a good practice to have two or more observers so that at least an estimation of the biases can be made.

Bias can enter the data whenever there is an opportunity for something other than the independent variable of interest to affect the outcomes in a systematic way. The techniques discussed in the first section of this chapter, such as randomization, counterbalancing, and so forth, should be built into the structure of the research to eliminate or reduce problems of bias.

Precision

The early sections of this chapter dealt with the notion of control over extraneous variables. What this control is actually all about is *control over variability in the dependent measures*. In the physical training example, we discussed the variability from one elderly individual to another on measures of cardiovascular functioning. The various control mechanisms discussed represented attempts to isolate that portion of the variability in cardiovascular status that could be attributable to participation in a physical training program. What the researcher is attempting to do may be expressed as the following ratio:

$$\frac{\text{Variability in cardiovascular status attributable to training program}}{\text{Variability in cardiovascular status attributable to age, sex, prior occupation, initial level of cardiovascular status}}$$

This ratio, though greatly simplified here, captures the essence of many statistical procedures. The researcher wants to make the variability in the numerator (the upper half) as large as possible relative to the variability in the denominator (the lower half) to demonstrate most clearly the relationship between program participation and cardiovascular functioning. The smaller the variability caused by extraneous variables such as age and sex, the easier it will be for the researcher to detect differences in cardiovascular functioning between those who did and those who did not participate in the physical training program. Designs that enable the researcher to reduce the variability caused by the extraneous variables are said to increase the precision of the research. As a purely hypothetical illustration of why this is so, we will attach some numerical values* to the ratio:

$$\frac{\text{Variability attributable to training program}}{\text{Variability attributable to extraneous variables}} = \frac{10}{4}$$

Now, if we can make the bottom number smaller, say from 4 to 2, then we will have a purer and more precise estimate of the effect of program participation on physical fitness.

How can a research design help to reduce the variability caused by extraneous variables? A randomized block design is one example of a design that increases the precision of an analysis. Let us say that we performed the physical fitness study as a true experiment, using two age groups. The total variability in cardiovascular functioning (i.e., the extent to which individuals had different heart rates and maximal oxygen consumption) can be conceptualized as having three components:

Total variability in cardiovascular status =
Variability attributable to program +
Variability attributable to age +
Variability attributable to other extraneous variables

This equation can be taken to mean that part of the reason why some individuals did well and others did less well on measures of cardiovascular functioning is that some participated in the training program and others did not; some people are older and some are younger; and other factors such as sex, prior occupation, and so forth had an effect.

The randomized block procedure allows us to segregate the variability that is the result of age and remove it from the variability resulting from all other extraneous variables. By doing this, the effect of the training program becomes greater, relative to the extraneous variability. Thus, we can say that the randomized block design has enabled

---

*The reader should not be concerned at this point with how these numbers can be obtained in a real analysis. The procedure will be explained at length in Chapter 21.

us to get a more precise estimate of the effect of participation in the training program. Research designs differ considerably in the sensitivity with which the treatment effects can be detected with statistical tools. Lipsey (1990) has prepared an excellent guide to assist researchers in enhancing the sensitivity of their research designs.

Power

We use power here to describe the ability of a research design to detect relationships among variables. Precision contributes to the power of a design. Power is also increased when a large sample is used. This aspect of power is discussed in Chapters 13 and 22.

One other aspect of a powerful design concerns the construction (in experimental research) or definition (in nonexperimental research) of the independent variable. For both statistical and theoretical reasons, results are clearer and more conclusive when the differences in the results between two groups are large. The researcher should generally aim to maximize group differences on the dependent variables by maximizing differences on the independent variable. In other words, the results are likely to be more clear-cut if the treatments can be made as different as possible. This advice is clearly more easily followed in experimental than in ex post facto research. Research manipulation allows the investigator to devise treatments that are distinct and as strong as time, money, ethics, and practicality permit. However, even in nonexperimental research, there are frequently opportunities to operationalize the independent variables in such a way that power to detect differences is enhanced.

≡ THE TIME DIMENSION

As mentioned in the first section of this chapter, the research design generally specifies when and how often data will be collected in a study. In many nursing research studies, data are collected at a single point in time. However, many studies involve data collection several times. Indeed, several designs involving multiple measurements have already been discussed, such as the pretest–posttest experimental design, the time series design, and the prospective design.

There are four situations in which it might be appropriate to design a study with multiple points of data collection:

1. Time-related processes. Certain research problems are concerned with phenomena that evolve over time. Examples include such phenomena as healing, learning, growth, recidivism, and physical development.
2. Time-sequenced phenomena. It is often important to correctly ascertain the temporal sequencing of phenomena. For example, if it is hypothesized that infertility results in depression, then it would be important to determine that the depression did not precede the fertility problem.
3. Comparative purposes. Sometimes a time dimension is useful for placing findings in a broader context, to determine if changes have occurred over time. For example, a study might be concerned with documenting trends in the incidence of child abuse over a 10-year period. Another example of collecting data over time for comparative purposes is a study using a time series design, in which the intent is to see if changes over time can reasonably be attributed to some intervention.
4. Enhancement of internal validity. As mentioned earlier in this chapter, some research designs capitalize on the use of a repeated measures design wherein subjects serve as their own controls to control for extraneous variables. Also, in nonequivalent control group designs, the collection of preintervention data allows the researcher to detect—and control for—any initial differences between groups.

Because of the importance of the time dimension in designing research, studies are often categorized in terms of how they deal with time. The major distinction is between cross-sectional and longitudinal designs.

Cross-sectional Designs

Cross-sectional studies involve the collection of data at one point in time. The phenomena under investigation are captured, as they manifest themselves, during one period of data collection. Surveys, for example, are often cross-sectional, and many field studies are cross-sectional in design.

Cross-sectional studies are especially appropriate for describing the status of phenomena or for describing relationships among phenomena at a fixed point in time. For example, in an experimental context, a researcher might seek to determine whether a stress-management program is effective in reducing tension headaches 2 weeks after completion of the program. In a nonexperimental context, a researcher might be interested in determining whether symptoms of irritability in menopausal women are correlated contemporaneously with physiologic symptoms.

However, cross-sectional designs are sometimes used for purposes such as the four described earlier, and in such instances the design is often much weaker than longitudinal designs. As one example, cross-sectional survey data are often used to infer a causal, temporal chain. For example, a researcher might test the hypothesis, using cross-sectional data, that a determinant of excessive alcohol consumption is low impulse control, as measured by a psychologic test. However, when both alcohol consumption and impulse control are measured concurrently, it is difficult to know which variable influenced the other, if either. Cross-sectional data can most appropriately be used to infer temporal sequencing under two circumstances: (1) when there is evidence or logical reasoning to ensure that one variable preceded the other (e.g., if gender were an independent variable in the study of alcohol consumption, then there would be no confusion over whether gender "came first") and (2) when there is a strong theoretical framework guiding the analysis, as in the case of many path analytic designs.

Cross-sectional studies can also be designed in such a way that processes evolving over time can be inferred, as when the measurements capture the process at different points in its evolution with different individuals. As an example, suppose we were interested in studying the changes in nursing students' attitude toward professionalism as they progress through a 4-year baccalaureate program. One way to investigate this issue would be to survey students when they are freshmen and survey them again every year until they graduate; this would be a longitudinal design. On the other hand, we could use a cross-sectional design by surveying members of the four classes at one point and then comparing the responses of the four groups. If seniors manifested more positive attitudes toward nursing professionalism than freshmen, it might be inferred that nursing students become increasingly socialized professionally by their educational experiences. To make this kind of inference, the researcher must assume that the senior students would have responded as the freshmen responded had they been questioned three years earlier, or, conversely, that freshmen students would demonstrate increased favorability toward professionalism if they were surveyed three years later.

The main advantage of cross-sectional designs in such situations is that they are practical: they are relatively economical and easy to manage. There are, however, a number of problems in inferring changes and trends over time using a cross-sectional design. The overwhelming number of social and technological changes that characterizes our society frequently makes it questionable to assume that differences in the behaviors, attitudes, or characteristics of different age groups are the result of the passage through time rather than the result of cohort or "generational" differences. In the nursing students example, seniors and freshmen may have different attitudes toward the nursing profession, independent of any experiences during their four years of education. In cross-sectional studies, there are frequently several rival hypotheses for any observed differences.

Longitudinal Designs

Research projects that are designed to collect data at more than one point in time are referred to as *longitudinal studies*. In previous chapters, various types of longitudinal studies were discussed, such as studies using a time series design. In this section we discuss several other types of longitudinal studies primarily to present new terminology and to acquaint students with alternative designs.

Trend studies are investigations in which samples from a general population are studied over time with respect to some phenomenon. Different samples are selected at repeated intervals, but the samples are always drawn from the same population. Trend studies permit researchers to examine patterns and rates of change over time and to predict future directions. For example, trend studies have been initiated to analyze the number of students entering nursing programs and to forecast future supplies of nursing personnel.

Cohort studies are a particular kind of trend study in which specific subpopulations are examined over time. Once again, different samples are selected at different points in time, but the samples are drawn from specific subgroups that are often age-related. For example, the cohort of women born from 1946 to 1950 may be studied at regular intervals with respect to health-care utilization. As another example, the cohort of nursing students receiving their bachelor's degree in the 1960s may be periodically surveyed to determine their employment/unemployment patterns.

A sophisticated design known as the *cross-sequential design* combines the features of cohort studies with a cross-sectional approach. In cross-sequential studies, two or more different age cohorts are studied longitudinally so that both changes over time and "generational" or cohort differences can be detected.

Panel studies differ from trend and cohort studies in that the *same* subjects are used to supply the data at two or more points in time. The term "panel," which is used almost exclusively in the context of longitudinal survey projects, refers to the sample of subjects involved in the study. Panel studies typically yield more information than trend studies because the investigator can usually reveal patterns of change and reasons for the changes. Because the same individuals are contacted at two or more points in time, the researcher can identify the subjects who did and did not change and then isolate the characteristics of the subgroups in which changes occurred. As an example, a panel study could be designed to explore over time the characteristics of people who were successfully able to quit smoking. Panel studies also allow the researcher to examine how conditions and characteristics at time 1 influence characteristics and conditions at time 2. For example, health outcomes at time 2 could be studied among individuals with different health-related practices at time 1. A panel study is intuitively appealing as an approach to studying change and temporal sequencing but is extremely difficult and expensive to manage. The most serious problem is the loss of participants at different points in the study—that is, the problem of attrition. Attrition is problematic for the researcher because those who drop out of the study may differ in important respects from the individuals who continue to participate; hence, both the internal and external validity of the study may be impaired.

Follow-up studies are quite similar in design to panel studies except that the term "follow-up studies" is usually associated with experiments or other types of nonsurvey research. Follow-up investigations are generally undertaken to determine the subsequent development of individuals who have a specified condition or who have received a specified intervention. For example, patients who have received a particular nursing intervention or clinical treatment may be followed up to ascertain the long-term effects of the treatment. To take a nonexperimental example, samples of premature babies may be followed up to assess their later perceptual and motor development. Studies that are referred to as "prospective" (Chapter 10) are generally either panel or follow-up studies.

In sum, longitudinal designs are appropriate for studying the dynamics of a variable or phenomenon over time. The number of data collection periods and the time intervals in between the data collection points depend on the nature of study. When change or development is rapid, numerous time points at short intervals may be required to document the pattern and make accurate forecasts.

Many nursing studies involve a time dimension. Table 12-3 presents a brief description of several nursing studies that have used different research designs to address time-related research questions.

☰ RESEARCH EXAMPLES

We conclude this chapter with examples of two research studies that highlight some of the points made. The first example illustrates a design that carefully controlled extraneous variables. The second example describes a study that used a twofold approach to looking at phenomena hypothesized to be affected by time, by using a cross-sequential design.

Example of a Randomized Block, Factorial Design

Johnson and her colleagues (1985) were interested in learning the effects of interventions that provided different mechanisms for patients to exert personal control over postoperative experiences. Their study was built on the premise that personal control can modify reactions to stressful experiences such as hospitalization. The factorial experiment they designed involved a 2 × 3 × 2 design. That is, they were interested in three different independent variables: (1) the presence or absence of concrete sensory information about the hospitalization experience; (2) three modes of instruction relating to coping strategies—a cognitive technique, a behavioral technique, or no specific instruction; and experimental and control information about postdischarge experiences. A total of 168 hysterectomy patients participated in the research and were randomly assigned to one of the treatment groups, in this case to one of 12 possible conditions. The dependent variables in this study included patients' ratings of pain; self-reported mood states such as anxiety and depression; ratings on a physical recovery index; and information from hospital records, such as medications used and length of hospitalization.

The investigators exerted strong control over the research situation through a number of techniques. First and foremost, subjects were randomly assigned to conditions. Through randomization, the researchers were able to maximize the likelihood that subjects in all treatment groups were as similar as possible with regard to all variables that could influence perceptions of the hospitalization experience. Second, the inves-

tigators introduced a blocking variable (race) in their design. By using race as a blocking variable (i.e., by randomly assigning black and white patients separately to experimental conditions), the researchers ensured that both racial groups would be proportionately represented in all conditions. Finally, the researchers exerted some control through homogeneity. By restricting the sample to hysterectomy patients, Johnson and her colleagues controlled patient gender and type of operation.

The results suggested that different strategies of introducing personal control had positive effects on different patient outcomes. For example, the behavioral coping strategy was associated with a reduction in patients' pain medication, but the cognitive coping strategy was associated with greater physical recovery during hospitalization.

Table 12-3. *Examples of Studies With a Time Dimension*

RESEARCH QUESTION	DESIGN	SAMPLE
What are the perceived stressors and strategies for coping used among renal transplant patients, and do these change over time? (Sutton & Murphy, 1989)	Cross-sectional	20 patients 0 to 23 months posttransplant 20 patients 24 to 48 months post-transplant
What are the trends in the academic achievement, values, and personal attributes of college freshmen aspiring to nursing careers from the 1960s to the 1980s? (Williams, 1988)	Trend study	Samples of 500 college freshmen surveyed in 1966, 1972, 1982, 1983, 1984, and 1985
What is the level of experienced burnout, depression, and substance abuse among nursing students, and are these related to year in school? (Haack, 1988)	Cross-sequential	283 sophomore, junior and senior nursing students over a 1-year period
What aspects of a nurse's job situation (e.g., workload, shift, and so forth) are predictive of job satisfaction? (Blegen & Mueller, 1987)	Panel study	370 nurses surveyed twice, 8 months apart
What are the factors associated with visiting and telephoning patterns of families of very low birthweight (VLBW) infants? (Brown et al., 1989)	Follow-up study	65 VLBW babies and their families, followed-up over a 6-week period

Example of a Cross-sequential Design

Mercer (1985) conducted a longitudinal study to explore the transition to the maternal role over the first year of a first-born infant's life. Her design was cross-sequential because, in addition to the fact that she gathered information longitudinally, she also followed the transition to the maternal role for three age groups—women who became mothers at age 15 to 19, 20 to 29, and 30 to 42. By using this design, she could examine how both time and maturation affected the process of role attainment.

The sample in Mercer's study consisted of 242 women, all of whom had delivered their first normal infant at a university-affiliated hospital. Interview data were obtained from subjects at 1, 4, 8, and 12 months postpartum. The interviews included a number of standardized measures, including such scales as Feelings About My Baby and Gratification in the Mothering Role.

By examining trends in the reporting of the subjects' feelings, the researcher was able to learn about the process of becoming a mother. Among the reported results was the finding that positive feelings about the baby and perceived maternal competency peaked at four months for mothers in all three age groups. Although the three age groups functioned at somewhat different levels, their patterns of functioning over the year were very similar, leading the researcher to conclude that the maternal role presented similar challenges for women at all ages and developmental levels.

≡ SUMMARY

The *research design* is the researcher's overall plan for answering the research question. The design indicates whether or not there is an intervention, and what the intervention is; the nature of any comparisons to be made; the methods to be used to control extraneous variables and enhance the study's interpretability; the setting in which the data collection will take place; and the timing of data collection activities.

A major function of most research designs is to control *extraneous variables,* that is, the unwanted or irrelevant variables in the research setting, or irrelevant characteristics of the participants, that could influence the results of the study. One important type of control relates to the *constancy of conditions* under which a study is performed. A number of aspects of the study, such as the environment, timing, communications, and the implementation of treatment, should be held constant or kept as similar as possible for each participant.

The most problematic and pervasive extraneous variables are intrinsic characteristics of the subjects. Several techniques are available to control such characteristics. First, the ideal method of control is through the random assignment of subjects to groups. Randomization effectively controls for all possible extraneous variables because it tends to produce groups in which individual variation is canceled out. Second, a homogeneous sample of subjects can be used such that there is no variability relating to characteristics that could affect the outcome of a study. Third, the extraneous variables can be built into the design of a study so that a direct assessment of their impact can be made. One such design that accomplishes this is the *randomized block design,* in which the extraneous variable is referred to as the *blocking variable.* The fourth approach, *matching,* is essentially an after-the-fact attempt to approximate a randomized block design. This procedure matches subjects (either through *pair-matching* or *balancing* groups) on the basis of one or more extraneous variables in an attempt to secure comparable groups. A fifth technique is to control extraneous variables by means of a statistical procedure known as *analysis of covariance.* Finally, in some types of studies subjects can be exposed to more than one level of a treatment and thus serve as their own controls. This sixth design, known as a *repeated measures design,* is efficient because it reduces the number of subjects required but may be unsuitable because of the potential problem of carry-over effects. Four of the procedures for controlling extraneous individual characteristics—homogeneity, blocking, matching, and matching, and analysis of covariance—share one disadvantage, and that is that the researcher must know which variables need to be controlled.

The control mechanisms reviewed here help to improve the *internal validity* of studies. Internal validity is concerned with the question of whether or not the results of a project are attributable to the independent variable(s) of interest or to other, extraneous factors. A number of plausible rival hypotheses, known as threats to the internal validity of a study, were discussed. These threats include *history, selection, maturation, testing, instrumentation,* and *mortality.*

External validity refers to the generalizability of the research findings to other individuals and other settings. A research study possesses external validity to the extent that the sample is representative of the broader population and to the extent that the study setting and experimental arrangements are representative of other environments. A useful distinction can be made between the *accessible population,* the population from which a sample is drawn, and the *target population,* which represents a larger group of individuals in whom the investigator is interested. The researcher should define the target population in terms of those characteristics that are present in the accessible population.

A research design must balance the need for internal and external validity to produce useful scientific results. In addition, a good design must be appropriate for the question being asked, free from bias, sufficiently powerful, and capable of enhancing statistical precision. Statistical *precision* refers to the sensitivity with which treatment effects, relative to the effects of extraneous variables, can be detected.

Research designers need to consider what time frame is best suited to their problem. *Cross-sectional studies* involve the collection of data at one point in time, whereas *longitudinal studies* collect data at two or more points in time. Research problems that involve trends, changes, or development over time or that intend to demon-

strate temporal sequencing of phenomena are best addressed through longitudinal designs. *Trend studies* investigate a particular phenomenon over time by repeatedly drawing different samples from the same general population. *Cohort studies* represent a type of trend study in which a particular subpopulation is studied over time with respect to some phenomenon. Longitudinal survey studies in which the *same* sample of subjects is questioned twice (or more often) are known as *panel studies. Follow-up studies* similarly deal with the same subjects studied at two or more points in time, and generally refer to those investigations in which subjects who have received a treatment or who have a particular characteristic of interest are followed up to study their subsequent development. Longitudinal studies are typically expensive, time consuming, and plagued with such difficulties as *attrition* (loss of subjects over time), but are often extremely valuable with respect to the information they produce.

≡ *STUDY SUGGESTIONS*

1. How do you suppose the use of identical twins in a research study can enhance control?

2. Suppose you were planning to conduct a non-experimental study concerning the effects of three types of ambulation devices (a cane, a walker, and a crutch) on feelings of control or security for people requiring such assistive devices. What types of extraneous variables relating to characteristics of the subjects would be important to consider and, if possible, control?

3. With respect to the preceding question, how would you go about controlling for the extraneous variables that you have identified?

4. Read a research report suggested under "Substantive References" in Chapters 9 through 11. Assess the adequacy of the control mechanisms used by the investigator and recommend additional ones if appropriate.

5. Suppose that you are studying the effects of range of motion exercises on radical mastectomy patients. You start your experiment with 50 experimental subjects and 50 control subjects. Your intervention requires the experimental subjects to come for daily sessions over a 2-week period, while control subjects come only once at the end of 2 weeks. Your final group sizes are 40 for the experimental group and 49 for the control group. The results of your study indicate that the experimental group did better in raising arm, affected side, above head level. What effects, if any, do you think the subject attrition might have on the internal validity of your study?

6. Suppose you wanted to study how nurses' attitudes toward death change as a function of years of nursing experience. Design a cross-sectional study to research this question, specifying the samples that you would want to include. Now design a longitudinal study to research the same problem. Identify the problems and strengths of each approach.

7. For each of the examples below, indicate the types of research approach that could be used to study the problem (e.g., experimental, quasi-experimental, and so forth); the type of approach you would recommend using; and how you would go about obtaining a sample, collecting data, and establishing control procedures.

  a. What effect does the presence of the newborn's father in the delivery room have on the mother's subjective report of pain?

  b. What is the effect of different types of bowel evacuation regimes on quadriplegics?

  c. Does the reinforcement of intensive care unit nonsmoking behavior in smokers affect postintensive care unit behaviors?

  d. Is the degree of change in body image of surgical patients related to their need for touch?

≡ SUGGESTED READINGS

METHODOLOGICAL REFERENCES

Beck, S.L. (1989). The crossover design in clinical nursing research. *Nursing Research, 38,* 291–293.

Braucht, G.H., & Glass, G.V. (1968). The external validity of experiments. *American Educational Research Journal, 5,* 437–473.

Burns, N., & Grove, S.K. (1987). *The practice of nursing research: Conduct, critique and utilization.* Philadelphia: W.B. Saunders. (Chapter 10)

Campbell, D.T., & Stanley, J.C. (1963). *Experimental and quasi-experimental designs for research.* Chicago: Rand McNally.

Collins, C., Given, B., & Berry, D. (1989). Longitudinal studies as intervention. *Nursing Research, 38,* 251–253.

Cook, T.D., & Campbell, D.T. (1979). *Quasi-experimentation: Design and analysis issues for field settings.* Chicago: Rand McNally.

Dayton, C.M. (1970). *The design of educational experiments.* New York: McGraw-Hill.

Given, B.A., Keilman, L.J., Collins, C., & Given, C.W. (1990). Strategies to minimize attrition in longitudinal studies. *Nursing Research, 39,* 184–186.

Hinshaw, A.S. (1979). Control by constancy: Will it work in clinical research? *Western Journal of Nursing Research, 1,* 142–145.

Kelly, J.R., & McGrath, J.E. (1988). *On time and method.* Newbury Park, CA: Sage.

Kempthorne, O. (1961). The design and analysis of experiments with some reference to educational research. In R.O. Collier & S.M. Elan (Eds.), *Research design and analysis* (pp. 97–126). Bloomington, IN: Phi Delta Kappa.

Kerlinger, F.N. (1973). *Foundations of behavioral research* (2nd ed.). New York: Holt, Rinehart & Winston. (Chapters 17–21)

Kirk, R.E. (1982). *Experimental design: Procedures for the behavioral sciences* (2nd ed.). Belmont, CA: Wadsworth.

Lipsey, M.W. (1990). *Design sensitivity: Statistical power for experimental research.* Newbury Park, CA: Sage.

Rosenthal, R. (1976). *Experimenter effects in behavioral research.* New York: Halsted Press.

Spector, P.E. (1981). *Research designs.* Beverly Hills, CA: Sage.

Weekes, D.P., & Rankin, S.H. (1988). Life-span developmental methods: Application to nursing research. *Nursing Research, 37,* 380–383.

Woods, N.F., & Catanzaro, M. (1988). *Nursing research: Theory and practice.* St. Louis: C.V. Mosby. (Chapters 8–11)

SUBSTANTIVE REFERENCES*

Baker, N.C., et al. (1984). The effect of type of thermometer and length of time inserted on oral temperature measurements of afebrile subjects. *Nursing Research, 33,* 109–111. [Constancy of conditions]

Blegen, M.A., & Mueller, C.W. (1987). Nurses' job satisfaction: A longitudinal analysis. *Research in Nursing and Health, 10,* 227–237. [Panel study]

Brown, L.P., York, R., Jacobsen, B., Gennaro, S., & Brooten, D. (1989). Very low birth-weight infants: Parental visiting and telephoning during initial infant hospitalization. *Nursing Research, 38,* 233–236. [Follow-up study]

DeWitt, S.C., & Matre, M. (1988). Nursing careers working with the elderly. *Western Journal of Nursing Research, 10,* 335–343. [Cross-sectional study]

Dunkelberger, J.E., & Aadland, S.C. (1984). Expectation and attainment of nursing careers. *Nursing Research, 33,* 235–240. [Panel study]

Foley, J., & Stone, G.L. (1988) Stress inoculation with nursing students. *Western Journal of Nursing Research, 10,* 435–448. [Randomization, blocking, repeated measures]

Greenleaf, N.P. (1983). Labor force participation among registered nurses and women in comparable occupations. *Nursing Research, 32,* 306–311. [Trend study]

Haack, M.R. (1988). Stress and impairment among nursing students. *Research in Nursing and Health, 11,* 125–134. [Cross-sequential design]

Harrison, T.M., Pistolessi, T.V., & Stephen, T.D. (1989). Assessing nurses' communication style: A cross-sectional study. *Western Journal of Nursing Research, 11,* 75–91. [Cross-sectional study]

Johnson, J.E., Christman, N.J., & Stitt, C. (1985). Personal control interventions: Short- and long-term effects on surgical patients. *Research in Nursing and Health, 8,* 131–145. [Factorial experiment, randomized block]

Kelley, S.J. (1990). Parental stress response to sexual abuse and ritualistic abuse of children in day-care centers. *Nursing Research, 39,* 25–29. [Matching]

Kirchhoff, K.T., Rebenson-Piano, M., & Patel, M.K. (1984). Mean arterial pressure readings: Variations with positions and transducer level. *Nursing Research, 33,* 343–345. [Repeated measures]

Kunnel, M.T., O'Brien, C., Munro, B.H., & Medoff-Cooper, B. (1988). Comparisons of rectal, femoral, axillary, and skin-to-mattress temperatures in stable neonates. *Nursing Research, 37,* 162–164. [Repeated measures]

Littlefield, V.M., Chang, A., & Adams, B.N. (1990). Participation in alternative care: Relationship to anxiety, depression, and hostility. *Research in Nursing and Health, 13,* 17–25. [Analysis of covariance]

Lu, Z., Metzger, B.L., & Therrien, B. (1990). Ethnic differences in physiological responses associated with the Valsalva maneuver. *Research in Nursing and Health, 13,* 9–16. [Homogeneity]

Mercer, R.T. (1985). The process of maternal role attainment over the first year. *Nursing Research, 34,* 198–203. [Cross-sequential design]

O'Brien, M.E. (1980). Hemodialysis regimen compliance and social environment. *Nursing Research, 29,* 250–255. [Panel study]

Reed, P.G. (1987). Spirituality and well-being in terminally ill hospitalized adults. *Research in Nursing and Health, 10,* 335–344. [Matching]

Rice, V.H., & Johnson, J.E. (1984). Preadmission self-instruction booklets, postadmission exercise performance, and teaching time. *Nursing Research, 33,* 147–151. [Randomized block]

Schraeder, B.D. (1986). Developmental progress in very low birth weight infants during the first year of life. *Nursing Research, 35,* 237–241. [Follow-up study]

Shaw, D.K., Deutsch, D.T., & Bowling, R.J. (1989). Efficacy of shoulder range of motion exercise in hospitalized patients after coronary bypass graft surgery. *Heart and Lung, 18,* 364–369. [Randomization]

Sutton, T.D., & Murphy, S.P. (1989). Stressors and patterns of coping in renal transplant patients. *Nursing Research, 46,* 46–49. [Cross-sectional study]

Thomas, S.A., & Friedman, E. (1990). Type A behavior and cardiovascular responses during verbalization in cardiac patients. *Nursing Research, 39,* 48–53. [Repeated measures]

*These studies illustrate some of the points made in this chapter. A comment in brackets after each citation designates the design feature of interest.

Wallston, B.S., Smith, R., Wallston, K., King, J., Rye, P., & Heim, C. (1987). Choice and predictability in the preparation for barium enemas: A person-by-situation approach. *Research in Nursing and Health, 10,* 13–22. [Blocking, randomization, analysis of covariance]

Williams, R.P. (1988). College freshmen aspiring to nursing careers: Trends from the 1960s to the 1980s. *Western Journal of Nursing Research, 10,* 94–97. [Trend study]

Yakel, M.E. (1989). Retention of cardiopulmonary resuscitation skills among nursing personnel: What makes the difference? *Heart and Lung, 18,* 520–525. [Randomized block]

Zebelman, E.S., & Olswang, S.G. (1989). Student career goal changes during doctoral education in nursing. *Journal of Nursing Education, 28,* 53–59. [Cross-sectional stduy]

13
Sampling Designs

Sampling is a complex and technical topic, to which entire texts have been devoted. At the same time, it is a topic whose basic features are familiar to us all. In the course of our daily activities, we gather knowledge, make decisions, and formulate predictions through sampling procedures. A nursing student may decide on an elective course for a semester by sampling two or three classes on the first day of the semester. Patients may generalize about the quality of nursing care as a result of their exposure to a sample of nurses during a 1-week hospital stay. We all come to conclusions about phenomena on the basis of exposure to a limited portion of those phenomena.

The scientist, too, generally derives knowledge from samples. For example, in testing the efficacy of a medication for asthma patients, a scientific researcher must come to some conclusion without administering the drug to every asthmatic. However, the scientist can rarely afford to draw conclusions based on a sample of only three or four subjects. Research methodologists have devoted considerable attention to the development of sampling plans that produce accurate and meaningful information. In this chapter we review some of these plans.

≡ BASIC SAMPLING CONCEPTS

Sampling is an indispensable step in the research process, and a step to which too little attention is typically paid. To understand the importance of sampling, the reader must first become familiar with the terms associated with sampling. Much of this terminology has been introduced in earlier chapters but will be explained in more detail here to avoid any possible confusion in subsequent discussions.

Populations

A *population* is the entire aggregation of cases that meet a designated set of criteria. For instance, if a nurse researcher were studying American nurses with doctorates, the population could be defined as all United States citizens who are registered nurses (RNs) and who have acquired a Ph.D., D.Sc.N., D.Ed., or other doctoral-level degree. Other possible populations might be all the male patients who had undergone surgery in one particular hospital during 1988, all the women in New York state who gave birth to a live baby during the past decade, all women older than age 60 who are under psychiatric care, or all the children in the United States with cystic fibrosis. As this list illustrates, a population may be broadly defined, involving millions of individuals, or may be narrowly specified to include only several hundred people.

The definition of population by no means restricts populations to human subjects. A population might consist of all of the hospital records on file in a particular hospital, or all of the blood samples taken from clients of a health maintenance organization (HMO), or all of the correspondence of Florence Nightingale. Populations may be defined in terms of actions, words, organizations, groups, and so on. Whatever the basic unit, the population always comprises the entire aggregate of elements in which the researcher is interested.

It is important in defining a population to be specific about the criteria for inclusion in the population. Consider a population defined as "American nursing students." Would this population include students in all three types of basic programs? Would part-time students be included? How about RNs returning to school for a bachelor's degree? Or those students who dropped out of school for a semester? Would foreign students enrolled in American nursing programs qualify? Insofar as possible, the researcher must consider the exact criteria by which it could be decided whether an individual person would or would not be classified as a member of the population in question. These criteria are sometimes referred to as *eligibility criteria*. The eligibility criteria identified in two nursing research projects are presented in Table 13-1.

In Chapter 12, a distinction between target and accessible populations was made. It is an important distinction for nurse researchers, who seldom have access to the entire target population about which they would like to draw conclusions. The *accessible population* is the aggregate of cases that conform to the designated criteria *and* that are accessible to the researcher as a pool of subjects for a study. The *target population* is the aggregate of cases about which the researcher would like to make generalizations. A target population might consist of all RNs currently employed in the United States, but the more modest accessible population might be restricted to employed RNs working in San Francisco. The utility of identifying both the target and accessible populations will be discussed in a later section of this chapter.

Samples and Sampling

Sampling refers to the process of selecting a portion of the population to represent the entire population. A *sample*, then, consists of a subset of the units that compose the population. In sampling terminology, the units that make up the samples and populations are usually referred to as elements. The *element* is the most basic unit about which information is collected. The element most typical in nursing research is individuals, but other entities can form the basis of a sample or population.

Samples and sampling plans vary considerably in quality. The overriding consideration in assessing a sample is its *representativeness*. A representative sample is one whose key characteristics closely approximate those of the population. If a population in a study of family-planning practices consists of 50% females, 25% of whom had used oral contraception, then a representative sample would reflect these attributes in the same proportions.

Unfortunately, there is no method for making certain that a sample is representative without obtaining the information from the entire population. Certain sampling procedures are less likely to result in biased samples than others, but there is never any guarantee of a representative sample. This may sound somewhat discouraging, but it must be remembered that the scientist always operates under conditions in which error is possible. An important role of the scientist is to minimize or control those errors, or at least to estimate the magnitude of their effects. With certain types of sampling plans it is possible to estimate through statistical procedures the *margin of error* in the data obtained from samples. Advanced textbooks such as those by Kish (1965) or Cochran (1963) elaborate on the procedures for making such estimates.

Sampling plans can be grouped into two categories: (1) probability sampling and (2) nonprobability sampling. *Probability sampling* involves some form of random selection in choosing the sampling units. The hallmark of a probability sample is that a researcher is in a position to specify the probability that each element of the population will be included in the sample. Probability sampling is the more respected of the two types of sampling plans because greater confidence can be placed in the representativeness of probability samples. In *nonprobability samples,* elements are selected by nonrandom methods. There is no way of estimating the probability that each element has of being included in a nonprobability sample, and there is no assurance that every element *does* have a chance for inclusion.

Strata

Sometimes it is useful to think of populations as consisting of two or more subpopulations or strata. A *stratum* refers to a mutually exclusive segment of a population established by one or more specifications. For instance, suppose our population consisted of all RNs currently employed in the United States. This population could be divided into two strata based on the gender of the nurse. Alternatively, we could specify three strata consisting of (1) nurses younger than 30, (2) nurses aged 30 to 45, and (3) nurses 46 or older. Within a sampling context, strata are often identified and used in the sample selection process to enhance the representativeness of the sample.

Table 13-1. *Eligibility Criteria as Specified in Nursing Studies*

PROBLEM STATEMENT	ELIGIBILITY CRITERIA
What is the relationship between new fathers' cardiovascular responses and their interactions with their newborn infants? (Jones & Thomas, 1989)	Infants at least 2,500 g at birth Mothers without complications during pregnancy or delivery Infant with a 5-minute Apgar score between 7 and 10 Fathers living with or married to mothers or expecting to see infants at least three times weekly
Can on–off differences in pulmonary artery pressures be attributed to blood volume status in acutely ill adults? (Lookinland, 1989)	Patient being treated with positive pressure volume-cycled ventilator Fraction of inspired oxygen <.50 Levels of positive and expiratory pressure <10 cm H_2O Placement of functional pulmonary artery and arterial catheters Patient without mitral disease or pulmonary hypertension

Sampling Rationale

Scientists work with samples rather than with populations because it is more economical and efficient to work with a small group of elements than with an entire set of elements. The typical researcher does not have the time or resources required to study all possible members of a population. The need for data in a specified period usually makes it imperative for the researcher to sample. Furthermore, it is usually unnecessary to gather information about some phenomenon from an entire population. It is almost always possible to obtain a reasonably accurate understanding of the phenomena under investigation by securing information from a sample. Samples, thus, are practical and efficient means of collecting data.

Still, despite all of the advantages of sampling, the data obtained from samples can lead to erroneous conclusions. Finding 100 willing subjects to participate in a research project seldom poses any difficulty at all to even a novice researcher. It is considerably more problematic to select 100 subjects who adequately represent the population. Biases in sample selection may be conscious or unconscious. *Sampling bias* refers to the systematic overrepresentation or underrepresentation of some segment of the population in terms of a characteristic relevant to the research question. Suppose a nurse researcher is investigating patients' responsivity to touch by nurses and decides to use as a sample the first 50 patients meeting certain criteria who are admitted to a specific hospital unit. Our fictitious researcher decides to omit Mr. Z from the sample because of his hostility to nurses. Mrs. X, who has just lost a spouse, is also excluded from the study out of consideration for her psychologic discomfort. The researcher has made conscious decisions to exclude certain types of individuals, and the decisions reflect personal biases rather than *bona fide* criteria for selection. Sampling bias is more likely to occur unconsciously than consciously, however. If a researcher studying nursing students systematically interviews every tenth student who enters the nursing school library, the sample will be strongly biased in favor of library-goers, even though the researcher may exert a conscientious effort to include every tenth entrant irrespective of the person's appearance, sex, or other characteristics.

The extent to which sampling bias is likely to cause concern is a function of the homogeneity of the population with respect to the attributes under investigation. If the elements in a population were all identical with respect to some critical attribute, then any sample would be as good as any other. Indeed, if the population were completely homogeneous, that is, exhibited no variability at all, then a single element would constitute a sufficient sample for drawing conclusions about the population. With regard to many physical or physiologic attributes, it may be safe to assume a reasonably high degree of homogeneity and to proceed in selecting a sample on the basis of this assumption. For example, the blood in a person's veins is relatively homogeneous. A single blood sample chosen haphazardly is usually adequate for clinical purposes. As another illustration, the physiology of laboratory rats is sufficiently similar that elaborate sampling procedures are unnecessary when testing physiologic processes with a sample of rats. For most human attributes, however, homogeneity is the exception rather than the rule. Variables, after all, derive their name from the fact that traits vary from one individual to the next. Age, income, religion, health condition, stress, attitudes, needs, habits—all of these attributes reflect the heterogeneity of humans. The researcher must be concerned with the problem of sampling bias to the degree that a population is heterogeneous on key variables. Whenever variation occurs in the population, then the same variation should be reflected in a sample.

≡ NONPROBABILITY SAMPLING

The nonprobability approach to selecting a sample is less likely than probability sampling to produce accurate and representative samples. Despite this fact, the vast majority of samples in most disciplines, including nursing research, are nonprobability samples. The three primary methods of nonprobability sampling of subjects are (1) convenience, (2) quota, and (3) purposive.

Convenience Sampling

Convenience sampling entails the use of the most conveniently available persons or objects for use as subjects in a study. The faculty member who distributes questionnaires to the nursing students in her or his class is using a convenience sample, or an *accidental sample,* as it is sometimes called. The nurse who conducts an observational study of husbands whose wives are delivering a baby at the local hospital is also relying on a convenience sample. The problem with convenience sampling is that available subjects might be atypical of the population with regard to the critical variables being measured.

Convenience samples do not necessarily comprise individuals known to the researchers. Stopping people at a street corner to obtain information on some issue is sampling by convenience. Sometimes a researcher seeking individuals with certain characteristics will place an advertisement in a newspaper or place signs in supermarkets, laundromats, community centers, or clinics. These approaches are subject to problems of bias, because people self-select themselves as pedestrians on certain streets or as volunteers in response to public notices.

Another type of convenience sampling is known as *snowball sampling* or *network sampling.* This approach is sometimes used when the research population consists of individuals with specific traits who are difficult to identify by ordinary means. Suppose a researcher were interested in studying mothers who had stopped breast-feeding their infants within one month of being released from a hospital. There are no lists or directories of people who meet these specifications. Therefore, the researcher might use a snowballing technique to get in touch with prospective subjects. Let us say that the researcher personally knows ten women who meet the designated criteria. These women are invited to participate and also asked to provide the names of any of their friends or acquaintances who also meet the criteria. The snowballing process continues until the desired sample size has been obtained. Like other types of accidental sampling, snowball sampling offers the researcher convenience at the risk of sample bias.

Convenience sampling is the weakest form of sampling. It is also the most commonly used sampling method in nursing studies. In cases in which the phenomena under investigation are fairly homogeneous within the population, the risks of bias may be minimal. In heterogeneous populations, there is no other sampling approach in which the risk of bias is greater.

If, in conducting a research study, you decide that there is no alternative to convenience sampling, you should take several steps to enhance the likelihood of achieving a representative sample. First, identify important extraneous variables. That is, identify the factors that influence the heterogeneity of the population with respect to the dependent variable. For example, in a study of the relationship between stress and health, a person's socioeconomic status is likely to be an important extraneous variable because poor people are likely to be less healthy and more stressed than more affluent ones. Then, decide how to account for this source of variation in the sampling design. One solution is to define the population such that variation resulting from extraneous variables is reduced. In the breast-feeding example, we might, for instance, restrict the sample to middle-class subjects. Alternatively, we could select the sample from communities known to differ in socioeconomic characteristics, so that our sample would be known to reflect the experiences of both lower- and middle-class subjects. In other words, if the population is known to be heterogeneous, we should take steps to either make it more homogeneous or to capture the full variation in the sample. Finally, we should attempt to gather information about the distribution of the research and extraneous variables in the population, so that general estimates of the direction and magnitude of any biases can be made. For example, if we know that 40% of the target population is of low income, but only 20% of the convenience sample is of low income, then it would be possible to make some inferences about the nature of biases in the results.

These recommended steps reinforce an earlier point: the function of research design (of which sampling design is a special case) is to control variability. Convenience sampling generally provides limited opportunity for such control. If convenience samples can be avoided, it is wise to do so. If not, the researcher should attempt some of the steps described above and should be cautious in analyzing and interpreting the resultant data.

Quota Sampling

Quota sampling is, like convenience sampling, a form of nonprobability sampling. Quota sampling goes one step beyond the suggestions made earlier in terms of efforts to use knowledge about the population to build some representativeness into the sampling plan. The *quota sample* is one in which the researcher identifies strata of the population and determines the proportions of elements needed from the various segments of the population. By using information about the composition of a population, the investigator can ensure that diverse segments are represented in the sample in the proportions in which they occur in the population. Quota sampling gets its name from the procedure of establishing "quotas" for the various strata from which data are to be collected.

Let us consider the example of a researcher interested in studying the attitudes of undergraduate nursing students toward the role of the industrial nurse. The accessible population is a single school of nursing that has an undergraduate enrollment of 1000 students. A sample size of 200 students is desired. The easiest procedure would be to use a convenience sample, by distributing questionnaires in classrooms or catching students as they enter or leave the library. The researcher may believe, however, that male and female students will have different attitudes toward the industrial nurse's role, as will members of the four different classes. A convenience sample could easily oversample and undersample these diverse population sectors. Table 13-2 presents some fictitious data showing the proportions of each stratum for the population and for a convenience sample. As this table shows, the convenience sample very seriously overrepresents freshmen and women, and underrepresents males and members of the sophomore, junior, and senior classes. In anticipation of a problem of this type, the researcher can guide the selection of subjects such that the final sample will include the correct number of cases from each stratum. Table 13-2 shows, in the bottom panel, the number of cases that would be required for each stratum in a quota sample for this example.

Table 13-2. *Numbers and Percentages of Students in Strata of a Population, Convenience Sample, and Quota Sample*

GROUP	GENDER	FRESHMEN	SOPHOMORES	JUNIORS	SENIORS	TOTAL
Population	Males	25(2.5%)	25(2.5%)	25(2.5%)	25(2.5%)	100(10%)
	Females	225(22.5%)	225(22.5%)	225(22.5%)	225(22.5%)	900(90%)
	Total	250(25%)	250(25%)	250(25%)	250(25%)	1000(100%)
Convenience sample	Males	2(1%)	4(2%)	3(1.5%)	1(.5%)	10(5%)
	Females	98(49%)	36(18%)	37(18.5%)	19(9.5%)	190(95%)
	Total	100(50%)	40(20%)	40(20%)	20(10%)	200(100%)
Quota sample	Males	5(2.5%)	5(2.5%)	5(2.5%)	5(2.5%)	20(10%)
	Females	45(22.5%)	45(22.5%)	45(22.5%)	45(22.5%)	180(90%)
	TOTAL	50(25%)	50(25%)	50(25%)	50(25%)	200(100%)

Table 13-3. *Students Willing to Consider Industrial Nurse Role*

SAMPLE	NUMBER IN POPULATION	NUMBER IN CONVENIENCE SAMPLE	NUMBER IN QUOTA SAMPLE
Freshmen males	2	0	0
Sophomore males	6	1	1
Junior males	8	1	2
Senior males	12	0	3
Freshmen females	6	2	1
Sophomore females	16	2	3
Junior females	30	4	7
Senior females	45	3	9
Number of willing students	125	13	26
Total number of students	1000	200	200
PERCENTAGE	12.5%	6.5%	13.0%

If we pursue this same example a bit further, the reader may perhaps better appreciate the dangers of inadequate representation of the various strata. Suppose that one of the key questions in this study was, "Do you think you might ever consider taking a position as an industrial nurse?" The percentage of students in the population who would respond "yes" to this inquiry is shown under "Number in Population" in Table 13-3. Of course, these values would never be known by the researcher; they are displayed to illustrate a point. Within the population, males and older students are more willing to consider the industrial nurse's role, yet these are the very groups that are underrepresented in the convenience sample. As a result, there is a sizable discrepancy between the population and sample values: nearly twice as many students are favorable toward the role of the industrial nurse (12.5%) than one would suspect based on the results obtained from the convenience sample (6.5%). The quota sample, on the other hand, does a reasonably good job of mirroring the viewpoint of the population. In actual research situations, the distortions introduced by convenience sampling may be much smaller than in this fictitious example but, conceivably, could be larger as well.

Quota sampling does not require sophisticated skills or an inordinate amount of time or effort. Many researchers who claim that the use of a convenience sample is unavoidable for their projects could probably design a quota sampling plan, and it would be to their advantage to do so. The characteristics chosen to form the strata are necessarily selected according to the researcher's judgment. The basis of stratification should be some variable that, in the estimation of the investigator, would reflect important differences in the dependent variable under investigation. Such variables as age, sex, ethnicity, socioeconomic status, educational attainment, medical diagnosis, and occupational rank are likely to be important stratifying variables in nursing research investigations.

Except for the identification of the strata and the proportional representation for each, quota sampling is procedurally quite similar to convenience sampling. Subjects are not recruited into the study according to any systematized scheme. The subjects in any particular cell constitute, in essence, a convenience sample from that stratum of the population. Referring back to the example in Table 13-2, the convenience sample of 200 students constituted a sample chosen "accidentally" from the population of 1000. In the quota sample, the 45 female seniors would constitute a convenience sample of the 225 female seniors in the population. Because of this fact, quota sampling shares many of the same weaknesses as convenience sampling. For instance, if a researcher is required by a sampling plan to interview ten males between the ages of 65 and 80, a trip to a nursing home might be the most convenient method of obtaining those subjects. Yet this approach would fail to give any representation to those many senior citizens who are living independently in the community. Despite its problems, quota sampling represents an important improvement over convenience sampling and should be considered by any researcher whose resources prevent the utilization of a probability sampling plan.

Purposive Sampling

Purposive or *judgmental sampling* derives from the belief that a researcher's knowledge about the population and its elements can be used to handpick the cases to be included in the sample. The researcher might decide to purposely select the widest possible variety of respondents or might choose subjects who are judged to be "typical" of the population in question or particularly knowledgeable about the issues under study. An underlying assumption in purposive sampling is that any errors of judgment will, in the long run, tend to balance out. Methodological research on this approach suggests, however, that this assumption may be unwarranted. Sampling in this subjective manner provides no external, objective method for assessing the typicalness of the selected subjects.

The purposive sampling method is not a generally recommended approach but can be used to advantage in certain limited instances. Newly developed instruments can be effectively pretested and evaluated with a purposive sample of divergent types of people. As another example, purposive sampling is often used when the researcher wants a sample of experts, as, for example, in conducting a needs assessment using the key informant approach or in doing a Delphi survey (see Chapter 17). Field researchers often use purposive sampling in their collection of data in the field.

The question of whether purposive samples tend to produce more accurate, representative data than convenience samples is open to conjecture. In a purposive sample, there is certainly a risk of conscious sample biases, but perhaps the necessity of making individual decisions minimizes the risk of unconscious biases. The same advice given earlier still pertains: purposive samples, like convenience samples, should be avoided if possible, particularly if the population is heterogeneous, and if they are unavoidable, the data should be treated with circumspection.

Evaluation of Nonprobability Sampling

We have stressed repeatedly the disadvantages of using nonprobability samples in scientific research. The difficulty stems from the fact that not every element in the population has a chance of being included in the sample. Therefore, it is likely that some segment of the population will be systematically underrepresented. If the population is homogeneous on the critical attributes, then systematic biases may be negligible. However, only a small fraction of the characteristics in which nurse researchers are interested are sufficiently homogeneous to render sampling bias an irrelevant consideration.

Why, then, are nonprobability samples used at all? Clearly, the advantage of this group of sampling designs lies in their practicality and economy. Probability sampling, which is discussed in the next section, requires skill, resources, time, and opportunity. In many situations, especially in studies of a clinical nature, the researcher may have no option but to use a nonprobability approach or to abandon the project altogether. Even hard-nosed research consultants would hesitate to advocate a total abandonment of one's ideas in the absence of a random sample. The researcher using a nonprobability sample out of necessity must be cautious about the inferences and conclusions drawn from the data. With care in the selection of the sample, a conservative interpretation of the results, and replication of the study with new samples, the researcher may find that nonprobability samples work reasonably well.

≡ *PROBABILITY SAMPLING*

The hallmark of *probability sampling* is the random selection of elements from the population. Random selection should not be confused with random assignment, which was described in connection with experimental research in Chapter 9. *Random assignment* refers to the process of allocating subjects to different experimental conditions on a random basis. Random assignment has no bearing on how the subjects participating in an experiment are selected in the first place. A *random selection process* is one in which each element in the population has an equal, independent chance of being selected. The four most commonly used probability sampling methods are (1) simple random, (2) stratified random, (3) cluster, and (4) systematic sampling.

Simple Random Sampling

Simple random sampling is the most basic of the probability sampling designs. Because the more complex probability sampling designs incorporate the features of simple random sampling, the procedures involved will be described here in some detail.

After the population has been identified and the eligibility criteria have been specified, it is necessary to establish what is known as a sampling frame. *Sampling frame* is the technical name for the actual list of the sampling units or elements from which the sample will be chosen. If nursing students attending Wayne State University constituted the accessible population, then a roster of those students would be the sampling frame. If the sampling unit were 400-bed (or larger) general hospitals in the United States, then a list of all such hospitals would be the sampling frame. In actual practice, a population may be defined in terms of an existing sampling frame

rather than starting with a population and then developing a list of sampling units. For example, if we wanted to use a telephone directory as a sampling frame, we would have to define the population as the residents of a certain community who are clients of the telephone company and who have a listed number. All members of a community do not own a telephone and others fail to have their numbers listed, so it would be inappropriate to consider a telephone directory to be the sampling frame for the entire community population.

Once a listing of the population elements has been developed or located, the elements must be numbered consecutively. A table of random numbers would then be used to draw a sample of the desired size. An example of a sampling frame with 50 individuals is presented in Table 13-4. Let us assume that a sample of 20 people is sufficient for our purposes. As in the case of random assignment, we would find a starting place in the table of random numbers by blindly placing our finger at some point on the page. To include all numbers between 1 and 50, two-digit combinations would be read. Suppose, for the sake of the example, that we began the random selection with the very first number in the random number table of Table 9-1 (in Chapter 9), which is 46. The person corresponding to the number, D. Abraham, is the first subject selected to participate in the study. Number 05, G. Espeland, is the second selection, and number 23, D. Young, is the third. This process would continue until the 20 required subjects were chosen. The selected elements are circled in Table 13-4.

It should be clear that a sample selected randomly in this fashion is not subject to the biases of the researcher. There is no chance for the operation of personal preferences. Despite the fact that systematic biases do not operate in a properly drawn random sample, there is no guarantee that the sample will be representative. Random selection does, however, guarantee that differences in the attributes of the sample and the population are purely a function of chance. The probability of selecting a markedly deviant sam-

Table 13-4. *Sampling Frame for Simple Random Sampling Example*

① N. Alexander	26. W. Bradford
2. S. Babiarz	27. J. Coyne
3. A. Condy	28. R. Donofrio
4. F. Doolittle	29. M. Elie
⑤ G. Espeland	30. D. Friedlander
⑥ B. Fernandez	㉛ J. Gueron
7. W. Glass	32. J. Healy
8. G. Holle	㉝ S. James
9. R. Ivry	㉞ G. Karl
10. P. Jackson	35. D. Long
11. T. Karasek	36. G. Mazula
12. M. Little	37. D. Navarro
⑬ W. McDuffy	㊳ J. O'Hara
⑭ D. Nunally	39. A. Patterson
15. G. Oliver	40. J. Quint
16. D. Pearson	41. J. Riccio
⑰ D. Queenan	42. C. Smith
⑱ S. Shurina	㊸ L. Traeger
19. B. Telasky	44. E. Vallejo
20. K. Upshaw	㊺ J. Wallace
㉑ J. Vega	㊻ D. Abraham
22. F. Walker	47. R. Bookwalter
㉓ D. Young	48. G. Cave
㉔ J. Zumbo	49. A. Demos
25. V. Askew	㊿ D. Edelstein

ple is normally quite low, and this probability decreases as the size of the sample increases.

Simple random sampling usually is a laborious process. The development of the sampling frame, enumeration of all the elements, and selection of the sample elements are time-consuming chores, particularly if the population is large. Imagine enumerating all of the telephone subscribers listed in the New York City telephone directory. If the elements can be arranged in computer-readable form, then the computer can easily be programmed to automatically select the sample. In actual practice, simple random sampling is not used frequently because it is a relatively inefficient procedure. Furthermore, it is often impossible to get a complete listing of every element in the population, so other methods may be required.

Stratified Random Sampling

Stratified random sampling is a variant of simple random sampling in which the population is first divided into two or more strata or subgroups. As in the case of quota sampling, the aim of stratified sampling is to obtain a greater degree of representativeness. Stratified sampling designs subdivide the population into homogeneous subsets from which an appropriate number of elements can be selected at random.

The stratification may be based on a wide variety of attributes, such as age, gender, occupation, and so forth. The chosen variable should be one that will result in internally homogeneous strata on the attributes about which information is being sought. The difficulty lies in the fact that the variables of interest may not be readily discernible or available. If one is working with a telephone directory, it would be risky to make decisions about a person's gender, and certainly age, ethnicity, or other personal information is not listed. One might be able to use the telephone exchange as an indicator of the area of residence, but perhaps the residential area would not be a relevant stratifying variable. Patient listings, student rosters, or organizational directories might contain the information needed for a meaningful stratification. Quota sampling does not have the same problem because the researcher can ask the prospective subject questions that determine his or her eligibility for a particular stratum. In stratified sampling, however, decisions about a person's status in a stratum must be made before a sample is chosen.

Various procedures for drawing a stratified sample have been used. The most common is to group together those elements that belong to a stratum and to select randomly the desired number of elements. The researcher may take either an equal number of elements from each stratum, or may decide to select unequal numbers, for reasons discussed later in this section. To illustrate the procedure used in the simplest case, suppose that the list in Table 13-4 consisted of 25 males (numbers 1 through 25) and 25 females (numbers 26 through 50). Using gender as the stratifying variable, we could guarantee a sample of ten males and ten females by randomly sampling ten numbers from the first half of the list and ten from the second half. As it turns out, our simple random sampling did result in ten elements being chosen from each half of the list, but this was purely by chance. It would not have been unusual to draw, say, seven names from one half and 13 from the other. Stratified sampling can guarantee the appropriate representation of different segments of the population.

In many cases, the stratifying variables will divide the population into unequal subpopulations. For example, if the person's race were used to stratify the population of U.S. citizens, the subpopulation of white persons would be larger than that of black and other nonwhite persons. In such a situation, the researcher might decide to select subjects in proportion to the size of the stratum in the population. This procedure is referred to as *proportional stratified sampling.* If an undergraduate population in a school of nursing consisted of 10% black students, 5% Hispanic students, and 85% white students, then a proportional stratified sample of 100 students, with racial/ethnic background as the stratifying variable, would consist of 10, 5, and 85 students from the respective subpopulations.

When the researcher is interested in understanding differences among the strata, proportional sampling may result in an insufficient base for making comparisons. In the previous example, would the researcher be justified in coming to conclusions about the characteristics of Hispanic nursing students based on only five cases? It would be extremely unwise to do so in most types of research. When random selection procedures are used, the probability of obtaining a representative sample increases as the sample size increases. For this reason, researchers often adopt a *disproportional sampling design* whenever interstratum comparisons are sought between strata of greatly unequal membership size. In the example, the sampling proportions might be altered to select 20 black students, 20 Hispanic students, and

60 white students. This design would ensure a more adequate representation of the viewpoints of the two racial/ethnic minorities. When disproportional sampling is used, however, it is necessary to make an adjustment to the data to arrive at the best estimate of overall population values. This adjustment process, known as *weighting,* is a simple mathematical computation that is described in detail in most texts on sampling.

Stratified random sampling offers the researcher the opportunity to sharpen the precision and representativeness of the final sample. When it is desirable to obtain reliable information about subpopulations whose membership is relatively small, stratification provides a means of including a sufficient number of cases in the sample by oversampling for that stratum. Stratified sampling may, however, be impossible if information on the critical variables is unavailable. Furthermore, a stratified sample requires even more labor and effort than simple random sampling, because the sample must be drawn from multiple enumerated listings.

Cluster Sampling

For many populations, it is simply impossible to obtain a listing of all of the elements. The population consisting of all full-time nursing students in the United States would be quite difficult to list and enumerate for the purpose of drawing a simple or stratified random sample. In addition, it would often be prohibitively expensive to sample nursing students in this way, because the resulting sample would include no more than one or two students per institution. If interviews were involved, the interviewers would have to travel to individuals scattered throughout the country. Because of these considerations, large-scale studies almost never use simple or stratified random sampling. The most common procedure for large-scale surveys is cluster sampling.

In *cluster sampling,* there is a successive random sampling of units. The first unit to be sampled is large groupings, or "clusters." In drawing a sample of nursing students, the researcher might first draw a random sample of nursing schools. Or, if a sample of nursing supervisors was desired, a random sample of hospitals might first be obtained. Usually, the procedure for selecting a general sample of citizens is to successively sample such administrative units as states, cities, districts, blocks, and then households.

The clusters can be selected either by simple or stratified methods. For instance, in selecting clusters of nursing schools it might be advisable to stratify on program type. The final selection from within a cluster may also be performed by simple or stratified random sampling.

Typically, cluster sampling proceeds through a series of different sampling units. One begins with the largest, most inclusive unit (such as a state); moving on to less inclusive units (such as counties, then hospitals); and then down to the most basic unit or element of the population (such as cardiac patients). Because of the successive stages of sampling, this approach is often referred to as *multi-stage sampling*.

For a specified number of cases, cluster sampling tends to contain more sampling errors than simple or stratified random sampling. Despite these disadvantages, cluster sampling is considerably more economical and practical than other types of probability sampling, particularly when the population is large and widely dispersed.

Systematic Sampling

The final type of sampling design to be discussed can be classified as either a probability or nonprobability sampling approach, depending on the exact procedure used. *Systematic sampling* involves the selection of every *k*th case from some list or group, such as every tenth person on a patient list, or every hundredth person listed in a directory of American Nurses' Association members. Systematic sampling is sometimes used to sample every *k*th person entering a bookstore, or passing down the street, or leaving a hospital, and so forth. In such situations, unless the population

is narrowly defined as consisting of all those people entering, passing by, or leaving, the sampling is nonprobability in nature. If college students were sampled systematically upon entering a bookstore, the resulting sample could not be called a random selection because not every student would have a chance of being selected.

Systematic sampling designs can, however, be applied in such a way that an essentially random sample is drawn. If the researcher has a list, or sampling frame, the following procedure can be adopted. The desired sample size is established at some number (n). The size of the population must be known or estimated (N). By dividing N by n, the sampling interval width (k) is established. The *sampling interval* is the standard distance between the elements chosen for the sample. For instance, if we were seeking a sample of 200 from a population of 40,000, then our sampling interval would be

$$k = 40,000/200 = 200$$

In other words, every 200th element on the list would be sampled. The first element should be selected randomly, using a table of random numbers. Let us say that we randomly selected number 73 from a table. The people corresponding to numbers 73, 273, 473, 673, and so forth would be included in the sample.

In actual practice, systematic sampling conducted in this manner is essentially identical to simple random sampling. Problems may arise if the list is arranged in such a way that a certain type of element is listed at intervals coinciding with the sampling interval. For instance, if every tenth nurse listed in a nursing personnel roster were a head nurse and the sampling interval was ten, then head nurses would either always or never be included in the sample. Problems of this type are not too common, fortunately. In most cases, systematic sampling is preferable to simple random sampling because the same results are obtained in a more convenient and efficient manner. Systematic sampling procedures can also be applied to lists that have been stratified.

Evaluation of Probability Sampling

Probability sampling is really the only viable method of obtaining truly representative samples. The superiority of probability sampling lies in its avoidance of conscious or unconscious biases. If all of the elements in the population have an equal probability of being selected, then the likelihood is high that the resulting sample will do a good job of representing the population.

A further advantage is that probability sampling allows the researcher to estimate the magnitude of sampling error. *Sampling error* refers to differences between population values (such as the average age of the population) and sample values (such as the average age of the sample). It is a very rare sample that is perfectly representative of a population and contains no sampling error on any of the attributes under investigation. Probability sampling does, however, permit estimates of the degree of expected error.

Probability sampling is at the heart of most statistical testing. Strictly speaking, it is inappropriate to apply inferential statistics to data obtained from nonprobability samples, although most researchers ignore this issue in their treatment of data. Chein (1976) has discussed this problem at some length, and the concerned reader would profit by reading this discussion.

The great drawback of probability sampling is its expense and inconvenience. Unless the population is very narrowly defined, it is usually beyond the scope of small-scale research projects to sample using a probability design. A researcher adopting a nonprobability sampling design might well be able to argue that the homogeneity of the attribute under consideration makes an elaborate sampling scheme unnecessary. This justification will probably be unacceptable, however, if psychologic, social, or economic attributes are being studied.

The *selection* of elements that is representative of the population does not guarantee the participation of all of those elements, however. Biased samples can result from probability sampling if certain segments of the population systematically refuse to cooperate. In sum, probability sampling is the preferred and most respected method of obtaining sample elements, but it may in some cases be impractical or unnecessary.

☰ *SAMPLE SIZE*

A major concern to beginning researchers is the number of subjects needed in a sample. There are some sophisticated methods for developing sample size estimates using a procedure known as *power analysis,* but some statistical knowledge is needed before this procedure can be explained. Below we offer guidelines to beginning researchers; the advanced student should review the discussion of power analysis in Chapter 22 or consult an advanced sampling or statistical text.

Although there are no simple formulas that indicate how large a sample is needed in a given study, we can offer a simple piece of advice: you should use the largest sample possible. The larger the sample, the more representative of the population it is likely to be. Every time a researcher calculates a percentage or an average based on sample data, the purpose is to estimate a population value. Smaller samples will tend to produce less accurate estimates than larger samples. In other words, the larger the sample, the smaller the sampling error.

Let us illustrate this notion with a simple example of, say, monthly aspirin consumption in a nursing home facility, as shown in Table 13-5. The population consists of 15 residents whose aspirin consumption averages 16 aspirins per month. Two simple random samples with sample sizes of two, three, five, and ten each have been drawn. Each sample average represents an estimate of the population, which is 16. Under ordinary circumstances, the population value would be unknown to us, and we would draw only one sample. With a sample size of two, our estimate might have been wrong by as many as eight aspirins in sample 1B—a 50% error. As the sample size increases, the averages not only get closer to the true population value, but the differences in the estimates between samples A and B get smaller as well. As the sample size increases, the probability of getting a markedly deviant sample diminishes. Large samples permit the principle of randomization to do the job for which it is designed: to counterbalance, in the long run, atypical values. The safest procedure in most circumstances is to obtain data from as large a sample as is economically and practically feasible.

However, large samples are no assurance of accuracy. When nonprobability sampling methods are used, even a large sample can harbor extensive bias. The famous example illustrating this point is the 1936 presidential poll conducted by the magazine *Literary Digest,* which predicted that Alfred M. Landon would defeat Franklin D. Roosevelt by a landslide. Approximately 2.5 million individuals participated in this poll—a rather substantial sample. Biases resulted from the fact that the sample was drawn from telephone directories and automobile registrations during a depression year when only the well-to-do had a car or telephone. Thus, a large sample cannot correct for a faulty sampling design. The researcher should make decisions about the sample size and design based primarily on how representative of the population the sample is likely to be.

Because practical constraints such as time, availability of subjects, and resources often limit the number of subjects included in nursing studies, many are based on relatively small samples. In a survey of nursing studies published over four decades (the 1950s to the 1980s), Brown and her colleagues (1984) found that the average sample size was under 100 subjects in all four decades, and similar results were reported in a more recent analysis (Moody et al., 1988). In many cases, a small sample is inappropriate and can lead to misleading results. However, in some cases, a small sample size may be justifiable. Below we discuss some considerations in deciding whether a small sample is appropriate.

Nature of the Investigation

When a researcher undertakes an in-depth, qualitative study, the sample of subjects used to generate data is typically small—usually well under 100 subjects. This is because the qualitative researcher is interested in studying some phenomenon intensively rather than extensively. Such studies are often descriptive, and serve to generate hypotheses and theory rather than to test them. Small samples are usually adequate to capture a full range of "themes" emerging in relation to the phenomenon of interest. Moreover, qualitative analysis is typically a time-con-

Table 13-5.   *Comparison of Population and Sample Values/Averages*

NUMBER IN GROUP	GROUP	VALUES (MONTHLY NUMBER OF ASPIRINS CONSUMED)	AVERAGE
15	Population	2, 4, 6, 8, 10, 12, 14, 16, 18, 20, 22, 24, 26, 28, 30	16.0
2	Sample 1A	6, 14	10.0
2	Sample 1B	20, 28	24.0
3	Sample 2A	16, 18, 8	14.0
3	Sample 2B	20, 14, 26	20.0
5	Sample 3A	26, 14, 18, 2, 28	17.6
5	Sample 3B	30, 2, 26, 10, 4	14.4
10	Sample 4A	22, 16, 24, 22, 2, 8, 14, 28, 20, 2	15.8
10	Sample 4B	14, 18, 12, 20, 6, 14, 28, 12, 24, 16	16.4

suming procedure that would become unwieldy with very large samples.

In quantitative studies, the researcher generally tests hypotheses using formal statistical procedures. Small samples are generally insufficiently powerful to provide a meaningful statistical test (and hence the use of power analysis to estimate sample size needs). Thus, whenever hypotheses are being tested, or when the researcher is interested in describing the extensiveness of some phenomenon (as is often the case in survey research), relatively large samples of subjects are generally needed.

Homogeneity of the Population

When the researcher has reason to believe that the population is relatively homogeneous with respect to the variables of interest, then a small sample may be adequate for research purposes. Let us demonstrate that this is so. The top half of Table 13-6 presents hypothetical population values for three different populations, with only ten people in each population. These values could reflect, for example, scores on a measure of anxiety. In all of the populations, the average anxiety score is 100. In population A, however, the individuals have fairly similar anxiety scores: the scores range in value from a low of 90 to a high of 110. In population B, the scores are more variable,

and in population C, the scores are more variable still: the scores range from 70 to 130.

The second half of Table 13-6 presents three sample values from the three populations. In the most homogeneous population (A), the average anxiety score for the sample is 98.33, which is close to the population value of 100. As the population becomes less homogeneous with regard to their anxiety scores, the average sample values less accurately reflect the population values. In other words, there is greater sampling error when the population is heterogeneous on the key variables. By increasing the sample size, the risk of sampling error would be reduced. For example, if sample C consisted of five values rather than three (say, all the even-numbered values), then the average would be closer to the population value (in this case, 102 rather than 91.67).

For clinical studies that deal with biophysiologic processes in which variation is limited, a small sample may adequately represent the population. For most nursing studies, however, it is probably safer to assume a fair degree of heterogeneity, unless there is evidence from prior research or from experience to the contrary.

Effect Size

Power analysis builds on the concept of effect size, a term that we mentioned briefly in

Table 13-6. *Three Populations of Different Homogeneity*

POPULATION	POPULATION VALUES	POPULATION AVERAGE
A	100 110 105 95 90 110 105 95 90 100	100
B	100 120 115 85 80 120 115 85 80 100	100
C	100 130 125 75 70 130 125 75 70 100	100

SAMPLE	SAMPLE VALUES	SAMPLE AVERAGE
A	110 90 95	98.33
B	120 80 85	95.00
C	130 70 75	91.67

connection with meta-analyses. *Effect size* is concerned with the strength of the relationship among research variables. If the researcher has reason to believe that the independent and dependent variables will be strongly interrelated, then a relatively small sample is generally adequate to demonstrate the relationship statistically. For example, if a researcher were testing a powerful new drug with human subjects, it might be possible to demonstrate the drug's effectiveness with a small number of subjects. Typically, however, interventions have modest effects, and variables are usually only moderately correlated with one another. When the researcher has no *a priori* reason for believing that relationships will be strong (i.e., when the effect size is expected to be modest), then relatively large samples are needed.

Attrition

In many situations, the number of subjects recruited to participate in a study declines during the course of the project. This is most likely to occur in longitudinal studies, especially if the time lag between data collection points is great; the population is a mobile or a hard-to-locate one; or the population is a high-risk, vulnerable one in which death or disability is likely to ensue. If resources are devoted to tracking down subjects in longitudinal studies, or if the researcher has an ongoing relationship with subjects (as might be true in many clinical studies), then the rate of attrition might be low. However, it is the rare longitudinal study that maintains the entire research sample. Therefore, in estimating sample size needs, the researcher should factor in anticipated loss of subjects from the sample. In many longitudinal studies, attrition rates of 20% or more are not uncommon.

Attrition problems are not restricted to longitudinal studies. Subjects who agree to cooperate in a study may be unable to participate for a number of reasons, such as death, deteriorating health condition, early discharge, or discontinued need for a particular intervention. Researchers should attempt to anticipate a certain amount of subject loss and to recruit subjects accordingly.

Other Considerations

Several other factors should be considered in deciding how large the research sample should be. These include the following:

Number of variables. In general, the greater the number of independent and extraneous variables, the larger the sample should be. If the research design can be laid out such that the number of "cells" can be determined, then the study should aim to have at least 20 to 30 subjects for each cell of the design. For example, a study of the effects of gender (male/female); race/ethnicity (white, black, Hispanic); and marital status (married/not married)—2 × 3 × 2—on success in an alcohol treatment program should ideally have at least 140 to 210 subjects. A power analysis might indicate that even more subjects should be included.

Subgroup analyses. A related point is that a researcher is sometimes interested in testing hypotheses not only for an entire population of subjects, but for specific subgroups as well. For example, a researcher might be interested in determining whether a structured exercise program is effective in improving infants' motor skills. After the researcher has tested this general hypothesis with a sample of infants, it might be useful to test whether the intervention is more effective for certain types of infants (e.g., very low birthweight infants) than for others. When a sample is divided to test for effects in specific subgroups, the sample must be large enough to support these divisions of the sample.

Sensitivity of the measures. Different measures vary in their ability to measure precisely the concepts under study. Biophysiologic measures are generally very sensitive—they measure phenomena accurately and they can often make fine discriminations in values. Measures that are psychologic in nature often contain a fair amount of "error" and are typically not very precise. In general, when the measuring tool is imprecise and susceptible to errors, larger samples are needed to adequately test hypotheses.

≡ *STEPS IN SAMPLING*

The steps to be undertaken in drawing a sample vary somewhat from one sampling design to the next. However, the general outline of procedures involved can be described. The first phase of the sampling process involves the identification of the target population and the specification of eligibility criteria. For example, the target population could consist of all RNs currently unemployed in the United States, or all diabetics, or all women who have had a miscarriage.

Unless the researcher has extensive resources at his or her disposal, access to the entire target population usually is impossible. Therefore, it is often useful to identify a portion of the target population that is accessible to the researcher. In essence, an accessible population is a sample from the larger target population. An accessible population might consist of unemployed RNs in the state of Ohio, or all diabetics under the care of a specific HMO, or women who had a miscarriage in a particular hospital in the past year.

Once the accessible population has been identified, the researcher must decide how the sample will be chosen and how large it will be. The sample size specification should consider the various aspects of the study that were discussed in the previous section. If the researcher can perform a power analysis to determine the desired number of subjects and it is appropriate to do so, it is highly recommended that a power analysis be undertaken. Similarly, if probability sampling is an option, that option should generally be exercised. The typical nurse researcher is not in a position to do either. In such a situation, we recommend using as large a sample as possible and taking steps to build representativeness into the design (e.g., by using quota sampling).

Once the sampling design has been specified, the next step is to recruit the subjects according to the designated plan (after any needed institutional permissions have been obtained) and ask them for their cooperation. It is generally important to record some information about all individuals approached, including those who refuse to participate. If possible, obtain background information such as age, gender, education, and occupation. This information may help you to estimate the extent of some of the biases in your results, by enabling you to compare the characteristics of individuals who agreed to participate with those of people who declined.

One final point concerns the interpretation of results. Ideally, the sample is representative of the accessible population, and the accessible population is representative of the target population. By using an appropriate sample size and sampling plan, the researcher can be reasonably confident that the first part of this ideal has been realized. A greater risk is involved in assuming that the second part of the ideal is also realized. Are the unemployed nurses of Ohio representative of all unemployed nurses in the United States? One can never be sure. The researcher must exercise judgment in assessing the degree of similarity.

There are, of course, no rules that a researcher can use as a guideline in making such judgments. The best advice is to be realistic and somewhat conservative. The researcher should interpret the findings and come to conclusions after asking: Is it reasonable to assume that the accessible population is representative of the target population? In what ways might they be expected to differ? How would such differences affect the conclusions? If the researcher decides that the differences in the two populations are too great, it would be prudent to identify a more restricted target population to which the findings could be meaningfully generalized.

☰ RESEARCH EXAMPLES

The overwhelming majority of nursing studies use convenience samples. However, an increasing number of investigations are using sophisticated sampling designs, including probability sampling. Table 13-7 presents some examples of nursing studies that used various methods of sampling. Below we describe a sampling plan of a nursing study in greater detail.

> Duxbury and her colleagues (1984) studied the effect of head nurse leadership style (as perceived by staff) on staff nurses' "burnout" and job satisfaction. The study focused on nurses working in neonatal intensive care units (NICUs). The aim was to distribute questionnaires to a national sample of nurses working in such units.
>
> The investigators began with a simple random sample of level III NICUs in the United States. From that random sample, a subsample of 20 NICUs was drawn, using judgmental procedures. The sample was selected to ensure that both high-turnover and low-turnover units would be represented in the study sample. Of the 20 NICUs selected, only 14 agreed to distribute the questionnaires to staff nurses.
>
> The final sample consisted of 283 RNs employed in staff nurse positions in the 14 NICUs. The method of distribution of questionnaires was not described in the report, but presumably all nurses meeting the study criteria in the 14 NICUs were asked to complete a questionnaire. Among those nurses to whom a questionnaire was given, 57.3% responded.

The investigators clearly took some steps to ensure that the results of their study would not be limited to a single institution or to several institu-

Table 13-7. *Examples of Sampling Designs Used in Nursing Studies*

PROBLEM STATEMENT	TYPE OF SAMPLING	DESCRIPTION OF SAMPLE
What is the relative predictive strength of self-help, uncertainty in illness, and social dependency on life quality among the chronically ill? (Braden, 1990)	Convenience	396 patients with a diagnosis of rheumatoid arthritis listed on a patient roster of an arthritis center in a southwestern community
Among experienced caregivers, what is the meaning of caring for severely demented nursing home patients? (Norberg & Asplund, 1990)	Purposive/quota	The three most experienced licensed practical nurses and the most experienced RN in each of 15 nursing homes; total of 60 care-givers
What are the perceptions of male nurses concerning role strain in the areas of community, colleagues, and patient care? (Egeland & Brown, 1988)	Simple random	367 male nurses from a list of all male nurses licensed and residing in Oregon
Is there significant variation in the personal characteristics of nurses (with regard to job satisfaction, powerlessness, and locus of control) in six types of hospitals? (Bush, 1988)	Multi-stage	171 nurses (a 10% random sample) from six hospitals differing in size, type, and governance (private versus nonprivate)
What is the relationship between delivery accommodations (traditional versus birthing room) and newborn Apgar scores? (Hutti & Johnson, 1988)	Stratified systematic	361 infants delivered in either an in-hospital birthing room or traditional delivery room in a tertiary care center, stratified (proportionately) by delivery accommodation
Does the perception of stress mediate the relationship between stressors and maternal identity? (Walker, 1989)	Stratified random	173 mothers randomly selected from birth announcements, stratified by infant age

tions in a single geographic area. Furthermore, although the questionnaire response rate was fairly low, the researchers instituted procedures to assess response bias. They compared the background characteristics of those nurses who completed the questionnaire with those of all who did not and found that, for the most part, there were few differences. However, the investigators did not indicate the extent to which the 14 NICUs were representative of all NICUs in the United States, in terms of turnover rate or other characteristics such as geographic location.

≡ SUMMARY

Sampling is the process of selecting a portion of the population to represent the entire population. A *population,* in turn, is the entire aggregate of cases that meet a designated set of *eligibility criteria*. In a sampling context, an *element* is the most basic unit about which information is collected.

The overriding consideration in assessing the adequacy of any sample is the degree to which it is representative of the population. Sampling plans vary in their ability to reflect adequately the population from which the sample was drawn. *Sampling bias* refers to the systematic overrepresentation or underrepresentation of some segment of the population. The greater the heterogeneity of the population with respect to the critical attributes, the greater the risk of sampling bias.

Sampling plans may be classified as either nonprobability or probability sampling. In *nonprobability sampling,* elements are selected by nonrandom methods. Convenience, quota, and purposive sampling are the principal nonprobability methods. *Convenience sampling* (sometimes called *accidental sampling*) consists of using the most readily available or most convenient group of subjects for the sample. A form of convenience sampling is *snowball* or *network sampling,* in which early sample members are asked to identify other potential subjects meeting the eligibility criteria. *Quota sampling* divides

the population into homogeneous *strata* or subpopulations to ensure representative proportions of the various strata in the sample. Within each stratum, the researcher selects subjects by convenience sampling. In *purposive sampling* (also referred to as *judgmental sampling*), subjects or objects are handpicked to be included in the sample, based on the researcher's knowledge about the population. Nonprobability sampling designs have the advantage of being convenient and economical. The major disadvantage of nonprobability sampling designs is their potential for serious biases.

Probability sampling designs involve the random selection of elements from the population. A *simple random sample* involves the selection of elements on a random basis from a *sampling frame* that enumerates all the elements. A *stratified random sample* divides the population into homogeneous subgroups from which elements are selected at random. *Cluster sampling* (also called *multi-stage sampling*) involves the successive selection of random samples from larger to smaller units by either simple random or stratified random methods. *Systematic sampling* is the selection of every *k*th case from some list or group. By dividing the population size by the desired sample size, the researcher is able to establish the *sampling interval,* which is the standard distance between the elements chosen for the systematic sample. Probability sampling designs are preferred to nonprobability methods because probability sampling designs tend to result in more representative samples and because they permit the researcher to estimate the magnitude of sampling error. Probability samples, however, are time-consuming, expensive, inconvenient, and, in some cases, impossible to obtain.

There is no simple equation that can be used to determine how large a sample is needed for a particular research project. If researchers cannot use *power analysis* to estimate the number of subjects needed for a study, they should use as large a sample as possible and practical, considering such factors as the nature of the study, the homogeneity of the population with respect to key variables, the risk of subject loss, and the anticipated magnitude of the relationships among key variables. In general, the larger the sample, the more representative of the population it is likely to be. Even a very large sample, however, does not guarantee representativeness if nonprobability sampling methods are used.

≡ *STUDY SUGGESTIONS*

1. Draw a simple random sample of 25 people from the sampling frame of Table 13-4 using the table of random numbers that appears in Table 9-1. Begin your selection by blindly placing your finger at some point on the table.
2. Suppose you have decided to use a systematic sampling design for a research project. The known population size is 4400 and the sample size desired is 200. What is the sampling interval? If the first element selected is 23, what would be the second, third, and fourth elements to be selected?
3. Read the article by Yarcheski and Mahon (1985) listed under "Substantive References." What were the successive clusters used to draw the sample?
4. Suppose a researcher is interested in studying the attitude of clinical specialists toward autonomy in the work situation. Suggest a possible target and accessible population. What strata might be identified by the researcher if quota sampling were used?
5. What type of sampling design was used to obtain the following samples?
   a. 15 people known by the researcher to have hypertension and 15 people known not to have hypertension
   b. the couples attending a particular prenatal class
   c. 100 nurses from a list of nurses registered in the state of Pennsylvania, using a table of random numbers
   d. 20 head nurses randomly selected from a random selection of ten hospitals located in one state
   e. every fifth article published in *Nursing Research* during the 1970s beginning with the first article

≡ *SUGGESTED READINGS*

METHODOLOGICAL REFERENCES

Babbie, E. (1973). *Survey research methods.* Belmont, CA: Wadsworth. (Chapters 5 & 6).

Brown, J.S., Tanner, C.A., & Padrick, K.P. (1984). Nursing's search for scientific knowledge. *Nursing Research, 33,* 26–32.

Chein, I. (1976). In C. Selltiz, L.S. Wrightsman, & S.W. Cook (Eds.), *Research methods in social relations* (3rd ed., pp. 512–540). New York: Holt, Rinehart & Winston.

Cochran, W.G. (1963). *Sampling techniques* (2nd ed.). New York: John Wiley and Sons.

Cohen, J. (1977). *Statistical power analysis for the behavioral sciences* (rev. ed.). New York: Academic Press.

Diekmann, J.M., & Smith, J.M. (1989). Strategies for accessment and recruitment of subjects for nursing research. *Western Journal of Nursing Research, 11,* 418–430.

Kish, L. (1965). *Survey sampling.* New York: John Wiley and Sons.

Levey, P.S., & Lemeshow, S. (1980). *Sampling for health professionals.* New York: Lifetime Learning.

Moody, L.E., Wilson, M.E., Smyth, K., Schwartz, R., Tittle, M., & VanCott, M.L. (1988). Analysis of a decade of nursing practice research: 1977–1986. *Nursing Research, 37,* 374–379.

Sudman, S. (1976). *Applied sampling.* New York: Academic Press.

Williams, B. (1978). *A sampler on sampling.* New York: John Wiley and Sons.

*SUBSTANTIVE REFERENCES**

Braden, C.J. (1990). A test of the self-help model: Learned response to chronic illness experience. *Nursing Research, 39,* 42–47. [Convenience sampling]

Bush, J.P. (1988). Job satisfaction, powerlessness, and locus of control. *Western Journal of Nursing Research, 10,* 718–731. [Multi-stage sampling]

Damrosch, S.P., & Strasser, J.A. (1988). A survey of doctorally prepared academic nurses on qualitative and quantitative research issues. *Nursing Research, 37,* 176–180. [Systematic sampling]

*A comment in brackets after each citation designates the sampling design feature of interest.

Dawson, C. (1985). Hypertension, perceived clinician empathy, and patient self-disclosure. *Research in Nursing and Health, 8,* 191–198. [Convenience sampling]

Duquette, A., Painchaud, G., & Blais, J. (1988). Reasons for nonparticipation in continuing education. *Research in Nursing and Health, 11,* 199–209. [Stratified random sampling]

Duxbury, M.L., Armstrong, G.D., Drew, G.D., & Henley, S.J. (1984). Head nurse leadership style with staff nurse burnout and job satisfaction in neonatal intensive care units. *Nursing Research, 33,* 97–101. [Purposive sampling]

Egeland, J.W., & Brown, J.S. (1988). Sex role stereotyping and role strain of male registered nurses. *Research in Nursing and Health, 11,* 257–267. [Simple random sampling]

Fuller, S.S., & Larson, S.B. (1980). Life events, emotional support, and health of older people. *Research in Nursing and Health, 3,* 31–39. [Simple random sampling]

Hanson, S. (1981). Single custodial fathers and the parent–child relationship. *Nursing Research, 30,* 202–204. [Quota sampling]

Hutti, M.H., & Johnson, J.B. (1988). Newborn Apgar scores of babies born in birthing rooms vs. traditional delivery rooms. *Applied Nursing Research, 1,* 68–71. [Stratified systematic sampling]

Jones, L. C., & Thomas, S.A. (1989). New fathers' blood pressure and heart rate: Relationships to interaction with their newborn infant. *Nursing Research, 38,* 237–241. [Convenience sampling]

Kelley, B.A. (1979). Nurses' knowledge of glycosuria testing in diabetes mellitus. *Nursing Research, 28,* 316–319. [Quota sampling]

King, I. (1984). Philosophy of nursing education: A national survey. *Western Journal of Nursing Research, 6,* 387–400. [Stratified random sampling]

Lookinland, S. (1989). Comparison of pulmonary vascular pressure based on blood volume and ventilator status. *Nursing Research, 38,* 68–71. [Quota sampling]

Mravinac, C.M., Dracup, K., & Clochesy, J.M. (1989). Urinary bladder and rectal temperature monitoring during clinical hypothermia. *Nursing Research, 38,* 73–76. [Convenience sampling]

Norberg, A., & Asplund, K. (1990). Caregivers' experience of caring for severely demented patients. *Western Journal of Nursing Research, 12,* 75–84. [Purposive/quota sampling]

Owen, B.D. (1989). The magnitude of low-back problem in nursing. *Western Journal of Nursing Research, 11,* 234–242. [Systematic sampling]

Penntengill, M.M., Knafl, K.A., Bevis, M.E., & Kirchhoff, K.T. (1988). Nursing research in midwestern hospitals. *Western Journal of Nursing Research, 10,* 705–717. [Stratified random sampling]

Reichelt, P.A. (1988). Public perception of nursing and strategy formulation. *Western Journal of Nursing Research, 10,* 472–476. [Stratified random sampling]

Walker, L.O. (1989). Stress process among mothers of infants: Preliminary model testing. *Nursing Research, 38,* 10–16. [Stratified random sampling]

Yarcheski, A., & Mahon, N.E. (1985). The unification model in nursing. *Nursing Research, 34,* 120–125. [Multi-stage sampling]

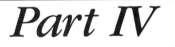

Part IV

Measure-ment and Data Collection

14
Interviews and Questionnaires

The concepts in which a researcher is interested must ultimately be translated into phenomena that can be observed and recorded. The tasks of defining the research variables and selecting or developing appropriate methods for collecting data are among the most challenging in the research process. Without high-quality data collection methods, researchers must always question the accuracy and robustness of the conclusions. As in the case of research designs and sampling plans, the researcher must often choose from an array of alternatives in deciding how to collect data.

Data collection methods vary along the following four important dimensions:

1. *Structure.* Research data are often collected according to a highly structured plan that indicates what information is to be gathered and exactly how to gather it. Sometimes, however, it is appropriate to impose a minimum of structure and to provide subjects with opportunities to reveal relevant information in a naturalistic way, as in the case of field studies.

2. *Quantifiability.* Data that will be subjected to statistical analysis must be gathered in such a way that they can be quantified. On the other hand, data that are to be analyzed qualitatively are typically collected in narrative form. Structured data collection approaches generally yield data that are more easily quantified. However, it is often possible and useful to quantify unstructured information as well.

3. *Researcher obtrusiveness.* Data collection methods differ in terms of the degree to which subjects are aware of their subject status. If subjects are fully aware of their role in a study, their behavior and responses might not be "normal." When data are collected unob-

277

trusively, however, ethical problems may emerge, as discussed in Chapter 3.

4. *Objectivity.* Some data collection approaches require more subjective judgment than others. Scientists generally strive for methods that are as objective as possible. However, in some research (especially, phenomenologically based research), the subjective judgment of the investigator is considered a valuable component of data collection.

Sometimes the nature of the research question will dictate where on these four continua the method of data collection will lie. For example, questions that require a field study will normally be low on all dimensions, whereas questions that require a survey will normally be high on all four. Often, however, the researcher has considerable latitude in selecting or designing a suitable data collection plan.

In addition to these four dimensions, nurse researchers must consider the form of data collection to use. Three types of approach have been used most frequently by nurse researchers: (1) self-report, (2) observation, and (3) physiologic measures. This chapter describes in detail options with respect to two types of self-report: interviews and questionnaires. Subsequent chapters in Part IV deal with other forms of self-report (standardized scales), as well as with observational methods, biophysiologic measures, and other less frequently used methods.

≡ *INTRODUCTION TO THE SELF-REPORT APPROACH*

In the human sciences, a good deal of information can be gathered by questioning people directly. If, for example, we are interested in learning about patients' perceptions of hospital care, patients' level of hunger or preoperative fears, or nursing students' attitudes toward gerontologic nursing, then we are likely to try to find answers by questioning a group of relevant people. For some research variables, alternatives to direct questions exist. However, the unique ability of humans to communicate verbally on a sophisticated level makes it unlikely that systematic questioning will ever be eliminated from the repertoire of data collection techniques. A recent analysis of published nursing studies spanning four decades revealed that the majority of nursing investigations involve data collected by means of self-reports (Brown et al., 1984).

The self-report method is strong with respect to its directness and versatility. If we want to know what people think, feel, or believe, the most direct means of gathering the information is to ask them about it. Perhaps the strongest argument that can be made for the self-report method is that it frequently yields information that would be difficult, if not impossible, to gather by any other means. Current behaviors can be directly observed, but only if the subject is willing to manifest them publicly. For example, it may be impossible for a researcher to observe such behaviors as child abuse, contraceptive practices, or drug usage. Furthermore, observers can only observe behaviors occurring at the time of the study; self-report instruments can gather retrospective data about activities and events occurring in the past, or gather projections about behaviors in which subjects plan to engage in the future. Information about feelings, values, opinions, and motives can sometimes be inferred through observation, but behaviors and feelings do not always correspond exactly. People's actions do not always indicate their state of mind. Here again, self-report instruments can be designed to measure psychologic characteristics through direct communication with the subject.

Self-reports are also versatile with respect to content coverage. People can be asked to report on facts about their personal background; facts about other people known to them; facts about events or environmental conditions; beliefs about what the facts are; attitudes, feelings, and opinions; reasons for opinions, attitudes, or behaviors; level of knowledge about conditions, situations, or practices; and intentions for future behaviors.

Despite these advantages, verbal report instruments share a number of weaknesses. The most serious issue is the question of the validity and accuracy of self-reports: How can we really be sure that respondents feel or act the way they say they do? How can we trust the information that respondents provide, particularly if the questions could potentially require them to reveal an unpopular position on a controversial issue or to admit to socially unacceptable behavior? Investigators often have no alternative but to assume that the majority of their respondents have been frank. Yet we all have a tendency to want to present ourselves in the best light, and this may conflict with the truth. Researchers who find it necessary or appropriate to gather self-report data should be cognizant of the limitations of this method and should be prepared to take these shortcomings into consideration when interpreting the results. Likewise, consumers of research reports should be alert to potential biases introduced when subjects are asked to describe themselves, particularly with respect to behaviors or feelings that our society judges to be wrong or unusual.

As noted in Chapter 11, self-report data can be gathered either orally by interview or in writing by questionnaire. Interviews (and, to a lesser extent, questionnaires) can vary considerably with respect to their degree of structure, as discussed in the following section.

≡ UNSTRUCTURED AND SEMISTRUCTURED SELF-REPORT TECHNIQUES

A researcher using a tightly structured approach always operates with a written document to guide the collection of data. With a non-oral format, the document is the questionnaire itself. With an oral format, the document is referred to as the *interview schedule. Standardized* or tightly *structured schedules* consist of a set of items in which the wording of both the question and the alternative responses is predetermined. When structured interviews or questionnaires are used, all subjects are asked to respond to exactly the same questions, in exactly the same order, and have the same set of options for their responses. In this

section we consider six approaches to collecting self-report data using unstructured or loosely structured methods.

Unstructured Interviews

When a researcher proceeds with no preconceived view of the content or flow of information to be gathered, he or she may conduct unstructured interviews with respondents (in self-report studies, subjects are generally referred to as *respondents* because they respond to the researcher's questions). *Unstructured interviews* are typically conversational in nature and are conducted in naturalistic settings. Their aim is to elucidate the respondents' perceptions of the world without imposing any of the researcher's views on them. A researcher using a completely unstructured approach may informally ask a broad question relating to the topic under investigation such as, "Tell me about what happened when you first learned you had AIDS [acquired immunodeficiency syndrome]?" Field studies generally rely heavily on unstructured interviews. Leininger (1984), for example, used unstructured interviews (as well as other methods) in her field study of the health-care values, beliefs, and practices of southern rural black and white cultures.

Focused Interviews

A researcher often wants to be sure that a given set of topics is covered in interviews with research subjects. In a *semistructured* or *focused interview,* the interviewer is given a list of areas or questions to be covered with each respondent; the list is referred to as a *topic guide.* The interviewer's function is to encourage participants to talk freely about all of the topics on the list and to record the responses (often on a tape recorder). For example, Kroska (1985) used a topic guide to study the role of "granny" midwives in rural Alabama.

A variant of the focused interview is the focus group interview, a technique that is becoming increasingly popular in the study of some health problems. In a *focus group interview,* a group of usually 10 to 15 individuals is assembled for a group discussion, led by an interviewer who is guided by a written series of questions or topics to be covered. The advantage of a group format is that it is efficient—the researcher obtains the viewpoint of many individuals in a short time. Its disadvantage is that some people are uncomfortable about expressing their views in front of a group. Morgan (1988) has developed guidelines for using focus group sessions for research purposes.

Life Histories

Life histories are narrative self-disclosures about a person's life experiences. Anthropologists frequently use the life history approach to learn about cultural patterns. With this approach, the researcher asks the respondents to provide, in chronological sequence, a narration of their ideas and experiences *vis-à-vis* some theme, either orally or in writing. Leininger (1985) has noted that comparative life histories are especially valuable for the study of the patterns and meanings of health and health care among elderly people. Her highly regarded essay provides a protocol for obtaining a life health-care history.

Critical Incidents

The *critical incidents technique* is a method of gathering information about people's behaviors by examining specific incidents relating to the behavior under investigation. The data for a critical incidents study are typically collected in a semistructured interview.

The technique, as the name suggests, focuses on a factual incident, which may be defined as an observable and integral episode of human behavior. The word "critical" means that the incident must have a discernible impact on some outcome; it must make either a positive or negative contribution to the accomplishment of some activity of interest.

An example should clarify the purpose of this technique. Suppose we were interested in

understanding why patients do not always follow their medication regimen and we wanted to develop teaching strategies to improve compliance. We might ask a sample of patients the following questions:

> Think of the last time you failed to take your medications as prescribed.
> > What led up to the situation?
> > Exactly what did you do?
> > Why did you feel it would be alright to miss taking the medicine?

The technique differs from other self-report approaches in that it focuses on something specific about which the respondent can be expected to "testify" as an expert witness. The primary concern is to collect one or more descriptions about factual incidents that can enlighten our understanding about why, and under what circumstances, people act the way they do. Clark and Lenburg (1980), for example, used the critical incidents technique to explore knowledge-informed behavior among nurses.

Diaries

Personal diaries have long been used as a source of data in historical research. It is also possible to generate new data for a nonhistorical study by asking subjects to maintain a diary over a specified period. The diaries may be completely unstructured; for example, individuals who have undergone an organ transplant could be asked simply to spend 10 minutes a day jotting down their thoughts and feelings. Frequently, however, subjects are requested to make entries into a diary regarding some specific aspect of their experience, sometimes in a semistructured format. For example, studies of the effect of nutrition during pregnancy on fetal outcomes frequently require subjects to maintain a complete diary of everything they ate over a 1- to 2-week period. Boyle (1985) used a Family Health Calendar over a 1-month period to collect information about how families prevent illness, maintain health, experience morbidity, and treat health problems.

Evaluation of Unstructured Approaches

Unstructured interviews are an extremely flexible approach to gathering data, and in many research contexts offer distinct advantages. In many clinical situations, for example, it may be appropriate to let individuals talk freely about their problems, allowing them to take much of the initiative in directing the flow of information. In general, unstructured interviews are of greatest utility, from a researcher's point of view, when a new area of research is being explored. In such situations, an unstructured approach may allow the investigator to ascertain what the basic issues or problems are, how sensitive or controversial the topic is, how easy it is to secure respondents' cooperation in discussing the issues, how individuals conceptualize and talk about the problems, and what range of opinions or behaviors exist that are relevant to the topic. Unstructured methods may also help elucidate the underlying meaning of a pattern or relationship repeatedly observed in survey research.

However, unstructured methods are extremely time consuming and demanding of the researcher's skill in analyzing and interpreting qualitative materials. Samples tend to be small because of the quantity of information produced, so it is often difficult to know whether findings can be generalized at all. Unstructured methods do not generally lend themselves to the rigorous testing of hypotheses concerning cause-and-effect relationships.

≡ RESEARCH EXAMPLES OF SEMISTRUCTURED AND UNSTRUCTURED SELF-REPORTS

An increasing number of published nursing studies are using unstructured or semistructured methods of self-reports to collect data. Table 14-1 briefly describes the research problem and data collection approach used in five such studies. A more detailed description of a study using semistructured interviews follows.

Table 14-1. *Examples of Nursing Studies Using Unstructured/Semistructured Self-Reports*

RESEARCH PROBLEM	SAMPLE	DATA COLLECTION APPROACH
What are the identity-management strategies used by children of gay fathers, and what are the factors that influence the use of these strategies? (Bozett, 1988)	19 children of gay fathers	Unstructured interviews
What types of upset are experienced by mothers of infants who received apnea monitoring for 1 to 17 months? (Nuttall, 1988)	74 mothers	Focused interviews
What are the traditional health beliefs and practices of black women and how are these beliefs and practices related to AIDS? (Flaskerud & Rush, 1989)	22 black women in five groups	Focus group interviews
What are the differences between mothers and nonmothers in developmental transitions over the life cycle? (Mercer et al., 1988)	50 mothers and 50 non-mothers	Life histories
What gastrointestinal (GI) symptoms do women experience across the menstrual phases and do the symptoms vary by dysmenorrhea/non-dysmenorrhea and use of oral contraceptives? (Heitkemper et al., 1988)	34 women	GI health diary

Aroian (1990) investigated the implications of migration and resettlement for emotional health and well-being in a sample of Polish immigrants who had resided in the United States for periods ranging from 4 months to 39 years. The study participants' initial and changing experiences during and following migration were explored to develop a model describing the migrants' psychologic adaptation. Migration and resettlement were treated as a process unfolding over time and presenting changing demands as well as evolving opportunities in America.

To fully explore this process, Aroian elected to conduct semistructured interviews (supplemented by a paper-and-pencil demographic questionnaire) with a sample of 25 Polish immigrants. Purposive sampling was used to stratify sample members according to three distinct waves of Polish migration. The interviews were guided by several broad questions, such as the following: "What prompted you to leave Poland?" "What is it like to be an immigrant?" "How has the experience of being an immigrant changed over time?" These broad questions were followed by more specific questions about the positive and negative aspects of migration and resettlement. All of the interviews were tape-recorded and transcribed verbatim.

Aroian found that loss and disruption, novelty, occupational adjustment, language accommodation, and subordination were predominant aspects of the migration and resettlement experience. Psychologic adaptation required the dual task of resolving grief over losses and disruption associated with leaving Poland, and of mastering various resettlement conditions in America. The model that emerged from Aroian's analysis may have implications for other types of major life change.

≡ STRUCTURED SELF-REPORT INSTRUMENTS

The majority of nurse researchers who collect self-report data use instruments with a moderate to high degree of structure. In developing structured instruments, a great deal of effort is usually devoted to the content, form, and wording of the questions being posed. This section provides some guidelines for the development and use of structured interview schedules and questionnaires.

Question Form

Structured instruments themselves vary in their degree of structure through their combination of open-ended and closed-ended questions. *Open-ended* questions (or *items,* as they are sometimes called) allow subjects to respond in their own words. The question, "What aspect of your professional relationship with physicians do you feel is most in need of improvement?" is an example of an open-ended question that might be used in a study investigating nurse–physician relationships. In questionnaires, the respondent is asked to give a written reply to open-ended items and, therefore, adequate space must be provided to allow full expression of opinions. In interviews, the interviewer is normally expected to quote the response verbatim or as closely as possible.

Closed-ended (or *fixed-alternative*) questions offer respondents a number of alternative replies from which the subjects must choose the one that most closely approximates the "right" answer. The alternatives may range from the simple yes–no variety ("Have you smoked a cigarette within the past 24 hours?") to rather complex expressions of opinion or behavior.

Both open- and closed-ended questions have certain strengths and weaknesses. Closed-ended items are difficult to construct but easy to administer and, especially, to analyze. With closed-ended questions, the researcher needs only to tabulate the number of responses to each alternative to gain some understanding about what the sample as a whole thinks about an issue. The analysis of open-ended items, on the other hand, is often difficult and time consuming. The procedure that is normally followed is the development of categories and the assignment of the open-ended responses to those categories. That is, the researcher essentially transforms the open-ended responses to fixed categories in a *post hoc* fashion so that tabulations can be made. This classification process takes considerable time and skill. Furthermore, because the ultimate classification decision lies in the hands of the researchers rather than the respondents, there is the possibility of inappropriate categorization resulting from misinterpretation of the responses or an inadequate classification system.

Closed-ended items are generally more efficient than open-ended questions in the sense that a respondent is normally able to complete more closed- than open-ended questions in a given amount of time. In questionnaires, subjects may be less willing to compose a written response than to simply check off or circle the appropriate alternative. With respondents who are unable to express themselves well verbally, closed-ended items have a distinct advantage. Furthermore, there are some types of questions that may seem less objectionable in closed form than in open form. Take the following example:

1. What was the gross annual income of your family last year?
2. In what range was your family's gross annual income last year?
   ( ) under $5,000
   ( ) $5,000 to $9,999
   ( ) $10,000 to $14,999
   ( ) $15,000 to $19,999
   ( ) $20,000 to $24,999
   ( ) $25,000 or over

The second question is more likely to be answered by respondents because the range of options allows them a greater measure of privacy than the blunter open-ended question.

These various advantages of the fixed-alternative question are offset by some corresponding shortcomings. The major drawback of closed-ended questions lies in the possibility of the researcher neglecting or overlooking some potentially important responses. It is often difficult to see an issue from multiple points of view. The omission of possible alternatives can, of course, lead to inadequate understanding of the issues and to outright bias if the respondents choose an alternative that misrepresents their position. When the researcher is unable to pretest the instrument thoroughly or when the area of research is relatively new, open-ended questions may be more suitable than closed-ended items for avoiding bias.

Another objection to closed-ended items is that they are sometimes considered too superficial. Open-ended questions allow for a richer and fuller perspective on the topic of interest, if the respondents are verbally expressive and cooperative. Some of this richness may be lost when the researcher later tabulates answers by developing a system of classification, but excerpts taken directly from the open-ended responses can be extremely valuable in a research report in imparting the "flavor" of the replies.

Finally, some respondents will often object to being forced into choosing from among responses that do not reflect their opinions precisely. Open-ended questions give a lot of freedom to the respondent and, therefore, offer the possibility of spontaneity, which is unattainable when a set of responses is provided.

The decisions to use open- and closed-ended questions are based on a number of important considerations such as the sensitivity of the topic, the verbal ability of the respondents, the amount of time available, and so forth. Combinations of both types are highly recommended to offset the strengths and weaknesses of each. Questionnaires typically use fixed-alternative questions predominantly to minimize the respondent's writing burden. Interview schedules, on the other hand, are more variable in their mixture of these two question types.

Question Wording

Unquestionably the most difficult aspect of constructing a schedule is the actual wording of the questions and, for closed-ended items, the wording of the alternative responses. In this section we discuss the problem of question wording and review four considerations that the researcher should bear in mind while designing the questions.

1. *Clarity.* It seems fairly obvious that the designer of a questionnaire or interview schedule should strive for clarity and unambiguity. A question that can be interpreted differently by different people is unlikely to produce meaningful information. Unfortunately clarity is more easily discussed than achieved. Even seemingly simple and straightforward questions may be ambiguous or open to various interpretations to respondents who do not have the same mind-set as the researcher. The question, "When do you usually eat your evening meal?" might bring forth such responses as "around 6 P.M.," "when my husband gets home from work," or "during the evening television news broadcast." The question itself contains no words that are technical or difficult but the question is unclear because the intent of the researcher is unapparent. The following suggestions might help you improve the precision of questions:

   - Clarify in your own mind the information that you are trying to obtain. If you are unclear about exactly what you want to find out, you can hardly expect respondents to guess your intentions.
   - Avoid long sentences or phrases.
   - Avoid "double-barreled" questions that contain two distinct ideas or concepts. The statement, "The mentally ill are essentially incapable of caring for themselves and should, therefore, be denied of any responsibilities or rights," might lead to conflicts of opinion in a single person, who might only agree with one part of the statement.
   - Avoid technical terms if more common terms are equally appropriate.
   - Try to state your questions in the affirmative rather than the negative.

2. *Ability of respondents to reply or give information.* A second important consideration is whether respondents can reasonably be expected to answer the questions accurately and meaningfully. Research participants are often reluctant to say, "I don't know" or "I don't understand." Therefore, the designer of the research instrument must give some thought to the characteristics of the sample in deciding whether to include certain questions and how to word them. The respondent may not be competent to answer questions for different reasons, each of which has implications for the wording of the question. In designing questions, researchers should consider the following:

   - Language. Try to use words that are simple enough for the *least* educated respondents in your sample. Do not assume that even members of your own profession will have extensive knowledge on all aspects of nursing and medical terminology.
   - Level of information. It should not be assumed that respondents will be aware of, or informed about, issues or questions in which you are interested. Furthermore, you should avoid giving the impression that respondents *ought* to have the information. Questions on complex or specialized issues can be worded in such a way that a respondent will be comfortable admitting ignorance. The following is one illustration: "Many people have not had an opportunity to learn much about the physiological side-effects of oral contraceptives, but some people have picked up information on this subject. Do you happen to know of any such side effects?" Such face-saving devices can be invaluable in making the respondent's lack of knowledge acceptable. Another approach is to preface a question by a short statement of explanation about terminology or issues.
   - Memory. You should not take for granted that respondents will be able to remember events, situations, or previous activities and feelings with a high degree of accuracy. To put respondents at ease, you

could preface a question requiring memory with a statement such as "For many of us, communications are so varied and rapid that it is difficult to remember very much in detail."

3. *Bias.* Bias is an extremely serious problem in verbal self-report instruments. Respondents, after all, can distort the results very easily by giving misinformation. The following techniques are useful in minimizing any biases that the researchers might inadvertently introduce themselves:

- Avoid leading questions that suggest a particular kind of answer. A question such as, "Do you agree that nurse–midwives play an indispensable role in the health team?" is not neutral.
- Avoid identifying a position or attitude with a prestigious person or group.
- State a range of alternatives within the question itself when possible. For instance, the question, "Do you normally prefer to get up early in the morning?" is more suggestive of the "right" answer than "Do you normally prefer to get up early in the morning or to sleep late, or does it depend on the circumstances?"

4. *Handling sensitive or personal information.* As researchers we must always keep in mind that respondents are doing us a favor by taking time to reply to our questions. Questionnaires and interviews always represent an intrusion on people's privacy. These instruments are not only time consuming but they are also designed to probe personal areas of the respondents' experience. On the other hand, many people are not only willing but happy to have the opportunity to express their views on certain topics. In any event, the researcher must strive to be courteous, considerate, and sensitive to the needs and rights of research participants. The following concepts might be kept in mind:

- For questions that deal with socially unacceptable behavior or attitudes (e.g., excessive drinking habits, premarital sexual behavior, noncompliance with physi-

cian's instructions, and the like), the researcher can usually elicit more frankness if the schedule creates an atmosphere of permissiveness or nonjudgment. The use of response alternatives may once again be useful in this regard because it is easier to merely check off having engaged in socially disapproved actions than to verbalize them in response to an open-ended question. Furthermore, the appearance of the behavior printed on an official-looking schedule is likely to make respondents aware that they are not alone in their behaviors or attitudes, so that admitting to them becomes less difficult.

- Impersonal wording of a question is often useful in minimizing embarrassment and encouraging honesty. To illustrate this point, compare these two statements with which respondents would be asked to agree or disagree: (1) "I am personally quite satisfied with the nursing care I received during my hospitalization." (2) "The quality of nursing care in this hospital is quite good." A respondent might feel more comfortable about admitting dissatisfaction with nursing care in the less personally worded second question.
- Politeness and encouragement help to motivate a respondent to cooperate. Include phrases such as "Would you mind ...," "We would appreciate ...," and "please" often.

Response Alternatives

If closed-ended questions are used, the researcher needs to make decisions about the form that the response alternatives will take. Below are four suggestions for preparing alternatives to closed-ended items.

1. *Coverage of alternatives.* The responses should adequately encompass all of the significant alternatives. If respondents are forced to choose a response from among op-

tions provided by the researcher, they should feel reasonably comfortable with the available options. As a safety measure, the researcher can have as one response option a phrase such as "Other—please specify."

2. *Overlapping responses.* The alternatives should be mutually exclusive.

3. *Ordering responses.* There should be some underlying rationale for the order in which the alternatives are presented to the respondent. Very often the options can be placed in order of decreasing or increasing favorability, agreement, or intensity. When the respondent is asked to choose from options that have no "natural" sequence or order, alphabetic ordering of the alternatives is less likely to "lead" the respondent to a particular response.

4. *Response length.* The response alternatives should not be too lengthy. One sentence or phrase for each alternative should almost always be sufficient to express a concept. In general, the response alternatives should be approximately equal in length.

Examples of Closed-Ended Questions

It is often difficult to create good-quality closed-ended questions because the researcher must pay careful attention not only to the wording of the question but also to the content, wording, and formatting of the fixed alternatives. Nevertheless, the analytic advantages of closed-ended questions make it compelling to include at least some on structured instruments. In this section we illustrate several types of closed-ended questions.

The simplest type of closed-ended questions requires the respondent to make a choice between two alternatives. *Dichotomous items,* as such questions are called, are considered most appropriate for gathering factual information, as in the following example:

Have you ever been hospitalized?

( ) Yes
( ) No

Dichotomous items often are considered too restrictive by respondents, who may resent being forced to see an issue as either yes or no. Graded alternatives are preferable for opinion or attitude questions because they give the researcher more information and because they give the respondent the opportunity to be more accurate. A range of alternatives provides more information in that the researcher can measure intensity of feeling as well as direction. Multiple-choice questions most commonly offer three to five alternatives, as in the following example:

How important is it to you to avoid a pregnancy at this time?

( ) Extremely important
( ) Very important
( ) Somewhat important
( ) Not at all important

A special type of multiple choice item is the "cafeteria" question, which asks respondents to select a response that most closely corresponds to their view. An example of this type is as follows:

People have different opinions about the use of estrogen replacement therapy for women in menopause. Which of the following statements best represents your point of view?

1. Estrogen replacement is so dangerous that it should be totally banned.
2. Estrogen replacement may have some undesirable side effects that suggest the need for caution in its use.
3. I am undecided about my views on estrogen replacement therapy.
4. Estrogen replacement has many beneficial effects that merit its availability and use.
5. Estrogen replacement is a powerful and ben-

eficial treatment that should be used by most menopausal women.

Rank-order questions ask respondents to rank their responses along a continuum, such as most favorable to least favorable (or most/least important, beneficial, familiar, and so forth). Rank-order questions can be quite useful but need to be carefully handled because they are often misunderstood by respondents. The following is an example:

People value different things about life. Below is a list of principles or ideas that are often cited when people are asked to name the things they value most. Please indicate the order of importance of these values to you by placing a "1" beside the most important, "2" beside the next most important, and so forth.

( ) Achievement and success
( ) Family relationships
( ) Friendships and social interaction
( ) Health
( ) Leisure and relaxation
( ) Money
( ) Religion and spirituality

Checklists are items that encompass several questions on a topic and require the same response format. Checklists are relatively efficient and easy for respondents to understand. Because checklists are difficult for an interviewer to read, they are used more frequently in self-administered questionnaires than in interviews.

A checklist is often a two-dimensional arrangement in which a series of questions is listed along one dimension (usually vertically) and response alternatives are listed along the other. It is this two-dimensional character that is being referred to when the term *matrix question* is used by some writers instead of the term "checklist." Figure 14-1 is an example of a checklist.

Instrument Format

The appearance and layout of the schedule may seem a matter of minor administrative importance. However, a poorly designed format can have substantive consequences if respondents (or interviewers) become confused, miss questions, or answer questions that they should have omitted. The format is especially important in the case of questionnaires because respondents who are unfamiliar with the researcher's intent will not

Here are some characteristics of birth-control devices that are of varying importance to different people. How important a consideration has each of these been for you in choosing a birth-control method?

	Of Very Great Importance	Of Great Importance	Of Some Importance	Of No Importance
1. Comfort				
2. Cost				
3. Ease of use				
4. Effectiveness				
5. Noninterference with spontaneity				
6. Safety to you				
7. Safety to partner				

Figure 14-1. *Example of a checklist.*

usually have an opportunity to ask questions. The following suggestions may assist the beginning investigator's efforts to lay out a schedule:

- Try not to compress too many questions into too small a space. An extra page of questions is better than a schedule that appears cluttered and confusing and that provides inadequate space for responses to open-ended questions.

- Set off the response options from the question or stem itself in formatting alternative responses. These options are usually aligned vertically. Respondents can be asked either to circle the appropriate answer or to place a check in the appropriate box, illustrated as follows as Methods A and B:

Are you a member of the American Nurses' Association?

1. yes	[ ] yes
2. no	[ ] no
Method A (Circling)	Method B (Checking)

- Give special care to formatting *filter questions,* which are designed to route respondents through different sets of questions depending on their response to earlier questions. Probably the least confusing approach is to set off questions appropriate to only a subset of respondents from the main series of questions, as the following shows:

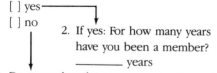

1. Are you a member of the American Nurses' Association?

    [ ] yes
    [ ] no

    2. If yes: For how many years have you been a member?
    _____ years

3. Do you subscribe to any nursing journals?

    [ ] yes
    [ ] no

There are alternative procedures, but they are more likely to lead to difficulties. Instructions such as, "Skip to question 3" might be misunderstood by some respondents. (However, "Skip to" instructions are commonly used in interview schedules because interviewers are generally thoroughly trained in the use of the instrument.) It is also best to avoid forcing all readers to go through inapplicable questions. That is, the question in the example could have been worded as follows: "If you are a member of the American Nurses' Association, for how long have you been a member?" The person who is not a member might not be sure how to handle this question and might be annoyed at having to read through material that is irrelevant.

Steps in Instrument Development

A careful, well-developed schedule cannot be prepared in minutes or even in hours. A researcher interested in designing a useful and accurate instrument must devote considerable time to analyzing the research requirements and attending to minute details. If a researcher is sloppy or haphazard in designing an instrument, little confidence can be placed in the obtained data. Imagine how wary you might be in using a piece of technical equipment—say a sphygmomanometer—that had been designed in haste and inadequately tested. The following seven steps are normally required to develop a sound self-report instrument:

PRELIMINARY DECISIONS

1. Decide whether to collect the data by means of interview or questionnaire. (The advantages and disadvantages of each are described in a later section.) Then, decide on the form the instrument will take. If the instrument is to be self-administered, the questions probably will be more structured and fewer open-ended questions will be included than if an interview were being used.

2. Next, decide on the type of information that needs to be collected. Instrument developers often decide in advance how many different *modules* or areas of questioning will be in-

cluded and approximately how much time should be devoted to each. For example, one module may focus on a person's stressful life events, another may focus on health-promoting activities, a third may focus on health symptoms, and a fourth may consist of background and demographic information. Then, within each module, decide on the concepts to be measured. If you are striving to develop an instrument of a fixed length (e.g., a 45-minute interview), you may need to prioritize concepts because there is often a tendency to want to ask more questions than time allows.

DRAFTING THE SCHEDULE

3. Do not develop the questions hastily. The content of the question needs to be matched to the most appropriate question type. Because there is a considerable variety of closed-question types, there is ample room for ingenuity and creativity. The wording of each question needs to be carefully monitored. However, you should not feel compelled to develop entirely original questions. Existing instruments on the same or a similar topic should be consulted. Particularly in the case of basic background information, it makes little sense for every questionnaire developer to struggle anew with the wording of virtually universal questions.

4. Because questions are seldom written in their order of presentation, decide how to sequence modules, as well as questions within modules. A questionnaire or interview schedule is not a random set of questions that the researcher creates arbitrarily. Some thought needs to be given to the sequencing of the questions to arrive at an order that is psychologically meaningful to respondents and encourages candor and cooperation. For example, the schedule should begin with questions that are interesting and motivating. The instrument also needs to be arranged in such a way that distortions and biases are minimized. The possibility that earlier questions will influence replies to the subsequent

questions is an ever present problem. Whenever both general and specific questions about a topic are to be included, the general question should be placed first to avoid putting ideas into people's heads. Once the questions have been ordered the instrument can be formatted.

5. Next, write an introduction and, for questionnaires, prepare instructions on how to complete the form. Every schedule should be prefaced by introductory comments about the nature and purpose of the study. In interviews, the introductory comments would normally be read to the respondents by the interviewer and incorporated into an informed consent form. In questionnaires, the introduction usually takes the form of a cover letter accompanying the instrument. The introduction should be given considerable care and attention, because it represents the first point of contact between the researcher and potential respondents. An example of a cover letter accompanying a mailed questionnaire is presented in Figure 14-2.

REVISING AND PRETESTING

6. When a first draft of the instrument is in reasonably good order, critically discuss it with individuals who are knowledgeable about the construction of questionnaires and with people who are familiar with the substantive content of your schedule. The instrument should also be reviewed by someone who is capable of detecting technical difficulties such as spelling mistakes, grammatical errors, and so forth. When these various people have provided feedback, a revised version of the instrument can be pretested.

7. Pretest the instrument. A *pretest* of an instrument is a trial run to determine, insofar as possible, its clarity, research adequacy, and freedom from bias. The pretest provides an opportunity for detecting at least gross inadequacies or unforeseen problems before going to the expense of a full-scale study. The pretest should be administered to individuals

Dear Mrs. _____:

We are conducting a study to examine how women who are approaching retirement age (age 55 to 65) feel about various issues relating to health and health care. This study, which is sponsored by the State Department of Health, will enable health-care providers to better meet the needs of women in your age group. Would you please assist us in this study by completing the enclosed questionnaire? Your opinions and experiences are very important to us and are needed to give an accurate picture of the health-related needs of women in the greater Middletown area.

Your name was selected at random from a list of residents in your community. The questionnaire is completely anonymous, so you are not asked to put your name on it or to identify yourself in any way. We therefore hope that you will feel comfortable about giving your honest opinions. If you prefer not to answer any particular question, please feel perfectly free to leave it blank. Please do answer the questions if you can, though, and if you have any comments or concerns about any question, just write your comments in the margin.

A postage-paid return envelope has been provided for your convenience. We hope that you will take a few minutes to complete and return the questionnaire to us—it should take only about 15 minutes of your time. To analyze the information in a timely fashion, we ask that you return the questionnaire to us by May 12.

Thank you very much for your cooperation and assistance in this endeavor. If you would like a copy of the summary of the results of this study, please check the box at the bottom of page 10.

Figure 14-2. *Fictitious example of a cover letter for a mailed questionnaire.*

who are similar to those who will ultimately participate in the study. Ordinarily, 10 to 20 pretested schedules should be sufficient, although more may be necessary if the instrument is complex and if the sample is heterogeneous. If extensive revisions are suggested by the reactions and responses to the pretest, a second pretest may be required. If minor revisions are sufficient, then the instrument should be given one final editing and can then be reproduced for the final administration.

≡ THE ADMINISTRATION OF SELF-REPORT INSTRUMENTS

Interview schedules and questionnaires require different skills and different considerations in their administration. The successful collection of the data is clearly as important to the research endeavor as is the design of the instruments. Both the quantity and the quality of the data gathered are influenced by the data collection procedures and the competencies of the research personnel. In this section we examine the problems involved in instrument administration and ways of handling those difficulties.

Collecting Interview Data

The quality of interview data depends to a great extent on the proficiency of the interviewers. Interviewers for large survey organizations receive extensive general training in addition to specific training for individual studies. Although this introductory book cannot adequately cover all of the principles of good interviewing, it can identify some of the major issues.

A primary task of the interviewer is to put respondents at ease so that they will feel comfortable in expressing their honest opinions. The respondents' personal reaction to the interviewer can seriously affect their willingness to participate. Interviewers, therefore, should always be neat (but not overdressed); punctual (if an appointment has been made); courteous; and friendly. The interviewer should strive to appear unbiased and to create a permissive atmosphere that encourages candor. The job of the interviewer is to serve as a neutral medium of communication. All opinions of the respondents should be accepted as natural—the interviewer should generally not express surprise, disapproval, or even approval.

When a structured interview schedule is being used, interviewers should follow the wording of the questions in the schedule precisely. Similarly, interviewers should not offer spontaneous explanations of what the questions mean. Repetitions of the questions are usually adequate to dispel any misunderstanding, particularly if the instrument has been properly pretested. The interviewer should not read the questions from the schedule. A naturalistic, conversational tone is essential in building rapport with respondents, and this tone is impossible to achieve if the questions are not thoroughly familiar to the interviewer.

When closed-ended questions with lengthy or complicated response alternatives are posed, the interviewer should hand the subjects a card that lists all of the options. Individuals cannot be expected to remember detailed unfamiliar material and are sometimes inclined to choose the last alternative if they cannot recall earlier ones. Closed-ended items can be recorded by checking or circling the appropriate alternative, but responses to open-ended questions need to be recorded in full or tape recorded for later transcription. The interviewer should not paraphrase or summarize the respondent's reply.

Interviewers typically find that obtaining complete and relevant responses to open-ended questions is not always an easy matter. Respon-dents often reply to seemingly straightforward questions with irrelevant discussions or partial answers, or they may say, "I don't know" to avoid giving their opinions on sensitive topics or to stall while they think over the question. In such cases, the job of the interviewer is to probe. The purpose of a *probe* is to elicit more useful information from a respondent than was volunteered during the first reply. A probe can take many forms: sometimes it involves a repetition of the original question and sometimes it is a long pause intended to communicate to respondents that they should continue. Frequently, it is necessary to encourage a more complete response by a nondirective supplementary question such as, "How is that?" The interviewer must be careful to use only *neutral* probes that do not influence the content of the subject's response. Box 14-1 gives some examples of neutral, nondirective probes that are used by professional interviewers in getting more complete responses to open-ended questions. The ability to probe well is perhaps the greatest test of an interviewer's skill. To know when to probe and how to select the best probes, the interviewer must comprehend fully the purpose of each question and the type of information being sought.

The guidelines for handling telephone interviews are essentially the same as those for face-to-face interviews, although additional effort usu-

---

BOX 14-1 EXAMPLES OF NEUTRAL, NONDIRECTIVE PROBES

Is there anything else?
Go on.
Are there any other reasons?
How do you mean?
Could you tell me more about that?
Why do you feel that way?
Would you tell me what you have in mind?
There are no right or wrong answers; I'd just like to get your thinking.
Could you please explain that?
Could you give me an example?

ally is required to build rapport over the telephone. In both cases, the interviewer should strive to make the interview a pleasant and satisfying experience in which respondents are made to feel as though the information they are providing is important.

Collecting Questionnaire Data

Self-administered questionnaires can be distributed in a number of ways. The most convenient procedure is to distribute the questionnaires to a group of respondents who complete the instrument together at the same time. This approach has the obvious advantage of maximizing the return rate and allowing the researcher to clarify any possible misunderstandings about the instrument. Group administrations are often possible in educational settings and might also be feasible in some hospital or community situations.

Personal presentation of questionnaires to individual respondents is another alternative. Personal contact with respondents has been found to have a positive effect on the rate of questionnaires returned. Furthermore, the availability of the researcher or an assistant can be an advantage in terms of explaining and clarifying the purposes of the study or particular items. This method may, however, be relatively time consuming and expensive if the questionnaires have to be delivered and picked up at respondents' homes. However, the distribution of questionnaires in a clinical setting is often inexpensive and efficient and likely to yield a high rate of completed questionnaires.

Questionnaires are often mailed to respondents. A problematic feature of this approach is that the *response rates* tend to be very low. When only a small subsample of respondents return their questionnaires, it may be unreasonable to assume that those who did respond were somehow "typical" of the sample as a whole. In other words, the researcher is faced with the possibility that those individuals who did not complete a questionnaire would, as a group, have answered the questions differently from those who did return the schedule. In such a situation, it may be inappropriate to generalize the results of the study to the target population.

If the response rate is high, the risk of serious response bias may be negligible. A response rate greater than 60% is probably sufficient for most purposes, but lower response rates are common. The researcher generally should attempt to discover how representative the respondents are, relative to the target population, in terms of basic demographic characteristics such as age, sex, marital status, and the like. This comparison might lead the researcher to conclude that respondents and nonrespondents are similar enough to assume the absence of serious biases. If demographic differences are found, the investigator will at least be in a position to make some inferences about the direction of the biases.

The response rate can be affected by the manner in which the questionnaires are designed and mailed. The physical appearance of the questionnaire can influence its appeal, so some thought should be given to the layout, quality and color of paper, method of reproduction, and typographic quality of the instrument. The standard procedure for distributing the questionnaire is to include with the schedule a cover letter and a stamped, addressed return envelope. Failure to enclose a return envelope could have a serious effect on the response rate. Also, you should be sure that both the main envelope and the return envelope carry sufficient postage.

The use of *follow-up reminders* has been found to be effective in achieving higher response rates for mailed questionnaires. This procedure involves the mailing of additional letters urging nonrespondents to complete and return their schedules. Follow-up letters or notices are typically sent two to three weeks after the initial mailing. A number of techniques have been adopted for follow-ups, the simplest being a letter of encouragement to nonrespondents. It is preferable, however, to enclose a second copy of the questionnaire with the reminder letter because most people will have misplaced the original copy. Telephone follow-ups can be quite success-ful, but they are costly and involve a considerable amount of time.

In the event that the questionnaire is anony-mous, the investigator may be unable to distin-guish respondents and nonrespondents for the purpose of sending follow-up letters. Although several techniques for dealing with this problem exist, the simplest procedure is to send out a follow-up letter to the entire sample, thanking those individuals who have already answered and asking others to cooperate.

As questionnaires are returned, the investi-gator should keep a log of the incoming receipts on a daily basis. Each questionnaire should be opened, checked for usability, and assigned an identification number. Such record-keeping will assist the researcher in assembling the results, monitoring the return rate, and making decisions about the timing of follow-up mailings and cutoff dates.

The problems associated with mailed ques-tionnaires are not ones that can be handled using interpersonal skills. Building rapport in a ques-tionnaire situation to enhance the response rate is a difficult chore and often depends on attention to details. Even though these procedural matters may seem trivial, the success of the project may depend on their careful execution.

☰ QUESTIONNAIRES VERSUS INTERVIEWS: AN ASSESSMENT

Self-administered questionnaires offer a number of advantages over personal interviews, but they have some drawbacks as well. Let us consider some of the following strong points of question-naires:

Questionnaires, relative to interviews, are gener-ally much less costly and require less time and energy to administer. Group-administered questionnaires are clearly the least expensive and time consuming of any procedure. With a fixed amount of funds or time, a larger and

more geographically diverse sample can usu-ally be obtained with mailed questionnaires than with interviews.

Questionnaires, unlike interview schedules, offer the possibility of complete anonymity. Some-times a guarantee of anonymity is crucial in obtaining candid responses, particularly if the questions are of a highly personal or sensitive nature. Anonymous questionnaires often result in a higher proportion of socially unacceptable responses (i.e., responses that place the re-spondent in an unfavorable light) than face-to-face interviews.

The absence of an interviewer ensures that there will be no interviewer bias. Ideally, an inter-viewer is a neutral agent through whom ques-tions and answers are passed. Studies have shown, however, that this ideal is difficult to achieve. Respondents and interviewers interact as humans, and this interaction can affect the subject's responses. This problem clearly is not present for questionnaires.

Despite these advantages, the strengths of interviews far outweigh those of mailed question-naires. It is true that interviews are costly, prevent respondent anonymity, and are subject to inter-viewer biases. Nevertheless, the numerous advan-tages described as follows have led many re-searchers to conclude that interviews are superior to questionnaires for most research pur-poses:

The response rate tends to be quite high in face-to-face interviews. Respondents are apparently more reluctant to refuse to talk to an inter-viewer who is directly in front of them than to discard or ignore a questionnaire. A well-de-signed and properly conducted interview study normally achieves a response rate in the vi-cinity of 80% to 90%. Because nonresponse is not a random process, low response rates may introduce serious biases.

There are many individuals who simply cannot fill out a questionnaire. Examples include young children and blind, elderly, illiterate, or uneducated individuals. Interviews, on the other hand, are normally feasible with most people.

Interviews offer some protection against ambiguous or confusing questions. The interviewer can determine whether questions have been misunderstood and can clarify matters. In questionnaires, items that are misinterpreted may go undetected by the researchers and the responses may, thus, lead to erroneous conclusions.

The information obtained from questionnaires tends to be somewhat more superficial than interview data partly because questionnaires ordinarily contain a preponderance of closed-ended items. Open-ended questions often engender resentment among questionnaire respondents, who dislike having to compose and write out a reply. Much of the richness and complexity of the human experience can be lost if closed-ended items are used exclusively. Furthermore, interviewers can enhance the quality of the self-report data through probing.

Respondents are less likely to give "don't know" responses or to leave a question unanswered in an interview situation than on questionnaires.

In an interview, the researcher has strict control over the order of presentation of the questions. Questionnaire respondents are at liberty to skip around from one section of the instrument to another. It is possible that a different ordering of questions from the one originally intended could bias the responses.

Interviews permit greater control over the sample in the sense that the interviewer knows whether or not the person being interviewed is the intended respondent. It is not unusual to have individuals who receive questionnaires pass the instrument on to a friend, relative, secretary, and so forth. This kind of activity can change the characteristics of the sample.

Finally, face-to-face interviews have an advantage in their ability to produce additional data through observation. The interviewer is in a position to observe or judge the respondents' level of understanding, degree of cooperativeness, social class, life style, and so forth. These kinds of information can be useful in interpreting the responses.

Many of the advantages of face-to-face interviews also apply to telephone interviews. Complicated or detailed schedules clearly are not well suited for telephone interviewing but, for relatively brief instruments, the telephone interview combines the economy and ease of administration of questionnaires with relatively high response rates.

≡ RESEARCH EXAMPLES: STRUCTURED SELF-REPORTS

Structured self-report instruments are the most commonly used method of collecting data for nursing research studies. Table 14-2 presents some examples of studies that have used structured interviews or questionnaires. A more detailed description of a questionnaire study follows.

Robarge and her colleagues (1982) studied whether extremely close birth spacing was an important risk factor in child abuse. They hypothesized that if spacing were a critical variable, as had been found in earlier studies, then twins ought to be especially at risk of being abused by their parents. To test this hypothesis, the investigators mailed questionnaires to a sample of mothers who recently had given birth. The questionnaires included 25 questions, designed to elicit information in five areas: (1) the mother's feelings about her pregnancy and delivery, (2) the mother's perceptions of her relationship with the baby or babies and other family members, (3) the mother's perception of difficulty in caring for the infant(s), (4) the mother's evaluation of infant health, and (5) the mother's perception of family and peer support. Questions on child abuse (the dependent variable) were not included on the questionnaires, because the investigators had access to records of reported child abuse through the county child protection agency. The questionnaires were mailed to mothers whose infants were delivered in a specific hospital and whose infants were at least six months old. To be eligible for the study, the mothers had to have given birth to twins whose birth weights exceeded 2000 grams and whose 5-minute Apgar score was at least 6. For each set of twins, two or three single birth infants (matched in terms of race, social class, maternal age, and birth date) were also included in the study as a comparison group. The sample consisted of mothers of 38 sets of twins and 97 comparison group mothers.

The questionnaire was pretested with a sample of similar patients to evaluate clarity, question relevancy, and ease of response. The finalized version of the questionnaire was mailed with a cover letter indicating that signature of the questionnaire was optional. However, the questionnaires were precoded so that the respondent could be identified and later matched to county child protection agency records. Eight weeks after the first mailing, a second questionnaire was mailed to those who had not responded to the first request. In a handful of cases, mothers who failed to respond but who attended the hospital clinic were personally requested to complete the questionnaire. The investigators also

Table 14-2. *Examples of Nursing Studies Using Structured Self-Reports*

RESEARCH PROBLEM	SAMPLE	DATA COLLECTION APPROACH	RESPONSE RATE
What factors are predictive of a nurse's intention to resign? (Choi et al., 1989)	792 registered nurses and licensed practical nurses in a large magnet hospital	Distributed questionnaires	98%
Are runners who report addictive behaviors at higher risk of physical injury than runners who report fewer addictive behaviors? (Rudy & Estok, 1989)	220 male and female marathon participants	Mailed questionnaires	45%
What are people's attributions about their weight outcomes (success or failure in weighing what they desire)? (Brubaker, 1988)	260 faculty and staff at (1) a small private college and (2) a large public university	Mailed questionnaires	64% (1) 97% (2)
How do patients with surgery for obesity rate their preoperative, hospitalization, and discharge experiences? (Bufalino et al., 1989)	123 obesity surgical patients	Mailed questionnaires	45%
What are the effects of social support on the health behavior practices of women during pregnancy? (Aaronson, 1989)	529 pregnant women	Telephone interviews and questionnaires	72%
What are the levels of satisfaction with and perceived barriers to health care among women enrolled in a Medicaid prepaid plan versus the regular fee-for-service Medicaid program? (Reis, 1990)	98 Medicaid participants	Personal interviews	89%

attempted to locate the addresses of any subjects who had moved after delivery.

Thus, these investigators took steps to ensure that their questionnaires were workable with the study population and initiated several activities to increase the rate of response to their mailed questionnaires. The final response rate was 61%; the supplementary steps taken by the investigators (such as the second mailing) boosted their response rate by approximately 50%.

Despite their efforts, the researchers were able to document response biases that underscore the difficulty with mailed questionnaires: in the entire original sample, there were nine reported cases of child abuse or neglect according to the child protective agency records, but only one of the nine mothers responded to the questionnaire. This systematic bias prevented the researchers from adequately testing their hypothesis.

☰ SUMMARY

A wide variety of data collection approaches are available to nurse researchers. Data collection methods vary along four important dimensions: (1) structure, (2) quantifiability, (3) research obtrusiveness, and (4) objectivity. Nurse researchers must consider these dimensions as well as the method of data collection to be used; the three principal data collection approaches are (1) self-report, (2) observation, and (3) biophysiologic measures. This chapter focused on self-reported data obtained through interviews or questionnaires.

The majority of nursing research studies involve the collection of *self-reported data*—that is, data obtained by directly questioning subjects regarding the desired information. The self-report method is strong with respect to its directness and versatility, but the major drawback is the potential for deliberate or unconscious distortions on the part of respondents.

Self-reported data are collected by means of an oral interview or written questionnaire. Self-

reports vary widely in terms of their degree of structure or standardization. Tightly structured methods provide little flexibility for respondents, and unstructured methods provide both respondent and interviewer latitude in the formulation of questions and answers. Several methods of collecting unstructured or loosely structured self-report data were described: (1) *unstructured interviews,* which are conversational discussions on the topic of interest, generally in naturalistic settings; (2) *semistructured* or *focused interviews,* in which the interviewer is guided by a broad *topic guide* of questions to be asked; (3) *focus group interviews,* which involve discussions with small groups about topics covered in a topic guide; (4) *life histories,* which encourage respondents to narrate, in chronological sequence, their life experiences *vis-à-vis* some theme; (5) *the critical incidents method,* which involves probes about the circumstances surrounding a behavior or incident that is critical to some outcome of interest; and (6) *diaries,* in which respondents are asked to maintain daily records about some aspects of their lives. Unstructured methods tend to yield data of considerable depth and are useful in gaining an understanding about little-researched phenomena. These methods, however, are time consuming, yield data that are difficult to analyze, and are often from small and perhaps unrepresentative samples.

Most self-report data in nursing studies are collected through structured interview schedules or questionnaires. Questions in the instrument also vary in their degree of structure. *Open-ended questions* permit respondents to reply to questions in their own words. *Closed-ended* (or *fixed-alternative*) *questions* offer a number of alternative responses from which respondents are instructed to choose.

One of the most problematic aspects of schedule construction is the wording of questions and response options. Several suggestions for question wording were offered under the general rubrics of clarity, respondents' ability to reply, biases, and the handling of sensitive or personal information. With regard to response alternatives, the major considerations dealt with were the adequate coverage of alternatives, overlapping responses, the ordering of responses, and response length.

Closed-ended questions can take a number of different forms. The simplest type of fixed alternative requires a choice between two options, such as yes—no; questions of this type are referred to as *dichotomous items. Multiple-choice questions* provide respondents with a range of alternatives. *"Cafeteria" questions* are a special type of multiple choice item in which respondents are asked to select a statement that best represents their view. Respondents are sometimes requested to *rank order* a list of alternatives along a continuum from (usually) most favorable to least favorable. A *checklist* groups together several questions that require the same response format and that can be answered by placing a check in the appropriate space on a *matrix.*

The construction of an interview schedule or questionnaire normally proceeds through a number of systematic steps. First, some preliminary decisions must be made: the researcher needs to decide whether the data will be collected through interviews or questionnaires, how structured the schedule should be, and what type of information should be collected. Next, the questions should be drafted and put into a suitable sequence, and an introduction or *cover letter* should be prepared. Finally, the draft of the instrument should be subjected to critical review and pretesting so that appropriate revisions can be made.

The collection of interview data depends quite heavily on the interpersonal skills of the interviewer. To secure participants' cooperation and trust, the interviewer must take pains to put people at ease. The interviewers should be thoroughly trained and familiar enough with the schedule so that they do not need to read questions from the schedule. When respondents give incomplete or irrelevant replies to a question, the interviewer must use a technique known as *probing* to solicit additional information.

Self-administered questionnaires can be distributed in various ways. Group administration to an intact group is the most convenient and economical procedure. The most common approach is to mail questionnaires to individuals at their home or place of work. The main problem with mailed questionnaires is that many people fail to respond to them, leading to the risk of a biased sample. A number of techniques, such as the use of *follow-up reminders,* are designed to increase the *response rate.*

Methods of direct questioning are probably indispensable as a means of collecting data on human subjects. These methods are open to a number of criticisms, particularly in regard to their validity and accuracy. On the whole, interviews suffer from fewer weaknesses than questionnaires. Questionnaires are less costly and time consuming than interviews, offer the possibility of anonymity, and do not run a risk of interviewer bias. However, interviews yield a higher response rate, are suitable for a wider variety of individuals, are less likely to lead to misinterpretations of questions, and provide richer data than questionnaires. The researcher with a limited budget and time constraints will have to consider these important advantages carefully.

≡ STUDY SUGGESTIONS

1. Identify which unstructured method(s) of self-report might be appropriate for the following research problems:
   a. What are the coping strategies of parents who have lost a child through sudden infant death syndrome (SIDS)?
   b. How do nurses in emergency rooms make decisions about their activities?
   c. What are the health beliefs and practices of Haitian immigrants in the United States?
2. Suppose you were interested in studying the experiences of young women suffering perimenstrual distress. Outline what you might do to collect data by means of a highly structured and highly unstructured self-report method.
3. Suggest ways of improving the following questions:

a. When do you usually administer your injection of insulin?

b. Would you disagree with the statement that nurses should not unionize?

c. Do you agree or disagree with the following statement: Alcoholics deserve more pity than scorn and should be encouraged to seek medical rather than spiritual assistance?

d. What is your opinion about the new health insurance bill recently passed by Congress?

e. Don't you think that the role of nurses ought to be expanded?

4. For the study outlined in Study Suggestion 2, develop two open-ended and two closed-ended questions.

5. The underutilization of nursing skills because of voluntary nonemployment is sometimes the cause of some concern. Suppose that you were planning to conduct a state-wide study concerning the plans and intentions of non-employed registered nurses in your state. Would you adopt an interview or questionnaire approach? How structured would your schedule be? Why?

6. Suppose that the investigation of nonemployed nurses were to be accomplished by means of a mailed questionnaire. Draft a cover letter to accompany the schedule.

≡ SUGGESTED READINGS

METHODOLOGICAL REFERENCES

Bradburn, N.M., & Sudman, S. (1979). *Improving interview method and questionnaire design*. San Francisco: Jossey-Bass.

Brown, J.S., Tanner, C.A., & Padrick, K. (1984). Nursing's search for scientific knowledge. *Nursing Research, 33,* 26–32.

Collins, C., Given, B., Given, C.W., & King, S. (1988). Interviewer training and supervision. *Nursing Research, 37,* 122–124.

Denzin, N.K. (1972). *The research act* (2nd ed.). New York: McGraw-Hill.

Dillman, D. (1978). *Mail and telephone surveys: The total design method*. New York: John Wiley.

Flanagan, J.C. (1954). The critical-incident technique. *Psychological Bulletin, 51,* 327–358.

Goldman, A.E., & McDonald, S.S. (1987). *The group depth interview: Principles and practice*. Englewood Cliffs, NJ: Prentice-Hall.

Gordon, R.L. (1980). *Interviewing: Strategy, techniques and tactics* (3rd ed.). Homewood, IL: Dorsey Press.

Institute for Social Research. (1976). *Interviewer's manual, Survey Research Center* (rev. ed.). Ann Arbor: University of Michigan.

Kingry, M.J., Fiedje, L.B., & Friedman, L.L. (1990). Focus groups: A research technique for nursing. *Nursing Research, 39,* 124–125.

Kornhauser, A., & Sheatsley, P.B. (1976). Questionnaire construction and interview procedure [Appendix B]. In C. Selltiz, L.S. Wrightsman, & S.W. Cook (Eds.), *Research methods in social relations* (3rd ed.). New York: Holt, Rinehart & Winston.

Krueger, R.A. (1988). *Focus groups: A practical guide for applied research*. San Mateo: Sage.

Leininger, M.M. (1985). Life-health-care history: Purposes, methods and techniques. In M.M. Leininger (Ed.), *Qualitative research methods in nursing*. New York: Grune & Stratton.

McCracken, G. (1988). *The long interview*. Newbury Park, CA: Sage.

Morgan, D.L. (1988). *Focus groups as qualitative research*. Newbury Park, CA: Sage.

Munhall, P.L., & Oiler, C.J. (Eds.). (1986). *Nursing research: A qualitative approach*. Englewood Cliffs, NJ: Prentice-Hall.

Oppenheim, A.N. (1966). *Questionnaire design and attitude measurement*. New York: Basic Books.

Payne, S. (1951). *The art of asking questions*. Princeton, NJ: Princeton University Press.

Schuman, H. (1981). *Questions and answers in attitude surveys: Experiments in questions form, wording and context*. New York: Academic Press.

Woods, N.F. (1981). The health diary as an instrument for nursing research. *Western Journal of Nursing Research, 3,* 76–92.

Woods, N.F., & Catanzaro, M. (1988). *Nursing Research: Theory and practice*. St. Louis, MO: C.V. Mosby. (Chapters 18 & 19).

Wykle, M.L., & Morris, D.L. (1988). The health diary. *Applied Nursing Research, 1,* 47–48.

SUBSTANTIVE REFERENCES

Unstructured/Semistructured Methods

Aroian, K.J. (1990). A model of psychological adaptation to migration and resettlement. *Nursing Research, 39,* 5–10.

Boyle, J.S. (1985). Use of the family health calendar and interview schedules to study health and illness. In M.M. Leininger (Ed.), *Qualitative research methods in nursing.* New York: Grune & Stratton.

Bozett, F.W. (1988). Social control of identity by children of gay fathers. *Western Journal of Nursing Research, 10,* 550–565.

Bramwell, L. (1984). Use of the life history in pattern identification and health promotion. *Advances in Nursing Science, 6,* 37–44.

Clark, N.M., & Lenburg, C.B. (1980). Knowledge-informed behavior and the nursing culture: A preliminary study. *Nursing Research, 29,* 244–249.

Cowles, K.V. (1988). Personal world expansion for survivors of murder victims. *Western Journal of Nursing Research, 10,* 687–699.

Flaskerud, J.H., & Rush, C.E. (1989). AIDS and traditional health beliefs and practices of black women. *Nursing Research, 38,* 210–215.

Heitkemper, M.M., Shaver, J.F., & Mitchell, E.S. (1988). Gastrointestinal symptoms and bowel patterns across the menstrual cycle in dysmenorrhea. *Nursing Research, 37,* 108–113.

Knafl, K.A., Hagle, M.E., Bevis, M.E., Faux, S.A., & Kirchhoff, K.T. (1989). How researchers and administrators view the role of the clinical nurse researcher. *Western Journal of Nursing Research, 11,* 583–592.

Kroska, R.A. (1985). Ethnographic research method: A qualitative example to discover the role of "granny" midwives in health services. In M.M. Leininger (Ed.), *Qualitative research methods in nursing.* New York: Grune & Stratton.

Leininger, M.M. (1984). *Care: The essence of nursing and health.* Thorofare, NJ: Charles B. Slack.

Mercer, R.T., Nichols, E.G., & Doyle, G.C. (1988). Transitions over the life cycle: A comparison of mothers and nonmothers. *Nursing Research, 37,* 144–151.

Miller, J.F. (1989). Hope-inspiring strategies of the critically ill. *Applied Nursing Research, 2,* 23–29.

Norberg, A., & Asplund, K. (1990). Caregivers' experience of caring for severely demented patients. *Western Journal of Nursing Research, 12,* 75–84.

Nuttall, P. (1988). Maternal responses to home apnea monitoring of infants. *Nursing Research, 37,* 354–357.

Savitz, J., & Friedman, M.I. (1981). Diagnosing boredom and confusion. *Nursing Research, 30,* 16–20.

Strumpf, N.E., & Evans, L.K. (1988). Physical restraint of the hospitalized elderly: Perceptions of patients and nurses. *Nursing Research, 37,* 132–137.

Tripp-Reimer, T. (1982). Barriers to health care: Variations in interpretation of Appalachian client behavior by Appalachian and non-Appalachian health professionals. *Western Journal of Nursing Research, 4,* 179–191.

Structured Methods

Aaronson, L.S. (1989). Perceived and received support: Effects on health behavior during pregnancy. *Nursing Research, 38,* 4–9.

Ailinger, R.L. (1988). Folk beliefs about high blood pressure in Hispanic immigrants. *Western Journal of Nursing Research, 10,* 629–636.

Benedict, S. (1989). The suffering associated with lung cancer. *Cancer Nursing, 12,* 34–40.

Broom, B.L. (1984). Consensus about the marital relationship during transition to parenthood. *Nursing Research, 33,* 223–228.

Brubaker, B.H. (1988). An attributional analysis of weight outcomes. *Nursing Research, 37,* 282–287.

Bufalino, J., Kolisetty, L., McCaskey, G.W., & Stratton, K.L. (1989). Surgery for morbid obesity: The patients' experiences. *Applied Nursing Research, 2,* 16–22.

Choi, T., Jameson, H., Brekke, M.L., Anderson, J.G., & Podratz, R.O. (1989). Schedule-related effects on nurse retention. *Western Journal of Nursing Research, 11,* 92–107.

Craft, M. (1981). Preferences of hospitalized adolescents for information providers. *Nursing Research, 30,* 205–211.

Green, G.J. (1988). Relationships between role models and role perceptions of new graduate nurses. *Nursing Research, 37,* 245–248.

Liebman, J.J., Hull, A.I., Blauner, M., Barker, J., Vignos, P., & Moskowitz, R.W. (1986). Identifying needs and community resources in arthritis care. *Public Health Nursing, 3,* 158–170.

Reis, J. (1990). Medicaid maternal and child health care:

Prepaid plans vs. private fee-for-service. *Research in Nursing and Health, 13,* 163–171.

Robarge, J.P., Reynolds, Z.B., & Groothuis, J.R. (1982). Increased child abuse in families with twins. *Research in Nursing and Health, 5,* 199–203.

Rudy, E.B., & Estok, P.J. (1989). Measurement and significance of negative addiction in runners. *Western Journal of Nursing Research, 11,* 548–558.

van Servellen, G. (1988). Nurses' perceptions of individualized care in nursing practice. *Western Journal of Nursing Research, 10,* 291–306.

Wilbur, J. & Dan, A.J. (1989). The impact of work patterns on psychological well-being of midlife nurses. *Western Journal of Nursing Research, 11,* 703–716.

Woods, N.F., Most, A., & Dery, G.K. (1982). Toward a construct of perimenstrual distress. *Research in Nursing and Health, 5,* 123–136.

15
Scales and Standardized Self-Report Measures

Self-report instruments such as those discussed in Chapter 14 frequently include one or more psychosocial scales. A *scale* is a device designed to assign a numerical score to individuals to place them along a continuum with respect to the attribute being measured. The purpose of psychosocial scales is to quantitatively distinguish among people in terms of the degree to which they can be characterized by some personal trait. Scales have been constructed to discriminate among people with different attitudes, fears, motives, perceptions, personality traits, and needs. Just as a thermometer is a scale that permits a quantitative differentiation between two different temperatures, so a scale that measures attitudes attempts to distinguish between individuals who are more or less favorable toward some concept.

In this chapter we will focus on scales that combine more than one measurement of an attribute to form a single composite score. We will discuss a number of different scaling approaches to assist researchers interested in devising their own measures. In a later section of this chapter we describe existing scales and other standardized self-report measures, together with procedures for locating them.

≡ METHODS OF SCALING PSYCHOSOCIAL TRAITS

Many of the sophisticated techniques developed by social psychologists for quantifying psychologic states have focused on the measurement of attitudes. These techniques are versatile and have proved to be quite useful to researchers in nursing and other disciplines. Our discussion, therefore, will focus on attitude scales,* although the procedures described have been profitably applied to other psychologic domains as well.

Likert Scales

The most common method of attitude measurement is the Likert scale, named after social psychologist Rensis Likert, who developed its use. A *Likert scale* consists of several declarative statements expressing a viewpoint on a topic. Respondents are asked to indicate the degree to which they agree or disagree with the opinion expressed in the statement. Table 15-1 presents a ten-item Likert scale for measuring attitudes toward the mentally ill. A number of features of the table are discussed in the following paragraphs; first let us briefly discuss the procedure for constructing a Likert scale.

The first step is to develop a large pool of items or statements that clearly state favorable and unfavorable attitudes toward the issue under consideration. Neutral statements or statements so extreme that virtually everyone would agree or disagree with them should be avoided. The aim is to spread out people with various attitudes along a continuum of favorability. Approximately equal numbers of positively and negatively worded statements should be chosen to avoid biasing the responses. It is also important to select only items that focus on one concept.† Usually 10 to 20 items are sufficient for a Likert scale.

There are differences of opinion concerning the appropriate number of response alternatives to use. Likert used five categories of agreement–disagreement, such as are shown in Table

---

*Among the earliest types of attitude scales were the Thurstone scales, named after the psychologist L.L. Thurstone, who developed them during the 1920s. The Thurstone approach to scaling is elaborate and time consuming, and has fallen into relative disuse. The interested reader can learn about the Thurstone technique in Selltiz, Wrightsman, and Cook (1976).

† It is possible to present statements relating to two or more concepts together in the same section of a questionnaire. However, it is important that separate scoring be performed for the various concepts. This distinction will hopefully become clearer in the subsequent discussion on scoring.

15-1. Some investigators prefer a seven-point scale, adding the alternatives "slightly agree" and "slightly disagree." There is also a diversity of opinion about the advisability of including an explicit category labeled "uncertain." Some researchers argue that the inclusion of this option makes the task less objectionable to people who cannot make up their minds or have no strong feelings about an issue. Others, however, feel that the use of this "undecided" category encourages fence-sitting, or the tendency to not take sides. Investigators who do not give respondents an explicit alternative for indecision or uncertainty proceed in principle as though they were working with a five- or seven-point scale, even though only four or six alternatives are given: nonresponse to a given statement is *scored* as though the neutral response were there and had been chosen.

After the items are administered to respondents, the responses to the Likert scale must be scored. Typically, the responses are scored in such a way that endorsement of positively worded statements, and nonendorsement of negatively worded statements, are assigned a higher score. Table 15-1 illustrates what this procedure involves. The first statement is phrased such that agreement is indicative of a favorable attitude toward the mentally ill.

The "+" in the first column of the table signifies that this is a positively worded item. We would, therefore, assign a higher score to a person agreeing with this statement than to someone disagreeing with it. Because the scale has a maximum of five points, we would give a "5" to someone strongly agreeing, "4" to someone agreeing, and so forth. The responses of two hypothetical respondents are shown by a $\sqrt{}$ or an X, and their score for each item is shown in the right-hand columns of the table. Person A, who agreed with the first statement, is given a score of 4, and Person B, who strongly disagreed, is given a score of 1.

The second item is negatively worded: someone who agreed with the statement would tend to have a negative attitude toward the mentally ill. For this question, the scoring must be *reversed,* assigning a score of "1" to those who strongly agree, and so forth. This reversal is necessary so that a high score will consistently reflect positive attitudes toward the mentally ill. When each item has been handled in this manner, a person's total score can be determined by adding together individual item scores. The arithmetic derivation of total scores in this manner has led to the term *summated rating scale,* which is sometimes used to refer to Likert-type scales. The total scores of the two hypothetical respondents to the items in Table 15-1 are shown at the bottom of that

Table 15-1.   *An Example of a Likert Scale to Measure Attitudes Toward the Mentally Ill*

DIRECTION OF SCORING*		RESPONSES†					SCORE	
		SA	A	?	D	SD	(√) Person A	(X) Person B
+	1. People who have had a mental illness can become normal, productive citizens after treatment.		√			X	4	1
−	2. People who have been patients in mental hospitals should not be allowed to have children.			X		√	5	3
−	3. The best way to handle patients in mental hospitals is to restrict their activity as much as possible.			X	√		4	2
+	4. Many patients in mental hospitals develop normal, healthy relationships with staff members and other patients.				√	X	3	2
+	5. There should be an expanded effort to get the mentally ill out of institutional settings and back into their communities.	√				X	5	1
−	6. Because the mentally ill can't be trusted, they should kept under constant guard.			X		√	5	2
−	7. There is really very little that can be done to help a person once they have had a mental disorder.			X		√	5	2
−	8. Too much money is being spent on research to help the mentally ill.	X				√	5	1
+	9. Mental illness could happen to anyone.	√			X		5	2
+	10. The condition of most facilities for the mentally ill is critically in need of improvement.	√		X			5	3
							46	19

Total Score for Person A = 46
Total Score for Person B = 19

* The researcher would not indicate the direction of scoring on a Likert scale administered to subjects. The scoring direction is indicated in this table for illustrative purposes only.

† SA, strongly agree; A, agree; ?, uncertain; D, disagree; SD, strongly disagree.

table. These scores reflect a considerably more positive attitude toward the mentally ill on the part of Person A compared with Person B.

Once the scoring is completed, the investigator developing a new scale should assess which items should be retained in the final scale and which should be discarded. A number of sophisticated procedures are available for accomplishing this selection task.* The researcher who lacks statistical skills can use a few basic criteria for eliminating nonuseful items. One issue is that the responses to items should reflect some variability. That is, some people should agree and others disagree with each statement. If variability is lacking, the item is not making a contribution toward a scale designed to discriminate among individuals on the basis of their attitudes. The researcher should also check to ensure that the *a priori* decision concerning the directionality of the item is justified. People who agree with positively worded statements should tend to get higher total scores than those who disagree. If the opposite is found to be the case, then the item should be reversed entirely and new total scores should be computed. If some items are endorsed about equally by those with high total scores and those with low total scores, then the item is probably irrelevant to the attitude being measured or ambiguously worded. Such items should be eliminated from the scale.

The fact that item responses are added together should indicate why it is inappropriate to score together responses relating to two or more different concepts. As an exaggerated example, if question 10 in Table 15-1 were replaced with the statement "Abortion should be available to all women seeking to terminate a pregnancy," it would make little sense to score the responses to this statement together with the other nine. It is unfortunately not always easy to tell which items are conceptually related. Complex topics often embrace a number of different dimensions and may need separately scored scales for each dimension. Statistical procedures such as factor

analysis are useful in this regard but are too complex to discuss here (advanced students can refer to Chapter 22). Beginning researchers who lack statistical expertise should use their logical skills to attempt to build scales that are *unidimensional,* that is, those having items that are all measuring the same thing.

Likert scales may appear to involve a lot of work and trouble but they are actually quite powerful. The summation feature of these scales makes it possible to make fine discriminations among individuals with different points of view. A single Likert question allows people to be put into only five (or seven) categories. A ten-item scale such as the one in Table 15-1 permits much finer gradations: from a minimum possible score of ten (10×1) to a maximum possible score of 50 (10×5).

Cumulative or Guttman Scales

A second method for measuring attitudes was developed by Louis Guttman during the 1940s. Like Likert scales, *Guttman scales* (also called *cumulative scales*) consist of a set of items with which respondents are asked to either agree or disagree. To construct a cumulative scale, a number of items of increasing intensity with regard to some attitude object are developed. Typically, the number of items is quite small: four or five items are common. The statements should form a homogeneous set relating to one (and only one) concept. The goal is to generate a hierarchy of items such that an individual who endorses an item of a given intensity should endorse *all* less-extreme items. The scoring procedure with cumulative scores is quite simple: a person is given a score equivalent to the number of items with which he or she agrees.

The following four items form a hypothetical cumulative scale:

1. A nursing research course at the undergraduate level should be available to students.
2. Students would very likely benefit from taking an undergraduate nursing research course.

---

* The advanced student who is developing a Likert scale for general use should consult a reference on psychometric procedures, such as *Psychometric Theory* by Nunnally (1978).

3. A nursing research course would be in the best interests of undergraduate students.
4. A course in nursing research should be mandatory for all undergraduate nursing students.

A person who *disapproved* of undergraduate nursing research courses would probably disagree with all four statements and would be assigned a score of 0. On the other hand, respondents who felt that such a course is essential in the undergraduate curriculum would probably agree with all four statements and would be assigned a score of four.

Guttman developed a procedure known as *scalogram analysis* for ascertaining whether the attitude under investigation really is unidimensional (i.e., measures a single concept). According to this procedure, if the cumulative scale is unidimensional, it should be possible to *reproduce* a person's response pattern based on the assigned score. For instance, in the nursing research course example, a score of "3" should signify that the individual endorsed items one, two, and three but not four. If the score of three were attained in any other way (say, by endorsing items one, three, and four) by a large number of respondents, then the scale is probably faulty. If an investigator can reproduce exactly the specific items with which a subject agreed by knowing the respondent's total score, the scale is said to exhibit a high degree of *reproducibility*. It is rare, in practice, to find a cumulative scale that is perfectly reproducible across all subjects, but close approximations are desirable. The function of scalogram analysis is to apply various statistical criteria in deciding whether a set of items may be appropriately regarded as approximating a unidimensional scale.

The Guttman technique offers an interesting approach to the measurement of attitudes but, like other techniques, has received its share of criticisms. One criticism is that the Guttman procedure offers no guidance for the selection or generation of items that are likely to form a cumulative scale. Furthermore, these scales do not permit fine discriminations among individuals:

the scores range from a low of zero to a high equal to the number of items, which is typically small. A number of other technical weaknesses have limited the usage of cumulative scales as attitudinal measures.

Semantic Differential

The *semantic differential* is a technique that is often used to measure attitudes. Osgood, Suci, and Tannenbaum (1957), who developed the semantic differential, describe it more generally as a technique for measuring the psychologic meaning of concepts or objects to an individual.

The building blocks of semantic differentials are *graphic rating scales*. With graphic rating scales, respondents are asked to give a judgment of something along an ordered dimension. The task is to place a √ at the appropriate point along the line that extends from one extreme of the characteristic or dimension in question to the other extreme. Graphic rating scales are *bipolar* in nature because they specify the two opposite ends of a continuum. The following is an example of an item that might be used in a questionnaire with discharged patients:

How would you rate the overall quality of your nursing care?
(Place a √ in the appropriate space on the scale.)

Very Poor | | | | | | | | Excellent
1 2 3 4 5 6 7

The semantic differential consists of a set of graphic rating scales. The respondent is asked to rate a given concept (e.g., primary-care nursing, integrated curriculum, or 4-day work schedule) on a series of bipolar rating scales. The scales consist of bipolar adjectives such as good–bad, important–unimportant, strong–weak, beautiful–ugly, and so forth. An example of the format for a complete semantic differential is shown in Figure 15-1. Seven scale points are most commonly used, as in this example, but five or nine might also be used.

The semantic differential has the advantage of being highly flexible and easy to construct. The

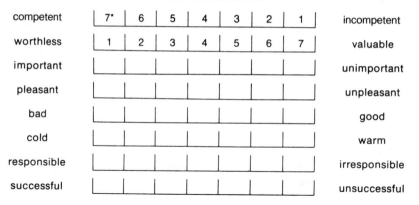

*The score values would not be printed on the form administered to actual subjects. The numbers are presented here solely for the purpose of illustrating how semantic differentials are scored.

Figure 15-1. *Example of a semantic differential.*

concept being rated can be virtually anything—a person, place, situation, abstract idea, controversial issue, and so forth. Furthermore, the concept can be a single word, a phrase, a sentence, or even a picture or sketch. Typically, several concepts are included on the same form so that comparisons can be made (if the same bipolar scales are used) across concepts. For instance, a researcher may be interested in contrasting the reactions of respondents to the concepts male nurse, female nurse, male physician, and female physician.

The researcher also has considerable freedom in constructing the bipolar scales. However, two considerations should guide the selection of the adjectives. First, the adjectives should be appropriate for the concepts being used and for the information being sought. The addition of the adjective pair tall–short in Figure 15-1 would add little understanding of how people react to the role of nurse practitioners. When the scales are used to rate two or more concepts, adjective pairs that were considered relevant for one concept may be inappropriate for another and may need to be discarded or replaced.

The second consideration in the selection of adjective pairs is the extent to which the adjectives are measuring the same dimension or aspect of the concept. Osgood and his colleagues (1957), through extensive research with semantic differ-

ential scales, found that adjective pairs tend to cluster along three principal and independent dimensions that they labeled (1) evaluation, (2) potency, and (3) activity. The most important group of adjectives are those that are evaluative, such as valuable–worthless, good–bad, fair–unfair, and so forth. Potency adjectives include strong–weak and large–small, and examples of activity adjectives are active–passive or fast–slow. The reason these three dimensions need to be considered separately is that a person's evaluative rating of a concept is independent of the activity or potency ratings of that concept. For example, two people who associate high levels of activity with the concept of nurse practitioner might have divergent views with regard to how valuable they perceive the concept of nurse practitioner. The researcher must decide whether to represent all three of these dimensions or whether only one or two are needed. Each dimension or aspect must be scored separately.

The scoring procedure for semantic differential responses is essentially the same as for Likert scales. Scores from one to seven are assigned to each bipolar scale response. Usually, the positively worded adjective is associated with higher scores, so that a √ to the extreme left for the competent–incompetent combination in Figure 15-1 would be scored "7," and a √ to the extreme right would be scored a "1." Note that in the figure, the direction of the adjective pairs has been randomly reversed to prevent response biases. Thus, for the next set of adjectives, worthless–valuable, a √ on the extreme *right* would be scored as "7." After proceeding in this fashion, subgroups of scale responses associated with the same dimension can be summed to yield a total score. Potentially, then, each concept could result in three scale scores (i.e., evaluation, potency, and activity) if adjective pairs representing these three dimensions are included. In Figure 15-1, only evaluative adjectives are listed, so that all scale responses could be added together.

Semantic differentials produce a large quantity of information with relatively little effort. The data from semantic differentials can be analyzed in a wide variety of ways. Different groups of respondents (e.g., males versus females) can be compared in terms of their ratings of a concept. The ratings of two or more different concepts also can be compared. Various sophisticated analytic techniques have also been devised expressly for handling semantic differential data. Although the semantic differential is versatile, respondents can become confused or bored with these questions and may manifest their discomfort by placing all of their check marks in the middle-scale position. Clear instructions are essential and an explicit example may be required.

Other Scaling Approaches

The techniques described are by far the most common methods of measuring attitudes currently in use. Other approaches do exist, however. The advanced student may want to refer to the references at the end of this chapter for a more extended discussion of advanced scaling procedures, such as ratio scaling, unfolding technique, multidimensional scaling, and multiple scalogram analysis.

The Problem of Response Sets

Scaling procedures are subject to several common problems, the most troublesome of which is referred to as *response sets*. The scale scores that represent individuals' attitudes toward some phenomenon are seldom entirely accurate and pure measures of the critical variable. A number of irrelevant factors are also being "measured" at the same time. Because these response-set factors can sometimes influence or bias responses to a considerable degree, investigators who construct scales must attempt to eliminate them or reduce their impact.

One influence on responses is a person's tendency to present a favorable image of himself or herself. The *social desirability* response set refers to the tendency of some individuals to misrepresent their attitudes by giving answers that are consistent with prevailing social mores. This problem is often difficult to combat. Subtle, indirect, and delicately worded questioning sometimes can help to alleviate this response bias. The creation of a permissive atmosphere and provisions for respondent anonymity also encourage frankness.

Extreme responses constitute another type of response set. This biasing factor results from the fact that some individuals consistently express their attitudes in terms of extreme response alternatives (e.g., "strongly agree"), and others characteristically endorse middle-range alternatives. This response style is a distorting influence in that extreme responses may not necessarily signify the most intense attitude toward the phenomenon under investigation. There appears to be little that a researcher can do to counteract this bias, although there are procedures for detecting its existence. There is some evidence that the distortion introduced by the extreme-response set is not powerful.

Some people have been found to agree with statements regardless of the content. In the research literature, these people are sometimes referred to as "yea-sayers"; the bias is known as the *acquiescence response set*. A less common problem is the opposite tendency for other individuals, called "nay-sayers," to disagree with statements independently of the question content. Although there apparently are some people for whom such tendencies are stable and enduring personality characteristics, acquiescence and its opposite counterpart can often be avoided or minimized by the simple strategy of *counterbalancing* positively and negatively worded statements.

The effects of response biases should not be exaggerated, but it is important that researchers who are constructing a scale give these issues some thought. If the investigator is developing a scale for general use by other researchers, it is recommended that evidence be gathered demonstrating that the scale is sufficiently free from the influence of response sets to measure the critical variable.

≡ EXISTING SCALES AND MEASURES

The preceding section described some of the principles underlying the construction of scales for measuring people's attitudes. In an emerging field such as nursing research, investigators will often find that no suitable scale exists to measure the concepts in which they are interested or that existing scales are in need of adaptation or improvement. In such a case, the researcher may be forced to develop a new scale or instrument. Nevertheless, the design and testing of an accurate and valid measure of personal traits or states is a difficult and time-consuming activity. Beginning researchers, in particular, should be careful to exhaust all other possibilities before developing a new instrument. Thousands upon thousands of existing scales and standardized instruments already exist, many of which have documentation concerning their accuracy, validity, response biases, and usages. This section describes general classes of psychosocial measures and provides clues on where to find them.

Attitude Scales

Because attitude scales were already treated extensively in the preceding section, we only mention a few sources for locating existing instruments in this section. For attitudinal variables that

are strictly related to nursing, the researcher should consult the various nursing indexes described in Chapter 6 or the books discussed in the concluding section of this chapter.

There are a number of more general concepts in which nurses share an interest with researchers from other disciplines. Examples of this second type of variable include attitudes toward death or attitudes toward alcoholics. Both the nursing and nonnursing indexes and abstracting services should be consulted for references to studies that have developed scales to measure such variables. *Psychological Abstracts* is particularly useful because it has separate sections entitled "Attitude Measurement" and "Attitude Measures." In addition, several useful anthologies of attitude scales have been prepared, including Robinson and Shaver's (1973) *Measures of Social Psychological Attitudes* and Shaw and Wright's (1967) *Scales for the Measurement of Attitudes*. These reference books present the actual items appearing on scales, together with a critique of the scale's technical adequacy. Another useful reference is Beere's (1979) *Women and Women's Issues: A Handbook of Tests and Measures*. Scales measuring the following kinds of attitudes are included in these sources: attitudes toward birth control, socialized medicine, death, old people, blindness, mentally retarded people, sexuality, abortion, and traditional sex roles.

Personality Measures

For the purpose of our discussion, we will define *personality* as the relatively enduring attributes of individuals that dispose them to respond in a certain way to their environment. A number of nursing research studies have used an instrument to assess the personality characteristics of such groups as practicing nurses, nursing faculty members, nursing students, and clients. For example, Levine and her associates (1988) used various personality tests to develop a psychologic profile of critical-care nurses and to determine which personality traits were most predictive of job satisfaction.

Literally hundreds of personality measures exist. Personality tests differ in their comprehensiveness (e.g., measurement of one versus multiple personality dimensions) and structure. The majority of instruments that nurse researchers have used are of the type known as a personality inventory. In a *personality inventory,* respondents are typically presented with a number of descriptive statements that they rate as either characteristic or uncharacteristic of them. For example, a tense individual would be likely to answer "yes" or "agree" to a statement such as, "I often worry about what the future holds for me." A person's score is usually calculated by summing the number of affirmative responses to statements relating to a trait. Major tests of this type include the California Psychological Inventory, the Sixteen Personality Factor Questionnaire, and Edwards Personal Preference Inventory.

Most of the tests we have discussed so far are intended to measure traits of psychologically healthy, normal individuals; however, several clinically oriented instruments measure different forms of psychopathology, such as paranoia, schizophrenia, and the like. The most commonly used measure of psychopathology is the Minnesota Multiphasic Personality Inventory.

Several references on psychologic measures offer thorough discussions and explicit information on available measures. Among these sources are Anastasi's (1988) sixth edition of *Psychological Testing;* the various *Mental Measurements Yearbooks,* published by the Buros Institute of Mental Measurements—for example, the ninth yearbook, edited by Mitchell (1985); the *Tests in Print* series by the Buros Institute—for example, *Tests in Print II* by Buros (1974); the *Test Critiques* series by the Test Corporation of America—for example, Volume 7 by Keyser and Sweetland (1988); and the *Handbook of Family Measurement Techniques* by Touliatos and his colleagues (1990). Additionally, information on many standardized testing instruments can be retrieved through a computerized literature search of the data base called *Mental Measurement Yearbook,* produced by the Buros Institute of Mental Measurements.

Intelligence, Developmental, and Achievement Tests

Occasionally, nurse researchers are interested in assessing the cognitive abilities and attainments of a group of subjects. For example, Froman and Owen (1989) used math and verbal scores on the Scholastic Aptitude Test to predict achievement in a baccalaureate nursing program and scores on the NCLEX-RN test.

Intelligence tests represent attempts to evaluate the general, global ability of individuals to perceive relationships and solve problems. Of the many such tests available, some have been developed for individual administration and others have been designed for group use. Also, a number of developmental tests are available for measuring the cognitive and motor development in young preschool children, such as the Denver Developmental Screening Test and Bayley's Scale of Infant Development. Good sources for learning more about ability and developmental tests are the Buros' books and the Anastasi (1988) text.

Nurse researchers are sometimes interested in tests of achievement. Achievement tests are designed to measure the subject's present level of proficiency or mastery of various areas of knowledge. Because both practicing nurses and nurse educators are involved, to differing degrees, in teaching, the measurement of instructional effectiveness is an area in which some nurse researchers are interested. Achievement tests are either standardized or specially constructed. Standardized tests are instruments that have been carefully developed and tested and that normally cover broad achievement objectives. The test constructors of such tests establish *norms,* which make possible the comparison of individuals and groups with a reference group. The National League for Nursing Achievement Tests are examples of standardized tests. For specific learning objectives, the researcher may be forced to construct a new test. The development of an achievement test that is objective, accurate, and valid is a laborious task. Ebel's (1986) book entitled *Essentials of Educational Measurement* is a useful reference for those readers interested in achievement test construction.

Other Types of Psychosocial Measures

In addition to measures of attitudes, personality, and cognitive functioning, there are numerous scales to measure other aspects of a person's psychosocial and health status. It is beyond the scope of this book to identify all psychosocial attributes that have attracted the interest of nurse researchers, but some attributes have received repeated attention because of their relevance to clinical nursing practice. Table 15-2 lists, in the first column, constructs that were studied in at least five nursing research investigations published in the 1980s and early 1990s. The second column provides references for some of these nursing studies, and the third column identifies the specific scale that was used to measure the construct. The methodological references at the end of this chapter should be useful in locating measures of other psychosocial variables not discussed in this chapter.

Another type of psychosocial measure that deserves special mention is the *visual analogue scale (VAS)*. *VASs* have come into increased use in clinical settings to measure subjective experiences, such as pain, nausea, dyspnea, fatigue, and so forth. The VAS is a straight line, the end anchors of which are labeled as the extreme limits of the sensation or feeling that is being measured. Subjects are asked to mark a point on the line corresponding to the amount of the sensation experienced. An example of a VAS is presented in Figure 15-2. Traditionally, the VAS line is 100 mm in length, which facilitates the derivation of a score from 0 to 100 through a simple measurement of the distance from one end of the scale to the subject's mark on the line. The line can be oriented horizontally or vertically; recent research suggests that the vertically oriented VAS produces more sensitive measures and is easier for subjects to use, but the horizontal VAS has been shown to produce a more uniform distribution of scores. The VAS has the advantage of being

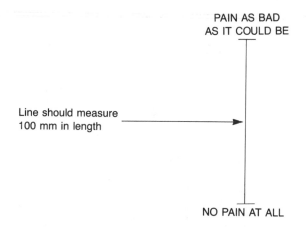

Figure 15-2. *Example of a visual analogue scale.*

easy to construct and avoids the pitfalls of language but may require a considerable amount of "teaching" before subjects understand what is expected of them. The VAS can be used to measure a wide variety of sensations but has most frequently been used in nursing studies to measure pain. For example, Hargreaves and Lander (1989) used a VAS to study the effect of transcutaneous electrical nerve stimulation on incisional pain caused by the procedure of cleaning and packing a surgical wound.

Instruments About Nursing Care and Patient Functioning

Nurse researchers have made tremendous strides over the past decade in developing instruments to evaluate nursing behaviors and competencies, as well as the behaviors, experiences, and affective states of people under their care. Excellent references for locating such measures are the book by Waltz, Strickland, and Lenz (1984) entitled *Measurement in Nursing Research* and the 1988 *Instruments for Clinical Nursing Research* edited by Frank-Stromberg. The instruments that have been developed by nurse researchers include highly structured scales that yield a quantified score as well as more loosely structured protocols for diagnosis and decision making. An important advantage of using or adapting a previ-

Table 15-2. *Examples of Concepts Frequently Measured With Psychosocial Scales in Nursing Studies*

CONCEPT	RESEARCH EXAMPLE REFERENCES	INSTRUMENT USED
Anxiety	Gennaro, 1988 Rudy & Estok, 1983 Littlefield et al., 1990	State-Trait Anxiety Inventory (STAI) Zuckerman's General Anxiety Scale Multiple Affect Adjective Checklist (MAACL)
Body image	Strang & Sullivan, 1985 Krouse & Krouse, 1982	Attitude Toward Body Image Scale Body Image Questionnaire
Coping	Gass & Chang, 1989 Herth, 1990	Lazarus Ways of Coping Scale Jalowiec Coping Scale
Depression	Robinson, 1989 Campbell, 1989 Upvall, 1990	Center for Epidemiological Studies Depression Scale (CES-D) Beck Depression Inventory (BDI) General Well-Being Scale
Family functioning	Stuifbergen, 1990 Mercer et al., 1988 Murata, 1990	Family Environment Scale (FES) Feethan Family Functioning Scale Family Adaptabililty & Cohesion Evaluation Scales (FACES)
Health locus of control	Itano et al., 1983 Weitzel, 1989	Health Locus of Control Scale Multidimensional Health Locus of Control Scale
Hope	Farran et al., 1990 Christman, 1990	Stoner Hope Scale Beck Hopelessness Scale
Locus of control	Thomas & Hooper, 1983 LaMontagne, 1984	Rotter I-E Scale Nowicki-Strickland Locus of Control Scale for Children
Mood states	Sime & Liberia, 1985 Bailie et al., 1988	Profile of Mood States (POMS) Profile of Mood States (POMS)
Morale/life satisfaction	Braden, 1990 Jackson, 1990	Index of Well-Being Life Satisfaction Index
Pain	Laborde & Powers, 1985 Zimmerman et al., 1989	McGill Pain Questionnaire McGill Pain Questionnaire
Psychosomatic symptoms	Moore et al., 1988 Murphy, 1988	Symptom Checklist-90 (SCL-90) Symptom Checklist-90 (SCL-90)
Self-esteem	Yarcheski & Mahon, 1989 Riffee, 1981	Rosenberg Self-Esteem Scale Coopersmith Self-Esteem Inventory
Social support	Aaronson, 1989 Primomo et al., 1990 Thomas and Hooper, 1983	Personal Resources Questionnaire (PRQ) Norbeck Social Support Questionnaire Interview for Social Interaction
Stress	Hall & Farel, 1988 VanOs et al., 1985 Norbeck & Anderson, 1989	Holmes-Rahe Social Readjustment Scale Schedule of Recent Experiences Life Events Questionnaire

ously developed measure is (in addition to ease and efficiency) that it facilitates the comparison of findings among studies and creates a greater potential for knowledge accumulation. Although we cannot list the many self-report instruments that have been developed specifically by or for nurses, Table 15-3 does provide some examples. This table gives the name of the instrument, the concepts it is designed to measure, and the source for the full description of the instrument.

≡ RESEARCH EXAMPLE

Heidrich and Cranley (1989) studied the effects of fetal movement, ultrasound scans, and amniocentesis on maternal–fetal attachment in normal pregnancies. Additionally, these investigators examined whether there was a relationship between women's perceptions of fetal growth and development on the one hand and maternal–fetal attachment on the other. The subjects in this study were 91 women who were in the second trimester of normal pregnancies. Women were categorized into one of three groups: an amniocentesis group (19 women); an ultrasound group (37 women); and a control group having neither procedure (35 women). Data were collected at two points in time, before and after the procedures. The mean gestational age at the first data collection time was 15.8 weeks and at the second, 19.9 weeks.

Heidrich and Cranley used various self-report instruments to measure their research variables, including an existing scale and a scale constructed specifically for this study. Maternal–fetal attachment, the dependent variable, was measured using the Maternal–Fetal Attachment Scale (MFA) created by Cranley herself in a previous study. The MFA is a 24-item Likert scale with demonstrated adequacy as a measure of maternal–fetal attachment. However, the investigators were unable to find a suitable scale to measure perceptions of fetal growth. Therefore, they developed a 10-item Likert-type scale called Perception of the Fetus (POF). Examples of the scale items are as follows: "My baby can swallow" and "My baby sleeps and wakes up now." Responses on the scale range from 1 to 5, with higher scores indicating a greater degree of perceived development. The investigators took steps to ensure that this new scale yielded accurate and valid scores.

The research indicated that women who reported feeling fetal movement early in the pregnancy had higher maternal–fetal attachment scores and higher scores on the POF. Ultrasound scans had no effect on either variable. Women who had amniocentesis had lower attachment scores before the procedure, but comparable attachment scores one month later. Maternal–fetal attachment and perceptions of fetal development were both found to increase between the two points of data collection for all three groups of women.

≡ SUMMARY

Scales are tools for quantitatively measuring the degree to which individuals possess or are characterized by target traits or attributes. Psychosocial scaling procedures have been most fully developed in connection with the measurement of attitudes.

The most common form of attitude measure is the Likert scale, or summated rating scale. Likert scales present the respondent with a series of items (normally between 10 and 20) that are worded either favorably or unfavorably toward some phenomenon. Respondents are asked to indicate their degree of agreement or disagreement with each statement. Five or seven response alternatives are typically used. The responses can then be combined to form a composite score, the aim of which is to signify the individual's position, relative to that of others, on the attitudinal favorability–unfavorability continuum. A total score is derived by the summation of scores assigned to all items, which in turn are scored according to the direction of favorability expressed.

Cumulative scales or Guttman scales are constructed with attitudinal statements with which respondents must agree or disagree. This type of scale uses a relatively small number of positively *or* negatively worded items that are graduated in terms of the intensity expressed. The aim is to select statements such that a person endorsing an item of a given intensity will also agree with all items of a lesser intensity. A person's score is equal to the total number of items endorsed. *Scalogram analysis* is applied to Guttman scales as a method of ascertaining their adequacy and unidimensionality. The analysis makes use of the concept of *reproducibility,* which is the degree to which knowledge of a person's score allows the investigator to designate which specific statements were approved.

The *semantic differential,* a procedure for measuring the meaning of concepts to individuals, has been used widely in the area of attitude measurement. The technique consists of a series of *graphic rating scales* on which respondents are asked to indicate their reaction toward some phenomenon. Normally 5 to 15 bipolar adjectival scales are included for each concept. The adjectives may be measuring an evaluation (good–bad); activity (active–passive); or potency (strong–weak) dimension. Scoring of the semantic differential proceeds in a fashion similar to that of Likert scales.

The researcher interested in constructing

Table 15-3. *Examples of Instruments for Measuring Nursing and Health-related Concepts*

NAME OF INSTRUMENT	CONCEPT MEASURED	REFERENCE
Bereavement Health Assessment	Changes in health after a major loss	Miles, 1985
Chronicity Impact and Coping Questionnaire	Parents' coping during child's long-term illness	Hymovich, 1984
Collaborative Practices Scale	Nurse–physician interaction in patient care	Weiss & Davis, 1985
Community Health Intensity Rating Scale	Classification of patient care requirements	Peters, 1988
Denyes Self-Care Agency Scale	Capability for self-care	Denyes, 1982
Health-Promoting Lifestyle Profile	Practice of health-promoting behaviors	Walker et al., 1987
Health Behavior Choice Scale	Practice of health behaviors	Laffrey, 1985
Health Self-Determinism Index	Motivation in health behavior	Cox, 1985
Hospital Stress Rating Scale	Patients' level of stress	Volicer & Bohannon, 1975
Meaning of Illness Questionnaire	Cognitive appraisal of an illness event	Browne, Bryne, Roberts, Streiner, Fitch, Corey, & Arpin, 1988
Nurse's Self-Description Form	Self-assessed nursing performance	Dagenais & Meleis, 1982
Patient Satisfaction Instrument	Patients' satisfaction with nursing care	Hinshaw & Atwood, 1982
Uncertainty in Illness Scale	Adults' uncertainty regarding their illness	Mishel, 1981

new psychologic measures must contend with a number of difficulties, some of which are referred to as *response-set* biases. This problem concerns the tendency of certain individuals to respond to items in characteristic ways, independently of the item's content. The *social desirability* response set is a bias stemming from a person's desire to appear in a favorable light. The *extreme-response* set results when a person characteristically endorses extreme response alternatives. Another type of response bias is known as *acquiescence,* which designates an individual's tendency to agree with statements regardless of their content. A converse problem arises less frequently when a person disagrees with most statements.

The researcher should give sufficient consideration to existing measures before embarking on a project to construct a new scale. The development of good instruments is both arduous and time consuming. Because literally thousands of previously developed and tested measures are available, some effort should be made to identify existing instruments that tap the variables of interest. Scales and tests that measure attitudes, personality traits, abilities, development, achievement, psychologic states, health behaviors, and nursing activities were discussed and sources for their location were identified in this chapter. Nurse researchers may also want to explore the use of *visual analogue scales* (VASs) for the measurement of subjective experiences such as pain and nausea.

≡ *STUDY SUGGESTIONS*

1. Below are 20 attitudinal statements that relate to attitudes toward menopause. Respond to these 20 statements and then score yourself in terms of overall favorability toward the menopause.
   1. Menopause is simply a normal period of biological development.
   2. I look forward to menopause as a relief from the nuisance of menstruation.

   3. I resent the thought of menopause.
   4. Menopause to me means the opportunity for greater freedom of sexual expression.
   5. I am ashamed to talk about the subject of menopause.
   6. I am indifferent to the thought of menopause.
   7. The idea of menopause frightens me a little.
   8. I dread the loss of my ability to reproduce.
   9. Menstruation makes me feel womanly, and I will regret its cessation.
   10. I am annoyed that menopause is a process over which I have no control.
   11. I am frightened by stories I have heard about the menopause.
   12. When I reach the menopause, I will consider myself an old woman.
   13. Menopause is a process about which I know very little.
   14. Menopause will give me a feeling of kinship with women of my age group.
   15. The thought of menopause revolts me.
   16. I am sure that when I reach the menopause I will not feel abnormal or peculiar.
   17. To me, menopause means that I will have reached a new level of maturity.
   18. I will want a lot of sympathy during the menopause.
   19. My life will probably change very little, if at all, because of menopause.
   20. I can talk freely about menopause with my friends or family.

2. From the 20 statements in question 1, select four that you feel might constitute a Guttman scale. Ask a friend to agree or disagree with the items. Are you able to perfectly reproduce your friend's score?

3. List ten pairs of bipolar adjectives that would be appropriate for rating *all* of the following concepts for a semantic differential scale: cigarettes, alcohol, marijuana, heroin, cocaine.

4. Using the references cited at the end of this

chapter, find the names of two or three instruments that measure a person's adjustment to illness.

5. Suppose that you were interested in studying the attitudes of men toward witnessing the birth of their children in a hospital delivery room. Develop five positively worded and five negatively worded statements that could be used in constructing a Likert scale for such a study.

≡ *SUGGESTED READINGS*

METHODOLOGICAL REFERENCES

Anastasi, A. (1988). *Psychological testing* (6th ed.). New York: Macmillan.

Batey, M.V. (1979). Acquiescent response set: A source of measurement error. *Western Journal of Nursing Research, 1,* 247–249.

Beere, C.A. (1979). *Women and women's issues: A handbook of tests and measures.* San Francisco: Jossey-Bass.

Buros, O.K. (1974). *Tests in print II.* Highland Park, NJ: Gryphon Press.

Cattell, J.B., & Warburton, F.W. (1967). *Objective personality and motivation tests.* Chicago: University of Illinois Press.

Chun, K.T., Cobb, S., & French, J.R.P., Jr. (1975). *Measures for psychological assessment.* Ann Arbor: Survey Research Center.

Davison, M.L. (1983). *Multidimensional scaling.* New York: John Wiley and Sons.

Ebel, R. (1986). *Essentials of educational measurement* (4th ed.). Englewood Cliffs, NJ: Prentice-Hall.

Edwards, A.L. (1982). *Techniques of attitude scale construction.* New York: Irvington.

Frank-Stromberg, M. (Ed.) (1988). *Instruments for clinical nursing research.* Norwalk, CT: Appleton and Lange.

Gift, A.G. (1989). Visual analogue scales: Measurement of subjective phenomena. *Nursing Research, 38,* 286–288.

Karoly, P. (1984). *Measurement strategies in health psychology.* New York: John Wiley and Sons.

Keyser, D.J., & Sweetland, R.C. (Eds.) (1988). *Test critiques.* (Vol. 7). Kansas City, MO: Test Corporation of America.

Lee, K.A., & Kieckhefer, G.M. (1989). Measuring human responses using visual analogue scales. *Western Journal of Nursing Research, 11,* 128–132.

Mitchell, J.V., Jr. (Ed.) (1985). The *ninth mental measurements yearbook.* Lincoln, NE: University of Nebraska Press.

Nunnally, J.C. (1978). *Psychometric theory.* New York: McGraw-Hill.

Osgood, C.E., Suci, G.J., & Tannenbaum, P.H. (1957). *The measurements of meaning.* Urbana, IL: University of Illinois Press.

Reeder, L.G., et al. (1976). *Handbook of scales and indices of health behavior.* Pacific Palisades, CA.: Goodyear.

Robinson, J.P., & Shaver, P.R. (1973). *Measures of social psychological attitudes* (rev. ed.). Ann Arbor: University of Michigan.

Selltiz, C., Wrightsman, L.S., & Cook, S.W. (1976). *Research methods in social relations* (3rd ed.). New York: Holt, Rinehart & Winston. (Chapter 12)

Shaw, M.E., & Wright, J.M. (1967). *Scales for the measurement of attitudes.* New York: McGraw-Hill.

Strickland, O.L., & Waltz, C. (1988). *Measurement of nursing outcomes: Vol. II. Measuring nursing performance.* New York: Springer.

Touliatos, J., Perlmutter, B.F., & Straus, M.A. (Eds.) (1990). *Handbook of family measurement techniques.* Newbury Park, CA: Sage.

Waltz, C.F., & Strickland, O.L. (1988). *Measurement of nursing outcomes: Vol. I. Measuring client outcomes.* New York: Springer.

Waltz, C.F., Strickland, O.L., & Lenz, E.R. (1984). *Measurement in nursing research.* Philadelphia: F.A. Davis.

Ward, M.J., & Felter, M.E. (1979). *Instruments for use in nursing education research.* Boulder, CO: Western Interstate Commission for Higher Education.

Ward, M.J., & Lindeman, C.A. (Eds.). (1978). *Instruments for measuring nursing practice and other health variables.* Washington, DC: U.S. Government Printing Office.

SUBSTANTIVE REFERENCES

*Studies With Original Scales**

Andreoli, K.G. (1981). Self-concept and health beliefs in compliant and noncompliant hypertensive pa-

*A comment in brackets after each citation designates the type of scale used.

tients. *Nursing Research, 30,* 323–328. [Likert scale]

Flagler, S. (1988). Maternal role competence. *Western Journal of Nursing Research, 10,* 274–290. [Semantic differential]

Glanz, D., Ganong, L., & Coleman, M. (1989). Client gender, diagnosis, and family structure. *Western Journal of Nursing Research, 11,* 726–735. [Semantic differential]

Heidrich, S.M., & Cranley, M.S. (1989). Effect of fetal movement, ultrasound scans, and amniocentesis on maternal–fetal attachment. *Nursing Research, 38,* 81–84. [Likert scale]

Jacobson, S.F. (1984). A semantic differential for external comparison of conceptual nursing models. *Advances in Nursing Science, 6,* 58–70. [Semantic differential]

Kramer, M., & Hafner, L.P. (1989). Shared values: Impact on staff nurse job satisfaction and perceived productivity. *Nursing Research, 38,* 172–177. [Likert scale]

Mahon, N.E., & Yarcheski, A. (1988). Loneliness in early adolescents: An empirical test of alternate explanations. *Nursing Research, 37,* 330–335. [Likert scale]

Walker, L.O. (1989). Stress process among mothers of infants: Preliminary model testing. *Nursing Research, 38,* 10–16. [Semantic differential]

Williams, R.A., & Wikolaisen, S.M. (1982). Sudden infant death syndrome: Parents' perceptions and responses to the loss of their infant. *Research in Nursing and Health, 5,* 55–61. [Likert scale]

Studies Using Existing Scales

Aaronson, L.S. (1989). Perceived and received support: Effects on health behavior during pregnancy. *Nursing Research, 38,* 4–9.

Bailie, V., Norbeck, J.S., & Barnes, L. (1988). Stress, social support, and psychological distress of family caregivers of the elderly. *Nursing Research, 37,* 217–222.

Braden, C.J. (1990). A test of the self-help model: Learned response to chronic illness experience. *Nursing Research, 39,* 42–47.

Brooten, D., Gennaro, S., Brown, L.P., Butts, P., Gibbons, A.L., Bakewell-Sachs, S., & Kumar, S.P. (1988). Anxiety, depression, and hostility in mothers of preterm infants. *Nursing Research, 37,* 213–216.

Burckhardt, C.S. (1985). The impact of arthritis on quality of life. *Nursing Research, 34,* 11–16.

Campbell, J.C. (1989). A test of two explanatory models of women's responses to battering. *Nursing Research, 38,* 18–24.

Christman, N.J. (1990). Uncertainty and adjustment during radiotherapy. *Nursing Research, 39,* 17–20.

Duffy, M.E. (1988). Determinants of health promotion in midlife women. *Nursing Research, 37,* 358–362.

Farran, C.J., Salloway, J.C., & Clark, D.C. (1990). Measurement of hope in a community-based older population. *Western Journal of Nursing Research, 12,* 42–59.

Froman, R.D., & Owen, S.V. (1989). Predicting performance on the National Council Licensure Examination. *Western Journal of Nursing Research, 11,* 334–346.

Gass, K.A., & Chang, A.S. (1989). Appraisals of bereavement, coping, resources, and psychosocial health dysfunction in widows and widowers. *Nursing Research, 38,* 31–36.

Gennaro, S. (1988). Postpartal anxiety and depression in mothers of term and preterm infants. *Nursing Research, 37,* 82–85.

Hall, L.A., & Farel, A.M. (1988). Maternal stress and depressive symptoms: Correlates of behavior problems in young children. *Nursing Research, 37,* 156–161.

Hanson, S. (1981). Single custodial fathers and the parent-child relationship. *Nursing Research, 30,* 202–204.

Herth, K. (1990). Relationship of hope, coping styles, concurrent losses, and setting to grief resolution in the elderly widower. *Research in Nursing and Health, 13,* 109–117.

Itano, J., Tanabe, P., Lum, J., Lamkin, L., Rizzo, E., Wieland, M., & Sato, P. (1983). Compliance of cancer patients to therapy. *Western Journal of Nursing Research, 5,* 5–16.

Jackson, B.B. (1990). Social support and life satisfaction of black climacteric women. *Western Journal of Nursing Research, 12,* 9–27.

Johnson, J.E., Christman, N.J., & Stitt, C. (1985). Personal control interventions. *Research in Nursing and Health, 8,* 131–145.

Krouse, H.J., & Krouse, J.H. (1982). Cancer as crisis: The critical elements of adjustment. *Nursing Research, 31,* 96–101.

Laborde, J.M., & Powers, M.J. (1985). Life satisfaction, health control orientation, and illness-related factors in persons with osteoarthritis. *Research in Nursing and Health, 8,* 183–190.

LaMontagne, L.L. (1984). Children's locus of control beliefs as predictors of preoperative coping behavior. *Nursing Research, 33,* 76–79.

Levine, C.D., Wilson, S., & Guido, G. (1988). Personality factors of critical care nurses. *Heart and Lung, 17,* 392–398.

Littlefield, V.M., Chang, A., & Adams, B.N. (1990). Participation in alternative care: Relationship to anxiety, depression, and hostility. *Research in Nursing and Health, 13,* 17–25.

Mercer, R.T., Ferketich, S.L., DeJoseph, J., May, K.A., & Sollid, D. (1988). Effect of stress on family functioning during pregnancy. *Nursing Research, 37,* 268–275.

Mishel, M.H., & Braden, C.J. (1988). Finding meaning: Antecedents of uncertainty in illness. *Nursing Research, 37,* 98–103.

Moore, I.M., Gilliss, C.L., & Martinson, I. (1988). Psychosomatic symptoms in parents two years after the death of a child with cancer. *Nursing Research, 37,* 104–107.

Murata, J.M. (1990). Father's family violence and son's delinquency. *Western Journal of Nursing Research, 12,* 60–74.

Murphy, S.A. (1988). Mental distress and recovery in a high-risk bereavement sample three years after an untimely death. *Nursing Research, 37,* 30–35.

Norbeck, J.S., & Anderson, N.J. (1989). Psychosocial predictors of pregnancy outcomes in low-income black, Hispanic, and white women. *Nursing Research, 38,* 204–209.

Primomo, J., Yates, B.C., & Woods, N.F. (1990). Social support for women during chronic illness. *Research in Nursing and Health, 13,* 153–161.

Riffee, D.M. (1981). Self-esteem changes in hospitalized school-age children. *Nursing Research, 30,* 94–97.

Robinson, K.M. (1989). Predictors of depression among wife caregivers. *Nursing Research, 38,* 359–363.

Rudy, E.B., & Estok, P.J. (1983). Intensity of jogging: Its relationship to selected physical and psychological variables in women. *Western Journal of Nursing Research, 5,* 325–336.

Ryden, M.B. (1984). Morale and perceived control in institutionalized elderly. *Nursing Research, 33,* 130–136.

Sime, A.M., & Libera, M.B. (1985). Sensation information, self-instruction and responses to dental surgery. *Research in Nursing and Health, 8,* 41–47.

Strang, V.R., & Sullivan, P.L. (1985). Body image attitudes during pregnancy and the postpartum period. *Journal of Obstetric, Gynecologic, and Neonatal Nursing, 14,* 332–337.

Stuifbergen, A.K. (1990). Patterns of functioning in families with a chronically ill parent. *Research in Nursing and Health, 13,* 35–44.

Thomas, P.D., & Hooper, E.M. (1983). Healthy elderly: Social bonds and locus of control. *Research in Nursing and Health, 6,* 11–16.

Upvall, M.J. (1990). A model of uprooting for international students. *Western Journal of Nursing Research, 12,* 95–107.

VanOs, D.K., Clark, C.G., Turner, C.N., & Herbst, J.J. (1985). Life stress and cystic fibrosis. *Western Journal of Nursing Research, 7,* 301–315.

Ventura, J.N. (1982). Parent coping behaviors, parent functioning, and infant temperament characteristics. *Nursing Research, 31,* 269–273.

Weitzel, M.H. (1989). A test of the health promotion model with blue collar workers. *Nursing Research, 38,* 99–104.

Yarcheski, A., & Mahon, N.E. (1989). A causal model of positive health practices: The relationship between approach and replication. *Nursing Research, 38,* 88–93.

Zimmerman, L., Pozehi, B., Duncan, K., & Schmitz, R. (1989). Effects of music in patients who had chronic cancer pain. *Western Journal of Nursing Research, 11,* 298–309.

Studies Using Visual Analogue Scales

Gaston-Johansson, F., Fridh, G., & Turner-Norvell, K. (1988). Progression of labor pain in primiparas and multiparas. *Nursing Research, 37,* 86–90.

Hargreaves, A., & Lander, J. (1989). Use of transcutaneous electrical nerve stimulation for postoperative pain. *Nursing Research, 38,* 159–161

Miller, K.M., and Perry, P.A. (1990). Relaxation technique and postoperative pain in patients undergoing cardiac surgery. *Heart and Lung, 19,* 136–145.

Steur, J., & Wewers, M.E. (1989). Cigarette craving and subsequent coping responses among smoking cessation clinic participants. *Oncology Nursing Forum, 16,* 193–198.

Webb, C.J., Stergios, D.A., & Rodgers, B.M. (1989). Patient-controlled analgesia as postoperative pain treatment for children. *Journal of Pediatric Nursing, 4,* 162–171.

Zimmerman, L., Pozehi, B., Duncan, K., & Schmitz, R. (1989). Effects of music in patients who had chronic cancer pain. *Western Journal of Nursing Research, 11,* 298–309.

References for Nursing and Health Related Instruments

Benner, P., & Benner, R. (1979). *The new nurse's work entry.* New York: Tiresias Press.

Browne, G.B., Byrne, C., Roberts, J., Streiner, D., Fitch, M., Corey, P., & Arpin, K. (1988). The Meaning of Illness Questionnaire: Reliability and validity. *Nursing Research, 37,* 368–373.

Cox, C.L. (1985). The Health Self-Determinism Index. *Nursing Research, 34,* 177–183.

Dagenais, F., & Meleis, A.I. (1982). Professionalism, work ethic and empathy in nursing. *Western Journal of Nursing Research, 4,* 407–422.

Denyes, M.J. (1982). Measurement of self-care agency in adolescents. *Nursing Research, 31,* 63–68.

Gortner, S.R., Hudes, M., & Zyzanski, S.J. (1984). Appraisal of values in the choice of treatment. *Nursing Research, 33,* 319–324.

Hinshaw, A.S., & Atwood, J.R. (1982). A Patient Satisfaction Instrument: Precision by replication. *Nursing Research, 31,* 170–175.

Hymovich, D.P. (1984). Development of the Chronicity Impact and Coping Instrument: Parent questionnaire (CICI:PQ). *Nursing Research, 33,* 218–222.

Ketefian, S. (1981). Moral reasoning and moral behavior among selected groups of practicing nurses. *Nursing Research, 30,* 171–176.

Laffrey, S.C. (1985). Health behavior choices as related to self-actualization and health conception. *Western Journal of Nursing Research, 7,* 279–300.

Miles, M.S. (1985). Emotional symptoms and physical health in bereaved parents. *Nursing Research, 34,* 76–81.

Mishel, M. (1981). The measurement of uncertainty in illness. *Nursing Research, 30,* 258–263.

Peters, D.A. (1988). Development of a community health intensity rating scale. *Nursing Research, 37,* 202–207.

Risser, N. (1975). Development of an instrument to measure patient satisfaction with nurses and nursing care in primary care settings. *Nursing Research, 24,* 45–52.

Volicer, B.J., & Bohannon, M.W. (1975). A hospital stress rating scale. *Nursing Research, 24,* 352–359.

Walker, S.N., Sechrest, K.R., & Pender, N.J. (1987). The health-promoting lifestyle profile: Development and psychometric characteristics. *Nursing Research, 36,* 76–81.

Weiss, S.J., & Davis, H.P. (1985). Validity and reliability of the Collaborative Practice Scales. *Nursing Research, 34,* 299–305.

Wolfer, J.A. (1973). Definition and assessment of surgical patients' welfare and recovery. *Nursing Research, 22,* 394–401.

16
Observational Methods

For certain types of research problems, an important alternative to self-reports for measuring variables of interest is direct observation of subjects' behavior and characteristics. Many kinds of information required by nurse researchers as evidence of nursing effectiveness or as clues to improving nursing practices can be obtained through direct observation. Suppose, for instance, we were interested in studying mental patients' methods of defending their personal territory, or children's reactions to the removal of a leg cast, or a patient's mode of emergence from anesthesia. Data relating to these phenomena could be collected by the direct observation of the relevant behaviors.

Scientific observation involves the systematic selection, observation, and recording of behaviors and settings relevant to a problem under investigation. Like self-report methods, observational methods can vary in terms of structure, from highly unstructured to highly structured approaches. Both structured and unstructured methods are discussed in this chapter. First, however, we present an overview of some general issues.

≡ *SELECTION OF PHENOMENA FOR OBSERVATION*

When a nurse researcher observes an event—such as a nurse administering an injection to a patient—he or she must have a clear idea about what is to be observed. A single incidence or occurrence encompasses a variety of aspects and dimensions. The researcher cannot absorb and record an infinite number of details and must, therefore, have some guidelines specifying the manner in which the observations are to be focused or edited.

The choice of the phenomena to be observed will be guided by the problem being investigated. However, even after the problem area is defined, there is a need for further specification and selection. Suppose we were interested in understanding how the educational preparation of nurses relates to their empathic behavior in administering injections to patients. We have now focused our attention on a specific dimension of nursing behavior, but how will we define and observe "empathic behavior?" We might select a number of alternatives, such as the frequency, content, or tone of the nurses' statements to the patients, or the nurses' facial expressions as they prepare and administer the injections, or their frequency and manner of touching the patients. Any of these behaviors, as well as several others, could be used as an observational measure of empathy among nurses. In this section, we will try to demonstrate the versatility of observational methods by pointing out some considerations for the selection of observable phenomena.

Phenomena Amenable to Observations

Nurse researchers usually make observational records of either human behaviors or the characteristics of individuals, events, environments, or objects. The following list of six observable phenomena is meant to be suggestive rather than exhaustive:

1. *Characteristics and conditions of individuals.* A broad variety of information about people's attributes and states can be gathered by direct observation. We refer not only to relatively enduring traits of individuals, such as their physical appearance, but also to more temporary conditions, such as physiologic symptoms that are amenable to observation. We include here physiologic conditions that can be observed either directly through the senses, or with the aid of observational apparatus, such as an x-ray. To illustrate this class of observable phenomena, the following could be used as dependent or independent vari-

ables in a nursing research investigation: the sleep or wake state of patients, the presence of edema in congestive heart failure, turgor of the skin in dehydration, the manifestation of decubitus ulcers, alopecia during cancer chemotherapy, or symptoms of infusion phlebitis in hospitalized patients.

2. *Verbal communication behaviors.* One of the most commonly observed types of human behavior is linguistic behavior. The content and structure of people's conversations are readily observable, easy to record, and, thus, are an obvious source of data. Among the kinds of verbal communications that a nurse researcher might be interested in observing are information-giving of nurses to patients, nurses' conversations with grieving relatives, exchange of information among nurses at change of shift report, the dialogue of residents in a nursing home, and conversations in a rural public health clinic.

3. *Nonverbal communication behaviors.* People communicate their fears, wants, and emotions in many ways other than just with words. For nursing researchers, nonverbal communication represents an extremely fruitful area for research because nurses are often called on to be sensitive to nonverbal cues. The kinds of nonverbal behavior amenable to observational methods include facial expressions; touch; posture; gestures and other body movements; and extralinguistic behavior (i.e., the manner in which people speak, aside from the content, such as the intonation, loudness, and continuity of the speech).

4. *Activities.* Many actions are amenable to observation and constitute valuable data for nursing researchers. Activities that serve as an index of health status or physical and emotional functioning are particularly important. As illustrations, the following kinds of activities lend themselves to an observational study: patients' eating habits and trends, bowel movements in postsurgical patients, self-grooming activities of nursing home residents, length and number of visits by friends and relatives to hospitalized patients, and ag-

gressive actions among children in the hospital playroom.

5. *Skill attainment and performance.* Nurses and nurse educators are constantly called on to develop skills among clients and students. The attainment of these skills is often manifested behaviorally, and in such cases, an observational assessment is appropriate. For example, a nurse researcher might want to observe the following kinds of behaviors: the ability of nursing students to properly insert a urinary catheter, the ability of stroke patients to scan a food tray if homonymous hemianopia is present, the ability of diabetics to test their urine for sugar and acetone, or the ability of a newborn to exhibit sucking behavior when positioned for breast-feeding.

6. *Environmental characteristics.* An individual's surroundings may have a profound effect on his or her behavior and, therefore, a number of studies have explored the relationship between certain observable attributes of the environment on the one hand and human beliefs, actions, and needs on the other. Examples of observable environmental attributes include the following: the noise levels in different areas of a hospital, the existence of architectural barriers in the homes of individuals with a disability, the color of walls in a nursing home, the laboratory facilities in a school of nursing, or the cleanliness of the homes in a community.

Units of Observation

In selecting behaviors, attributes, or situations to be observed, the investigator must decide what constitutes a unit. There are two basic approaches, which are perhaps best considered as the end points of a continuum. The *molar approach* entails observing large units of behavior and treating them as a whole. For example, psychiatric nurse researchers might engage in a study of patient mood swings. An entire constellation of verbal and nonverbal behaviors might be construed as signaling aggressive behaviors, and

another set might constitute passive behaviors. At the other extreme, the *molecular approach* uses small and highly specific behaviors as the unit of observation. Each movement, action, gesture, or phrase is treated as a separate entity, or perhaps broken down into even smaller units. The choice of approaches depends to a large degree on the nature of the problem and the preferences of the investigator. The molar approach is more susceptible to observer errors and distortions because of the greater ambiguity in the definition of the units. On the other hand, in reducing the observations to more concrete and specific elements, the investigator may lose sight of the activities that are at the heart of the inquiry.

≡ THE OBSERVER/OBSERVED RELATIONSHIP

The observer–researcher can interact with individuals in the observational setting to varying degrees. The issue of the relationship between the observer and those observed is an important one, and one that has stirred much controversy. The most important aspects of this issue are intervention and concealment. The decisions a researcher makes in establishing a strategy for handling these considerations should be based on an understanding of the ethical and methodological implications.

In observational studies, intervention may involve an experimental intervention of the type described in Chapter 9 on experimental designs. For example, a nurse researcher may observe patients' postoperative behaviors following an intervention designed to improve the patients' ability to cough and breathe after surgery. However, in observational studies, the researcher sometimes intervenes to structure the research setting, without necessarily introducing an experimental treatment, that is, without manipulating the independent variable. This approach is sometimes referred to as the use of *directed settings.* For instance, researchers sometimes "stage" a situation to provoke specific behavioral patterns. Certain events or activities are rare in naturalistic settings and, therefore, it becomes inexpedient to await their manifestation. Investigators in such studies typically make every attempt to maintain the outward appearance of a natural event. For example, a large number of social psychologic investigations have studied the behavior of bystanders in crisis or emergency situations. Crises are not very common and their occurrence is unpredictable. Therefore, to observe the determinants of helping behavior (or lack of it) among onlookers, investigators have created "emergencies." Such studies are considered high on the intervention dimension.

Studies in which the researcher intervenes to elicit behaviors of interest may be practical when there is little opportunity to observe activities or events as they unfold naturalistically. However, such studies are sometimes criticized on the grounds of artificiality and may suffer from serious problems of external validity.

The second dimension that concerns the relationship between the observer and the observed is the degree to which subjects are aware of the observation and their subject status. In naturalistic settings, researchers are often concerned that their presence, if known, would alter the behaviors under observation. In some situations, therefore, observers may adopt a completely passive role, attempting insofar as possible to become unobtrusive bystanders. The problem of behavioral distortions owing to the known presence of an observer has been called a reactive measurement effect or, more simply, *reactivity*.

One approach to minimizing the problem of reactivity is to make the observations without the subjects' knowledge, through some type of concealment. For example, a nurse could monitor patients' conversations surreptitiously by means of the call system located at the nurses' station. In laboratory environments or in some "directed settings," concealed observations can be accomplished through the use of one-way mirrors.

Concealment offers the researcher a number of distinct advantages, even beyond the reduction of reactivity. Some individuals might deny a researcher the privilege of observing

them altogether, so that the alternative to concealed observation might be no observation at all. Total concealment, however, may be difficult to attain except in highly structured or active observational settings. Furthermore, concealed observation, without the knowledge and consent of those observed, is ethically problematic (see Chapter 3).

A second situation is one in which the subjects are aware of the researcher's presence but may not be aware of the investigator's underlying motives. This approach offers the researcher the opportunity of getting more in-depth information than is usually possible with total concealment. Also, because the researcher is not totally concealed, there may be fewer ethical problems. Nevertheless, the issues of subject deception and failure to obtain informed voluntary consent remain thorny ones. Furthermore, a serious drawback of this second approach is the possibility that the interaction between the observer and the observed will alter the subjects' behavior. Even when the observed individuals are unaware of being participants in a research study, there is always a risk that the researcher's presence will alter their normal activities, mannerisms, or conversations.

The researcher will be confronted with methodological, substantive, or ethical issues at every point along the concealment and intervention dimensions. Some of these problems will be irrelevant in particular projects, but the careful investigator should assess the relative weaknesses of an approach against the possible advantages it might offer.

≡ OBSERVATIONAL METHODS: UNSTRUCTURED OBSERVATIONS

Field research (see Chapter 11) usually involves the collection of unstructured or loosely structured observational data. The aim of field research is typically to understand the behaviors and experiences of people as they actually occur in naturalistic settings. Therefore, the field researcher's aim is to observe and record information about people and their environments with a minimum of structure and researcher-imposed interference.

The gathering of observational data in field settings is often referred to as *participant observation*. In such research, the investigator participates in the functioning of the social group under investigation and strives to observe and record information within the contexts, structures, and symbols that are relevant to the group members. Although it is beyond the scope of this book to describe in detail the methods used in participant observation research, we describe some of the salient issues. Textbooks on field research methods, such as that by Schatzman and Strauss (1982), should be consulted for a more thorough elaboration of methods.

The Observer–Participant Role

The role that an observer plays in the social group under investigation is important because the social position of the observer determines what he or she is likely to see. That is, the behaviors that are likely to be available for observation will depend on the observer's position in a network of relations.

Leininger (1985) has noted that the observer's role typically evolves through a sequence of four phases:

1. Primarily observation
2. Primarily observation with some participation
3. Primarily participation with some observation
4. Reflective observation

In the initial phase, the researcher observes and listens to those under study to obtain a broad view of the situation. This phase allows both observers and subjects to "size up" each other, to become acquainted, and to become more comfortable in interacting. In phase 2, observation is enhanced by a modest degree of participation. As the researcher participates more actively in the activities of the social group, the reactions of people to specific researcher behaviors can be more

systematically studied. In phase 3, the researcher strives to become a more active participant, learning by the actual experience of "doing" rather than just watching and listening. In phase 4, the researcher reflects on the total process of what transpired and how people interacted with and reacted to the researcher.

The observer must overcome at least two major hurdles in assuming a satisfactory role *vis-à-vis* subject–informants. The first is to gain entrée into the social group under investigation; the second is to establish rapport and develop trust within the social group. Without gaining entrée, the study cannot proceed; but without the trust of the group, the researcher will typically be restricted to what Leininger (1985) refers to as "front stage" knowledge, that is, information that is distorted by the group's protective facades. The goal of the participant observer is to "get back stage"—to learn about the true realities of the group's experiences and behaviors.

Clearly, interpersonal skills play an important role in overcoming both these hurdles. Wilson (1985) has noted that successful participant observation research may require researchers to "go through channels, cultivate relationships, contour [their] appearances, withhold evaluative judgments, and be as unobtrusive and charming as possible" (p. 376).

Gathering and Recording Unstructured Observational Data

During the initial phase of a field study, it is often useful to gather some written or pictorial descriptive information that provides an overview of the environment. In an institutional setting, for example, it may be helpful to obtain a floor plan, an organizational chart, an annual report, and so on. Then, a preliminary personal tour of the site should be undertaken to gain familiarity with the ambience of the site and to note major activities, social groupings, transactions, and events.

The next step is to identify a meaningful way to sample observations and to select observational locations. Sampling by time and by event are common strategies for observational sampling (these strategies are discussed later in this chapter). It is generally useful to use a combination of positioning approaches in selecting observational locations. *Single positioning* means staying in a single location for a period to observe behaviors and transactions in that location. *Multiple positioning* involves moving around the site to observe behaviors from different locations. *Mobile positioning* involves following a person throughout a given activity or period.

Because participant observers cannot spend a lifetime in one site and because they cannot be in more than one place at a time, observation is almost always supplemented with information obtained in unstructured interviews or conversations. For example, an informant may be asked to describe what went on in a meeting that the observer was unable to attend, or informants may be asked to describe an event that occurred before the observer entered the field. In such a case, the informant functions as the observer's observer.

The participant observer typically places few restrictions on the types of data collected, in keeping with the goal of minimizing observer-imposed meanings and structure. Given this aim, the most common forms of record-keeping in participant observation studies are logs and field notes. A *log* is a daily record of events and conversations. *Field notes* may include the daily log but tend to be much broader, more analytic, and more interpretive than a simple listing of occurrences. Field notes represent the participant observer's efforts to record information and also to synthesize and understand the data.

Field notes are sometimes categorized according to the purpose they will serve during the analysis and integration of information. *Observational notes* are objective descriptions of events and conversations; information such as time, place, activity, and dialogue are recorded as completely and objectively as possible. *Theoretical notes* are interpretive attempts to attach meaning to observations. *Methodological notes* are instructions or reminders about how subsequent observations will be made. *Personal notes* are comments about the researcher's own feelings during the research process. Table 16-1 presents some examples of all four types of field notes from a fictitious study of an *in vitro* fertilization (IVF) treatment facility.

The success of any participant observation study depends highly on the quality of the logs and field notes. It is clearly essential to record observations while the researcher is still in the process of collecting information, because the memory is bound to fail if there is too long a delay. On the other hand, the participant observer cannot usually perform the recording function by openly carrying a clipboard, pens, and paper, because this action would undermine the observer's role as an ordinary participant of the group. The researcher, therefore, must develop the skill of making detailed mental notes that can later be committed to paper or recorded on tape. Alternatively, the observer can try to jot down unobtrusively a phrase or sentence that will later serve as a reminder of an event, conversation, or impression. At a later point—preferably as soon as possible—the observer can utilize the brief notes and mental recordings to develop the more extensive field notes. The use of portable computers with word processing capabilities can greatly facilitate the recording and organization of notes in the field.

Evaluating Unstructured Observation

Unstructured observation is a method of collecting research data that has both strong opponents and proponents. Those researchers who support the use of unstructured methods point out that these techniques usually provide a deeper and richer understanding of human behaviors and social situations than is possible with more standardized procedures. Participant observation is particularly valuable, according to this view, for its ability to "get inside" a particular situation and lead to a more complete understanding of its complexities. Furthermore, unstructured observational approaches are inherently flexible and, therefore, permit the observer greater freedom to reconceptualize the problem after becoming more familiar with the situation. Advocates of qualitative observational research also claim that structured, quantitatively oriented methods are too mechanistic and superficial to render a meaningful account of the intricate nature of human behavior.

Critics of the unstructured approach point out a number of methodological shortcomings. Observer bias and observer influence are prominent difficulties. Not only is there a concern that the observer may lose objectivity in recording actual observations, there is also the question that the observer will inappropriately sample events and situations to be observed. Once the researcher begins to participate in a group's activities, the possibility of emotional involvement becomes a salient issue. The researcher in the new "member" role may fail to attend to many scientifically relevant aspects of the situation or may develop a myopic view on issues of importance to the group. Participant observation techniques, thus, may be an unsuitable approach to study problems when one suspects that the risks of identification are strong. Memory distortions represent another possible source of inaccuracy. Finally, unstructured observational methods depend more on the observational and interpersonal skills of the observer than do highly structured techniques. A highly skilled and sensitive observer can develop extremely valuable knowledge about human experiences in much the same way that a talented novelist does. However, talent of this kind is uncommon and may be difficult to cultivate.

There is obviously no "right" or "wrong"

Table 16-1. *Example of Field Notes: Study of an In Vitro Fertilization (IVF) Facility*

Observational notes	Couple A entered the center for the first time at around 7 PM on a Tuesday evening. Mrs. A sat very stiffly on the chair next to the receptionist's desk, and Mr. A sat beside her. Both parties looked uncomfortable and tense. There was little interaction between them until they were called in for the initial consultation. While in the waiting area, Mrs. A picked up several magazines, thumbed through them absently, and then put them down again. Mr. A spent most of the time smoking cigarettes, staring at the ceiling or at the entrance to the office. Couple A spent approximately 15 minutes in the waiting area. When their name was called, Mrs. A jumped as though startled and then moved quickly toward the door. She turned back once to make sure Mr. A was following, and when she saw that he was just rising, motioned for him to follow her.
Theoretical notes	Tension is a common feature among couples waiting for their initial consultation. However, the tension seems to stem from different sources and manifests itself in different ways. Some couples seem not to be persuaded that IVF is right for them; these couples seem embarrassed and tend not to communicate with one another. The source of tension seems to stem less from conflict about whether to try IVF but rather from the fear of disappointment. These couples tend to engage in continuous *sotto voce* discussions about what they've heard about IVF while waiting for their intake.
Methodological notes	I decided yesterday to make more systematic observations of couples immediately after they complete their initial interview. This decision was spurred by an incident yesterday in which both partners left the office in tears.
Personal notes	My progress in understanding what these couples seeking IVF treatment are going through is very uneven. Two days ago, I was confident that patterns were falling into place. But this afternoon, a little girl in the waiting room (an adopted daughter of a couple undergoing treatment) made me painfully aware of how much more complex the phenomenon of infertility and its social and psychologic meanings really are.

answer to the question of which approach should be adopted. The researcher should choose an approach that, given the research problem and the researcher's own skills and interests, is most likely to yield meaningful and useful data. On the whole, it would appear that unstructured observational methods are extremely profitable for exploratory research in which the investigator wishes to establish an adequate conceptualization of the important variables in a social setting or wants to develop a set of hypotheses. The more rigorous observational methods, discussed in the following section, are probably better suited in most cases to the testing of research hypotheses.

☰ *OBSERVATIONAL METHODS: STRUCTURED OBSERVATIONS*

Structured observational methods differ from unstructured techniques in the specificity of behaviors or events selected for observation, in the advanced preparation of record-keeping forms, and in the kinds of activities in which the observer engages. The observer utilizing a structured observational procedure may still have ample room for making inferences and exercising judgment but is restrained with regard to the kinds of phenomena that will be watched and recorded. The creativity of structured observation lies not in the observation itself but, rather, in the formulation of a system for accurately categorizing, recording, and encoding the observations and sampling the phenomena of interest. Because structured techniques depend on plans developed before observation, they are not considered appropriate when the investigator has limited or no knowledge about the phenomena under investigation.

Categories and Checklists

The most common approach to making structured observations of ongoing events and behaviors consists of the construction of a category system to which the observed phenomena can be assigned. A *category system* represents an attempt to designate in a systematic or quantita-

tive fashion the qualitative behaviors and events transpiring within the observational setting.

CONSIDERATIONS IN USING CATEGORY SYSTEMS

One of the most important requirements of a category system is the careful and explicit definition of the behaviors and characteristics to be observed. Each category should be explained in detail with an operational definition so that observers will have relatively clear-cut criteria for assessing the occurrence of the phenomenon in question. For example, Borgatta (1962) presented a category system for the observation of verbal communication and social interaction involving two or more individuals. The Interaction Process Score system involves 18 categories of interactive behavior. Category 4, which designates the observed subject's "acknowledgement, understanding, or recognition" within a social interaction, is defined as follows:

> This category includes all passive indicators of having understood or recognized the communication directed toward the recipient. The most common score for this category is a nod or saying "Uhuh," "Yes," "O.K.," "Mum," "Right," "Check," "I see," "That may be, but . . . ." In general, items are scored into this category if they indicate the acceptance of an item of communication, but this does not require agreement with the communication, the presence of which would place the response in Category 5. (Borgatta, 1962, p. 273)

In developing or selecting a categorization scheme, the researcher must make a number of important decisions. One decision concerns the exhaustiveness of the phenomena to be observed and the number of categories to be included. Some category systems, such as Borgatta's interaction procedure, are constructed such that *all* observed interactive behaviors can be classified into one (and only one) category. Another example of an exhaustive system is the Downs and Fitzpatrick (1976) observation tool for analyzing body position and motor activity in mobile subjects. Their instrument was developed with the objective that all postural and motor behavior could be classified into one of their categories.

A contrasting technique is to develop a nonexhaustive system in which only particular types of behavior are categorized. For example, Gill and colleagues (1984) used a more restrictive category system for the observation of crying behaviors in newborn infants. Their system categorizes 25 different crying behaviors, but noncrying behaviors are not included. As another example, if we were observing the aggressive behavior of autistic children, we might develop such categories as "strikes another child," "kicks or hits walls/floors," "calls other children names," "throws objects around the room," and so forth. In this restricted category system, many behaviors (all those that are nonaggressive) would not be classified. Such nonexhaustive systems are adequate for many research purposes. However, they run the risk of providing data that are difficult to interpret. When a large number of observed behaviors are unclassified, the investigator may have difficulty in placing the categorized behaviors into a proper perspective.

Virtually all category systems require that some inferences be made on the part of the observer, but there is considerable variability on this dimension. The Downs and Fitzpatrick (1976) observational instrument for body position and motor activity consists of a category system that requires only a modest amount of inference. For example, total body position is classified in one of six relatively straightforward categories: (1) upright, (2) lying down, (3) leaning, (4) sitting, (5) leaning over, and (6) kneeling. On the other hand, a category system such as the Abnormal Involuntary Movement Scale (AIMS) requires considerably more inference. The AIMS system, which was developed by the National Institute for Mental Health and used in a study by Whall and associates (1983) for detecting tardive dyskinesia associated with the prolonged use of neuroleptic drugs, contains such categories as "global judgments" and "trunk movements." Even when such categories are accompanied by detailed definitions and descriptions, there is clearly a heavy inferential burden placed on the observer. The decision con-

cerning how much observer inference is appropriate depends on a number of factors, including the research purposes and the skills of the observers. Beginning researchers are advised to construct or use category systems that require only a moderate degree of inference. In general, category systems that use molecular units of behavior tend to require less inference than those that use molar units.

Once a category system has been developed or selected, the researcher can proceed to construct a *checklist,* which is the instrument used by the observer to record observed phenomena. Whether one constructs a new category system or uses a well-developed method, the system should be subjected to pilot runs to assess its suitability for the intended study.

CHECKLISTS FOR EXHAUSTIVE SYSTEMS

When an observer uses an exhaustive system (i.e., when all behaviors of a certain type—such as verbal interaction—are observed and recorded), the researcher must be especially careful to define the categories in such a way that the observers know when one behavior ends and a new one begins. Another essential feature of exhaustive systems is that the referent behaviors should be mutually exclusive. If overlapping categories are not eliminated, then the observer may have difficulty in deciding how to classify a particular observation. The underlying assumption in the use of such a category system is that behaviors, events, or attributes that are allocated to a particular category are equivalent to every other behavior, event, or attribute in that same category.

The checklist is generally formatted with the list of behaviors or events from the category system on the left and space for tallying the frequency or duration of occurrence of behaviors on the right. In complex social situations with multiple actors, the right-hand portion may be divided into panels according to characteristics of the actors (e.g., nurse/physician; male patients/female patients) or by individual subjects' names or identification numbers.

The task of the observer using this approach

is to place all behaviors in only one category for each element. By *element,* we refer here to either a unit of behavior, such as a sentence in a conversation, or to a time interval. To illustrate, suppose that we were interested in studying the problem-solving behavior of a group of public health workers developing a maternal–child health program in a rural area. We might construct a category system such as the following: (1) information seeking, (2) information giving, (3) problem describing, (4) suggestion proposing, (5) suggestion opposing, (6) suggestion supporting, (7) summarizing, and (8) miscellaneous. The observer would be required to classify every group member's contribution—using, for example, each sentence as the element—to the problem-solving process in terms of one of these eight categories. By employing such a system, it would be possible to analyze, for example, the relationship between a group member's role, status, or characteristics on the one hand and the types of problem-solving behaviors engaged in on the other.

The second manner in which this approach can be used is to categorize the relevant behaviors at regular time intervals. The observational system for analyzing motor activity developed by Downs and Fitzpatrick (1976) uses 15-second time intervals as the basic recording unit. That is, the observer is expected to record all body positions and movements occurring within a 15-second period. Checklists based on exhaustive category systems are demanding of the observer, because the recording task is continuous.

CHECKLISTS FOR NONEXHAUSTIVE SYSTEMS

The second approach, which is sometimes referred to as a *sign system,* begins with a listing of categories of behaviors that may or may not be manifested by the subjects. The observer's task is to watch for instances of the behaviors on the list. When a behavior occurs, the observer either places a check mark beside the appropriate behavior to designate its occurrence or makes a cumulative tally of the number of times the behavior was witnessed. The product of this type of

endeavor is a kind of demography of events transpiring within the observational period. With this type of checklist, the observer does not classify *all* the behaviors or characteristics of the individuals being observed but rather identifies the occurrence and frequency of particular behaviors. A hypothetical example of a checklist using the sign system for describing patients' ability to perform selected activities of daily living is presented in Table 16-2.

Rating Scales

Structured observations can be recorded in a number of ways other than through the use of category systems and checklists. The major alternative is to use rating scales. A *rating scale* is a tool that requires the observer to rate some phenomenon in terms of points along a descriptive contin-

Table 16-2. *Example of Categories for a Sign Analysis*

ACTIVITY	FREQUENCY
Eating behaviors	
Eats with hand	
Eats with spoon or fork	
Cuts soft food	
Cuts meat	
Drinks from a straw	
Drinks from a cup or glass	
Hygiene	
Washes hands or extremities	
Brushes teeth	
Cleans fingernails	
Brushes or combs hair	
Shaves	
Dressing skills	
Fastens or unfastens buttons	
Fastens or unfastens snaps	
Pulls zipper up or down	
Ties or unties shoelace	
Puts on or takes off eyeglasses	
Fastens or unfastens buckle	
Puts in or takes out dentures	

uum. The ratings usually are quantified during the subsequent analysis of the observational data.

Rating scales normally are used in one of two ways. The observer may be required to make ratings of behavior or events at frequent intervals throughout the observational period in much the same way that a checklist would be used. Alternatively, the observer may use the rating scales to summarize an entire event or transaction after the observation is completed. Postobservation ratings require the observer to integrate a number of activities and to judge which point on a scale most closely resembles the interpretation given to the overall situation. For example, suppose that we were interested in comparing the behaviors of nurses working in intensive care units with those of nurses in other units. After 15-minute observation sessions, the observer might be asked to rate the perceived anxiety level of the nursing staff in each unit as a whole, or that of individual members. The rating scale item might take the following form:

According to your perceptions, how tense were the nurses in the observed unit?

1. extremely relaxed
2. rather relaxed
3. somewhat relaxed
4. neither relaxed nor tense
5. somewhat tense
6. rather tense
7. extremely tense

The same information could be solicited using a graphic rating scale format:

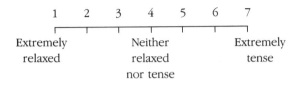

Visual analogue scales (see Chapter 15) may also be used to secure global observational ratings.

Rating scales can also be used as an extension of checklists wherein the observer records not only the occurrence of some behavior but also some qualitative aspect of it, such as its mag-

nitude or intensity. The Downs and Fitzpatrick (1976) instrument for motor activity once again provides a good example. Their category scheme comprises eight body movement categories: (1) head active, (2) right arm active, (3) left arm active, (4) both arms active, (5) right leg active, (6) left leg active, (7) both legs active, and (8) both arms and legs active. Observers must both classify the subjects' activity in terms of these categories *and* rate the intensity of the movement on a three-point scale: (1) minimally active, (2) moderately active, and (3) very active. When rating scales are coupled with a category scheme in this fashion, considerably more information about the phenomena under investigation can be obtained. The disadvantage of this approach is that it places an immense burden on the observer, particularly if there is an extensive amount of activity.

Constructing Versus Borrowing Structured Observational Instruments

The development, testing, refining, and retesting of a new category scheme or rating scale may require weeks or even months of effort, particularly if the system is intended to be used in a variety of settings and with a variety of subjects. In some cases, a researcher may have no alternative but to design new observational instruments. For example, the researcher may be investigating a relatively new area or may be expanding an area of inquiry with a new population of subjects for whom existing tools may be inappropriate. However, as in the case of self-report instruments, we encourage researchers to fully explore the literature for potentially usable observational instruments.

Many observational systems have been constructed with the intent of being applied to a variety of research situations. Generalized systems, such as those of Downs and Fitzpatrick and Borgatta described earlier, should be scrutinized before proceeding to design a new system. The use of an existing system not only saves a considerable amount of work but also facilitates comparisons among investigations.

A few source books describe available observational checklists for certain research applications. For example, the reference books by Frank-Stromberg (1988) and Strickland and Waltz (1988), which describe instruments for measuring variables of relevance to nursing, include some observational instruments. Perhaps the best source for such tools, however, is the current research literature on the topic of interest. For example, if you wanted to conduct an observational study of maternal–infant bonding behavior, a good place to begin is by reviewing recently completed research on this or similar topics to get clues about how "maternal bonding" was operationalized. Table 16-3 provides examples of some concepts of interest to nurse researchers for which observational instruments have been developed and lists the appropriate references for locating them.

Observational Sampling

Structured observational methods rarely involve the recording of all behaviors or activities that occur in a given situation. The investigator must often decide how and when the system will be applied. Observational sampling methods represent a mechanism for obtaining representative examples of the behavior being observed without having to observe for prolonged periods.

The most frequently used system is the *time-sampling method*. This procedure involves the selection of periods during which the observations will occur. The time frames may be systematically selected (e.g., every 30 seconds at 2-minute intervals) or may be selected at random. As a hypothetical example, suppose we were studying the interaction patterns of mothers and their handicapped children. Some of the mothers have received specific preparation from a community health nurse for dealing with their conflict over the child's dependence–independence needs, and a control group of mothers has not received this intervention. To examine the effects of this special program, the behavior of the mothers and children are observed in a playground setting. During a 1-hour observation period, we decide to sample behaviors rather than to observe the entire session. For the sake of simplicity, let us say that 3-minute observations will be made. If we use a systematic sampling approach, we would observe for 3-minutes, then cease observing for a prespecified period, say 3 minutes. Using this scheme, a total of ten 3-min-

Table 16-3. *Examples of Observational Category Systems Used by Nurse Researchers*

NAME OF INSTRUMENT	CONCEPT(S) MEASURED	SOURCE
Home Observation for Measurement of the Environment (HOME)	Child-rearing environments	Elardo et al., 1977
Index of Activities of Daily Living (ADL)	Level of independence of the chronically ill or aged	Katz & Akpom, 1976
Nonverbal Behavior Worksheet	Nonverbal behavior of patients	McCorkle, 1974
Nurse Practitioner Rating Form	Performance in the nurse practitioner role	Prescott et al., 1981
Oral Assessment Guide	Oral cavity condition	Eilers et al., 1988
Parent–Child Communication	Parent–child interaction	O'Brien, 1980
Quality of Patient Care Scale (QualPacs)	Quality of nursing care	Wandelt & Ager, 1974
Recovery Room Activity Schedule	Behavior observed in the recovery room	Elms, 1972
Sleep Status Observation Form	Sleep/wake behaviors	McFadden & Giblen, 1971

ute observations would be made. A second approach is to randomly sample 3-minute periods from the total of 20 such periods in an hour. The decision with regard to the length and number of periods for creating a suitable sample must be influenced by the aims of the research. In establishing time units, one of the most important considerations is determining a psychologically meaningful time frame. A good deal of pretesting and experimentation with different sampling plans is essential in developing or adapting observational strategies.

Event sampling is a second system for obtaining a set of observations. This approach selects integral behaviors or events of a prespecified type for observation. Event sampling requires that the investigator either have some knowledge concerning the occurrence of events or be in a position to await their occurrence. Examples of "integral events" that may be suitable for event sampling include shift changes of nurses in a hospital, cast removals of pediatric patients, epileptic seizures, and cardiac arrests in the emergency room. This sampling approach is preferable to time sampling when the events of principal interest are infrequent throughout the day and are at risk of being missed if specific time-sampling frames are established. In addition, event sampling has the advantage that the observation treats situations in their entirety rather than fragmenting them into discontinuous segments. Still, when behaviors and events are relatively frequent, time sampling does have the virtue of enhancing the representativeness of the observed behaviors. Time sampling and event sampling can sometimes be profitably combined.

Training Observers

Observational methods are more vulnerable to human perceptual errors than virtually any other data collection procedure. If people are to become good "instruments" for collecting observational data, then they must be trained to observe in such a way that accuracy is maximized and biases are minimized. The training of observers is a crucial phase in the preparation of a study and should not be neglected. Even when the

investigator who designed the study does most or all of the observations, training and "dry runs" are essential.

The observers must be familiarized thoroughly with the aims of the project, the nature of the behaviors or events to be observed, the sampling strategy, and the formal instrument. For large projects that involve more than one or two observers, it is wise to produce an *observer's manual* with detailed instructions and examples. When category systems are used, the observers should memorize the scheme, because they are typically called on to record observations virtually simultaneous with the occurrence of the observed behaviors. Training sessions are useful for clarifying any ambiguities, for explaining how to deal with marginal cases, and for alerting the observers to the need to perceive familiar behaviors within the constraints imposed by the observation schedule.

After this initial training, the observers are ready for a trial use of the instrument. The setting during this trial period should resemble as closely as possible the settings that will be the focus of the final observations. Sometimes it may be possible to use role-playing techniques to simulate events and behaviors. This approach has the advantage that the trainees can interrupt the interaction to ask questions if difficulties arise. Thorough discussions of the trial experience are recommended to address any problems and to allow the observers an opportunity to make suggestions for improving the instruments' efficiency or quality. During a practice session, the comparability of the observers' recordings should be assessed. That is, two or more observers should watch a trial event or situation, and the notations on the checklist or rating scales should be compared. This procedure is referred to as an evaluation of *interrater reliability* and will be described more fully in Chapter 18.

Structured Observations by Nonresearch Personnel

The research we have discussed thus far involves situations in which the researcher (or an observer assistant) observes ongoing events or behaviors of relevance to the research problem and then codes information relating to what has been seen in some specified period. Other forms of observational data-gathering methods provide more global information about the characteristics and behaviors of individuals. Often such methods involve asking nonresearch personnel to summarize on structured scales their knowledge of a person or group, based on their own observations. This method has much in common (in terms of format and scoring procedures) with the self-report scales described in Chapter 15; the primary difference is that the person completing the scale describes the attributes and behaviors of people other than themselves. For example, a mother might be asked to describe the temperament of her infant, staff nurses might be asked to evaluate the functional capacity of nursing home residents, or a nursing supervisor might be asked to assess the nursing competency of nurses on the unit. As with self-report instruments, a researcher might decide to construct his or her own behavior rating scale for a specific research purpose, or might choose to use or adapt an existing scale.

Some of the references cited in Chapter 15 and at the end of this chapter identify observational instruments. Table 16-4 lists several such global rating scales that have been used in nursing studies.

The use of nonresearch personnel to provide observational data has a number of practical advantages. It is an economical method compared with using trained observers. For example, an observer might have to watch children for hours or days to fully describe the nature and intensity of certain behavior problems when a parent or teacher could readily do this. In some situations, the behaviors of interest might never be capable of observation by an outsider, because of reactivity problems, because they occur in private situations, or because they constitute rare events (e.g., sleepwalking). Also, self-report data cannot be obtained for some populations such as infants, the mentally retarded, or the very old.

On the other hand, such methods may have all of the same problems as self-report scales (such as response set biases) in addition to the problem of observer bias. Nonresearch observers are typically "untrained" and interob-

Table 16-4. *Examples of Behavioral Rating Scales That Can Be Completed by Nonresearch Personnel*

NAME OF INSTRUMENT	CONCEPTS(S) MEASURED	SOURCE
Nursing Rating Scale (nurses)*	Psychopathologic disturbance in hospitalized psychiatric patients	Hargreaves, 1968
Child Health Questionnaire (teachers)	Psychologic health of grade school children	Butler, 1975
Infant Characteristics Questionnaire (parents)	Infant temperament	Bates et al., 1979
Eyberg Child Behavior Inventory (parents)	Children's conduct problems	Eyberg & Ross, 1978
Blank Infant Tenderness Scale (mothers)	Infants' need for tenderness	Blank, 1985
Parents' Perception of Uncertainty Scale (parents)	Children's uncertainty in illness	Mishel, 1983
Ibe Behavioral Checklist (nurses)	Patients' level of dependence	Clough & Derdiarian, 1980
Six-Dimension Scale of Nursing Performance (supervisors)	Nursing performance	Schwirian, 1978

* Parentheses indicate people normally asked to complete the instrument.

server reliability cannot usually be determined. Thus, this approach has a number of problems but will inevitably continue to find many research applications because, in many cases, there are no alternatives.

☰ *MECHANICAL AIDS IN OBSERVATIONS*

Our discussion has focused thus far on those types of observations that are made by observers directly through the use of their sensory organs. There are observational studies in which this is not the case. In this section, we look at mechanical devices or other equipment that can be used either as an extension of the human senses or as a means of securing permanent records of observational data.

The health-care field has a rich store of devices and equipment designed to make available to observers conditions or attributes that are ordinarily imperceptible. Nasal speculums, stethoscopes, bronchoscopes, radiographic and imaging equipment, ultrasound technology, and a myriad of other medical instruments make it possible for health-care personnel to gather observational information concerning the health status and bodily functioning of patients.

In addition to equipment for enhancing physiologic observations, several mechanical devices are available for recording behaviors and events. These techniques make possible categorization at a later time. When the behavior of interest is primarily auditory, tape recordings can be obtained and used as a permanent observational record. Transcripts from such recordings can then be prepared to facilitate the classification process. Other technological instruments to aid auditory observation have been developed, such as laser devices that are capable of recording sounds by being directed on a window to a room, and voice tremor detectors that are sensitive to stress.

When a visual record is desired, motion picture films or videotapes are suitable media. Both of these techniques—and particularly videotapes—have gained increased acceptability as their advantages have become apparent. Films and videotapes, in addition to being permanent, offer the possibility of capturing complex behaviors that would elude categorization by an on-the-spot observer. Visual records are also capable of capturing finer units of behavior, such as micromomentary facial expressions, than the naked eye. Videotapes and films offer the possibility of checking the accuracy of the coders and, thus, are quite useful as an aid to training. Finally, it is often easier to conceal a camera than a human observer, and in some situations, this feature would constitute a major advantage. Film records also have a number of drawbacks, some of which are fairly technical, such as lighting requirements, lens limitations, and so forth. Other serious problems result from the fact that the camera angle adopted could present a lopsided view of an event or situation. The ability of films and videotapes to capture complex or fleeting behaviors is at once an advantage and a disadvantage. The analysis of motion picture records, frame by frame, can become a complicated and time-consuming process. Still, for many applications permanent visual records offer unparalleled opportunities to expand the range and scope of observational studies.

Also of interest is the growing technology for assisting with the encoding and recording of observations made directly by on-the-spot observers. For example, there is equipment that permits the observer to enter observational data directly into a computer as the observation occurs, and in some cases, the equipment can be used to record physiologic data concurrently. Such a system used in one nursing study is described in a research example at the end of this chapter.

☰ *EVALUATION OF OBSERVATIONAL METHODS*

The field of nursing is well-suited to observational research: observation has always been an integral part of the nursing process. Observational methods have both weaknesses and strengths, however, as is the case for so many approaches to obtaining data on humans. The investigator about to embark on a research project should carefully weigh both the negative and positive aspects of this approach before collecting data.

Advantages of Observational Methods

One of the main reasons for using observational methods is that it may be impossible to obtain the desired information in any other way. Self-report measures such as questionnaires and interviews are often inadequate for dealing with activities and behaviors of which individuals may themselves be unaware or unable to describe. For certain research questions, there simply may be no acceptable substitute for observation.

Observational methods have an intrinsic appeal with respect to their ability to capture directly a record of behaviors and events. Furthermore, there is virtually no other data collection method that can provide the depth and variety of information as observation. With this approach, humans—the observers—are used as "measuring instruments," and provide a uniquely sensitive and intelligent (if fallible) tool.

Although we have used examples in this chapter that may suggest that observational methods are most suitable for descriptive or naturalistic studies, the techniques described here are quite flexible and may be appropriately used for both experimental and nonexperimental research. Both laboratory and field studies have put observational methods to creative and skillful use. Within the area of nursing research, observational methods have broad applicability for clinical inquiries, as well as for educational and administrative studies.

Disadvantages of Observational Methods

Some of the problems with which an observational researcher must contend were described in our discussion of the observer/observed rela-

tionship. These problems include possible ethical difficulties, reactivity of the observed when the observer is conspicuous, and lack of consent to being observed. Observational data are clearly vulnerable to many distortions and biases. Human perceptual errors and inadequacies are a continuous threat to the quality of obtained information. Observation and interpretation are demanding tasks, requiring attention, sensation, perception, and conception. To accomplish these activities in a completely objective fashion is probably impossible, although structured category systems and sampling procedures help to reduce observer subjectivity. A number of factors interfere with objective observations: emotions, prejudices, attitudes, and values may result in faulty inference; personal interest and commitment may color what is seen in the direction of what the observer wants to see; anticipation of what is to be observed may affect what is observed; and hasty decisions before adequate information is collected may result in erroneous classifications or conclusions.

Several types of observational biases are especially common. One bias is referred to as the *enhancement of contrast effect*. The observer may tend to distort the observation in the direction of dividing the content into clear-cut entities. The converse effect—a bias toward *central tendency*—occurs when extreme events are distorted toward a middle ground. A series of biases are in a category described as *assimilatory*. The observer may tend to distort observations in the direction of identity with previous inputs. This bias would have the effect of miscategorizing information in the direction of regularity and orderliness. Assimilation to other "objects" also occurs: expectations and attitudes of the observer are the most common.

Rating scales are susceptible to several distinct types of error. The *halo effect* refers to the tendency of the rater to be influenced by one characteristic in rating other unrelated characteristics. For example, if we formed a very positive general impression of a person, we would probably be likely to rate that person as "intelligent," "loyal," and "dependable" simply because these traits are positively valued. Rating scales may reflect the personality traits of the observer. The *error of leniency* is the tendency for the observer to rate everything positively and the *error of severity* is the contrasting tendency to rate too harshly.

Needless to say, these biases are much more likely to operate when a high degree of observer inference is required by the observational tasks. The careful construction and pretesting of checklists and rating scales, the development of an adequate sampling plan, the proper training of observers, and interrater comparisons are techniques that can play an important role in minimizing or estimating these problematic biases. Although the degree of observer bias is not necessarily a function of the degree of structure imposed on the observation, the difficulty with unstructured methods is that it is generally more difficult to assess the extent of bias.

≡ RESEARCH EXAMPLES

Table 16-5 presents several examples of observational studies conducted by nurse researchers. Two other examples that illustrate observational research in greater detail follow.

Table 16-5. *Examples of Observational Studies*

RESEARCH PROBLEM	TYPE OF OBSERVATION	PHENOMENA OBSERVED
Are existing observer-rated functional assessment instruments for the elderly adequately comprehensive? (Travis, 1988)	Unstructured	Activities, characteristics, and conditions of the elderly in institutions
What is the nature of the interactions between migrant farmworkers and health care providers? (Jezewski, 1990)	Participant observation	Interactions during migrant farmworker clinic sessions
What patterns of sex or gender role behavior do nurses exhibit when enacting their professional role? (Katzman & Roberts, 1988)	Participant observation	Nurse–physician interactions
Are there differences in the task behaviors performed by nursing personnel working within the team nursing, total patient care nursing, and primary nursing patient care organization systems? (Clark & Zornow, 1989)	Structured	Nursing activities
What are the times in infants' feeding cycles at which performance on a neurobehavioral evaluation is optimal? (Medoff-Cooper & Brooten, 1987)	Structured	Reflexes, movement, and tone; mental status; and behavioral responses in newborns
Does the attachment behavior of mothers to their infants differ depending on whether the infants are handicapped or not? (Capuzzi, 1989)	Structured	Attachment and responsiveness of mothers during feeding
What type of supplemental information (i.e., that unavailable from memory or on computer) is sought by cardiovascular nurses? (Corcoran-Perry & Graves, 1990)	Structured	Information-seeking of nurses

Unstructured Observation

Cohen (1982) studied the birthing beliefs and practices of the Black Caribs of Central America as a participant observer. During seven months of fieldwork, she talked with villagers and observed their behaviors with regard to pregnancy, delivery, postpartum care, and immediate infant care. Mechanical equipment (e.g., camera and tape recorder) was used occasionally, but the primary means of recording observations was through written field notes that were analyzed and cataloged every evening. During the course of the fieldwork, Cohen increased her participation in the birthing activities of the village. She assisted in the delivery of three infants, at the invitation of the village midwife, and eventually helped one woman single-handedly in the delivery of her baby.

Cohen's report summarized the process of prenatal care, labor, delivery, and postpartum care of Black Carib village women. Cohen noted the numerous differences that exist between birthing practices in the village compared with standard North American practices. For example, the Carib mother is encouraged by the midwife to walk during the entire course of labor. Women deliver in a squatting position and delivery occurs in the home, attended by friends and relatives. Forceps are not used and no medications are given to ease the pain of labor. Based on her research, Cohen encouraged self-examination of some American practices, such as birth positioning.

Structured Observation

White and her colleagues (1983) tested whether a tape-recorded bedtime story read by a parent would help to ease separation anxiety and facilitate falling asleep among hospitalized children whose parents were not rooming-in. A sample of 18 children aged 3 to 8 (seven of whom had a tape-recorded story read by a parent; the control children had no special treatment) were observed for three nights during the falling asleep period (event sampling) for 15 minutes. The investigators used an exhaustive structured instrument called the Falling Asleep Inventory that encompassed 54 behaviors in which the child could engage during the observation session. Examples include "eye rubbing," "verbally seeking assistance," and "getting out of bed." The inventory was designed for use with the Senders Signals and Receivers (SSR) system, an observational and data management system that permitted automatic entry into a computer of observational codes relating to the children's falling asleep behaviors. Rather than using manual recording forms, observers entered codes for observed behaviors into an SSR keyboard. Duration and sequence of entries were automatically incorporated into the encoding system. The observer recorded when a given behavior began, who exhibited the behavior, what the action was, and what the object of the behavior was (e.g., the nurse). For example, the following code entered onto the keyboard would mean that the child began to stroke a toy:

$$+ \qquad 05 \qquad ST \qquad 06$$

Findings from this research indicated that children who had stories read to them had a tendency to fall asleep sooner, exhibit more sleepy behaviors, and display fewer active behaviors than the control group children. The investigators concluded that hospitalized children who hear a recorded bedtime story use self-soothing behaviors to cope with the separation experience.

However, in a more recent study, White and other researchers (1990) used the same SSR system to test alternative strategies to promote night sleep in hospitalized children and obtained different resutls. The SSR system was used to measure three dependent variables: length of sleep onset latency, incidence of distress, and self-soothing behaviors. In this study, the researchers found that the presence of a parent or a parent-recorded story was associated with longer sleep onset latency and a greater incidence of distress. The researchers concluded that the results of the more recent study were likely to be more valid, and that the discrepancy in the findings were probably attibutable to the fact that a larger sample was used in the later study.

☰ *SUMMARY*

Observational methods are techniques for acquiring information for research purposes through the direct observation and interpretation of phenomena in the environment. A wide variety of human activity and experience can be researched using observational methods.

In any observational setting—whether it be in a natural field situation or laboratory setup—the observer cannot possibly attend to every behavior or event. Therefore, the investigator usually specifies in advance the nature of the phenomena to be observed. The researcher must also select an appropriate *unit of observation*. The *molar approach* entails the observation of large segments of behaviors and events as integral units. The *molecular approach,* on the other hand, treats small, specific actions as separate entities.

The investigator must make decisions concerning the relationship between the observer and the subjects. The decisions relate primarily to the dimensions of *concealment* and *intervention*. Concealment refers to the degree to which the observed people are aware that they are being observed or that they are the subjects of a research study. The problem of behavioral distortions stemming from the presence of an observer (known as *reactivity*) is a major reason for making concealed observations. Intervention refers to the degree to which the investigator structures the observational setting in line with research demands as opposed to being a passive observer.

Like self-reports, observational data vary on a structured/unstructured dimension. Field studies generally collect observational data that are unstructured, using a procedure known as participant observation. *Participant observation* is a method that has been used extensively by anthropologists and sociologists as a means of understanding cultures, institutions, and social groups. The participant observer endeavors to obtain information about the dynamics of the social group within the subject's own frame of reference, without imposing a preconceived structure based on the researcher's world view.

In participant observation studies, the researcher must pay careful attention to his or her role in the social group under study, because the behaviors available for observation will generally be contingent on the role. The researcher must first gain entrée into the group and then develop the trust of group members to get at the "back stage" realities of the group's experiences.

In the initial phase of a participant observation study, the researcher is primarily an observer and gathers a preliminary understanding of the site. As time passes, the researcher typically becomes a more active participant and also develops a plan for sampling events and selecting observational positions. The observer usually combines *single positioning, multiple positioning,* and *mobile positioning*. The final phase of the research involves reflective observation about the activities that transpired.

Participant observation places few restrictions on the type or amount of data collected. *Logs* of daily events and *field notes* are the major methods of recording data. Field notes have multiple purposes and may be categorized as *observational notes, theoretical notes, methodological notes,* and *personal notes*.

Proponents of the participant observation approach claim it represents both a source of data *and* a basis for understanding what the data mean. Although unstructured methods can yield extremely rich and useful information, particularly when used by insightful observers, they are nevertheless subject to a number of methodological difficulties. The most prominent difficulties are observer bias in sampling, recording, and interpreting phenomena; observer influence (reactivity); and observer identification with the observed group.

Structured observational methods impose a number of constraints on the observer for the purpose of maximizing observer accuracy and objectivity and for obtaining an adequate representation of the phenomena of interest. Two types of record-keeping forms are used most commonly by observers in structured situations. *Checklists* are tools for recording the appearance or frequency of prespecified behaviors, events, or characteristics. Checklists are based upon the development of *category systems* for encoding the observed phenomena. The researcher constructing a category system must make a number of decisions concerning its exhaustiveness, generality, inference requirements, and training demands. One type of checklist is based on the *sign system* and is used as a demographic record of the types of behavior that occurred during the observational session. A second format is used to exhaustively analyze ongoing events and activities.

Rating scales are the second most common record-keeping tool for structured observations. The observer using a rating scale is required to rate some phenomenon according to points along a dimension that is typically bipolar (e.g., passive/aggressive or excellent health/poor health). Ratings are generally made either during the observational setting at specific intervals (e.g., every five minutes) or after the observation is completed.

Most structured observations make use of some form of *sampling plan* for selecting the behaviors, events, and conditions to be observed. The most frequently used approach is *time sampling,* which involves the specification of the duration and frequency of both the observational periods and the intersession intervals. *Event sampling* selects integral behaviors or events of a special type for observation.

It is crucial that observers be properly trained. The training should include thorough familiarization with the research aims and sensitization to perceiving common occurrences in an unusual way. The category scheme (if one is used for recording information) should be memorized and trial runs made with the instrument before the observers proceed to make the observations.

Technological advances have greatly augmented the researcher's capacity to collect, record, and preserve observational data. Such devices as tape recorders, movie cameras, videotape cameras, laser devices, and so forth permit behaviors and events to be categorized after their occurrence.

Perhaps the greatest strength of observation is that it allows for the collection of data that would be impossible to obtain in any other way. Important descriptive information about behavioral patterns and the human condition can be made available to scientific researchers through direct observation. The methods outlined in this chapter are flexible and can be applied to a wide variety of research problems and designs.

On the other hand, the researcher using observational techniques must be aware of their limitations. In addition to problems of an ethical nature, observation is subject to a variety of biasing effects. The greater the degree of observer inference and judgment, the more likely it is that perceptual errors and distortions will occur.

≡ *STUDY SUGGESTIONS*

1. Suppose you were interested in observing the behavior of fathers in the delivery room during the birth of their first child. Identify the observer/observed relationship along the concealment and intervention dimensions that you would recommend adopting for such a study and defend your recommendation. What are the possible drawbacks of your approach and how might you deal with them?

2. Would a psychiatric nurse researcher be well suited to conduct a participant observation study of the behavior of psychiatric nurses and their interactions with clients? Why or why not?

3. A nurse researcher is planning to study temper tantrums displayed by hospitalized children. Would you recommend using a time-sampling approach? Why or why not?

4. Suppose you were interested in studying pain-related behaviors using observational methods. Develop some categories of behavior that could be used for classifying the observations.

5. Below are a list of problem statements. Indicate which of these problems could be studied by using some form of observational

method. For each problem that is amenable to observation, specify whether you think a structured or unstructured approach would be preferable.

a. Does team nursing versus primary nursing affect the type of communication patterns between nurses and patients?

b. Is there a relationship between prenatal instruction and delivery room behaviors of primiparas?

c. Is the number of hours of direct clinical practice for student nurses related to their performance on the licensure examination?

d. Do the attitudes of nurses toward abortion affect the quality of care given to abortion patients?

e. Do industrial alcohol programs have a positive impact on on-the-job accident rates?

f. Is the touching behavior of nurses related to their ethnic or cultural background?

≡ SUGGESTED READINGS

METHODOLOGICAL REFERENCES

General References

Byerly, E.L. (1976). The nurse researcher as participant–observer in a nursing setting. In P.J. Brink (Ed.), *Transcultural nursing: A book of readings.* Englewood Cliffs, NJ: Prentice-Hall.

Dowrick, P., & Biggs, S.J. (Eds.). (1983). *Using video: Psychological and social applications.* New York: John Wiley and Sons.

Frank-Stromberg, M. (Ed.). (1988). *Instruments for clinical nursing research.* Norwalk, CT: Appleton & Lange.

Godsmith, J.W. (1981). Methodological considerations in using videotape to establish rater reliability. *Nursing Research, 30,* 124–127.

Gold, R.L. (1971). Roles in sociological observations. In B.J. Franklin & H.W. Osborne (Eds.), *Research methods: Issues and insights* (pp. 255–267). Belmont, CA: Wadsworth.

Jackson, B.S. (1973). Participant observation in nursing research. *Supervisor Nurse, 4,* 30–40.

Kerlinger, F. (1986). *Foundations of behavioral research* (3rd ed.). New York: Holt, Rinehart & Winston.

LaFrance, M. (1981). Observational and archival data [Chapter 11]. In L.H. Kidder (Ed.), *Selltiz, Wrightsman, and Cook's research methods in social relations.* New York: Holt, Rinehart & Winston.

Leininger, M. (1985). Ethnography and ethnonursing: Models and modes of qualitative data analysis. In M. Leininger (Ed.), *Qualitative research methods in nursing.* New York: Grune & Stratton.

Lofland, J., & Lofland, L. (1984). *Analyzing social settings: A guide to qualitative observation and analysis.* Belmont, CA: Wadsworth.

McCall, G.J., & Simmons H.L. (Eds.). (1969). *Issues in participant observation: A text and reader.* Reading, MA: Addison-Wesley.

Morrison, E.F., Phillips, L.R., & Chal, Y.M. (1990). The development and use of observational measurement scales. *Applied Nursing Research, 3,* 73–86.

Pearsall, M. (1965). Participant observation as role and method in behavioral research. *Nursing Research, 14,* 37–42.

Schatzman, L., & Strauss, A. (1982). *Field research: Strategies for a natural sociology* (2nd ed.). Englewood Cliffs, NJ: Prentice-Hall.

Strickland, O.L., & Waltz, C. (Eds.). (1988). *Measurement of nursing outcomes.* New York: Springer.

Ward, M.J., & Lindemann, C. (Eds.). (1979). *Instruments for measuring nursing practice and other health care variables.* Hyattsville, MD: Department of Health, Education and Welfare.

Wilson, H.S. (1985). *Research in nursing.* Menlo Park, CA: Addison-Wesley. (Chapter 13).

References to Observational Instruments

Bates, J.E., Freeland, C.A., & Lounsbury, M.L. (1979). Measurement of infant difficultness. *Child Development, 50,* 794–803.

Blank, D.M. (1985). Development of the Infant Tenderness Scale. *Nursing Research, 34,* 211–216.

Borgatta, E.F. (1962). A systematic study of interaction process scores, peer and self-assessments, personality and other variables. *Genetic Psychology Monographs, 65,* 219–291.

Butler, A.C. (1975). The Child Health Questionnaire. *Psychology in the Schools, 12,* 153–160.

Clough, D.H., & Derdiarian, A. (1980). A behavioral checklist to measure dependence and independence. *Nursing Research, 29,* 55–58.

Downs, F., & Fitzpatrick, J.J. (1976). Preliminary investigation of the reliability and validity of a tool for the assessment of body position and motor activity. *Nursing Research, 25,* 404–408.

Eilers, J., Berger, A.M., & Peterson, M.C. (1988). Development, testing and application of the Oral Assessment Guide. *Oncology Nursing Forum, 15,* 325–330.

Elardo, R., Bradley, R., & Caldwell, B. (1977). A longitudinal study of the relationship of infants' home environment to language development at age three. *Child Development, 48,* 595–603.

Elms, R.R. (1972). Recovery room behavior and postoperative convalescence. *Nursing Research, 21,* 390–397.

Eyberg, S.M., & Ross, A.W. (1978). Assessment of child behavior problems: The validation of a new inventory. *Journal of Clinical Child Psychology, 7,* 113–116.

Gill, N.E., White, M.A., & Anderson, G.C. (1984). Transitional newborn infants in a hospital nursery: From first oral cue to first sustained cry. *Nursing Research, 33,* 213–217.

Hargreaves, W.A. (1968). Systematic nursing observation of psychopathology. *Archives of General Psychiatry, 18,* 518–531.

Katz, S., & Akpom, A. (1976). A measure of primary socio-biologic functions. *International Journal of Health Services, 6,* 493–508.

McCorkle, R. (1974). The effects of touch on seriously ill patients. *Nursing Research, 23,* 125–132.

McFadden, E.H., & Giblin, E. (1971). Sleep deprivation in patients having open-heart surgery. *Nursing Research, 20,* 249–254.

Mishel, M.H. (1983). Parents' perception of uncertainty concerning their hospitalized child. *Nursing Research, 32,* 324–330.

O'Brien, R.A. (1980). Relationship of parent—child and self-differentiation. *Nursing Research, 29,* 150–156.

Prescott, P.A., et al. (1981). The Nurse Practitioner Rating Form. *Nursing Research, 30,* 223–228.

Schwirian, P.M. (1978). Evaluating the performance of nurses. *Nursing Research, 27,* 347–351.

Wandelt, M.A., & Ager, J.W. (1974). *Quality Patient Care Scale.* New York: Appleton-Century-Crofts.

Whall, A.L., et al. (1983). Development of a screening program for tardive dyskinesia: Feasibility issues. *Nursing Research, 32,* 151–156.

*Substantive References**

Capuzzi, C. (1989). Maternal attachment to handicapped infants and the relationship to social support. *Research in Nursing and Health, 12,* 161–167. [Structured observation]

Clark, M.F., & Zornow, R.A. (1989). Nursing organizing systems: A comparative study. *Western Journal of Nursing Research, 11,* 757–764. [Structured observation]

Cohen, F.S. (1982). Childbirth belief and practice in a Garifuna (Black Carib) village on the north coast of Honduras. *Western Journal of Nursing Research, 4,* 193–208. [Unstructured observation]

Corcoran-Perry, S., & Graves, J. (1990). Supplemental-information-seeking behavior of cardiovascular nurses. *Research in Nursing and Health, 13,* 119–127. [Structured observation]

Gill, N.E., Behnke, M., Conlon, M., McNeely, J.B., & Anderson, G.C. (1988). Effect of nonnutritive sucking on behavioral state in preterm infants before feeding. *Nursing Research, 37,* 347–350. [Structured observation]

Harrell, J.S., & Damon, J.F. (1989). Prediction of patients' need for mouth care. *Western Journal of Nursing Research, 11,* 748–756. [Structured observation]

Harrison, M.J. (1990). A comparison of parental interactions with term and preterm infants. *Research in Nursing and Health, 13,* 173–179. [Structured observation]

Hutchinson, S.A. (1987). Toward self-integration: The recovery process of chemically dependent nurses. *Nursing Research, 36,* 339–343. [Unstructured observation]

Jezewski, M.A. (1990). Culture brokering in migrant farmworker health care. *Western Journal of Nursing Research, 12,* 497–513. [Unstructured observation]

Jones, L.C., & Thomas, S.A. (1989). New fathers' blood pressure and heart rate: Relationships to interaction with their newborn infant. *Nursing Research, 38,* 237–241. [Structured observation]

Katzman, E.M., & Roberts, J.I. (1988). Nurse—physician conflicts as barriers to the enactment of nursing roles. *Western Journal of Nursing Research, 10,* 576–590. [Unstructured observation]

Kerr, J.A.C. (1985). Space use, privacy, and territoriality. *Western Journal of Nursing Research, 7,*

---

*A comment in brackets after each citation designates the observational method of interest.

199–219. [Structured and unstructured observation]

Medoff-Cooper, B., & Brooten, D. (1987). Relation of the feeding cycle to neurobehavioral assessment in preterm infants. *Nursing Research, 36,* 315–317. [Structured observation]

Niemeier, D.F. (1983). A behavioral analysis of staff–patient interactions in a psychiatric setting. *Western Journal of Nursing Research, 5,* 269–277. [Unstructured observation]

Salyer, J., & Stuart, B.J. (1985). Nurse–patient interaction in the intensive care unit. *Heart and Lung, 14,* 20–24. [Structured observation]

Schoenhofer, S.O. (1989). Affectional touch in critical care nursing. *Heart and Lung, 18,* 146–154. [Structured observation]

Taylor, S.G., Pickens, J.M., & Geden, E.A. (1989). Interactional styles of nurse practitioners and physicians regarding patient decision-making. *Nursing Research, 38,* 50–55. [Structured observation]

Travis, S.S. (1988). Observer-rated functional assessments for institutionalized elderly. *Nursing Research, 37,* 138–143. [Unstructured observation]

Whall, A.L., Booth, D.E., Kosinski, J., Donbroski, D., Zajul-Krupa, I., & Weissfeld, L. (1989). Tardive dyskinetic movements over time. *Applied Nursing Research, 2,* 128–134. [Structured observation]

White, M.A., Wear, E., & Stephenson, G. (1983). A computer-compatible method for observing falling asleep behavior of hospitalized children. *Research in Nursing and Health, 6,* 191–198. [Structured observation]

White, M.A., Williams, P.D., Alexander, D.J., Powell-Cope, G.M., & Conlon, M. (1990). Sleep onset latency and distress in hospitalized children. *Nursing Research, 39,* 134–139. [Structured observation]

17
Biophysiologic and Other Data Collection Methods

The majority of nursing research studies involve the collection of data by means of methods discussed in the preceding chapters—interviews, questionnaires, psychosocial scales, and observational methods. However, other methods of measuring research variables are of interest to nurse researchers, and several of these are reviewed in this chapter. The most important alternative method is the use of biophysiologic measures.

≡ BIOPHYSIOLOGIC MEASURES

The trend in nursing research has been toward increased clinical, patient-centered investigations, and this trend is likely to continue in years to come. One result of this trend is an expanded use of measures to assess the physiologic status of subjects. In this section, we discuss a particular class of measures, namely those physiologic and physical variables that require specialized technical instruments and equipment for their measurement and, generally, specialized training for the interpretation of results.

Settings in which nurses operate are typically filled with a wide variety of technical instruments for measuring physiologic functions. It is beyond the scope of this book to describe in any detail the many kinds of biophysiologic measures available to nurse researchers. Our objective is to present an overview of potential criterion measures for clinical nursing studies, to illustrate their usage in a research context, and to direct the interested reader to more comprehensive sources for further information.

Even these objectives are not easily achieved. We have unavoidably omitted many tests and measures that would be of great interest to clinical researchers in nursing. A unique difficulty we faced in preparing this section (as opposed to Chapters 14–16) is that here we are concerned with instrument identification rather than instrument development. Nurse researchers *do* design their own observational instruments and interview schedules, and it is possible to present general guidelines for developing such measuring tools. It is unlikely that many nurse researchers will develop technical apparatus and electronic instruments. Thus, just as it was impossible to catalog all available psychosocial instruments, it is likewise impractical to adequately cover all physiologic measures. Still, we believe that a consideration of physiologic tools is extremely important, and thus we have accepted incompleteness and the inevitability of being outdated by rapid technological advances.

A good many variables that are of interest in clinical research do not require biophysiologic instrumentation for their measurement. Data on physiologic functioning can often be gathered by self-report or through direct observation (or through observation enhanced by special equipment such as x-rays); these methods were described in previous chapters. For instance, the presence or absence or intensity of physiologic activity or dysfunction is often amenable to observational methods. Examples include such phenomena as vomiting, cyanosis, postcardiotomy delirium, edema, and wound status. Other biophysiologic data can be gathered by asking people directly. Examples of possible self-report measures include time of first postoperative voiding, assessment of pain, ratings of fatigue, and reports of nausea. This section focuses on phenomena that require the use of specialized technical apparatus that yield quantitative measures.

Purposes of Using Biophysiologic Measures

Clinical nursing studies often involve specialized equipment and instruments both for creating independent variables (e.g., an intervention using biofeedback equipment) and for measuring dependent variables. For the most part, our discussion focuses on the use of biophysiologic measures as dependent variables.

The majority of nursing studies in which biophysiologic measures have been used fall into one of four classes. The first involves the study of basic physiologic processes that have relevance for nursing care. Such studies often involve subjects who are healthy and normal or some subhuman animal species. For example, Lu and colleagues (1990) studied ethnic differences in cardiovascular indices at rest and across the Valsalva maneuver. Thomas and Friedmann (1990) examined blood pressure and heart rate responses of Type A versus Type B cardiac patients during routine, nonthreatening verbalization.

A second class of studies includes explorations of the ways in which nursing actions affect the health outcomes of patients. For example, Kirchhoff and her colleagues (1990) examined the necessity of restricting ice water for patients with acute myocardial infarction by examining the effects of small and moderate amounts of ingested ice water on the electrocardiograms (ECGs) of myocardial infarction patients. Osborne (1984) investigated whether there were differences in the cardiovascular responses of patients ambulated 32 versus 56 hours after coronary artery bypass surgery.

The third class of studies concerns an evaluation of a specific nursing procedure or intervention. These studies differ from the studies in the second class in that they generally involve a hypothesis stating that a new nursing procedure will result in improved biophysiologic outcomes among patients. For example, MacVicar and her colleagues (1989) evaluated the effects of an aerobic exercise training program on the functional capacity of women receiving chemotherapy for breast cancer. Levesque and coworkers (1984) evaluated the recovery outcomes of cholecystectomy patients who participated in a preadmission teaching program.

A fourth class of studies in which biophysiologic measures have been used focuses on the improvement in measuring and recording physiologic information that is normally gathered by nurses. For example, Heidenreich and Giuffre

(1990) studied the appropriateness of the axillary site for temperature measurement in postoperative patients. Another team of nurse researchers (Preusser et al., 1989) conducted a study to determine the minimum discard sample required to obtain an accurate blood gas sample.

The physiologic phenomena that interest nurse researchers run the full gamut of available measures. Some of these measures are discussed in the following section.

Types of Biophysiologic Measures

Physiologic measurements can be classified in one of two major categories. *In vivo measurements* are those that are performed directly within or on living organisms themselves. One example of an *in vivo* measure is blood flow determination through radiography. An *in vitro measurement,* by contrast, is performed outside of the organism's body, as in the case of measur-

ing serum potassium concentration in the blood drawn from a patient.

IN VIVO MEASURES

In vivo measures often involve the use of highly complex instrumentation systems. An *instrumentation system* is the apparatus and equipment used to measure one or more attributes of a subject and the presentation of that measurement data in a manner that humans can interpret. Organism-instrument systems involve up to six major components: (1) stimulus; (2) subject; (3) sensing equipment; (4) signal-conditioning equipment; (5) display equipment; and (6) recording, data processing, and transmission equipment. These components and their interrelationships are presented in Figure 17-1. The role of each component is briefly described as follows:

1. *Stimulus.* Many physiologic measurements require some type of external stimulus. The

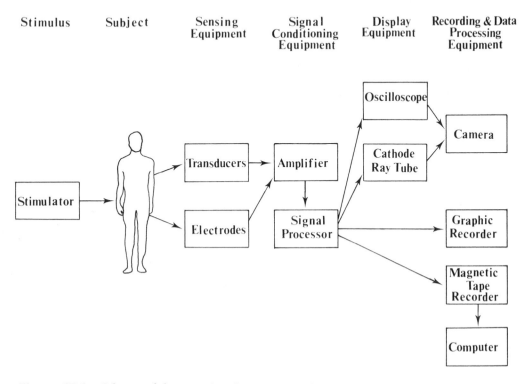

Figure 17-1. *Schema of the organism–instrument system.*

stimulation may be engendered by another human, as in the case of requests for deep and rapid breathing by the patient when recording electrical activity from the brain. The stimulus may also be produced by electrical or mechanical equipment, such as an external pacemaker and cardiac defibrillator.

2. *Subject.* The bodies of humans (and other organisms) consist of chemical, electrical, mechanical, thermal, hydraulic, pneumatic, and other systems interacting with each other and with the outside world. Communication of the human organism with the external environment consists of various inputs (e.g., sensory inputs, inspired air, or liquid and food intake) and outputs (e.g., speech, body movements, expired air, or wastes). The majority of these inputs and outputs are easily amenable to measurements. The major bodily systems—circulatory, respiratory, and so forth—also communicate with each other internally, as do smaller subsystems, such as organs and cells. Biomedical instrumentation constitutes the tools for measuring the information communicated by these diverse elements.

3. *Sensing equipment.* Sensing equipment normally consists of one or more transducers. Generally defined, a *transducer* is a device that converts one form of energy into another. Transducers are used in organism-instrument systems to measure physical phenomena by producing an electrical signal proportional to these phenomena. Electrical signals permit presentations of the desired physiologic information in a highly useful form. With an electrical analog of the critical physiologic event, the scientist can store the event on magnetic tape for later inspection and analysis.

   A few examples of methods used to convert a physiologic characteristic into electrical output should suffice to illustrate the underlying principles. A *displacement transducer* converts volume displacement of some element into an electrical signal. A fluid column blood pressure transducer operates on a displacement principle by converting fluid pressure into force, which is then converted to linear displacement. *Temperature transducers* are exemplified by the thermistor, which is an element whose resistance varies proportionately with temperature. To measure *bioelectric potentials* produced by the heart, brain, or other organs, a transducer consisting of two electrodes is used. *Electrodes* are devices for converting bioelectric (ionic) potentials into electronic potentials. In sum, the transducer plays a key role in instrumentation systems designed to make biophysical measurements.

4. *Signal-conditioning equipment.* Signal-conditioning or signal-processing equipment is used to amplify or modify the transducer's electrical signal. Both the input to and the output from signal-conditioning equipment are electrical signals. However, the output signal usually is modified in some respect to prepare the signals for operating display and recording equipment. Physiologic signals acquired by transducers are typically below 10 millivolts in amplitude and must, therefore, be amplified to be compatible with display units and recorders. In virtually all physiologic measurements, two signals are produced by the subject: (1) the key physiologic signal, such as the electrocardiographic signal, and (2) an interference signal. An important function of signal-conditioning equipment is to reject the interference signal and to amplify the desired physiologic signal.

5. *Display equipment.* Display devices convert the modified electrical signals into visual or auditory output. The most common display device is the oscilloscope. An *oscilloscope* is a device that allows for the visual observation of the wave form of a signal. It is used to display and measure the time, phase, voltage, or frequency of a physiologic signal. The information is presented on a *cathode ray tube*. The face of the display is typically calibrated in centimeters with voltage (amplitude) on the ordinate (the vertical plane) and time on the abscissa (horizontal plane). With sophisticated equipment, a television screen that shows interpretation of the various physi-

ologic functions being monitored is often available.

6. *Recording, data processing, and transmission equipment*. For research purposes, it is usually necessary to obtain a permanent record of the physiologic measurements for subsequent scrutiny and analysis. The recording equipment can either be a unit separate from the display device or integrated with it. A *strip recorder* is an example of a device that both displays electrical potentials and provides a permanent record of them. Other devices supplement oscilloscopes or other display units. For example, a signal may often be stored on magnetic tape. The use of a magnetic tape recorder or other computer-linked equipment has the advantage of permitting information to be transmitted and replayed for convenient and detailed analysis.

Not all instrumentation systems involve all six components. Some systems, such as an electronic thermometer, are quite simple; other systems are extremely complex. For example, there are some electronic monitors that, although they are miniaturized and can be put into place during ambulation, yield simultaneous measures of such physiologic variables as cardiac responsivity, respiratory rate and rhythm, core temperature, and muscular activity.

In vivo instruments have been developed to measure all bodily functions, and technological improvements continue to advance our ability to measure biophysiologic phenomena more accurately, more conveniently, and more rapidly than ever before. It is impossible to catalog all such instruments, but Table 17-1 presents a list of some commonly used instruments and the variables they measure, according to six physiologic systems.

Table 17-1. *Examples of Instruments for* In Vivo *Measurements*

BODILY FUNCTION	VARIABLE	EXAMPLE(S) OF INSTRUMENTATION
Circulatory	Blood pressure	Sphygmomanometer/stethoscope
	Blood volume	Plethysmograph
	Blood flow velocity	Laser Doppler velocimeter
	Cardiac potential	Electrocardiograph (ECG); cardiac ultrasound Holter monitor
Respiratory	Respiratory volume	Spirometer
	Respiratory air flow	Spirometer; pneumotachometer
	Oxygen consumption	Max Planck respirometer; Douglas bag technique
Neurological	Systemic body temperature	Thermometer; thermo-couple; thermistor
	Skin surface temperature	Infrared thermometer
	Bioelectric brain potential	Electroencephalograph (EEG)
	Tumors	Nuclear magnetic resonance (tomography)
Musculoskeletal	Muscular contractions	Myograph
	Electrical muscular potential	Electromyograph (EMG)
	Muscle tremors	Accelerometer; tromometer
	Muscle strength	Dynamometer
	Motor response	Steadiness tester; pursuit rotor
	Range of motion	Goniometer; actometer
	Reaction time	Chronoscope
Gastrointestinal	Gastric motility	Pressure transducer/Dynograph recorder
	Electrical potential of stomach muscles	Electrogastrograph (EGG)
	Gastrointestinal activity	Endoradiosones
Genitourinary	Renal obstruction	Renal arteriograph
	Prostatic obstruction	Ureteral pressure profile

The uses to which such instruments have been put by nurse researchers is richly diverse and impressive. Table 17-2 presents examples of research questions that have been posed by nurse researchers relating to the six physiologic systems, together with a list of the physiologic variables measured. Of course, most nurse researchers who have gathered physiologic data have used data from two or more physiologic systems. For example, it is common for nurses to use data on vital signs (e.g., temperature, heart rate, or blood pressure) in their investigations. It is also common for nurses to combine informa-

tion from *in vivo* measures with that from *in vitro* measures.

IN VITRO MEASURES

With *in vitro* measures, data are gathered from subjects by extracting some physiologic material from subjects and subjecting it to laboratory analysis. Nurse researchers may or may not be involved in the extraction of the material; however, the analysis is normally done by highly specialized laboratory technicians. Generally, each laboratory establishes a range of normal values for each measurement, and this information is

Table 17-2. *Examples of Nursing Research Studies Using* In Vivo *Measures*

RESEARCH PROBLEM	MEASUREMENTS	REFERENCE
Do patients who receive colloid therapy after cardiac surgery require smaller fluid volumes to achieve and maintain hemodynamic stability than patients receiving crystalloid therapy?	Circulatory function: diastolic and systolic blood pressure, pulmonary artery pressures, pulmonary capillary wedge pressure, heart rate	Ley et al., 1990
What are the effects of progressive muscle relaxation on dyspnea and anxiety in patients with chronic obstructive pulmonary disease?	Respiratory function, respiratory rate, forced vital capacity, forced expiratory volume	Renfroe, 1988
What are the relationships among three temperatures measured concurrently in the urinary bladder, rectum, and pulmonary artery of cardiac surgical patients being rewarmed following induced hypothermia?	Neurological function: core body temperature	Mravinac et al., 1989
Can a digital test of pelvic muscle strength be reliably used to evaluate the effectiveness of a pelvic muscle exercise program for older women with urinary incontinence?	Musculoskeletal function: pelvic muscle strength, vaginal myography	Brink et al., 1989
What is the effect of nasogastric tube feedings administered at three different temperatures on gastric motility and total gastrointestinal transit time?	Gastrointestinal function: gastric motility, intragastric pressure	Kagawa-Busby et al., 1980
What variables are related to the employment potential of patients receiving hemodialysis?	Genitourinary function: mean arterial pressure	Ferrans & Powers, 1985

critical for interpreting the results of laboratory tests.

Several classes of laboratory analysis have been used in studies by nurse researchers. These include

- *Chemical measurements,* such as the measure of hormone levels, sugar levels, or potassium levels
- *Microbiologic measures,* such as bacterial counts and identification

- *Cytologic or histologic measures,* such as tissue biopsies

Because nurse researchers as a rule are not responsible for the analysis of *in vitro* extractions, it is unnecessary to explain relevant instrumentation or procedures and it is impossible to catalog the thousands of laboratory tests available. However, to give students a flavor of how *in vitro* measures have been used by nurse researchers, we present some examples in Table 17-3. Labora-

Table 17-3. *Examples of Nursing Research Studies Using* In Vitro *Measures*

TYPE OF TEST	RESEARCH PROBLEM	MEASUREMENT
Blood tests	Are changes in plasma beta-endorphin–like immunoreactivity during pregnancy and labor associated with alterations in self-reports of pain? (Cahill, 1989)	Plasma beta-endorphin–like levels
	What is the relationship between Type A behavior patterns and physiologic risk factors for cardiovascular disease in school-age children? (Hayman, Meininger et al., 1988)	Total cholesterol, low-density lipoprotein cholesterol, high-density lipoprotein cholesterol, tryglycerides, apolipoprotein B
Urine tests	What is the relationship between stress, social support, and risk among low-income pregnant women? (Kemp & Hatmaker, 1989)	Urinary catecholamine levels
	What is the relationship between antineoplastic exposure by nurses and urinary mutagen levels? (Caudell et al., 1988)	Urine mutagenicity level
Sputum culture	Does the type of tracheotomy care affect postoperative pulmonary infection? (Harris & Hyman, 1984)	Growth of specific organism changes under normal colonization
Umbilical cord culture	Does sibling contact affect the colonization rates of neonates? (Kowba & Schwirian, 1985)	Bacterial colonization rates (staphylococcus and group B Streptococcus)
Hand culture	Do latex and vinyl procedure gloves differ in terms of integrity and bacterial penetration under in-use conditions? (Korniewicz et al., 1989)	Culture of *Serratia marcescens*
Gastrointestinal aspirates	Can *p*H values of aspirates from feeding tubes be used to differentiate among gastric, intestinal, and respiratory placement? (Metheny et al., 1989)	Acidity levels of aspirates from feeding tubes
Cell histology	What is the effect of the epidermal growth factor on wound healing in a pig model? (Gill & Atwood, 1981)	Histologic measurements of the migration of keratinocytes over the wound; mitotic index

tory analyses of blood and urine samples are the most frequently used *in vitro* measures in nursing investigations.

Selecting a Biophysiologic Measure

For nurses unfamiliar with the hundreds of biophysiologic measures available in institutional settings, the selection of one or more appropriate measures of important research variables may pose a real challenge. There are, unfortunately, no comprehensive handbooks to guide interested researchers to the measures, instruments, and interpretations that might be required in collecting physiologic data. Among the best sources of information on measures that might be useful are original research articles on a problem similar to your own, a review article on the central phenomenon under investigation, manufacturers' catalogs, and exhibits of manufacturers at professional conferences.

Obviously, the most basic issue to address in selecting a physiologic measure is whether the measure will yield good information about the research variable under investigation. In some cases, the researcher will need to consider whether the variable should be measured by observation or self-report instead of (or in addition to) using biophysiologic equipment or apparatus. For example, stress could be measured by asking people questions (e.g., using the State–Trait Anxiety Inventory); by observing their behavior during exposure to stressful stimuli; or by measuring heart rate, blood pressure, or levels of adrenocorticotropic hormone in urine samples.

Several other considerations should be kept in mind in selecting a biophysiologic measure, several of which have been noted by Lindsey and Stotts (1989). These include the following:

- Is the equipment or laboratory analysis you will need readily available to you? If not, can it be borrowed, rented, or purchased?

- If equipment must be purchased, is it affordable? Can funding be acquired to cover the purchase (or rental) price?

- Can you operate the required equipment and interpret its results, or will you need training? Are there resources available to help you with operation and interpretation?

- Will you encounter any difficulties in obtaining permission to use the necessary equipment from an Institutional Review Board or other institutional authority?

- Does the measure need to be direct (e.g., a direct measure of blood pressure by way of an arterial line) or is an indirect measure (e.g., blood pressure measurement by way of a sphygmomanometer) sufficient?

- Will continuous monitoring be necessary (for example, ECG readings) or is a point-in-time measure adequate?

- Will your activities during data collection permit you to be recording data simultaneously or will you need an instrument system with recording equipment (or a research assistant)?

- Will a mechanical stimulus be needed to get appropriate or meaningful measurements? Does available equipment include the required stimulus?

- Will a single measure of your dependent variable be sufficient or is it preferable to operationalize your research variable using multiple measures? If multiple measures are better, what burden does this place on you as a researcher and on patients as research subjects?

- Are your measures likely to be influenced by *reactivity* (i.e., the subjects' awareness of their subject status)? If so, can alternative or supplementary nonreactive measures be identified, or can the extent of reactivity bias be assessed?

- Can your research variable be measured using a noninvasive procedure or is an invasive procedure required?

- Is the measure you plan to use sufficiently accurate and sensitive to variation?

- Are you thoroughly familiar with rules and

safety precautions, such as grounding procedures, especially when using electrical equipment?

The difficulty in choosing biophysiologic measures for nursing research investigations lies not in their shortage, or in their questionable utility, or in their inferiority to other methods. Indeed they are plentiful, often highly reliable and valid, and extremely useful in clinical nursing studies. However, great care must be exercised in selecting appropriate instruments or laboratory analyses with regard to practical, ethical, medical, and technical considerations.

Evaluation of Biophysiologic Measures

A major strength of biophysiologic measures is their objectivity. *Objectivity* refers to the degree of agreement between the final "scores" assigned by two independent observers. Nurse A and Nurse B, reading from the same spirometer output, are likely to record the same or highly similar tidal volume measurements for a patient. Furthermore, barring the possibility of equipment malfunctioning, two different spirometers are likely to produce identical tidal volume readouts.

Another advantage of physiologic measurements is the relative precision and sensitivity that they normally offer. By "relative," we are implicitly comparing physiologic instruments with devices for obtaining various psychologic measurements, such as self-report measures of anxiety, pain, attitudes, and so forth. Patients are unlikely to be able to deliberately distort measurements of physiologic functioning. Furthermore, researchers are generally quite confident that physiologic instrumentation provides measures of those variables in which they are interested: thermometers can be depended on to measure temperature and not blood volume, and so forth. This characteristic may seem so obvious as to render its mention unnecessary. However, for nonphysiologic measurements, the question of whether a measuring tool is really measuring the target concept is a continuously perplexing problem.

In comparison with other types of data collection tools, the equipment for obtaining physiologic measurements is rather costly. However, because such equipment is generally available in hospital settings, the costs to nurse researchers may be quite small or nonexistent.

Physiologic measures also have some disadvantages. For example, the highly technical nature of the equipment may constitute a difficulty, because the failure of nonengineers to understand the limitations of the instruments may result in greater faith in their accuracy than is warranted.

A problem that physiologic measures share with other data collection approaches is the effect that the measuring tool itself has on the variables it is attempting to measure. The presence of a sensing device such as a transducer can change the variable of interest. For instance, a flow transducer located in a blood vessel partially blocks that vessel and, hence, alters the pressure-flow characteristics being measured. Some researchers have erroneously assumed that physiologic measures are unobtrusive, based on the argument that the patients are unaware of the research purposes to which the measurements will be applied. From the body's point of view, however, physiologic measures are rarely unobtrusive.

Another difficulty is that there are normally interferences that create artifacts in physiologic measurements. For example, "noise" generated within a measuring instrument interferes with the signal being produced. The subject may also create artifactual signals, particularly when the subject's movements result in movements of the sensing devices. Many transducers are highly sensitive to motion and may produce signal variations that confound or obscure variations from the critical variable.

Despite the presentation in Tables 17-1 and 17-2 in terms of bodily functions, there is clearly a high degree of interaction among the major physiologic systems. These interrelationships can result in problems if the stimulation of one system leads to responses in other systems. Sometimes such responses are unpredictable and poorly understood, resulting in a confounding of effects that is difficult to unravel. Measuring devices themselves can produce interactions in other systems.

Energy must often be applied to the organism when making the physiologic measurements. The energy requirements mean that extreme caution must continually be exercised to avoid the risk of damaging cells by high energy concentrations. Any researcher utilizing electrical equipment should be thoroughly familiar with safety rules and considerations such as grounding specifications.

Research Example

Beckman (1990) studied the temperature- and glucose-regulating abilities of a sample of infants during the first 24 hours of life. Because pregnancies that extend beyond 42 weeks of gestation have been found to have a higher risk of uteroplacental insufficiency than do pregnancies delivered earlier, Beckman compared the regulating abilities of 63 postterm infants (over 42 weeks gestation) with those of 88 term infants (38 to 41 weeks). Gestational age was confirmed by ultrasound, clinical estimation, and Ballard assessment.

The infants' axillary temperatures were assessed using an electronic thermometer upon admission to the recovery room, hourly for the first four hours of life, and every eight hours for the remaining 24 hours. Capillary glucose was assessed using a CHEMSTRIP® hourly for the first four hours of age and before each feeding for the first 24 hours. When there were signs of hypoglycemia (a glucose reading of 40 mg/gl or below) the glucose was rechecked 30 minutes after feeding and, in some cases, a serum glucose level was drawn.

Beckman found that the two groups of infants differed in a number of respects. Postterm infants weighed more than term infants and were more likely to experience meconium-stained amniotic fluid, wasting, and peeling skin. However, differences between the two groups in terms of temperature and glucose regulation were gener-

ally small and determined to be of little clinical significance. The results for both groups were well within the normal range.

≡ RECORDS AND AVAILABLE DATA

Thus far we have examined a number of data collection strategies for which it was assumed that the researcher would be responsible for actually collecting the data and, in some cases, developing the data collection instruments. However, it is not always necessary for a researcher to collect fresh data. A wealth of data is gathered for nonresearch purposes and can be fruitfully exploited to answer research questions. Nurse researchers are particularly fortunate in the amount and quality of existing data available to them for exploration. Hospital records, patient charts, physicians' order sheets, care plan statements, and so forth all constitute rich data sources to which nurse researchers may have access.

Data Sources

The places where a nurse researcher is likely to find useful records are too numerous to list here, but a few suggestions might be helpful. Within a hospital or other health-care setting, excellent records are kept routinely and systematically. In addition to medical and nursing records, hospitals maintain financial records, personnel records, nutritional records, and so forth. Educational institutions maintain various records. For example, most schools of nursing have permanent files on their students. Public school systems also keep records, but the smaller school systems are less likely to keep extensive and accurate records than the larger ones. Industries and businesses normally maintain a variety of records that might interest industrial nurse researchers, such as information on employees' absenteeism, health status, on-the-job accidents, job performance ratings, alcoholism or drug problems, and so forth. The state and federal governments also maintain records that have been used frequently by researchers. In addition to institutional records, personal documents such as diaries and letters should be considered as possible data sources.

Advantages and Disadvantages of Using Records

The use of information from records is advantageous to the researcher for several reasons. The most salient advantage of existing records is that they are an economical source of information. The collection of data is often the most time consuming and costly step in the research process. The use of preexisting records also permits an examination of trends over time, if the information is of the type that is collected repeatedly. Problems of reactivity and response biases may be completely absent when the researcher obtains information from records. Furthermore, the investigator does not have to be concerned with obtaining cooperation from participants.

On the other hand, because the researcher has not been responsible for the collection and recording of information, he or she may be unaware of the limitations, biases, or incompleteness of the records. Two of the major sources of bias in records are *selective deposit* and *selective survival*. If the records available for use do not constitute the entire set of all possible such records, the investigator must somehow deal with the question of how representative the existing records are. Many record-keepers intend to maintain an entire universe or set of records rather than a sample but may fail to adhere to this ideal. The lapses from the ideal may be the result of some systematic biases, and the careful researcher should attempt to learn just what those biases might be.

An additional problem with which researchers must contend is the increasing reluctance of institutions to make their records available for scientific studies. The Privacy Act, a federal regulation enacted to protect individuals against possible misuses of records, has made hospitals, agencies, schools, and industrial organizations sensitive to the possibility of legal action from individuals who feel that their right to privacy has been violated. The major issue here is the divulgence of an individual's identity. If records are maintained with an identifying number rather than a name, permission to use the records may be readily granted. However, most institutions *do* maintain records by their clients' names. In such a situation, the researcher may need the assistance of personnel at the institution to maintain client anonymity, and some organizations may be unwilling to use their personnel for such purposes.

A number of other difficulties in the use of records for research purposes may be relevant. Sometimes the records have to be verified in terms of their authenticity, authorship, or accuracy, a task that may be difficult to execute if the records are old. The researcher using records must be prepared to deal with forms and file systems that he or she does not understand. Codes and symbols that had meaning to the record-keeper may have to be "translated" to be usable. In using records to study trends, the researcher should always be alert to the possibility of changes in record-keeping procedures. For example, does a dramatic increase or decrease in the incidence of sudden infant death syndrome reflect changes in the causes or cures of this problem, or does it reflect a change in diagnosis or record-keeping?

These considerations suggest that, although existing records may be plentiful, inexpensive, and accessible, they should not be used without paying attention to potential problems and weaknesses.

Research Example

Davis and Nomura (1990) were concerned about the appropriate frequency for assessing patients' vital signs following surgery. They noted that hospitals typically have protocols governing the frequency of this monitoring, but that the frequencies specified vary considerably from hospital to hospital, and that such variations appear to be based on tradition rather than on scientific data. The purpose of their investigation was to determine whether the protocol in effect in one specific hospital (a 450-bed acute-care hospital in a large urban area) was appropriate for class I surgical patients. The protocol in effect was q 15 minutes × 4, q ½ hour × 2, q 1 hour × 1, and q 4 hours × 4.

Various hospital records were obtained for 250 surgical patients who were determined to be class I by an anesthesiologist. Charts of patients over a 1-year period for those undergoing five different types of surgical procedures were randomly selected. Data were gathered from the admit/discharge sheet; surgical permit; anesthesia record; recovery room record; unit record of temperature, pulse, respiration, and blood pressure; intake/output sheet; medication record; doctor's progress notes; and nurses' notes.

The investigators' analysis focused primarily on the timing of vital signs outside abnormal parameters and the occurrence of abnormal signs and symptoms such as nausea and vomiting and urinary retention. The pattern of findings revealed a dramatic reduction in vital signs outside normal parameters between the first and second hour postoperative, with few signs occurring at hour 4 or beyond. Newly occurring abnormal vital signs appeared in only 2% of the sample in hour 3 on the unit, and none of these patients had recurrences in the following hour. Based on this analysis, the protocol in the hospital in which the study was conducted was changed. Unless otherwise ordered by the physician, the new frequency is q 15 minutes × 1, q 30 minutes × 2, q 1 hour × 1, q 4 hours × 4.

≡ Q METHODOLOGY

Q methodology is the term used by William Stephenson (1975) to refer to a constellation of substantive, statistical, and psychometric concepts relating to research on individuals. Q methodology utilizes a procedure known as the *Q sort,* which involves the sorting of a deck of cards according to specified criteria.

Q Sort Procedures

In a Q sort, the subject is presented with a set of cards on which words, phrases, statements, or other messages are written. The subject is then asked to sort the cards according to a particular dimension, such as approval–disapproval, most like me–least like me, or highest priority–lowest priority. The number of cards to be sorted is typically between 60 and 100. Usually, the subject sorts the cards into 9 or 11 piles, with the number of cards placed in each pile determined by the researcher. A common practice is to have the subjects distribute the cards such that fewer cards are placed at either of the two extremes and more cards are placed toward the middle. Table 17-4 shows a hypothetical distribution of 60 cards, with the specification of the number of cards to be placed in each of the nine piles.

The sorting instructions as well as the objects to be sorted in a Q sort investigation vary according to the requirements of the research. Attitudes can be studied by asking subjects to sort statements in terms of agreement and disagreement or approval and disapproval. The researcher can study personality by developing cards on which personality characteristics are described. The subject can then be requested to sort items on a very much like me–not at all like me continuum. Self-concept can be explored by comparing responses to this "like me" dimension to responses elicited when the instructions are to sort cards according to what subjects consider ideal personality traits. Q sorts can be used to great advantage in studying individuals in depth. For example, subjects could be asked to sort traits as they apply to themselves in different roles such as employee, parent, spouse, friend, and so forth. The technique can also be used to gain information concerning how individuals see themselves, as they perceive others see them, as they believe others would like them to be, and so forth. Other applications include asking patients to rate nursing behaviors on a continuum of most helpful–least helpful; asking nursing students to rate aspects of their educational preparation along a most useful–least useful continuum; and asking cancer patients to rate various aspects of their treatment in terms of a most distressing–least distressing dimension.

The number of cards in a Q sort varies

according to the research problem. However, it is unwise to use fewer than 50 or 60 items, because it is difficult to achieve stable and reliable results with a smaller number. On the other hand, 100 to 200 cards are normally considered the upper limit, inasmuch as the task becomes tedious and difficult with larger numbers.

The analysis of data obtained through Q sorts is a somewhat controversial matter. The options range from the most elementary, descriptive statistical procedures such as rank orderings, averages, and percentages to highly complex procedures such as factor analysis. *Factor analysis,* a procedure designed to reveal the underlying dimensions or common elements in a set of items, is described in Chapter 22. Some researchers insist that factor analysis is essential in the analysis of Q sort data.

Evaluation of Q Methodology

Q methodology can be a powerful methodological tool but, like other data collection techniques, has a number of drawbacks as well. On the plus side, we have seen that Q sorts are extremely versatile and can be applied to a wide variety of problems. Unlike many other clinical approaches, we find in Q methodology an objective and (usually) reliable procedure for the intensive study of an individual. Q sorts have been used effectively to study the progress of people during different phases of therapy, particularly psychotherapy. The requirement that individuals place a predetermined number of cards in each pile virtually eliminates response set biases that often characterize responses to written scale items. Furthermore, the task of sorting cards may

be more agreeable to some subjects than completing a paper-and-pencil instrument.

On the other hand, it is difficult and time consuming to administer Q sorts to a large sample of individuals. Without a sizable sample, it becomes problematic to generalize the results of the study. The sampling problem is further compounded by the fact that Q sorts cannot normally be administered through the mail, thereby resulting in difficulties in obtaining a geographically diverse sample of subjects. Some critics have argued that the forced procedure of distributing cards according to the researcher's specifications is artificial and actually excludes information concerning how the subjects would ordinarily distribute their opinions.

Another criticism of Q sort data relates to permissible statistical operations. Most statistical tests and procedures assume that responses to items are independent of one another. Likert-type scales exemplify items that are totally independent: a person's response of agree–disagree to one item does not in any way restrict responses to other items. Techniques of this type are known as *normative measures.* Normative measures can be interpreted by comparing individual scores with the average score for a group. The Q sort technique is a *forced-choice procedure,* wherein a person's response to one item depends on, and is restricted by, responses to other items. Referring to Table 17-4, a respondent who has already placed two cards in category 1 ("approve of least") is not free to place another item in this same category.* Such forced-choice approaches

---

*Subjects are usually told, however, that they can move cards around from one pile to another until the desired distribution is obtained.

Table 17-4. *Example of a Distribution of Q-Sort Cards*

	APPROVE OF LEAST							APPROVE OF MOST	
Category	1	2	3	4	5	6	7	8	9
Number of cards	2	4	7	10	14	10	7	4	2

produce what is known as *ipsative measures*. With ipsative measures, the average of a group is an irrelevant point of comparison, because the average is identical for all individuals. With a nine-category Q sort such as shown in Table 17-4, the average "value" of the sorted cards will always be five. (The average value of a *particular item* can be meaningfully computed and compared among individuals or groups, however.) Strictly speaking, ordinary statistical tests of significance are inappropriate for use with nonindependent ipsative measures. In practice, many researchers feel that the violation of assumptions in applying standard statistical procedures to Q sort data is not a serious transgression, particularly if the number of items is large.

Research Example

Harrison, Pistolessi, and Stephen (1989) used a Q sort in a cross-sectional study of communication styles among nursing students. The aim of the study was to address two questions: (1) Does the communication style of students differ as a function of experience or educational level? (2) Are nursing students with more experience or education better communicators?

To address these questions, all of the sophomore, junior, and senior nursing students in a liberal arts college were administered the Communication Styles Q-Set (CSQS). The CSQS is a set of 100 cards, each containing a statement describing an aspect of interpersonal behavior. Examples of statements include, "Finishes sentences for others," and "Listens intently and carefully." Respondents were given the following instruction to guide them: "Imagine that you are on the job interacting with a client. Use the cards to describe the behaviors you would use to communicate with that client." Each card had to be sorted into one of nine categories, from 1, "least characteristic of me in that situation," to 9, "most characteristic of me in that situation." The forced-choice distribution for the nine categories were 5, 8, 12, 16, 18, 16, 12, 8, and 5.

The results indicated that students with nursing experience were more likely than those without experience to say they realize when others do not understand them and that they are sensitive to others' feelings; they were less likely to characterize their communication as involving gossiping, blaming, and deception. However, communication effectiveness, a measure devised by comparing self-reported patterns of communication to patterns considered appropriate by faculty, was not found to be different for students in the three different classes, or for students differing in nursing experience.

≡ DELPHI TECHNIQUE

The method known as the Delphi technique was developed by a research and development organization (the Rand Corporation) as a tool for short-term forecasting. This technique uses self-report questionnaires, but the procedures for data collection and analysis differ from normal survey procedures.

Delphi Procedures

The *Delphi technique* requires the cooperation of a panel of experts who are asked to complete a series of questionnaires. The information solicited in the instruments typically relates to the expert's opinions, predictions, or judgment concerning a specific topic of interest. The Delphi technique differs from other surveys in several respects. First, the Delphi technique consists of several rounds of questionnaires. Each of the cooperating experts is asked to complete three or more instruments. This multiple iteration approach is used as a means of effecting group consensus of opinion—without the necessity of face-to-face committee work. A second feature is the use of feedback to members of the panel. Responses to each round of questionnaires are analyzed, summarized, and returned to the experts with a new questionnaire. The experts can then reformulate their opinions with the knowledge of the group's viewpoint in mind. The process of response–analysis–feedback–response usually is repeated three times until a general consensus is obtained.

Evaluation of the Delphi Technique

The Delphi technique is a relatively efficient and effective method of combining the expertise of a large group of individuals to obtain information for planning and prediction purposes. The experts are spared the necessity of being brought together for a formal meeting, thus saving considerable time and expense for the panel members. Another advantage is that any one persuasive or prestigious expert cannot have an undue influence on the opinions of others, as could happen in a face-to-face situation. Each panel member is on an equal footing with all others. Anonymity probably encourages a greater frankness of opinion than might be expressed in a formal meeting. The feedback–response loops allow for multichanneled communication without any risk of the members being sidetracked from their mission.

At the same time, it must be conceded that the Delphi technique is both costly and time consuming for the researcher. Experts must be solicited, questionnaires prepared and mailed, responses analyzed, results summarized, new questionnaires prepared, and so forth. The cooperation of the panel members may wane in later rounds of the questionnaire mailings. The problem of sample bias through nonresponse is a constant threat, though probably less severe than through ordinary questionnaire procedures. On the whole, the Delphi technique represents a significant methodological tool for solving problems, planning, and forecasting.

Research Example

Melnyk (1990) conducted a study using the Delphi technique as the first phase of a project to operationalize the concept of "barriers to care." A panel of 12 individuals was selected for their knowledge of the health-care system. In the first round, panel members were asked to list circumstances of daily life and characteristics that make it difficult for people to obtain care for health problems. The panel submitted a total of 226 suggestions, representing approximately 150 distinctive barriers.

The two most frequently cited barriers were long waiting time at the time of the appointment (mentioned seven times) and fear of the diagnosis (five times).

The items were then grouped into loose categories for ease of contrast and comparison. Examples of the categories include the provider/patient relationship, patient attitudes and beliefs, cost/finances, location/distance/transportation, the appointment system, and physical facilities at the service site. In the second round, panelists were directed to refine the list of barriers to ensure that each was specific, appropriate, and unique. This task was guided by criteria established by the investigator. As a result of responses in the second round, 13 items were deleted and 50 items were combined with others, leaving 81 remaining items.

In the third and final round, panelists were asked to indicate which of the barriers applied to preventive care, to illness care, or to both. Almost all items were judged to apply to both preventive and illness care. The panelists were also invited to suggest further deletions or changes in wording to the 81 items. The results of these three rounds of questioning were used as the basis for the development of a survey questionnaire administered to a large sample from a well population.

≡ *PROJECTIVE TECHNIQUES*

Questionnaires, interview schedules, and psychologic tests and scales normally depend on the respondents' capacity for self-insight or willingness to share personal information with the researcher. *Projective techniques* include a variety of methods for obtaining psychologic measures with only a minimum of cooperation required of the person. Projective methods give free play to the subjects' imagination and fantasies by providing them with a task that permits an almost unlimited number and variety of responses. The rationale underlying the use of projective techniques is that the manner in which a person organizes and reacts to unstructured stimuli is a reflection of the person's needs, motives, attitudes, values, or personality characteristics. A stimulus of low structure is sufficiently ambiguous that respondents can "read in" their own interpretations and in this way provide the researcher with information about their perception of the world. In other words, people project part of themselves into their interaction with phenomena, and projective techniques represent a means of taking advantage of this fact.

Types of Projective Techniques

Projective techniques are highly flexible, because virtually any unstructured stimuli or situation can be used to induce projective behaviors. One class of projective methods utilizes pictorial materials. One particularly useful *pictorial device* is the Thematic Apperception Test (TAT). The TAT materials consist of 20 cards that contain pictures. The subject is requested to make up a story for each picture, inventing an explanation of what led up to the event shown, what is happening at the moment, what the characters are feeling and thinking, and what kind of outcome will result. The responses are then scored according to some scheme for the variables of interest to the researchers. The TAT and other similar instruments have been used in a variety of contexts. Variables that have been measured by TAT-type pictures are achievement motivation, need for affiliation, parent–child relationships, attitude toward minority groups, creativity, religious commitment, attitude toward authority, and fear of success.

Verbal projective techniques present subjects with an ambiguous verbal stimulus rather than a pictorial one. Verbal methods can be categorized into two classes, according to the type of response elicited: (1) association techniques and (2) completion techniques. *Word-association methods* present subjects with a series of words, to which subjects respond with the first thing that comes to mind. The word list often combines both neutral and emotionally tinged words, which are included for the purpose of detecting impaired thought processes or internal conflicts. The word-association technique has also been used to study creativity, interests, and attitudes.

The most common completion technique is *sentence completion*. The person is supplied with a set of incomplete sentences and is asked to complete them in any desired manner. This approach is frequently used as a method of measuring attitudes or some aspect of personality. Some examples of incomplete sentences include the following:

When I think of a nurse practitioner I think . . . .
The thing I most admire about nurses is . . . .
A good nurse should always . . . .

The sentence stems are designed to elicit responses toward some attitudinal object or event in which the investigator is interested. Responses are typically categorized or rated according to a prespecified plan.

A third class of projective measures falls into a category known as *expressive methods*. These techniques encourage self-expression, in most cases, through the construction of some product out of raw materials. The major expressive methods are play techniques, drawing and painting, and role-playing. The assumption is that people express their feelings, needs, motives, and emotions by working with or manipulating various materials.

Evaluation of Projective Measures

Projective measures are among the most controversial in the behavioral sciences. Critics point out that projective techniques generally are incapable of being scored objectively. A high degree of inference is required in gleaning information from projective tests, and the quality of the data depends heavily on the sensitivity and interpretive skill of the investigator or analyst. It has been pointed out that the interpretation of the responses by the researcher is almost as projective as the subjects' reactions to original stimuli.

Another problem with projective techniques is that there have been difficulties in demonstrating that they are, in fact, measuring the variables that they purport to measure. If a pictorial device is used to score aggressive expressions, can the researcher be confident that individual differences in aggressive responses really reflect underlying differences in aggressiveness?

Projective techniques have supporters as well as critics in the research community. People have advocated using projective devices, arguing that they probe the unconscious mind, encompass the whole personality, and provide data of a breadth and depth unattainable by more traditional methods. One useful feature of projective instruments is that they are less susceptible to faking than self-report measures. Another strength is that it is often easier to build rapport and gain the subject's interest with a projective measure than with a questionnaire or scale. Finally, some projective techniques are particularly useful with special groups, such as children or people with speech and hearing defects. Nevertheless, the use of projective techniques for research applications appears to be associated with more disadvantages than advantages.

Research Example

Walker (1988) investigated patterns of stress and mechanisms of coping among children whose siblings were cancer patients. Various projective techniques—puppet play, cartoon storytelling, and a sentence completion test—were used to collect data from the children, whose average age was 9.5 years. The puppet play entailed pretending that the puppet's brother was sick, and asking the children what the puppet was feeling, and what the puppet might do about those feelings. The cartoon scenes depicted a possible stressful situation, using animal characters. For each of four cartoons, the children were asked how the animal might feel and what that animal might do. The sentence completion test involved 16 incomplete sentences relating to loss, harm, threat, and challenge stressors. For example, one sentence on loss was, "My best friend just moved, so I . . . ." Children were asked to complete the sentence with what they might do.

The children's responses to these various techniques were analyzed to discover major themes. For example, three major themes of stress were detected: (1) loss, (2) fear of death, and (3) change. Three domains of cognitive coping strategies and three more of behavioral coping strategies were also identified, enabling the investigator to construct a preliminary taxonomy of coping responses.

≡ VIGNETTES

The final data collection alternative we will examine are called vignettes.

The Uses of Vignettes

Vignettes are brief descriptions of an event or situation to which respondents are asked to react. The descriptions can either be fictitious or based on fact, but are always structured to elicit information about respondents' perceptions, opinions, or knowledge about some phenomenon under study. The vignettes are often written, narrative descriptions, but researchers have also begun to use videotaped vignettes that portray a specific situation. The questions posed to respondents following the presentation of the vignettes may either be open-ended (e.g., How would you recommend handling this situation?) or closed-ended (e.g., On the nine-point scale below, rate how well you believe the nurse in this story handled the situation). Normally, the number of vignettes included in a study ranges from four to ten.

The purpose of the study in which vignettes are used is sometimes not revealed to subjects. This technique has sometimes been used as an indirect measure of attitudes, prejudices, and stereotypes through the use of embedded or hidden descriptors. For example, a researcher interested in exploring attitudes toward, or stereotypes of, male nurses could present subjects with a series of vignettes describing fictitious nurses in terms of, say, their education, family background, nursing experience, and so forth. For each vignette, the nurse would be described as a male half the time (at random) and as a female the other half.

The subjects could then be asked to describe the fictitious nurses in terms of likableness, friendliness, cheerfulness, effectiveness, and so forth. Any differences in the subjects' descriptions presumably result from attitudes toward appropriate sex-role behavior.

Evaluation of Vignettes

Vignettes are often an economical means of eliciting information about how people might behave in situations that would be difficult to observe in daily life. For example, we might want to assess how patients would react to or feel about nurses with different types of personalities and personal styles of interaction. In clinical settings, it would be difficult to expose patients to many different nurses, all of whom have been evaluated as having different personalities. Another advantage of vignettes is that it is possible to experimentally manipulate the stimuli (the vignettes) by randomly assigning vignettes to groups, as in the example about male nurses. Furthermore, vignettes often represent an interesting task for subjects. Finally, vignettes can be incorporated into mailed questionnaires and are therefore an inexpensive data collection strategy.

Vignettes are handicapped by some of the same problems as other self-report techniques. The principal problem is that of response biases. If a respondent describes how he or she would react in a situation portrayed in the vignette, how accurate is that description of the respondent's actual behavior? Thus, although the use of vignettes can be profitable, researchers should consider how to minimize or at least assess potential response biases.

Research Example

Flaskerud (1984) used vignettes to explore cultural and role differences in perceptions of problematic behavior. She incorporated ten vignettes into an interview schedule that was administered to members of six different minority groups (Chinese-Americans, Mexican-Americans, Filipino-Americans, Native Americans, Black Americans, and Appalachians) and to mental health professionals in three states. The ten vignettes each told in lay language a short fictitious story of a person experiencing problems. Following each vignette, respondents were asked three questions: (1) What do you think of this person's behavior? (2) Do you think anything should be done about it? (3) If so, what? None of the vignettes or questions specifically suggested a mental illness or a psychiatric treatment response.

The analyses of responses indicated substantial differences between minority group members and mental health professionals, both in the labels attached to the problematic behaviors and in the recommended strategy for managing the behaviors. The mental health professionals tended to perceive the behaviors as symptoms of mental illness and advised psychiatric treatment. The minority groups "viewed the behavior from a broader perspective that encompassed spiritual, moral, somatic, psychological, and metaphysical components" (p. 196). The investigator concluded that health professionals need to be sensitive to culturally relevant explanations of behavior and should design culture-compatible interventions.

☰ SUMMARY

This chapter reviewed several data collection strategies that are used less frequently than those described in Chapters 14–16. For certain research problems, these alternative techniques—and especially biophysiologic measures—may be strong candidates as methods of collecting data.

The trend in nursing research is toward increasing numbers of clinical, patient-centered investigations in which biophysiologic indicators of patients' health status are used as dependent variables. Although it is beyond the scope of this book to describe physiologic equipment in detail, many examples of instruments and laboratory tests used in nursing studies were described. Particular attention was paid to the *instrumentation systems* used for *in vivo measurements* (those performed within or on living organisms). The components of an organism-instrument system are the stimulus, subject, sensing equipment, signal-conditioning equipment, display equipment, and recording equipment. Examples of instrumentation used to assess the functioning of six bodily systems were presented. Blood tests and urine tests are the most frequently used *in vitro measurements* (those performed outside the organism's body), but examples of other chemical, microbiologic, and histologic analyses were described. Despite the clear-cut utility of biophysiologic measures for nursing science, great care must be taken in selecting such measures with regard to practical, technical, and ethical considerations.

One of the greatest advantages of using physiologic measures is their objectivity and validity. Independent researchers are apt to obtain the same results using the same measure. Disadvantages associated with the use of physiologic instrumentation are the possible malfunctioning of the equipment, safety problems, and artifacts that interfere with the system.

Existing *records* are often used by researchers in the conduct of scientific investigations. Such records provide an economical source of information. In using records, the researcher should try to determine how representative and accurate they are. Two major sources of bias in records are (1) *selective deposit* and (2) *selective survival.*

Q sorts involve having the subject sort a set of statements into piles according to specified criteria. Attitudes, personality, and self-concept are some of the traits that may be measured by Q methodology. The procedure may be used to study an individual in depth or to rate groups of individuals. One limitation in using Q sorts is that it produces *ipsative measures* wherein the average across cards is an irrelevant basis of comparison, inasmuch as the *forced-choice approach* produces the same average for all subjects. This differs from other techniques that produce *normative measures* because each choice is independent of other choices.

The *Delphi technique* is a method in which several rounds of questionnaires are mailed to a panel of experts. Feedback from previous questionnaires is provided with each new questionnaire. This technique is used for problem solving, planning, and forecasting.

Projective techniques encompass a variety of data collection methods that rely on the subject's projection of psychologic traits or states in response to vaguely structured stimuli. *Pictorial methods* present a picture or cartoon and ask the subject to describe what is happening, what led up to the event, or what kind of action is needed. *Verbal methods* present the subject with an ambiguous verbal stimulus rather than a picture. The two categories of verbal methods are (1) *word association* and (2) *sentence completion. Expressive methods* take the form of *play, drawing,* or *role-playing.*

Vignettes are brief descriptions of some event, person, or situation to which respondents are asked to react. Vignettes are often incorporated into questionnaires or interview schedules. They may be used to assess respondents' hypothetical behaviors, opinions, and perceptions.

≡ *STUDY SUGGESTIONS*

1. Formulate a research problem in which each of the following could be used as the measurements for the dependent variable:
   a. Blood pressure
   b. Electromyograms
   c. Thermograms
   d. Blood sugar levels
2. Identify some of the *in vivo* or *in vitro* measures you might use to address the following research questions:
   a. Does clapping the lungs before suctioning result in better patient outcomes than suctioning without clapping?
   b. What is the effect of various bed positions on the development of respiratory acidosis or alkalosis?
   c. What are the cardiovascular effects of administering liquid potassium chloride in three different solutions (orange juice, fruit punch, cranberry juice)?

d. What is the rate of respiratory increase for designated decreases in the *p*H level of cerebrospinal fluid?

3. Suppose that you were interested in studying the following variables: professionalism in nurses, fear of death in patients, achievement motivation in nursing students, job satisfaction among industrial nurses, fathers' reactions to their newborn infants, and patients' needs for affiliation. Describe at least two ways of collecting data relating to these concepts, using the following approaches:
   a. Vignettes
   b. Verbal projective techniques
   c. Pictorial projective techniques
   d. Records
   e. Q sorts

≡ *SUGGESTED READINGS*

METHODOLOGICAL REFERENCES

Biophysiologic References

Abbey, J. (Guest Ed.). (1978). Symposium on bioinstrumentation for nurses. *Nursing Clinics of North America, 13,* 561–640.

Bauer, J.D., Ackermann, P.G., & Toro, G. (1982). *Clinical laboratory methods* (9th ed.). St. Louis: C.V. Mosby.

Cromwell, L., Weibell, F.J., & Pfeiffer, E.A. (1980). *Biomedical instrumentation and measurements* (2nd ed.). Englewood Cliffs, NJ: Prentice-Hall.

Ferris, C.D. (1980). *Guide to medical laboratory instruments.* Boston: Little, Brown.

Fischbach, F. (1988). *A manual of laboratory diagnostic tests* (3rd ed.) Philadelphia: J.B. Lippincott.

Lindsey, A.M. (1984). Research for clinical practice: Physiological phenomena. *Heart and Lung, 13,* 496–507.

Lindsey, A.M., & Stotts, N.A. (1989). Collecting data on biophysiologic variables. In H.S. Wilson, *Research in nursing* (2nd ed.) Menlo Park, CA: Addison-Wesley.

Pagana, K.D., & Pagana, T.J. (1990). *Diagnostic testing and nursing implications: A case study approach* (3rd ed.) St. Louis: C.V. Mosby.

Weiss, M.D. (1973). *Biomedical instrumentation.* Philadelphia: Chilton Book Company.

Widmann, F.K. (1983). *Clinical interpretation of laboratory tests* (9th ed.). Philadelphia: F.A. Davis.

Other Data Collection Methods

Anastasi, A. (1988). *Psychological testing* (6th ed.). New York: Macmillan. (Chapter 19)

Angell, R.C., & Freedman, R. (1953). The use of documents, records, census materials, and indices. In L. Festinger & D. Katz (Eds.), *Research methods in the behavioral sciences* (pp. 300–326). New York: Holt, Rinehart & Winston.

Block, J. (1961). *The Q-Sort method in personality assessment and psychiatric research.* Springfield, IL: Charles C Thomas.

Couper, M.R. (1984). The Delphi technique: Characteristics and sequence model. *Advances in Nursing Science, 7,* 72–77.

Flaskerud, J.H. (1979). Use of vignettes to elicit responses toward broad concepts. *Nursing Research, 28,* 210–212.

Kerlinger, F.N. (1986). *Foundations of behavioral research* (3rd ed.). New York: Holt, Rinehart & Winston.

Lanza, M.L. (1988). Development of a vignette. *Western Journal of Nursing Research, 10,* 346–351.

Linstone, H., & Turoff, M. (1975). *The Delphi technique and applications.* Reading, MA: Addison-Wesley.

Semeomoff, B. (1976). *Projective techniques.* New York: John Wiley and Sons.

Simpson, S. H. (1989). Use of Q-sort methodology in cross-cultural nutrition and health research. *Nursing Research, 38,* 289–290.

Stephenson, W. (1975). *The study of behavior: Q technique and its methodology.* Chicago: University of Chicago Press.

Tetting, D.W. (1988). Q-sort update. *Western Journal of Nursing Research, 10,* 757–765.

Waltz, C.F., Strickland, O.L., & Lenz, E.R. (1984). *Measurement in nursing research.* Philadelphia: F.A. Davis. (Chapter 9)

Wittenborn, J. (1961). Contributions and current status of Q methodology. *Psychological Bulletin, 58,* 132–142.

SUBSTANTIVE REFERENCES

Biophysiologic Studies

Beckman, C.A. (1990). Postterm pregnancy: Effects on temperature and glucose regulation. *Nursing Research, 39,* 21–24.

Brink, C., Sampselle, C., Wells, T., Diokno, A., & Gillis, G. (1989). A digital test for pelvic muscle strength in older women with urinary incontinence. *Nursing Research, 38,* 196–199.

Cahill, C.A. (1989). Beta-endorphin levels during pregnancy and labor: A role in pain modulation? *Nursing Research, 38,* 200–203.

Caudell, K.A., Vredevoe, D.L. Dietrich, M.F., Caudell, T., Hoban, M., & Block, J. (1988). Quantification of urinary mutigens in nurses during potential antineoplastic agent exposure. *Cancer Nursing, 11,* 41–50.

Ferrans, C., & Powers, M. (1985). The employment potential of hemodialysis patients. *Nursing Research, 34,* 273–277.

Gill, B.P., & Atwood, J.R. (1981). Reciprocy and helicy used to relate mEGF and wound healing. *Nursing Research, 30,* 68–72.

Harris, R.B., & Hyman, R.B. (1984). Clean vs. sterile tracheotomy care and level of pulmonary infection. *Nursing Research, 33,* 80–85.

Hayman, L.L. Meininger, J.C., Stashinko, E., Gallagher, P., & Coates, P. (1988). Type A behavior and physiological cardiovascular risk factors in school-age twin children. *Nursing Research, 37,* 290–296.

Heidenreich T. & Giuffre M. (1990). Postoperative temperature measurement. *Nursing Research, 39,* 153–155.

Kagawa-Busby, K.S., et al. (1980). Effects of diet temperature on tolerance of enteral feedings. *Nursing Research, 29,* 276–280.

Kemp, V.H., & Hatmaker, D.D. (1989). Stress and social support in high-risk pregnancy. *Research in Nursing and Health, 12,* 331–336.

Kirchhoff, K., Holm, K., Foreman, M., & Rebenson-Piano, M. (1990). Electrocardiographic response to ice water ingestion. *Heart and Lung, 19,* 41–48.

Korniewicz, D.M., Laughton, B., Butz, A., & Larson, E. (1989). Integrity of vinyl and latex gloves. *Nursing Research, 38,* 144–146.

Kowba, M.D., & Schwirian, P.M. (1985). Direct sibling contact and bacterial colonization in newborns. *Journal of Obstetric Gynecologic, and Neonatal Nursing, 14,* 418–423.

Levesque, L., et al. (1984). Evaluation of a presurgical group program given at two different times. *Research in Nursing and Health, 7,* 227–236.

Ley, S.J., Miller, K., Skov, P., & Preisig, P. (1990). Crystalloid versus colloid fluid therapy after cardiac surgery. *Heart and Lung, 19,* 31–40.

Lu, Z., Metzger, B.L., & Therrien, B. (1990). Ethnic differences in physiological responses associated with the Valsalva maneuver. *Research in Nursing and Health, 13,* 9–15.

MacVicar, M., Winningham, M., & Nickel, J. (1989). Effect of aerobic interval training on cancer patients' functional capacity. *Nursing Research, 38,* 348–351.

Meier, P. (1988). Bottle- and breast-feeding: Effects on transcutaneous oxygen pressure and temperature in preterm infants. *Nursing Research, 37,* 36–41.

Metheny, N., Williams, P., Wiersema, L., Wehrle, M., Eisenberg, P., & McSweeney, M. (1989). Effectiveness of pH measurements in predicting feeding tube placement. *Nursing Research, 38,* 280–285.

Mravinac, C.M., Dracup, K., & Clochesy, J.M. (1989). Urinary bladder and rectal temperature monitoring during clinical hypothermia. *Nursing Research, 38,* 73–76.

Osborne, D. (1984). Cardiovascular responses of patients ambulated 32 and 56 hours after coronary artery bypass surgery. *Western Journal of Nursing Research, 6,* 321–324.

Preusser, B., Lash, J., Stone, K., Winningham, M., Gonyon, D., & Nickel, J. (1989). Quantifying the minimum discard sample required for accurate arterial blood gases. *Nursing Research, 38,* 276–279.

Renfroe, K.L. (1988). Effect of progressive relaxation on dyspnea and state anxiety in patients with chronic obstructive pulmonary disease. *Heart and Lung, 17,* 408–413.

Thomas, S.A., & Friedmann, E. (1990). Type A behavior and cardiovascular responses during verbalization in cardiac patients. *Nursing Research, 39,* 48–53.

*Studies Using Other Data Collection Methods**

Aaronson, L.S., & MacNee, C.L. (1989). The relationship between weight gain and nutrition in pregnancy. *Nursing Research, 38,* 223–227. [Records]

Albrecht, S.A., & London, W.P. (1990). Season of birth and laterality of breast cancer. *Nursing Research, 39,* 118–119. [Records]

Brown, L.P., York, R., Jacobsen, B., Gennaro, S., & Brooten, D. (1989). Very low birth-weight infants: Parental visiting and telephoning during

*A comment in brackets after each citation designates the data collection strategy of interest.

initial infant hospitalization. *Nursing Research, 38,* 233–236. [Records]

Burokas, L. (1985). Factors affecting nurses' decisions to medicate pediatric patients after surgery. *Heart and Lung, 14,* 373–379. [Vignettes]

Davidson, R.A., & Lauver, D. (1984). Nurse practitioner and physician roles. *Research in Nursing and Health, 7,* 3–9. [Vignettes]

Davis, M.J., & Nomura, L.A. (1990). Vital signs of class I surgical patients. *Western Journal of Nursing Research, 12,* 28–41. [Records]

Dennis, K.E. (1990). Patients' control and the information imperative: Clarification and confirmation. *Nursing Research, 39,* 162–166. [Q-sorts]

Dennis, K.E., Howes, D.G., & Zelauskas, B. (1989). Identifying nursing research priorities: A first step in program development. *Applied Nursing Research, 2,* 108–113. [Delphi survey]

Devine, E.C., & Werley, H.H. (1988). Test of the nursing minimum data set: Availability of data and reliability. *Research in Nursing and Health, 11,* 97–104. [Records]

Flaskerud, J.H. (1984). A comparison of perceptions of problematic behavior by six minority groups and mental health professionals. *Nursing Research, 33,* 190–197. [Vignettes]

Ganong, L.H., Coleman, M., & Riley, C. (1988). Nursing students' stereotypes of married and unmarried pregnant clients. *Research in Nursing and Health, 11,* 333–342. [Vignettes]

George, T.B. (1982). Development of the self-concept of nurse in nursing students. *Research in Nursing and Health, 5,* 191–197. [Projective technique]

Gershan, J.A., et al. (1990). Fluid volume deficit: Validating the indicators. *Heart and Lung, 19,* 152–156. [Delphi survey]

Harrison, T.M., Pistolessi, T.V., & Stephen, T.D. (1989). Assessing nurses' communication style: A cross-sectional study. *Western Journal of Nursing Research, 11,* 75–91. [Q sort]

Holm, K., Cohen, F., Dudas, S., Medema, P.G., & Allen, B.L. (1989). Effect of personal pain experience on pain assessment. *Image, 21,* 72–75. [Vignettes]

Hughes, K.K., & Young, W.B. (1990). The relationship between task complexity and decision-making consistency. *Research in Nursing and Health, 13,* 189–197. [Vignettes]

Hutti, M.H., & Johnson, J.B. (1988). Newborn Apgar scores of babies born in birthing rooms vs. traditional delivery rooms. *Applied Nursing Research, 1,* 68–71. [Records]

Martell, L.K., Imle, M., Horwitz, S., & Wheeler, L. (1989). Information priorities of new mothers in a short-stay program. *Western Journal of Nursing Research, 11,* 320–327. [Q sort]

McGee, R., Powell, M., Broadwell, D., & Clark, J. (1987). A Delphi survey of oncology clinical nurse specialist competencies. *Oncology Nursing Forum, 14,* 29–45. [Delphi technique]

Melnyk, K. (1990). Barriers to care: Operationalizing the variable. *Nursing Research, 39,* 108–112. [Delphi technique]

Munroe, D.J. (1990). The influence of registered nurse staffing on the quality of nursing home care. *Research in Nursing and Health, 13,* 263–270. [Records]

Taylor, A.G., Skelton, J.A., & Butcher, J. (1984). Duration of pain condition and physical pathology as determinants of nurses' assessments of patients in pain. *Nursing Research, 33,* 4–8. [Vignettes]

Ventura, M., & Walegora-Serafin, B. (1981). Setting priorities for nursing research. *Journal of Nursing Administration, 11,* 30–34. [Delphi technique]

Walker, C.L. (1988). Stress and coping in siblings of childhood cancer patients. *Nursing Research, 37,* 208–212. [Projective technique]

Wood, S.P. (1983). School-aged children's perceptions of the causes of illness. *Pediatric Nursing, 9,* 101–104. [Projective technique]

18

Criteria for Assessing and Selecting Measuring Tools

Chapters 14 through 17 reviewed a variety of methods for collecting research data—that is, for measuring the research variables. In this chapter, we discuss criteria for selecting and evaluating measuring tools.

An ideal measuring instrument is one that results in measures that are relevant, accurate, unbiased, sensitive, unidimensional, and efficient. These requirements are rather stringent. For most of the concepts of interest to nurse researchers, there are few, if any, data collection procedures that match this ideal. Measures that are physical or physiologic in nature have a much higher chance of success in attaining these goals than measures that are psychologic or behavioral, but no measurement tools are perfect.

Inasmuch as measurement plays such a central role in the research process, scientists have developed a number of techniques for evaluating the quality of their instruments, which we review in this chapter. We turn first, however, to basic concepts from the theory of measurement error.

≡ *ERRORS OF MEASUREMENT*

The measurement of attributes does not occur in a vacuum. Both the procedures involved in applying the measurement and the object being measured are susceptible to numerous influences that could alter the resulting information. Some of the factors that impinge on the measurement process can be controlled to a certain degree, and attempts should always be made to do so; however, it must be recognized that scores obtained from most measuring tools are fallible.

Components of Scores

If an instrument is not perfectly accurate, then the measures it yields can be said to contain a certain degree of error. Conceptually, an *ob-*

served or *obtained score* can be decomposed into two parts—(1) an error component and (2) a true component. This can be written symbolically as follows:

$$\text{Obtained score} = \text{True score} \pm \text{Error}$$
$$\text{or}$$
$$X_O = X_T \pm X_E$$

The first term in this equation represents the actual, observed score for some measurement. For example, it could represent a patient's systolic blood pressure, a nursing student's score on a scale measuring attitude toward death, a woman's fear of the labor and delivery experience as indicated in a Q sort, and so forth. The "X_T" stands for the true value that would be obtained if it were possible to arrive at an infallible measure. The *true score* is a hypothetical entity—it can never be known because measures are *not* infallible—though its value can be estimated. The final term in the equation is the *error of measurement*. The difference between true and obtained scores is the result of factors that affect the measurement and, therefore, result in distortions.

Decomposing obtained scores in this fashion brings to light an important point. When a researcher measures an attribute of interest, he or she is also *measuring* attributes that are not of interest. The true score component is what one hopes to isolate; the error component is a composite of other factors that are also being measured, contrary to the desires of the researcher. This concept can be illustrated with an exaggerated example. Suppose a researcher were measuring the weight of ten people on a spring scale. As each subject stepped on the scale, our fictitious researcher places a hand on the subject's shoulder and applies some pressure. The resulting measures (the X_Os), will all be biased in an upward direction because the scores reflect the influence of both the subject's actual weight (X_T) and the researcher's pressure (X_E). Other errors of measurement probably affected the observed scores as well.

Errors of measurement are problematic because they represent an unknown quantity and also because they are variable. In our example of the careless weight measurer, the amount of pressure applied would undoubtedly vary from one subject to the next. In other words, the proportion of true score component in an obtained score varies from one person to the next.

If this example appears too contrived, consider the evaluation of nursing knowledge as measured by the national licensure examination. Perhaps some individuals did not sleep enough the night before the examination; other individuals may misunderstand the directions for responding; yet others may arrive at the test site late. Therefore, the obtained scores reflect not only nursing knowledge, but also represent "measures" of alertness, comprehension of directions, punctuality, and dozens of other attributes. Some major influences on measurements are described in the next section.

Sources of Measurement Error

Many factors contribute to errors of measurement. Among the most common are the following seven factors:

1. *Situational contaminants.* Scores can be affected by the conditions under which they are produced. The subject's awareness of an observer's presence (the reactivity problem) is one source of bias. The anonymity of the response situation, the friendliness of the researchers, or the location of the data gathering can all affect a subject's responses. Other environmental factors such as the temperature, humidity, lighting, time of day, and so forth can represent sources of measurement error.

2. *Response set biases.* A number of relatively enduring characteristics of the respondents can interfere with accurate measures of the target attribute. Response sets such as social desirability, extreme responses, and acquiescence are potential problems in self-report measures, particularly in psychologic scales (see Chapter 15).

3. *Transitory personal factors.* The scores of an

individual may be influenced by a variety of temporary personal states such as fatigue, hunger, anxiety, mood, and so forth. In some cases these factors can affect a measurement directly, as in the case of anxiety affecting a measurement of pulse rate. In other cases, temporary personal factors can alter individuals' scores by influencing their motivation to cooperate, act "naturally," or do their best.

4. *Administration variations.* Alterations in the methods of collecting data from one subject to the next could result in variations in obtained scores that have little to do with variations in the target attribute. If observers alter their coding categories or definitions, if interviewers improvise the wording of a question, if test administrators change the test instructions, or if some physiologic measures are taken before a feeding and others are taken postprandially, then measurement errors can potentially occur.

5. *Instrument clarity.* If the directions for obtaining measures are vague or poorly understood, then scores may reflect this ambiguity and misunderstanding. For example, questions in a self-report instrument may sometimes be interpreted differently by different respondents, leading to a distorted measure of the critical variable. Observers may miscategorize observations if the classification scheme is unclear. The training of observers, interviewers, and other research personnel can reduce this source of error but may not eliminate it completely.

6. *Response sampling.* Sometimes errors are introduced as a result of the sampling of items used to measure an attribute. For example, a nursing student's score on a 100-item test of general nursing knowledge will be influenced to a certain extent by *which* 100 questions are included on the examination. A person might get 95 questions correct on one test but only get 90 right on another similar test.

7. *Instrument format.* Several technical characteristics of an instrument can influence the obtained measurements. Open-ended questions may yield information different from closed-ended questions. Oral responses to a specific question may be at odds with responses to a written form of the same question. The ordering of questions within an instrument may also influence responses.

This list represents a sampling of the sources of measurement error with which a researcher must deal. Other common problems will come to light in other sections of this chapter.

≡ *RELIABILITY*

The reliability* of a measuring instrument is a major criterion for assessing its quality and adequacy. Essentially, the *reliability* of an instrument is the degree of consistency with which it measures the attribute it is supposed to be measuring. If a scale gave a reading of 120 pounds for a person's weight one minute, and a reading of 150 pounds in the next minute (barring any tampering with the instrument or subject), we would naturally be wary of using that scale because the information would be unreliable. The less variation an instrument produces in repeated measurements of an attribute, the higher its reliability. Thus, reliability can be equated with the stability, consistency, or dependability of a measuring tool.

Another way of defining reliability is in terms of accuracy. An instrument can be said to be reliable if its measures accurately reflect the "true scores" of the attribute under investigation. This definition links reliability to the issues raised in the discussion of measurement error. We can make this relationship clearer by stating that an instrument is reliable to the extent that errors of measurement are absent from obtained scores. A reliable measure is one that maximizes the true score component and minimizes the error component. The greater the error, the greater the unreliability.

---

*The discussion of reliability presented here is based entirely on classical measurement theory. Readers concerned with assessing the reliability of instructional measures that can be classified as mastery-type or criterion-referenced should consult Thorndike and Hagen (1977).

These two ways of approaching the concept of reliability (consistency and accuracy) are not so different as they might at first appear. The errors of measurement that impinge on an instrument's accuracy also affect its consistency. The example of the scale that produced variable weight readings should clarify this point. Suppose that the true weight of a subject is 125 pounds, but that two independent measurements yielded 120 and 150 pounds. In terms of the equation presented in the previous section, we could express the measurements as follows:

$$120 = 125 - 5$$
$$150 = 125 + 25$$

The values of the errors of measurement for the two trials are -5 and $+25$, respectively. These errors produced scores that are both inconsistent and inaccurate. We must conclude that our fictitious spring scale is highly unreliable.

Scientists can place little confidence in their findings if the instruments they use are of questionable reliability. Therefore, it has become a customary procedure for developers of new instruments to estimate the reliability of their tools before making them available for general use. Such an evaluation is often referred to as a *psychometric assessment* of an instrument. Instruments that are psychologic or behavioral in nature are in particular need of psychometric testing. However, an instrument's reliability is not a fixed entity. *The reliability of an instrument is not a property of the instrument, but rather of the instrument when administered to a certain sample under certain conditions.* A scale developed to measure dependence in hospitalized adults in the United States may be unreliable for use with hospitalized adults in Mexico, or for hospitalized adolescents, or for the elderly in nursing homes, and so forth.

What are the implications of this fact for researchers? First, in selecting a measuring tool, one should always learn about the characteristics of the group with whom or for whom the instrument was developed. If the original group was similar to the researcher's target group, then the reliability estimate provided by the scale devel-oper is probably a reasonably good index of the instrument's accuracy and consistency for the new study. Other things being equal, one should always choose a measure with demonstrated high reliability. However, the prudent scientist is not satisfied with an instrument that will "probably" be reliable in his or her study. The recommended procedure is to compute estimates of reliability whenever data are collected for a scientific investigation. For physiologic measures that are relatively impervious to random fluctuations stemming from personal or situational factors, this procedure may be unnecessary. However, observational tools, self-report measures, tests of knowledge or ability, and projective tests—all of which are highly susceptible to errors of measurement—should be subjected to a reliability check as a routine step in the research process. The interpretation of a study's findings can be greatly affected by the knowledge that the instruments were reliable or were unreliable.

The reliability of a measuring tool can be assessed in several different ways. The method chosen depends to a certain extent on the nature of the instrument but also on the aspect of the reliability concept that is of greatest interest. Three aspects that have received major quantitative attention are (1) stability, (2) internal consistency, and (3) equivalence.

Stability

The *stability* of a measure refers to the extent to which the same results are obtained on repeated administrations of the instrument. The estimation of reliability here focuses on the instrument's susceptibility to extraneous factors from one administration to the next.

Assessments of the stability of a measuring tool are derived through procedures that evaluate *test–retest reliability*. The researcher administers the same test to a sample of individuals on two occasions and then compares the scores obtained. The comparison procedure is performed objectively by computing a *reliability coefficient,* which is a numerical index of the magnitude of the test's reliability.

We must pause at this point to briefly explain the concepts underlying the statistic known as the *correlation coefficient.** We have pointed out repeatedly in this text that a scientist often strives to detect and explain the relationships among phenomena: Is there a relationship between patients' gastric acidity levels and incidents of emotional upset? Is there a relationship between body temperature and perceptions of the passage of time? The correlation coefficient is an important tool for quantitatively describing the magnitude and direction of a relationship. The computation of this index does not concern us here. It is more important to understand how to "read" a correlation coefficient.

Two variables that are obviously related to one another are the height and weight of individuals. Tall people tend, on the average, to be heavier than short people. Light persons tend, on the whole, to be shorter than heavy persons. We would say that the relationship were perfect if the tallest person in the world were the heaviest, the second tallest person were the second heaviest, and so forth. The correlation coefficient summarizes how "perfect" a relationship is. The possible values for a correlation coefficient range from a −1.00 through 0.0 to +1.00. If height and weight were perfectly correlated, then the correlation coefficient expressing this relationship would be 1.00. Because the relationship does exist but is not perfect, the correlation coefficient is probably in the vicinity of .50 or .60. The relationship between height and weight would be described as a *positive relationship* because increases in height tend to be associated with increases in weight.

When two variables are totally unrelated, the correlation coefficient is equal to zero. One might anticipate that a woman's dress size is unrelated to her intelligence. Large women are as likely to perform well on tests of ability as small women. The correlation coefficient summarizing such a relationship would presumably be in the vicinity of 0.0.

*Computational procedures and additional information concerning correlation coefficients (Pearson's *r*) are presented in Chapter 20.

Correlation coefficients running from 0.0 to −1.00 express what is known as *inverse* or *negative relationships.* When two variables are inversely related, increments in one variable are associated with decrements in the second variable. Suppose that there is an inverse relationship between a nurse's age and attitude toward abortion. This means that, on the average, the *older* the nurse, the *less* favorable the attitude. If the relationship were perfect (i.e., if the oldest nurse had the least favorable attitude and so on), then the correlation coefficient would be equal to −1.00. In actuality, the relationship between age and abortion attitudes is probably quite modest—in the vicinity of −.20 or −.30. A correlation coefficient of this magnitude describes a weak relationship wherein older nurses tend to be unfavorable and younger nurses tend to be favorable toward abortion, but a "crossing of lines" is not unusual. That is, many younger nurses oppose abortion and many older nurses support it.

Now we are prepared to discuss the use of correlation coefficients to compute reliability estimates. In the case of test–retest reliability, a sample of subjects is exposed to the administration of the instrument on two occasions. Let us say we are interested in the stability of a scale to measure nurses' leadership potential. Because leadership potential might be presumed to be a fairly enduring attribute in individuals, we would expect a measure of it to yield consistent scores on two separate testings. As a check on the instrument's stability, the scale is administered to a sample of ten people three weeks apart. Some fictitious data for this example are presented in Table 18-1. It can be seen that, generally, the differences in the scores on the two testings are not large. The reliability coefficient for test–retest estimates is the correlation coefficient between the two sets of scores. In this example, the computed reliability coefficient is .95, which is quite high.

The value of the reliability coefficient theoretically can range between −1.00 and +1.00, just as in the case of other correlation coefficients. A negative coefficient would have been obtained in the leadership potential example if persons who

Table 18-1. *Fictitious Data for Test–Retest Reliability of a Leadership Potential Scale*

SUBJECT NUMBER	TIME 1	TIME 2	
1	55	57	
2	49	46	
3	78	74	
4	37	35	
5	44	46	
6	50	56	
7	58	55	
8	62	66	
9	48	50	
10	67	63	$r = .95$

had the highest scores in leadership potential at time 1 had the lowest scores at time 2. In practice, reliability coefficients normally range between 0.0 and 1.00. The higher the coefficient, the more stable the measure. For most purposes, reliability coefficients above .70 are considered satisfactory. In some situations, a higher coefficient may be required, or a lower one may be considered acceptable.

The test–retest method is a relatively easy and straightforward approach to estimating reliability. It is a method that can be used with self-report, observational, and physiologic measures. However, the test–retest approach has certain disadvantages. One problem is that many traits of interest do change over time, independently of the stability of the measure. Attitudes, behaviors, moods, knowledge, physical condition, and so forth can be modified by intervening experiences between the two testings. The procedures used to estimate stability confound changes resulting from random fluctuations and those resulting from true modifications in the attribute being measured. Still, there are many attributes that are relatively enduring characteristics for which a test–retest approach is suitable. The example of leadership potential is one such attribute.

Stability estimates suffer from other problems, however. One possibility is that the subjects' responses or observer's coding on the second administration will be influenced by the memory of their responses/coding on the first administration, regardless of the actual values on the second day. This memory interference will result in a spuriously high reliability coefficient. Another difficulty is that subjects may actually change as a result of the first administration. Finally, people may not be as careful using the same instrument a second time. If they find the procedure boring on the second occasion, then the responses could be haphazard, resulting in a spuriously low estimate of stability.

In summary, the test–retest approach is a procedure for estimating the stability of a measure over time. On the whole, reliability coefficients tend to be higher for short-term retests than for long-term retests (i.e., those greater than one or two months) because of actual changes in the attribute being measured. Stability indexes are most appropriate for relatively enduring characteristics such as personality, abilities, or certain physical attributes such as height.

Internal Consistency

Psychosocial scales are often evaluated in terms of their internal consistency. Ideally, scales designed to measure an attribute are composed of a set of items, all of which are measuring the critical attribute and nothing else. On a scale to measure the decision-making abilities of nurses, it would be inappropriate to include an item that is a better measure of empathy than skill in decision making. An instrument may be said to be *internally consistent* or *homogeneous* to the extent that all of its subparts are measuring the same characteristic.

The internal consistency approach to estimating an instrument's reliability is probably the most widely used method among researchers today. The reason for the popularity of the procedures is not only that they are economical (they require only one test administration) but also that they are the best means of assessing one of the most important sources of measurement error in psychosocial instruments, the sampling of items.

One of the oldest methods for assessing

internal consistency is the *split-half* technique. In this approach, the items composing a test are split into two groups, scored independently, and the scores on the two half-tests are used to compute a correlation coefficient. To illustrate this procedure, the fictitious scores from the first administration of the leadership potential scale are reproduced in the second column of Table 18-2. For the sake of simplicity, we will say that the total instrument consists of 20 questions. To compute a split-half reliability coefficient, the items must be divided into two groups of ten. Although a large number of possible "splits" is possible, the most widely accepted procedure is to use odd items versus even items. One half-test, therefore, consists of items 1, 3, 5, 7, 9, 11, 13, 15, 17, and 19, and the even-numbered items compose the second half-test. The scores on the two halves for our example are shown in the third and fourth columns of Table 18-2. The correlation coefficient describing the relationship between the two half-tests is an estimate of the internal consistency of the leadership potential scale. If the odd items are measuring the same attribute as the even items, then the reliability coefficient should be high. The correlation coefficient computed on the fictitious data is .67.

The correlation coefficient computed on split-halves of a measure tends to systematically underestimate the reliability of the entire scale.

Other things being equal, longer scales are more reliable than shorter ones. The correlation coefficient computed on the data in Table 18-2 is an estimate of reliability for a ten-item instrument, not a 20-item instrument. To overcome this difficulty, a formula has been developed for adjusting the correlation coefficient to give an estimate of reliability for the entire test. The correction equation, which is known as the *Spearman-Brown prophecy formula,* is as follows:

$$r^1 = \frac{2r}{1 + r}$$

where r = the correlation coefficient computed on the split halves

r^1 = the estimated reliability of the entire test

Using the formula, the reliability for our hypothetical 20-item measure of leadership potential would be

$$r^1 = \frac{(2)\,(.67)}{1 + .67} = .80$$

The split-half technique is easy to use and eliminates most of the problems associated with

Table 18-2. *Fictitious Data for Split-Half Reliability of a Leadership Potential Scale*

SUBJECT NUMBER	TOTAL SCORE	ODD-NUMBERS SCORE	EVEN-NUMBERS SCORE	
1	55	28	27	
2	49	26	23	
3	78	36	42	
4	37	18	19	
5	44	23	21	
6	50	30	20	
7	58	30	28	
8	62	33	29	
9	48	23	25	
10	67	28	39	$r = .67$

the test–retest approach. However, the split-half technique is handicapped by the fact that different reliability estimates can be obtained by using different "splits"; that is, it makes a difference whether one uses an odd–even split, a first half––second half split, or some other method of dividing the items into two groups. For this reason the split-half approach is increasingly being replaced by formulas that compensate for this deficiency.

The two most widely used methods are *coefficient alpha* (or *Cronbach's alpha*) and the *Kuder-Richardson formula 20* (abbreviated KR-20). It is beyond the scope of this text to explain in detail the application of these formulae. However, because coefficient alpha is perhaps the single most useful index of reliability available, the reader is urged to consult Cronbach (1984) or Nunnally (1978).*

Both the coefficient alpha and KR-20 produce a reliability coefficient that can be interpreted in the same fashion as other reliability coefficients described here. That is, the normal range of values is between 0.0 and +1.00, and higher values reflect a higher degree of internal consistency. Coefficient alpha (and KR-20, which is actually a special case of the more general coefficient alpha used with dichotomous items) is preferable to the split-half procedure because it gives an estimate of the split-half correlation for *all possible* ways of dividing the measure into two halves.

In summary, indices of homogeneity or internal consistency estimate the extent to which different subparts of an instrument are equivalent in terms of measuring the critical attribute. The split-half technique frequently has been used to estimate homogeneity, but the coefficient alpha is a preferable method. None of these approaches considers fluctuations over time as a source of unreliability.

Equivalence

A researcher may be interested in estimating the reliability of a measure by way of the *equivalence* approach under one of two circumstances: (1) when different observers or researchers are using an instrument to measure the same phenomena at the same time or (2) when two presumably parallel instruments are administered to individuals at about the same time. In both situations, the aim is to determine the consistency or equivalence of the instrument(s) in yielding measurements of the same traits in the same subjects.

In Chapter 16, "Observational Methods," it was pointed out that a potential weakness of this data collection approach is the fallibility of the observer. The greater the interpretive burden on the observer, the higher is the risk of observer error or bias. The accuracy of observer ratings and classifications can be enhanced by careful training, the development of clearly defined and nonoverlapping categories, the use of a small number of categories, and the use of behaviors that tend to be molecular rather than molar. Even when great care is taken to design an observational system that minimizes the possibility of error, the researcher should assess the reliability of the instrument. In this case, the instrument includes both the category system developed by the researcher and the observer making the measurements.

Interrater (or *interobserver*) *reliability* is estimated by having two or more trained observers watching some event simultaneously and independently recording the relevant variables according to a predetermined plan or coding system. The resulting records can then be used to compute an index of equivalence or agreement. Several procedures for arriving at such an index are possible. For certain types of observational data, correlation techniques may be suitable. That is, a correlation coefficient may be computed to

*The coefficient alpha equation, for the advanced student, is as follows:

$$r = \frac{k}{k-1}\left[1 - \frac{\Sigma \sigma_i^2}{\sigma y^2}\right]$$

where:

r = the estimated reliability

k = the total number of items in the test

σ_i^2 = the variance of each individual item

σy^2 = the variance of the total test scores

Σ = the sum of

demonstrate the strength of the relationship between one observer's ratings and another's.

Another procedure is to compute reliability as a function of agreements, using the following equation:

$$\frac{\text{Number of agreements}}{\text{Number of agreements + disagreements}}$$

This simple formula unfortunately tends to overestimate observer agreements. If the behavior under investigation is one that observers code for absence or presence every, say, 10 seconds, then by chance alone the observers will agree 50% of the time. Other approaches for estimating interrater reliability may be of interest to advanced students. Guilford (1964) has described the use of such techniques as analysis of variance, intraclass correlations, and rank-order correlations to assess the reliability of observational measures.

The second situation in which the equivalence of measures is evaluated is when two alternative, parallel forms of a single instrument are available. This type of research problem is unlikely to present itself frequently in nursing research, except perhaps in an educational context. For example, alternate forms of a test of nursing knowledge might be needed. In such a case, the two forms should be administered to a sample of individuals in immediate succession, randomly alternating the order of presentation of the forms. The correlation coefficient between the two sets of scores would be an index of reliability of equivalence. This procedure is adopted to determine whether the two instruments are, in fact, measuring the same attribute. The researcher uses this technique to assess the errors of measurement resulting from errors in item sampling.

Interpretation of Reliability Coefficients

The reliability coefficients computed according to the procedures just described can be used as an important indicator of the quality of an instrument. A measure that is unreliable interferes with an adequate testing of a researcher's hypotheses. If data fail to confirm a research prediction, one possibility is that the measuring tools were unreliable—not necessarily that the expected relationships do not exist. There is no standard for what an acceptable reliability coefficient should be. If a researcher is only interested in making group-level comparisons, then coefficients in the vicinity of .70 or even .60 would probably be sufficient. By group-level comparisons, we mean that the investigator is interested in comparing the scores of such groups as male versus female, nurse versus physician, smoker versus nonsmoker, and so forth. However, if measures were to be used as a basis for making decisions about individuals, then the reliability coefficient should be .90 or better. For instance, if a score on a test were to be used as a criterion for admission to a graduate nursing program, then the accuracy of the test is of critical importance to both individual applicants and the school of nursing.

The reliability coefficient has a special interpretation that should be briefly explained without elaborating on technical details. This interpretation relates to the earlier discussion of decomposing an observed score into an error and true component. Suppose that we have just administered to 50 nurses a scale that measures empathy. It would be expected that the scores would vary from one nurse to another, because some nurses are more empathic than others. Some of the variability in scores is "true" variability, reflecting real individual differences in the attribute being measured; some of the variability, however, is error. Thus,

$$V_O = V_T + V_E$$

where V_O = observed total variability in scores
V_T = true variability
V_E = variability owing to random errors

A reliability coefficient is directly associated with this equation. *Reliability is the proportion of true variability to the total obtained variability,* or

$$r = \frac{V_T}{V_O}$$

If, for example, the reliability coefficient were .85, then 85% of the variability in obtained scores could be said to represent "true" individual differences, and 15% of the variability would reflect random, extraneous fluctuations. Looked at in this way, it should be a bit clearer why instruments with reliabilities of .60 or lower are risky to use.

Knowledge of the reliability of an instrument is useful to researchers not only because it helps them to interpret results, but also because it suggests whether modifications to the instrument are necessary. Instrument developers should be aware of the following issues in improving their measures:

- The reliability of psychosocial scales is partly a function of their length or number of items. To improve the reliability, more items tapping the same concept should be added.
- In observational scales, reliability can often be improved by greater precision in the definitions associated with a category system or through increased observer training.
- The reliability of an instrument is related in part to the heterogeneity of the sample with which it is used. The more homogeneous the sample (i.e., the more similar their scores), the lower the reliability coefficient will be. This is because instruments are designed to measure differences among those being measured. If the sample is homogeneous, then it is more difficult for the instrument to reliably discriminate among those who possess varying degrees of the attribute being measured.

- Reliability estimates vary according to the procedure used to obtain them. The researcher should determine the aspect of reliability (stability, internal consistency, or equivalence) that is most relevant to the attribute and instrument under consideration.

Table 18-3 illustrates different forms of reliability evaluations that nurse researchers have used to assess instruments that they or others developed.

≡ VALIDITY

The second important criterion by which an instrument's psychometric adequacy is evaluated is its validity. *Validity* refers to the degree to which an instrument measures what it is sup-

Table 18-3. *Examples of Reliability Assessments by Nurse Researchers*

INSTRUMENT	TYPE OF RELIABILITY	RELIABILITY COEFFICIENT	REFERENCE
Quality of Life Scale (QOLS)— a 15-item self-report scale	Test–retest (3 weeks) Test–retest (6 weeks) Cronbach's alpha	.84 .76 .89	Burckhardt et al., 1989
Health-Related Hardiness Scale (HRHS)—a 34-item self-report scale	Test–retest (6 months) Cronbach's alpha	.76 .91	Pollock & Duffy, 1990
Chronic Pain Experience Instrument (CPEI)—a 16-item self-report scale	Test–retest (2 weeks) Cronbach's alpha	.77 .89	Davis, 1989
Digital test for pelvic muscle strength—an observational rating scale	Test–retest (6 weeks) Interrater reliability	.65 .90	Brink et al., 1989
Oral Assessment Guide—an observational rating scale	Interrater reliability	.91	Eilers et al., 1988

posed to be measuring. When an instrument to measure nurses' "burnout" has been developed, how can its designer really know that the resulting scores validly reflect "burnout" and not some other concept, such as job satisfaction? Problems of validity relate to the question, Are we really measuring the attribute we think we are measuring?

Like reliability, validity has a number of different aspects and assessment approaches. Unlike reliability, however, the validity of an instrument is extremely difficult to establish. Solid evidence supporting the validity of most psychologically oriented measures is rarely available. There are no formulas or equations that can easily be applied to the scores of the hypothetical "burnout" scale to estimate how good a job the scale is doing in measuring the critical variable.

The reliability and validity of an instrument are not totally independent qualities of an instrument. *A measuring device that is unreliable cannot possibly be valid.* An instrument cannot validly be measuring the attribute of interest if it is erratic, inconsistent, and inaccurate. An unreliable tool would be "measuring" too many other factors associated with random error to be considered a valid indicator of the target variable. However, an instrument can be reliable without being valid. Suppose we had the idea to measure anxiety in patients by measuring the circumference of their wrists. We could obtain highly accurate, consistent, and precise measurements of the wrist circumferences, but such measures would not be valid indicators of anxiety. Thus, the high reliability of an instrument provides no evidence of its validity for an intended purpose; the low reliability of a measure *is* evidence of low validity.

The methodological literature abounds with terms relating to different facets of the validity question. The classification system adopted here focuses on three types of validity: (1) content, (2) criterion-related, and (3) construct validity.

Content Validity

Content validity is concerned with the sampling adequacy of the content area being meas-

ured. Content validity is of most relevance to individuals designing a test to measure knowledge in a specific content area. In such a context, the validity question being asked is, How representative are the questions on this test of the universe of all questions that might be asked on this topic? Suppose we were interested in testing the knowledge of a group of lay people concerning the seven danger signals of cancer identified by the American Cancer Society. To be representative, or content valid, the questions on the test would have to include items from each of the seven danger signals or "CAUTION":

*C*hange in bowel or bladder habits
A sore that does not heal
*U*nusual bleeding or discharge
*T*hickening or lump in breast or elsewhere
*I*ndigestion or difficulty in swallowing
*O*bvious change in wart or mole
*N*agging cough or hoarseness

The issue of content validity sometimes arises in conjunction with measures of attributes other than knowledge, such as in attitudinal measures. For example, Frank-Stromberg (1989) made efforts to incorporate features of content validity in developing her Reaction to the Diagnosis of Cancer Questionnaire. She began by asking 340 cancer patients the following open-ended question: "What do you remember of your feelings when first told you had cancer?" Prevalent themes that emerged in the responses to this question were then incorporated into items in the scale, thus reflecting the major content areas experienced by cancer patients.

The content validity of an instrument is necessarily based on judgment. There are no completely objective methods of assuring the adequate content coverage of an instrument. Experts in the content area may be called on to analyze the items to see if they represent adequately the hypothetical content universe in the correct proportions. The researcher developing a test or scale, in writing or selecting items for inclusion in an instrument, should aim to build in content validity by careful planning and the careful execution of a prespecified plan.

Criterion-related Validity

The *criterion-related* approach to validity assessment is a pragmatic one. The researcher attempting to establish the criterion-related validity of an instrument is not seeking to ascertain how well the tool is measuring a particular theoretical trait. The emphasis is on establishing the relationship between the instrument and some other criterion. The instrument, whatever abstract attribute it is measuring, is said to be valid if its scores correlate highly with some criterion. For example, if a measure of birth control use among sexually active teenage girls correlates highly with subsequent premarital pregnancies, then the birth control measure could be described as having good validity. In terms of the criterion-related validation approach, the key issue is whether the instrument is a useful predictor of subsequent behaviors, experiences, or conditions.

The essential component of the criterion-related approach to validation is the availability of a reasonably reliable and valid criterion with which the measures on the target instrument can be compared. This is, unfortunately, seldom easy. If we were developing an instrument to predict the nursing effectiveness of nursing students, we might use subsequent supervisory ratings as our criterion. However, how can we be sure that these ratings are themselves valid and reliable? In fact, the supervisory ratings might themselves be in need of validation. Usually the researcher must be content with less than perfect criteria.

Once the criterion is selected, the validity can be assessed easily and straightforwardly. The scores on the "predictor" instrument are correlated with scores on the criterion variable. The magnitude of the correlation coefficient is a direct estimate of how valid the instrument is, according to this method of validation. To illustrate, suppose a team of nurse researchers developed a scale to measure professionalism among nurses. They administer the instrument to a sample of nurses and at the same time ask the nurses to indicate how many articles they have published. The publications variable was chosen as one of many potential objective criteria of professionalism. Fictitious data are presented in Table 18-4. The correlation coefficient of .83 indicates that the "professionalism scale" is a reasonably good predictor of the number of published articles a nurse has written. Whether the scale is really measuring professionalism is a somewhat different issue—an issue that is the concern of construct validation discussed in the next section.

Sometimes a distinction is made between two types of criterion-related validity. The distinction is not a very important one, but the terms are used frequently enough to warrant their mention.

Table 18-4. *Fictitious Data for Criterion-Related Validity Example*

SUBJECT	SCORE ON PROFESSIONALISM SCALE	NUMBER OF PUBLICATIONS	
1	25	2	
2	30	4	
3	17	0	
4	20	1	
5	22	0	
6	27	2	
7	29	5	
8	19	1	
9	28	3	
10	15	1	$r = .83$

Predictive validity refers to the adequacy of an instrument in differentiating between the performance or behaviors of individuals on some future criterion. When a school of nursing correlates the incoming Scholastic Aptitude Test (SAT) scores of students with subsequent grade point averages, the predictive validity of the SATs for nursing school performance is being evaluated. *Concurrent validity* refers to the ability of an instrument to distinguish individuals who differ in their present status on some criterion. For example, a psychologic test to differentiate between those patients in a mental institution who can and cannot be released could be correlated with current behavioral ratings of health-care personnel. The difference between predictive and concurrent validity, then, is the difference in the timing of obtaining measurements on a criterion.

Validation by means of the criterion-related approach is most often used in applied or practically oriented research. Criterion-related validity is helpful in assisting decision makers by giving them some assurance that their decisions will be effective, fair, and, in short, valid.

Construct Validity

Validating an instrument in terms of *construct validity* is one of the most difficult and challenging tasks that a researcher faces. The instrument designer adopting this approach is concerned with the questions, What is this measuring device really measuring? Is the abstract concept under investigation being adequately measured with this instrument? Unlike criterion-related validity, construct validity is more concerned with the underlying attribute than with the scores that the instrument produces. The scores are of interest only insofar as they constitute a valid basis for inferring the degree to which a subject possesses some characteristic. Unfortunately, the more abstract the concept, the more difficult it is to establish the construct validity of the measure; at the same time, the more abstract the concept, the less suitable it is to validate a measure by the criterion-related approach. Actually, it is really not just a question of suitability, but also of feasibility. What

objective criterion is there for such concepts as empathy, grief, role conflict, or separation anxiety?

Despite the obstacles and difficulties encountered in assessing the construct validity of instruments, this activity is a vital component of scientific progress. The constructs in which scientists are interested must be measured, and they must be reliably and validly measured. The significance of construct validity is in its linkage with theory and theoretical conceptualization. In validating a measure of death anxiety, we would probably be less concerned with the adequate sampling of items or in relating the resultant scores to a criterion than with the extent to which the measure corresponds to a theory of death anxiety that is acceptable to us.

Construct validation can be approached in several ways, but there is always an emphasis on logical analysis and the testing of relationships predicated on the basis of theoretical considerations. Constructs are usually explicated in terms of other concepts; therefore, the researcher should be in a position to make predictions about the manner in which the construct will function in relation to other constructs. One common approach to construct validation is the *known-groups technique*. In this procedure, groups that are expected to differ on the critical attribute because of some known characteristic are administered the instrument. For instance, in validating a measure of fear of the labor experience, one might contrast the scores of primiparas and multiparas. Because one would expect that women who had never given birth would experience more fears and anxiety than women who had already had children, one might question the validity of the instrument if such differences did not emerge. There is not necessarily an expectation that the differences would be very great. It would be expected that some primiparas would feel no anxiety at all, and some multiparas would express some fears. On the whole, however, it would be anticipated that some group differences would be reflected in the scores. As another example of the known-groups technique, consider the example of validating a measure concerning limitations in functional ability. One might choose people with emphysema and people without emphysema to validate the instrument. The validity of the instrument might be questioned if differences in scores between the two groups did not occur, because one would expect that people with emphysema would have experienced limitations in functional ability.

A significant advance in the area of construct validation is the procedure developed by Campbell and Fiske (1959) known as the *multitrait–multimethod matrix method.* This procedure makes use of the concepts of convergence and discriminability. *Convergence* refers to evidence that different methods of measuring a construct yield similar results. Different approaches to measurement should converge on the construct. *Discriminability* refers to the ability to differentiate the construct being measured from other similar constructs. Campbell and Fiske argued that evidence of both convergence and discriminability should be brought to bear in the construct validity question.

To help explain the multitrait–multimethod approach, fictitious data from a study to validate a "need for autonomy" measure are presented in Table 18-5. In using this approach, the researcher must measure the critical concept by two or more methods. Suppose we measured "need for autonomy" in a sample of graduate nursing students by having the students respond to a self-report sum-

mated rating scale (the measure we are attempting to validate); having nursing faculty rate each student after observing the student in a task designed to elicit different degrees of autonomy; and having the students write out stories in response to a pictorial (projective) stimulus depicting an autonomy-relevant situation. A second requirement of the multitrait–multimethod approach is that we must also measure constructs from which we wish to differentiate the key construct, using the same measuring methods. In the current example, suppose that we decided to differentiate "need for autonomy" from "need for affiliation." The two concepts are related: one would expect, on the average, that people who exhibited a high degree of "need for autonomy" would be relatively low in terms of "need for affiliation." The point of including both concepts in a single validation study is to gather evidence that the two concepts are, in fact, distinct rather than two different labels for the same underlying attribute.

The numbers in Table 18-5 represent the correlation coefficients between the scores on the six different measures (two traits × three methods). For instance, the coefficient of −.38 at the intersection of A1−B1 expresses the relationship between the self-report scores on the need for autonomy and need for affiliation measures. It will be recalled that a minus sign before the correlation coefficient signifies an inverse relation-

Table 18-5. *Multitrait–Multimethod Matrix*

		METHOD 1		METHOD 2		METHOD 3	
Method	*Traits*	A_1	B_1	A_2	B_2	A_3	B_3
Method 1	A_1	(.88)					
	B_1	−.38	(.86)				
Method 2	A_2	.60	−.19	(.79)			
	B_2	−.21	.58	−.39	(.80)		
Method 3	A_3	.51	−.13	.55	−.12	(.74)	
	B_3	−.14	.49	−.17	.54	−.32	(.72)

Traits: A, need for autonomy trait; B, need for affiliation trait.
Methods: 1, self-report summated scale; 2, observational rating; 3, projective test.

ship. In this case, the − .38 tells us that there was a slight tendency for people scoring high on the need for autonomy scale to score low on the need for affiliation scale. The numbers in parentheses along the diagonal of this matrix are the reliability coefficients.

Various aspects of the multitrait–multimethod matrix have a bearing on the construct validity question. The most direct evidence (convergence) comes from the correlations between two different methods for measuring the same trait. In the case of A1–A2, the coefficient is .60, which is reasonably substantial. Convergent validity should be sufficiently large to encourage further scrutiny of the matrix. Second, the convergent validity entries should be higher (in terms of absolute magnitude*) than those correlations between measures that have neither method nor trait in common. That is, A1–A2 should be greater than A2–B1 or A1–B2. Inspection of the table reveals that, indeed, .60 surpasses the "heterotrait–heteromethod" values of − .21 and − .19. This requirement is a minimum one which, if failed, should cause the researcher to have serious doubts about the validity of the measures. Third, the convergent validity coefficients should be greater than the coefficients between measures of different traits by a single method. Once again, the matrix in Table 18-5 fulfills this criterion: A1–A2 (.60) and A2–A3 (.55) are higher than A1–B1 (− .38), A2–B2 (− .39) and A3–B3 (− .32). The last two requirements provide some evidence for discriminant validity.

The multitrait–multimethod approach can be extended to include more traits and more methods. The difficulty is in administering a large number of measures to a sample of subjects. Also, the evidence is seldom as clear-cut as in this contrived example and, therefore, additional measures may create undesirable confusion. The full matrix as exemplified in Table 18-5 represents a valuable and perhaps unparalleled tool for exploring the validity of instruments. The re-

searcher should not abandon attempts to utilize the concepts underlying the procedure even when the full model is not feasible. Perhaps in some cases only an A1–B1 type of combination is possible, whereas in others, A1–A2–A3 would be manageable. Without any doubt, the execution of any portion of the model is better than no effort to estimate construct validity, and generally is preferable to a content validity approach for the great majority of concepts of interest to nursing researchers.

In addition to the known-groups technique and the multitrait–multimethod procedure there are other approaches to construct validation. For example, many researchers assess an instrument's construct validity through predictive modeling or by examining relationships based on theory, which are really variants of the known-groups approach. A researcher might reason as follows:

- according to theory, construct X is positively related to construct Y;
- instrument A is a measure of construct X and instrument B is a measure of construct Y;
- scores on A and B are correlated positively, as predicted by the theory;
- therefore, it is inferred that A and B are valid measures of X and Y.

This logical analysis is fallible and does not constitute proof of construct validity but is important as a type of evidence, nevertheless.

Another approach to construct validation employs a statistical procedure known as factor analysis. Although factor analysis, which will be discussed in Chapter 22, is computationally complex, it is conceptually rather simple. *Factor analysis* is essentially a method for identifying clusters of related variables. Each cluster, called a *factor,* represents a relatively unitary attribute. The procedure is used to identify and group together different measures of some underlying attribute. In effect, factor analysis constitutes another means of looking at the convergent and discriminant validity of a large set of measures.

In summary, construct validation uses both logical and empirical procedures. Like content

---

*The absolute magnitude refers to the value without a plus or minus sign. A value of − .50 is of a higher absolute magnitude than + .40.

validity, construct validity requires a judgment pertaining to what the instrument is measuring. Unlike content validity, however, the logical operations required by construct validation are typically linked to a theory or conceptual framework. Construct and criterion-related validity share an empirical component, but in criterion-related validity there is usually a pragmatic, objective criterion with which to compare a measure, rather than a second measure of an abstract theoretical construct.

Interpretation of Validity

Like reliability, validity is not an all-or-nothing characteristic of an instrument. An instrument cannot really be said to possess or lack validity; it is a question of degree. Furthermore, although we have referred to the process of testing the validity of an instrument as "validation," it is inappropriate to speak of the process as yielding proof of validity. Like all tests of hypotheses, the testing of an instrument's validity is not "proved," "established," or "verified," but rather supported to a greater or lesser degree by evidence.

Strictly speaking, a researcher does not validate the instrument *per se* but rather some application of the instrument. A measure of anxiety may be valid for presurgical patients on the day before an operation but may not be valid for nursing students on the morning of a final examination. Of course, some instruments may be valid for a wide range of uses with different types of samples, but each use requires new supporting evidence. In a sense, validation is a never-ending process. The more evidence that can be gathered that an instrument is measuring what it is supposed to be measuring, the more confidence researchers will have in its validity.

Nurse researchers have become increasingly sophisticated in assessing the validity of measures. Table 18-6 presents some examples of measures that have been subjected to a validation process by nurse researchers.

Table 18-6. *Examples of Validity Assessments by Nurse Researchers*

INSTRUMENT	TYPE OF VALIDITY	PROCEDURE	REFERENCE
The UCLA Loneliness Scale	Construct	Factor analysis Theoretical modeling	Mahon & Yarcheski, 1990
What Being the Parent of a New Baby is Like Scale-Revised (WPL-R)	Construct	Factor analysis Known groups Theoretical modeling	Pridham & Chang, 1989
	Content	Open-ended questions to target group	
MS-Related Symptom Checklist	Content	Review by experts	Gulick, 1989
	Criterion	Prediction of level of functioning	
	Construct	Factor analysis Theoretical modeling	
McCloskey-Mueller Satisfaction Scale	Construct	Factor analysis Theoretical modeling	Mueller & McCloskey, 1990
	Criterion	Scores on other satisfaction scales	
Clinical Neurological Assessment Tool	Construct	Factor analysis	Crosby & Parsons, 1989
	Criterion	Scores on Glasgow Coma Scale	

≡ *OTHER CRITERIA FOR ASSESSING MEASURES*

Reliability and validity are the two most important aspects to consider in evaluating a measuring instrument. If a measure can be shown to be reasonably reliable and valid for a specific purpose, then the researcher can have some assurance that the results of a study will be meaningful. High reliability and validity are a necessary, though insufficient, condition for good scientific research.

Sometimes a researcher needs to consider other qualities of an instrument in addition to its validity and reliability. These additional criteria are by no means a substitute for reliability and validity but may in some cases be equally important. Indeed, several of these qualities are directly related to the issues raised in the preceding two sections. In many research situations, however, the criteria discussed as follows may be irrelevant or unimportant.

Efficiency

Instruments of comparable reliability and validity may still differ in their efficiency. An instrument that requires 10 minutes of a subject's time to measure his or her coping capacity is efficient in comparison with an instrument to measure the same attribute that requires 30 minutes to complete. One aspect of efficiency is the number of items incorporated in an instrument. Long instruments tend to be more reliable than shorter ones. There is, however, a point of diminishing returns. As an example, consider a 40-item scale to measure feelings of guilt among parents of handicapped children. Let us say that we find a reliability of .94 for the scale, using coefficient alpha as our index of internal consistency. Using the Spearman-Brown formula, we can estimate how reliable the scale would be with only 30 items:

$$r^1 = \frac{kr}{1 + [(1 - k)r]} = \frac{.75\,(.94)}{1 - [.25\,(.94)]} = .92,$$

where k is the factor by which the instrument is being incremented or decreased; in this case, $k = 30 \div 40 = .75$.

As this calculation shows, a 25% reduction in the length of the instrument resulted in this case in a negligible decrease in reliability, from .94 to .92. Most researchers probably would be willing to sacrifice a modest amount of reliability in exchange for the opportunity to substantially reduce the subjects' response burden.

Efficiency is more characteristic of certain types of data collection procedures than others. In a questionnaire or interview, closed-ended questions are more efficient than open-ended items. Self-report scales tend to be less time consuming than projective instruments for a comparable amount of information. Of course, a researcher may decide that other advantages (such as depth of information) offset a certain degree of inefficiency. Other things being equal, however, it is desirable to select as efficient an instrument as possible.

Sensitivity

The sensitivity of an instrument affects how small a variation in an attribute can be reliably detected and measured. A yardstick marked off with only three divisions for feet would result in a highly insensitive measure of a person's height. The yardstick could be made more sensitive to variations in height by subdividing each foot into 12 equal sections for inches, and the process could be continued until a sufficiently sensitive measuring tool were obtained for the purposes needed. Unfortunately, it is not quite this easy to increase the sensitivity of most instruments.

The sensitivity of an instrument determines how discriminating its measurements will be between individuals with differing amounts of an attribute. Using the yardstick marked off in feet only, it would be impossible to discriminate between a person who is 5'8" tall and one who is 6'3" tall: both would be measured as 6', measuring to the nearest foot. There are statistical procedures that permit a researcher to enhance the sensitivity of paper-and-pencil measures by assessing the degree to which each item is contributing to the instrument's power to make discriminations. These *item analysis techniques* are described in detail in texts on measurement and psychometric theory. Several references are noted at the end of this chapter.

The sensitivity of an instrument is most likely to become an issue in certain kinds of situations. When changes in the level of an attribute are being closely monitored, as in the case of many physiologic measurements, then it is important to use a sensitive device. If important decisions are to be based on the measures resulting from an instrument, then the sensitivity of the instrument could have serious consequences. Experimenters must also be concerned with the sensitivity of measuring tools whenever the treatments they are introducing are not markedly different from their control conditions. In the nursing research literature, there are many examples of studies in which differences between conditions were not detected. Part of the difficulty in many nursing intervention studies is that new interventions are compared with older interventions, rather than with no intervention at all. When experimental and control conditions are not maximally different—as must often be the case in nursing research—then highly sensitive instruments may be required to detect differences in the effects of the treatments.

Other Criteria

There is no need to elaborate in detail on the few remaining qualities that should be considered in assessing a measuring tool. Most of the following ten criteria are actually aspects of the reliability/validity issues:

1. *Objectivity.* There should be as little room as possible for disagreements between two or more independent researchers applying the instrument to measure the same phenomenon.
2. *Comprehensibility.* The subject or the researcher should be able to comprehend the behaviors required to secure accurate and valid measures.
3. *Balance.* The instrument designer should strive for a balanced measure to minimize response set biases and to facilitate content validity.
4. *Speededness.* For most types of instruments, the researcher should be sure that adequate time is allowed to obtain complete measurements without rushing the measuring process.
5. *Unidimensionality.* A measuring tool should be designed to produce separate scores for unitary, isolatable concepts.
6. *Range.* The instrument should be capable of achieving a meaningful measure from the smallest expected value of the variable to the largest.
7. *Linearity.* A researcher normally strives to construct measures that are equally accurate and sensitive over the entire range of values.
8. *Signal-to-noise ratio.* In physiologic measures, it is important to use instruments and procedures that maximize the signal reading and minimize the interference noise.
9. *Reactivity.* The instrument should, insofar as possible, avoid affecting the attribute that is being measured.
10. *Simplicity.* Other things being equal, a simple instrument is more desirable than a complex instrument inasmuch as complicated measures run a greater risk of having errors.

It is probably fair to say that the development of adequate measuring tools is the single most pressing problem in the field of nursing research—as it is in such fields as education, psychology, sociology, and other disciplines concerned with human behavior. One of the greatest challenges facing this generation of nurse researchers is the construction and utilization of reliable, valid, and sensitive criterion measures of outcomes of relevance to nursing. Given the improbability of ever finding *the* perfect criterion measure, researchers should often use *multiple criterion measures,* each of whose measurement strengths complement one another.

≡ *ASSESSMENT OF QUALITATIVE DATA COLLECTION METHODS*

The methods of assessment described in this chapter apply primarily to structured data collection instruments that yield quantitative scores. For the most part, these procedures cannot be meaningfully applied to such qualitative materials as unstructured interview responses or narrative descriptions from a participant observer's field notes. However, this does not imply that qualitative researchers are unconcerned with the concepts of reliability and validity. The central question underlying the two concepts is this: Do the data collected by the researcher reflect the "truth"? Certainly, qualitative researchers are as eager as quantitative researchers to have their findings reflect the true state of human experience. (Indeed, some qualitative researchers argue that their techniques are superior to others in their ability to really shed light on human behavior and experience.)

Although qualitative methodologists have been less concerned with the issues of reliability and validity than quantitative methodologists, there is a growing interest in addressing these issues. Among the various strategies recommended, perhaps the most important rest on a principle known as triangulation. *Triangulation* refers to the use of multiple referents to draw conclusions about what constitutes the "truth."

Denzin (1989) has identified four basic types of triangulation:

Data triangulation: The use of multiple data sources in a study (e.g., interviewing multiple key informants about the same topic).

Investigator triangulation: The use of multiple individuals to collect and analyze a single set of data.

Theory triangulation: The use of multiple perspectives to interpret a single set of data.

Methodological triangulation: The use of multiple methods to address a research problem (e.g., observation, interviews, or inspection of documents).

The purpose of using triangulation is to provide a basis for convergence on truth. In other words, by using multiple methods and perspectives, it is hoped that "true" information can be sorted out from "error" information. In the final analysis, this is not conceptually different from the process of estimating reliability and validity by quantitative researchers. The reader interested in a further discussion of reliability and validity in qualitative research would be well-advised to consult LeCompte and Goetz (1982) or Kirk and Miller (1985).

≡ *FACTORS TO CONSIDER IN SELECTING MEASURING TOOLS*

In Part IV of this book, we have discussed a number of different methods for measuring concepts of interest to nurse researchers. These methods have varied with regard to type of measurement approach—self-report, observational method, biophysiologic measure, projective technique, and so on. We have also noted that data collection methods vary along several dimensions, such as structure, quantifiability, researcher obtrusiveness, and objectivity. All of these aspects of measures must be considered in selecting an approach that will yield the best possible information for a specific research problem.

In this chapter, we have discussed other factors to consider in developing a data collection strategy. Researchers should strive to use a measurement approach that will yield valid and reliable indicators of the constructs being studied. Thus, one important task in selecting measures for a study is to search for evidence of the psychometric adequacy of measures under consideration.

However, the selection of a specific measure is rarely based exclusively on the basis of a psychometric assessment. Many other factors may guide the choice of measures. Below are six issues that often affect the researcher's decisions in designing a data collection plan.

1. *Resources.* Resource constraints sometimes make it impossible to use "ideal" measures.

Costs may be associated with the measure directly (e.g., some psychologic tests must be purchased from publishers). Costs are often associated with the length of time required to administer the measure, if research personnel must be paid to collect the data. Also, if the data collection procedures are considered burdensome, it may be necessary to pay a respondent stipend. All of the associated costs of data collection should be carefully considered, especially if the use of time-consuming or expensive measures means that the investigator will be forced to cut costs elsewhere (e.g., by using a smaller sample).

2. *Availability and familiarity.* In selecting measures, the researcher may want to consider how readily available or accessible various tools are, especially if they are biophysiologic in nature. Relatedly, data collection strategies with which the researcher is familiar or has had experience are generally preferable to new measures because administration is generally smoother and more efficient in such cases.

3. *Norms and comparability.* A researcher may find it desirable to select a measure for which there are relevant norms. *Norms* indicate the "normal" values and distribution of values on the measure with respect to a specified population. For example, most standardized tests (such as the SAT) have national norms. The availability of norms is often useful because they offer, in essence, a built-in comparison group. For similar reasons, a researcher may decide that it is useful to adopt a specific instrument because it was used in other similar studies and therefore offers a supplementary basis for putting the study findings in context. Indeed, when a study is a replication by intention, it often becomes essential to use the same instruments as were used in the original study, even if higher quality measures are available.

4. *Administration issues.* An important consideration often relates to the instrument's requirements for obtaining valid and accurate

measures. For example, in obtaining information about the developmental status of children, the researcher might want to consider whether the administration of a given measure requires the skills of a professional psychologist or whether a "lay" interviewer with adequate training can obtain high-quality data. Another administration issue concerns constraints on where the data must be collected. Certain instruments may require or assume stringent conditions with regard to the time of administration, privacy of the setting, and so on. In such a case, requirements for obtaining valid measures must match the characteristics of the intended research setting.

5. *Population appropriateness.* The measure should be chosen with the characteristics of the target population in mind. Characteristics of special importance include the age of the subjects, their intellectual abilities or reading skills, and their cultural or ethnic background. If the subjects include members of minority groups, the measures should not be culturally biased, to the extent possible, especially if racial or ethnic comparisons would be made. If non–English-speaking subjects are included in the sample, then the selection of a measure may be based, in part, on the availability of a translated version of the measure.

6. *Reputation.* Instruments designed to measure the same construct often differ in the kinds of reputations they enjoy among specialists working in a field, even if they are comparable with regard to psychometric qualities. Therefore, a researcher selecting an instrument should seek the advice of knowledgeable individuals, preferably ones with personal, direct experience in using the instruments.

In summary, the selection of appropriate measures for a research project is a challenging task that involves the consideration of many theoretical, methodological, and practical factors, as well as ethical ones. It is a task to which researchers should devote considerable attention, diligence, and creativity.

≡ RESEARCH EXAMPLE

Phillips and colleagues (1989) developed an instrument designed to identify caregivers who are at high risk of providing poor-quality care to a dependent elderly person in the home: the Beliefs About Caregiving Scale (BACS).

The instrument was developed on the basis of a theoretical model that emerged in a qualitative study of family caregivers. Concepts and themes that were discovered in the qualitative study formed the basis for the construction of items. The five major constructs were (1) Monitoring, (2) Testing, (3) Assessing/Nurturing, (4) Enmeshment, and (5) Dogmatism. A separate subscale of the BACS was developed for each of these constructs.

The original version of the BACS consisted of 98 Likert-type items with four response alternatives. Examples of items included the following: Punishing the elder when he or she deliberately makes a mess is something a caregiver must do (Monitoring); A caregiver has the responsibility of making sure the elder does not embarrass himself or herself (Assessing); and, The way an elder looks is a reflection of the caregiver (Enmeshment).

Four studies were undertaken to refine and test the BACS. Each of the first three studies involved three stages of psychometric testing. In stage 1 of study 1, the internal consistency (estimated using Cronbach's alpha) for the total scale was greater than .80, but the subscale reliability estimates were all below .70. In stage 2, item analysis procedures were used to delete items that did not contribute to internal consistency or stability. This process yielded a 47-item instrument that had an alpha of .89 and a test–retest coefficient of .72. In stage 3, the subscales were reconstructed using a procedure known as *cluster analysis,* a statistical technique that is similar to factor analysis. This analysis revealed that no discrete dogmatism subscale emerged; a four-subscale structure was supported by the analysis.

The alphas for the four subscales were found to be low, leading the researchers to undertake steps to improve the internal consistency in later studies. For example, for study 3, all items were rewritten to reflect a more personalized view of caregiving. For example, the item from the Monitoring Subscale previously cited was changed to the following: "Punishing my elder when s/he deliberately makes a mess is something I must do." These and other refinements in the first three studies led to the final version of the BACS, which had 28 items and (as determined by a factor analysis) two subscales (Testing/Monitoring and Assessing/Nurturing). The reliability of the total final scale was .89 and the two subscales had alphas that exceeded .80.

Study 4 focused on the construct validity of the BACS. The researchers administered the BACS and several other scales to a sample of subjects and constructed a multitrait–monomethod (only one method of assessment) matrix. The other scales included such measures as dogmatism, adaptability, social desirability, and depression. This analysis provided evidence for the construct validity of the BACS, particularly for the Monitoring Subscale and the total BACS. The researchers concluded that the scale may be useful for identifying caregivers at high risk of providing poor-quality care.

These researchers demonstrated extreme diligence in assessing the psychometric adequacy of their instrument and of taking incremental steps to improve it. Efforts such as these will benefit other researchers and clinical staff by increasing their confidence in the scale's usefulness.

≡ SUMMARY

Few, if any, measuring instruments used by researchers are pure or infallible. *Obtained scores*—that is, the actual measurements obtained through the administration of the instruments—can be decomposed into two parts—(1) a true score and (2) an error component. The *true score* is a hypothetical entity that represents the value that would be obtained if it were possible to arrive at a "perfect" measure. The error component, or *error of measurement,* represents the inaccuracies present in the measurement process. Sources of measurement error include situational contaminants, response set biases, transitory personal factors, and several others.

One important characteristic of a measuring tool is its *reliability,* which refers to the degree of consistency or accuracy with which an instrument measures an attribute. The higher the reliability of an instrument, the lower the amount of error present in the obtained scores. Several empirical methods assess various aspects of an instrument's reliability. The *stability* aspect, which concerns the extent to which the instrument yields the same results on repeated administrations, is evaluated by *test–retest* procedures. The *internal consistency* or *homogeneity* aspect of reliability refers to the extent to which all of the instrument's subparts or items are measuring the same attribute. Internal consistency may be evaluated using either the *split-half reliability* technique or *Cronbach's alpha* method. When the focus of a reliability assessment is on establishing *equivalence* between observers in rating behaviors, estimates of *interrater reliability* may be obtained. The reliability of an instrument is partly a function of its length, the adequacy of the sampling of items, the heterogeneity of the groups to which the instrument was administered, and the procedure used for obtaining the reliability estimate. Most of the methods of estimating reliability rely on the calculation of a *reliability coefficient,* an index that reflects the proportion of true variability in a set of scores to the total obtained variability. Reliability coefficients generally range in value from a low of .00 to 1.00, with higher values reflecting increased reliability.

Validity refers to the degree to which an instrument measures what it is supposed to be measuring. *Content validity* is concerned with the sampling adequacy of the content being measured. *Criterion-related validity* focuses on the relationship or correlation between the instrument and some outside criterion. *Construct validity* refers to the adequacy of an instrument in measuring the abstract construct of interest. One approach to assessing the construct validity of a measuring tool is the *known groups technique,* which contrasts the scores of groups that are presumed to differ on the attribute. Another construct validity approach is the *multitrait–multimethod matrix* technique, which is based on the concepts of convergence and discriminability. *Convergence* refers to evidence that different methods of measuring the same attribute yield similar results. *Discriminability* refers to the ability to differentiate the construct being measured from other similar concepts.

Although high reliability and validity are essential criteria for assessing the quality of an instrument, other characteristics of the tool may also be important. Other criteria for evaluating a measuring tool include its efficiency, sensitivity, objectivity, comprehensibility, balance, speededness, unidimensionality, range, linearity, signal-to-noise ratio, frequency response, reactivity, and simplicity.

Triangulation is the process most frequently used to establish the worth of qualitative data collection approaches. Four types of triangulation have been identified: (1) data triangulation, (2) investigator triangulation, (3) theoretical triangulation, and (4) methodological triangulation. Given the fallibility of data collection methods, the use of *multiple criterion measures* (a form of methodological triangulation) is being increasingly advocated. Such triangulation might profitably involve the use of both qualitative and quantitative methods in a single study.

In selecting a data collection strategy, the researcher is guided by numerous considerations. In addition to the *psychometric adequacy* of a measuring tool (i.e., evidence of its validity and reliability), the researcher may be guided by such factors as cost constraints, accessibility of the instruments, personal familiarity with the instruments, the availability of *norms* or comparison information, administrative considerations, the appropriateness of the instrument for the target population, and the instrument's reputation.

≡ STUDY SUGGESTIONS

1. Explain in your own words the meaning of the following correlation coefficients:
   a. The relationship between intelligence and grade point average was found to be .72.
   b. The correlation coefficient between age and gregariousness was −.20.
   c. It was revealed that patients' compliance with nursing instructions was related to their length of stay in the hospital ($r = -.50$).
2. Suppose the split-half reliability of an instrument to measure attitudes toward contraception was .70. Calculate the reliability of the full scale by using the Spearman-Brown formula.
3. If a researcher had a 20-item scale whose reliability was .60, approximately how many items would have to be added to achieve a reliability of .80?
4. An instructor has developed an instrument to measure knowledge of research terminology. Would you say that more reliable measurements would be yielded before or after a year of instruction on research methodology, using the exact same test, or would there be no difference? Why?
5. What aspects of the multitrait–multimethod matrix that follows identify weaknesses in the measures?

	Traits	Method 1		Method 2	
		A_1	B_1	A_1	B_1
Method 1	A_1	(.40)			
	B_1	.38	(.65)		
Method 2	A_2	.36	.50	(.80)	
	B_2	.19	.48	.25	(.75)

6. What types of groups do you feel might be useful to use for a known-groups approach to validating a measure of emotional maturity; attitudes toward alcoholics, territorial aggressiveness; job motivation; and subjective pain?

≡ SUGGESTED READINGS

METHODOLOGICAL REFERENCES

Armstrong, G.D. (1981). The intraclass correlation as a measure of interrater reliability of subjective judgments. *Nursing Research, 30,* 314–315.

Brinberg, D., & McGrath, J.E. (1985). *Validity and the research process.* Beverly Hills, CA: Sage.

Campbell, D.T., & Fiske, D.W. (1959). Convergent and discriminant validation by the multitrait–multimethod matrix. *Psychological Bulletin, 56,* 81–105.

Cronbach, L.J. (1984). *Essentials of psychological testing* (4th ed.). New York: Harper & Row.

Denzin, N.K. (1989). *The research act* (3rd ed.). New York: McGraw-Hill.

Ebel, R.L. (1979). *Essentials of educational measurement* (3rd ed.). Englewood Cliffs, NJ: Prentice-Hall.

Garvin, B.J., Kennedy, C.W., & Cissna, K.N. (1988). Reliability in category coding systems. *Nursing Research, 37,* 52–55.

Guilford, J.P. (1964). *Psychometric methods* (2nd ed.) New York: McGraw-Hill.

Holm, K., & Kavanagh, J. (1985). An approach to modifying self-report instruments. *Research in Nursing and Health, 8,* 13–18.

Horn, B.J. (1980). Establishing valid and reliable criteria: A researcher's perspective. *Nursing Research, 29,* 88–90.

Kerlinger, F.N. (1986). *Foundations of behavioral research* (3rd ed.). New York: Holt, Rinehart & Winston.

Kirk, J., & Miller, M.L. (1985). *Reliability and validity in qualitative research.* Beverly Hills, CA: Sage.

LeCompte, M.D., & Goetz, J.P. (1982). Problems of reliability and validity in ethnographic research. *Review of Educational Research, 52,* 31–60.

Lynn, M.R. (1986). Determination and quantification of content validity. *Nursing Research, 35,* 382–385.

Murdaugh, C. (1981). Measurement error and attenuation. *Western Journal of Nursing Research, 3,* 252–256.

Norbeck, J.S. (1985). What constitutes a publishable report of instrument development? *Nursing Research, 34,* 380–382.

Nunnally, J. (1978). *Psychometric theory.* New York: McGraw-Hill.

Ryan, J.W., Phillips, C.Y., & Prescott, P.A. (1988). Interrater reliability: The underdeveloped role of rater training. *Applied Nursing Research, 1,* 148–150.

Thorndike, R.L., & Hagen, E. (1977). *Measurement and evaluation in psychology and education* (4th ed.). New York: John Wiley and Sons.

Tilden, V.P., Nelson, C.A., & May, B.A. (1990). Use of qualitative methods to enhance content validity. *Nursing Research, 39,* 172–175.

Waltz, C.F., Strickland, O.L., & Lenz, E.R. (1984). *Measurement in nursing research.* Philadelphia: F.A. Davis. (Chapter 5).

Washington, C.C., & Moss, M. (1988). Pragmatic aspects of establishing interrater reliability in research. *Nursing Research, 37,* 190–191.

Zeller, R.A., & Carmines, E.G. (1980). *Measurement in the social sciences.* New York: Cambridge University Press.

SUBSTANTIVE REFERENCES*

Brink, C.A., Sampselle, C.M., Welles, T.J., Diokno, A.C., & Gillis, G.L. (1989). A digital test for pelvic muscle strength in older women with urinary incontinence. *Nursing Research, 38,* 196–199. [Interrater reliability, criterion-related validity, known-groups approach]

Browne, G.B., Byrne, C., Roberts, J., Streiner, D., Fitch, M., Corey, P., & Arpin, K. (1988). The meaning of illness questionnaire: Reliability and validity. *Nursing Research, 37,* 368–373. [Test–retest reliability, interrater reliability, construct validity]

Burckhardt, C.S., Woods, S.L., Schultz, A.A., & Ziebarth, D.M. (1989). Quality of life of adults with chronic illness: A psychometric study. *Research in Nursing and Health, 12,* 347–354. [Test–retest reliability, internal consistency reliability, construct validity: convergent and discriminant validity, known groups approach]

Cox, C.L. (1985). The Health Self-Determinism Index. *Nursing Research, 34,* 177–183. [Cronbach's alpha, content validity, discriminant validity]

Cox, C.L., Cowell, J.M., Marion, L.N., & Miller, E.H. (1990). The Health Self-Determinism Index for Children. *Research in Nursing and Health, 13,* 237–246. [Test–retest reliability, internal consistency reliability, content validity, criterion-related validity, construct validity]

Crosby, L., & Parsons, L.C. (1989). Clinical neurologic assessment tool: Development and testing of an instrument to index neurologic status. *Heart and Lung, 18,* 121–129. [Internal consistency reliability, construct validity, criterion-related validity]

Davis, G.C. (1989). Measurement of the chronic pain experience: Development of an instrument. *Research in Nursing and Health, 12,* 221–227. [Test–retest, internal consistency, construct validity: factor analysis, exploratory modeling]

Eilers, J., Berger, A.M., & Petersen, M.C. (1988). Development, testing and application of the Oral Assessment Guide. *Oncology Nursing Forum, 15,* 325–330. [Interrater reliability, content validity]

Ferrans, C.E., & Powers, M.J. (1985). Quality of life index: Development and psychometric properties. *Advances in Nursing Science, 8,* 15–24. [Test–retest reliability; internal consistency: Cronbach's alpha, content validity, criterion-related validity]

Frank-Stromberg, M. (1989). Reaction to the diagnosis of cancer questionnaire: Development and psychometric evaluation. *Nursing Research, 38,* 364–369. [Test–retest, Cronbach's alpha, construct validity: factor analysis, content validity]

Gulick, E.E. (1989), Model confirmation of the MS-related symptom checklist. *Nursing Research, 38,* 147–153. [Content validity, construct validity, concurrent and predictive validity, internal consistency reliability, test–retest reliability]

Lasky, P., et al. (1985). Developing an instrument for the assessment of family dynamics. *Western Journal of Nursing Research, 7,* 40–57. [Internal consistency reliability: Cronbach's alpha, content validity, construct validity]

Mahon, N.E., & Yarcheski, A. (1990). The dimensionality of the UCLA Loneliness Scale in early adolescents. *Research in Nursing and Health, 13,* 45–52. [Construct validity]

Mueller, C.W., & McCloskey, J.C. (1990). Nurses' job satisfaction: A proposed measure. *Nursing Research, 39,* 113–117. [Test–retest reliability, internal consistency reliability, criterion-related validity, construct validity]

Mynatt, S. (1985). Empathy in faculty and students in different types of nursing preparation programs. *Western Journal of Nursing Research, 7,* 333–348. [Interrater reliability]

Phillips, L.R., Rempusheski, V., & Morrison, E. (1989). Developing and testing the Beliefs About Care-

*A comment in brackets after each citation designates the assessment procedure of interest.

giving Scale. *Research in Nursing and Health, 12,* 207–220. [Cronbach's alpha, test–retest reliability, item analysis, construct validity, content validity]

Pollock, S.E., & Duffy, M.E. (1990). The Health-Related Hardiness Scale: Development and psychometric analysis. *Nursing Research, 39,* 218–222.

[Test–retest reliability, internal consistency reliability, construct validity]

Pridham, K.F., & Chang, A.S. (1989). What Being the Parent of a New Baby is Like: Revision of an instrument. *Research in Nursing and Health, 12,* 323–329. [Test–retest reliability, internal consistency reliability, construct validity]

19
Quantitative Measurement

Not all nursing research studies involve the collection of quantitative data, but the majority do. Even studies that use narrative sources of information, such as unstructured interviews or historical documents, often convert some or all of the information to quantified expression. This chapter discusses some of the basic principles of measurement and quantification, in preparation for a discussion on statistical analysis.

The measurement process and the problems it entails are central concerns of the researcher using the scientific approach. Hypotheses are tested through the collection of data, and data are gathered by measuring those variables designated in the hypotheses. This sounds straightforward, and sometimes it is. The measurement of someone's height is easy enough, but how about the measurement of pain, or loneliness, or empathy? The rules for measuring such attributes are neither unanimously agreed upon nor intuitively obvious. The rules for measuring a person's height are not unanimously agreed upon either, but most people accept either the "inches–feet–yards" or metric conventions. Analogous conventions for measuring social and psychologic variables do not exist, nor are they likely to be developed. Most social scientists agree that measurement constitutes the most perplexing and enduring problem in the research process. Because much of nursing research deals with social or psychologic phenomena, the measurement problem in nursing research is a major concern.

Measurement may be defined as follows: "Measurement consists of rules for assigning numbers to objects to represent quantities of attributes" (Nunnally, 1978, p. 2). In our private lives, we develop our own "rules" for measuring things, but as researchers we must either adopt well-specified rules (as in the case of measuring body temperature in Fahrenheit degrees) or explicitly formulate new ones. Let us consider various aspects of the definition of measurement and the measurement process.

≡ ASPECTS OF QUANTITATIVE MEASUREMENT

Abstraction and Measurement

When we measure something, it is not the object itself that is measured. Rather, we measure abstract attributes or characteristics of the object. The researcher uses the term "concepts" in referring to abstractions of interest. The measurement procedures constitute, in short, the operational definitions of the concepts.

Before measuring the abstractions in which we are interested, it is useful to consider thoroughly the nature of the critical attribute. We should ask ourselves, first, if the attribute really exists. As in the case of all abstractions, we are dealing with human conceptualizations. That is, the abstractions represent a structure that humans impose on objects, and these abstractions may or may not be appropriate or relevant dimensions to consider. The ways in which we normally describe people may not be matched in reality by attributes that can be measured. Is there really such a phenomenon as "women's intuition" or "superego strength"?

A second aspect of the problem is that our abstraction may not be "pure"; that is, it may be a conglomerate of several interrelated concepts rather than a unitary attribute. This problem is an important one for measurement purposes. A good measurement tool should yield a quantitative score for one unitary, isolated attribute. If the concept is complex, then several measures may be required to produce data relating to its various facets. Consider for a moment the concept of creativity. Creativity is a term with which we are all familiar and that we use in normal speech, but scientists have had difficulties in dealing with this construct, partly because it is elusive and partly

because it manifests itself in vastly different ways in different kinds of people. Is creativity in a nurse researcher similar in any way to creativity in a novelist? The researcher seeking a measuring tool should consider if a more modest abstraction might not, in fact, be easier to define and defend. Perhaps instead of dealing with "creativity," the researcher would be advised to focus more narrowly on one aspect of creativity, such as fluidity of verbal expression.

Quantification and Measurement

Quantification is intimately associated with measurement. An often-quoted statement by early American psychologist L.L. Thurstone advances a position assumed by many researchers: "Whatever exists, exists in some amount and can be measured." The notion underlying this statement is that attributes of objects are not constant—they vary from day to day, from situation to situation, or from one person to another. This variability is capable of a numerical expression that signifies *how much* of an attribute is present in the object. Quantification is used to communicate that amount.

The purpose of assigning numbers, then, is to differentiate between persons or objects that possess varying degrees of the critical attribute. If Nurse X is a more effective nurse than Nurse Y, then Nurse X should have a higher "score" for effectiveness than Nurse Y. The crucial problem is determining *how much* higher the score should be to accurately reflect the differences that exist.

Rules and Measurement

Numbers must be assigned to objects according to specified rules rather than haphazardly. Quantification in the absence of rules would be meaningless. The rules for measuring temperature, weight, blood pressure, and other physical attributes are familiar to us. Rules for measuring many variables for nursing research studies, however, have to be invented. Whether the data are collected by way of observation, self-report questionnaire, or some other method, the researcher must specify under what conditions and according to what criteria the numerical values are to be assigned to the characteristic of interest.

As an example, suppose we were studying attitudes toward traditional sex roles and asked nurses to express their extent of agreement with the following statement:

> Basically, women are too emotional and dependent to be placed in positions of authority.
> [ ] Strongly agree
> [ ] Agree
> [ ] Slightly agree
> [ ] Undecided
> [ ] Slightly disagree
> [ ] Disagree
> [ ] Strongly disagree

The responses to this question can be quantified by developing a system for assigning numbers to them. It should be stressed that *any* rule would satisfy the definition of measurement. We could assign the value of 30 to "strongly agree," 27 to "agree," 20 to "slightly agree," and so on, but there is no apparent justification for doing so. Therefore, in measuring attributes, we must strive not only to develop rules, but also to develop good, meaningful rules. A simplified scheme of assigning a 1 to "strongly agree" and a 7 to "strongly disagree" is probably the most defensible procedure for the question at hand. This "rule" would quantitatively differentiate, in increments of one point, between people who have seven different reactions to the statement.

In developing a new set of rules for measuring attributes, the researcher seldom knows in advance if his or her rules really are the best possible. In essence, a new set of measurement rules constitutes a researcher's hypothesis concerning how an attribute functions and varies. The adequacy of the hypothesis—that is, the worth of the measuring tool—needs to be assessed, using procedures described in the preceding chapter.

Measurement and Reality

The concepts we use and the rules we develop to quantify those concepts must be linked to the real world. To state this requirement somewhat more technically, the measurement procedures must be isomorphic to reality. The term *isomorphic* signifies equivalence of or similarity between two phenomena. A measurement tool cannot be of scientific utility unless the measures resulting from it have some rational correspondence with reality.

Perhaps the isomorphism criterion strikes the reader as self-evident. Yet researchers continuously face the risk that their instruments are not accurately and validly reflecting real-world phenomena. Failures to meet the requirement for isomorphism generally stem from inadequate conceptualization or definition of attributes, inappropriate rules for assigning numbers to objects, or both of these deficiencies.

To illustrate this point, suppose the Scholastic Aptitude Test (SAT) is administered to ten people, who obtain the following scores on the verbal portion of the test: 345, 395, 430, 435, 485, 505, 550, 575, 620, 640. These values are shown at the top of Figure 19-1. Let us further suppose that "in reality" the true scores of these same ten people in terms of a hypothetical perfect test of verbal scholastic aptitude would be as follows: 355, 380, 430, 465, 470, 500, 550, 610, 590, 665. These values are shown at the bottom of Figure 19-1. This figure shows that, although not perfect, the obtained test scores came fairly close to representing the "true" scores of the ten subjects. Two actual scores matched exactly the hypothetical true scores, and no score was off by more than 40 points. Only two individuals (H and I) were improperly ordered as a result of the actual test. This example illustrates a measure whose isomorphism with reality can be considered high, but improvable.

The researcher almost always works with fallible measures. Instruments that measure psychologic concepts are less likely to correspond to "reality" than physical measures, but few instru-

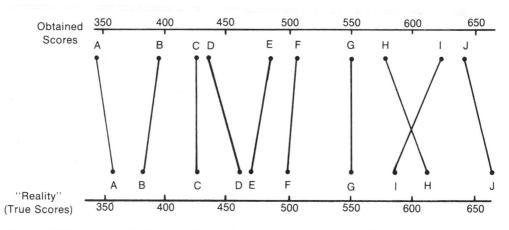

Figure 19-1. *Relationship between obtained and true scores for a hypothetical set of test scores.*

ments are immune from error. A person's "true score" on an attribute can never be known, of course, but reliability procedures can be used for estimating the instrument's success in satisfying the isomorphism criterion.

≡ ADVANTAGES OF MEASUREMENT

What exactly does measurement accomplish that nonmeasurement does not? In this section, we examine some answers to the question of what the function of measurement is in science. Before noting the major advantages of measurement, consider what researchers would work with in its absence. What would happen, for example, if there were no measures of body temperature, blood pressure, or respiratory volume? All that would be left is intuition, guesses, personal judgment, and subjective evaluations. With this thought in mind, many of the advantages described in the following section should be apparent.

Objectivity

One of the principal strengths of measurement is that it removes much of the guesswork in gathering scientific data. An objective measure is one that can be independently verified by other researchers. For example, two people measuring the weight of a subject using the same scale would be likely to get identical or highly similar results. Not all scientific measures are completely objective, but most are likely to incorporate rules for minimizing subjectivity.

In addition to the objectivity that is often built into the measure itself, quantification enhances objectivity in another respect. The numerical results of measurement are amenable to analytic procedures in which subjectivity is all but nonexistent. With purely qualitative information, the organization and analysis are likely to be judgmental. Of course, one of the strengths of qualitative research is that the human mind is capable of making remarkably astute judgments. Nevertheless, even in qualitative research investigators normally take steps to avoid subjective biases and distortions.

Precision

Quantitative measures make it possible to obtain reasonably precise information. Instead of describing John as "rather tall," we can depict him as a man who is 6'1" tall. If we chose, or if the research requirements demanded it, we could obtain even more precise height measurements. Because of the possibility for precision, the researcher's task of differentiating among objects that possess different degrees of an attribute becomes considerably easier.

Communication

Measurement constitutes a language of communication. Science is not a private enterprise, engaged in solely to amuse or satisfy the curiosity of isolated researchers. Communication among scientists is essential if a knowledge base is to be developed. Inasmuch as numbers are less vague than words, quantitative measurement does a reasonably good job of communicating information to a broad audience of people. If a researcher reported that the average oral temperature of a sample of postoperative patients was "somewhat high," different readers might develop different conceptions about the physiologic state of the sample. However, if the researcher reported an average temperature of 99.5°F, there is no possibility of ambiguity and misinterpretation.

☰ *LEVELS OF MEASUREMENT*

Scientists have developed a system for categorizing different types of measures. This classification system is important because the analytic operations that can be performed on data depend on the measurement level used. Four major classes, or levels, of measurement have been identified: (1) nominal measurement, (2) ordinal measurement, (3) interval measurement, and (4) ratio measurement.

Nominal Measurement

The lowest level of measurement is referred to as *nominal measurement*. This level involves the assignment of numbers to simply classify characteristics into categories. For many qualitative attributes, we can do no more than to perform this sorting function. Examples of variables amenable to nominal measurement include gender, race, religion, eye color, blood type, nationality, and medical diagnosis.

The numbers assigned in nominal measurement are not intended to convey any quantitative implications. If we establish a rule to classify males as 1 and females as 2, the numbers in and of themselves have no meaning. The number 2 here clearly does not mean "more than" or "better than" 1. It would be perfectly acceptable to reverse the code and use 1 for females and 2 for males. The numbers are merely symbols that represent two different values of the gender attribute. Indeed, instead of numerical symbols we could as easily have chosen alphabetical symbols such as *M* and *F*. We recommend, however, thinking in terms of numerical categories because the subsequent analysis of data will be simplified if such a procedure is adopted when a computer is used.

Nominal measurement provides no information about an attribute except that of equivalence and nonequivalence. If we were to "measure" the gender of Tom, Mary, Susan, and Jim, we would—according to our rule—assign them the codes, 1, 2, 2, and 1, respectively. Tom and Jim are considered equivalent, at least with respect to the target attribute, but are not equivalent to the other two subjects.

The basic requirements for measuring attributes on the nominal scale are that the classifications must be mutually exclusive and collectively exhaustive. For example, if we were measuring ethnicity, we might establish the following scheme: 1 = whites, 2 = blacks, 3 = Hispanics. Each subject must be classifiable into one and only one of these categories. The requirement for collective exhaustiveness would not be met if, for example, there were several individuals of Asian descent in the sample.

The numbers used in nominal measurement cannot be treated mathematically. Although it might make perfectly good sense to determine the average weight of a sample of subjects, it is meaningless to calculate the average gender of a sample. However, the elements assigned to each category can be enumerated, and statements can be made concerning the frequency of occurrence in each class. In a sample of 50 patients, we might find 30 males and 20 females. We could also say that 60% of the subjects were male and 40% were female. However, no further mathematical operations would be meaningful with data from nominal measures.

It might strike some readers as odd to think of the categorization procedure we have been describing as measurement. If our definition of measurement is recalled, however, it can be seen that nominal measurement does, in fact, involve the assignment of numbers to attributes according to rules. The rules are not sophisticated, to be sure, but they are rules nonetheless.

Ordinal Measurement

The next level in the measurement hierarchy is ordinal measurement. *Ordinal measurement* permits the sorting of objects on the basis of their standing relative to each other on a specified attribute. This level of measurement goes beyond a mere categorization: the attributes are *ordered* according to some criterion. If a researcher were to rank order subjects from the heaviest to the lightest, or if subjects were classified into three groups based on their daily amount of exercise— (1) under 15 minutes, (2) 15 to 30 minutes, (3) more than 30 minutes—then we would say that an ordinal level of measurement had been used.

The fundamental difference between nominal and ordinal measurement is that with ordinal measurement information concerning not only equivalence but also concerning relative standing or ordering among objects is implied. When we assign numbers to a person's religious affiliation, the numbers have no inherent meaning or significance. We could develop a scheme whereby Roman Catholics were assigned to category 1, Jews to 2, Protestants to 3, and all others to 4. This nominal measuring scheme is absolutely arbitrary. Now, consider this scheme for measuring a client's ability to perform activities of daily living: (1) completely dependent, (2) needs another person's assistance, (3) needs mechanical assistance, (4) completely independent. In this case, the measurement is ordinal. The numbers are not arbitrary—they signify incremental ability to perform the activities of daily living. The individuals assigned a value of four are equivalent to each other with regard to their ability to function *and,* relative to those in all the other categories, have more of that attribute.

Ordinal measurement does not, however, tell us anything about how much greater one level of an attribute is than another level. We do not know if being completely independent is "twice as good" as needing mechanical assistance, nor do we know if the difference between needing another person's assistance and needing mechanical assistance is the same as that between needing mechanical assistance and being completely independent. Ordinal measurement only tells us the relative ranking of the levels of an attribute.

As in the case of nominal scales, the types of mathematical operations permissible with ordinal-level data are rather restricted. Averages are generally meaningless with rank-order measures. Frequency counts, percentages, and several other statistical procedures to be discussed in Chapter 20 are appropriate for analyzing ordinal-level data.

Interval Measurement

Interval measurement occurs when the researcher can specify both the rank ordering of objects on an attribute and the distance between those objects. Interval scales have numerical values, the distances between which represent equal distances in the attribute being measured. Most psychologic and educational tests are based on interval scales. The SAT is an example of this level of measurement. A score of 550 on the SAT is higher than a score of 500, which in turn is higher than 450. In addition to providing this rank-order information, a difference between 550 and 500 on the test is presumably equivalent to the difference between 500 and 450.

Interval measures, then, are more informative than ordinal measures. One piece of information that interval measures fail to provide is the absolute magnitude of the attribute for any particular object. The Fahrenheit scale for measuring temperature illustrates this point. A temperature of 60° is 10° warmer than 50°. A 10° difference similarly separates 40° and 30°, and the two differences in temperature are equivalent. However, it cannot be said that 60° is twice as hot as 30°, or three times as hot as 20°. The Fahrenheit scale, then, is not a measure of temperature in absolute units. The assignment of numbers to temperature on the Fahrenheit scale involves an arbitrary zero point. Zero on the thermometer does not signify a total absence of heat. In interval scales, there is no real or rational zero point.

The use of interval scales greatly expands the researcher's analytic possibilities. The intervals between numbers can be meaningfully added and subtracted: the interval between 10° and 5° is 5°, or $10 - 5 = 5$. This same operation could not be performed with ordinal measures. Because of this capability, interval-level data can be averaged. It is perfectly reasonable, for example, to compute an average daily temperature for hospitalized patients from whom temperature readings are taken four times a day. Most sophisticated statistical procedures require that measurements be made on an interval scale.

Ratio Measurement

The highest level of measurement is the ratio scale. *Ratio scales* are distinguished from interval scales by virtue of having a rational, meaningful zero. Measures on a ratio scale provide information concerning the rank ordering of objects on the critical attribute, the intervals between objects, and the absolute magnitude of the attribute for the object. Many physical measures provide ratio-level data. A person's weight, for example, is measured on a ratio scale, because zero weight is an actual possibility. It is perfectly acceptable to say that someone who weighs 200 pounds is twice as heavy as someone who weighs 100 pounds.

Because ratio scales have an absolute zero, all arithmetic operations are permissible. One can meaningfully add, subtract, multiply, and divide numbers on a ratio scale. Consequently, all of the statistical procedures suitable for interval-level data are also appropriate for ratio-level data. Ratio measurement constitutes the measurement ideal for scientists but is probably an unattainable

ideal for the vast majority of attributes of a psychologic nature.

Comparison of the Levels

The four levels of measurement presented in this section constitute a hierarchy, with ratio scales at the pinnacle and nominal measurement at the base. The basic characteristics of each level have been discussed, but several additional points should be mentioned.

The researcher generally should strive to construct measuring instruments on as high a level of measurement as possible, especially for measures that will be used for dependent variables. This guideline is based on two considerations: (1) higher levels of measurement generally yield more information and (2) they are amenable to more powerful and sensitive analytic procedures than lower levels. When one moves from a higher to a lower level of measurement, there is always an information loss. Let us demonstrate that this is so with an example relating to data on the weight of a sample of individuals. Table 19-1 presents fictitious data for ten subjects. The second column shows the ratio-level data, that is, the actual weight in pounds. The ratio measure gives us complete information concerning the absolute weight of each subject and the differences in weights between all pairs of subjects.

In the third column, the original data have been converted to interval measures by assigning a score of 0 to the lightest individual (Katy), the score of 5 to the person 5 pounds heavier than the lightest person (Amy), and so forth. Note that the resulting scores are still amenable to addition and subtraction; the differences in pounds are equally far apart, even though they are at different parts of the scale. The data no longer tell us, however, anything about the absolute weights of the people in this sample. Katy, the lightest individual, might be a 10-pound infant or a 200-pound Weight Watcher.

In the fourth column of Table 19-1, ordinal measurements were assigned by rank ordering the sample from the lightest, who was assigned the score of 1, to the heaviest, who was assigned the score of 10. Now even more information is missing. The data provide no indication of how much heavier Nathan is than Katy. The difference separating them might be as little as 5 pounds or as much as 150 pounds.

Finally, the fifth column presents nominal measurements in which all subjects were classified as either "heavy" or "light." The criterion applied in categorizing individuals was arbitrarily set as a weight either greater than 150 pounds (2), or less than/equal to 150 pounds (1). The available information is very limited. Within any one category, there are no clues as to who is heavier than whom. With this level of measurement Nathan, Corey, and Richard are considered equivalent. They are equivalent with regard to the attribute heavy/light as defined by the classification criterion.

This example illustrates that at every successive level in the measurement hierarchy there is a loss of valuable information. It also illustrates another point: when one has information at one level, one can always manipulate the data to arrive at a lower level, but the converse is not true. If we were only given the nominal measurements, it would be impossible to reconstruct the actual weights. Researchers seldom collapse information to arrive at lower-level data, but it is important to recognize the greater flexibility possible with ratio and interval measures than with ordinal and nominal measures.

Although it is generally preferable to use the highest possible level of measurement, there are exceptions to this guideline. For example, researchers sometimes use people's scores on interval- or ratio-level measures to create groups, and sometimes group membership is more meaningful or interpretable than continuous scores. For example, for some research and clinical purposes, it may be more relevant to designate infants as being of low birthweight or normal birthweight (nominal level) than to use actual birthweight values (ratio level).

It is not always a straightforward task to identify the level of measurement for a particular instrument. Usually, nominal measures and ratio scales are discernible with little difficulty, but the distinction between ordinal and interval measures is more problematic. Some methodologists argue that most psychologic measures that are treated as interval measures are really only ordinal measures. The majority of writers seem to believe that, although such instruments as Likert scales produce data that are, strictly speaking, ordinal level, the distortion introduced by treating them as interval measures is too small to warrant an abandonment of powerful statistical analyses.

≡ RESEARCH EXAMPLE

As shown in the examples presented in Table 19-2, nurse researchers have operationalized their re-

Table 19-1. *Fictitious Data for Four Levels of Measurement*

SUBJECTS	RATIO-LEVEL	INTERVAL-LEVEL	ORDINAL LEVEL	NOMINAL LEVEL
Nathan	180	70	10	2
Katy	110	0	1	1
Corey	165	55	8	2
Lauren	130	20	5	1
Richard	175	65	9	2
Amy	115	5	2	1
Claire	125	15	4	1
Jesse	150	40	7	1
Thomas	145	35	6	1
Megan	120	10	3	1

search variables at every level of measurement. The following more detailed example illustrates the use of multilevel measures within a single study.

Halm (1990) conducted a quasi-experimental study to examine the effectiveness of support groups in reducing the anxiety of family members during a relative's critical illness. Her study included a variety of measures and encompassed every level of measurement.

The independent variable (a dichotomous nominal-level variable) was the subjects' group status. The control group relatives received conventional bedside support from nurses during visiting hours or condition reports. The relatives in the experimental group received conventional bedside support and also attended a support group to share feelings and experiences in coping with illness. As a check on the internal validity of the study, the two groups of subjects were compared in terms of such background variables as age (ratio level); sex (nominal level); socio-economic status (ordinal level); distance of their residence to the hospital (ratio level); and religion (nominal level). The two groups of relatives were also compared in terms of patient characteristics, such as type of surgical procedure (nominal level) and length of stay in hospital (constructed to be ordinal level). The two groups were similar on these and other extraneous variables.

The major dependent variable was anxi-

Table 19-2. *Examples of Variables Measured at Different Levels of Measurement*

LEVEL	*CONCEPT/MEASURE*	*REFERENCE*
Nominal	Behavior pattern (Type A/Type B)	Thomas & Friedmann, 1990
	Patient status (patient/spouse of patient)	Miller et al., 1990
	Type of solution for intravenous replacement fluid (crystalloid versus colloid)	Ley et al., 1990
	Cancer site (genitourinary/other)	Christman, 1990
	Occupationally related lower back pain (presence/absence)	Owen, 1989
	Type of delivery (vaginal/cesarean)	Fortier, 1988
Ordinal	Children's behavior problems (0, 1–3; 4+)	Schraeder et al., 1990
	Foreign students' level of contact with Americans (little, medium, a lot)	Upvall, 1990
	Pulmonary edema (5-point rating scale)	Ley et al., 1990
	Stage of cancer (I, II, III, or IV)	Christman, 1990
	Change in activities of daily living (none to large amount)	Owen, 1989
Interval	Children's learning skills (Mullen Scales of Early Learning)	Schraeder et al., 1990
	Depression (General Well-Being Scale)	Upvall, 1990
	Compliance with medical regimen (Health Behavior Scale)	Miller et al., 1990
	Symptom severity (Symptom Distress Scale)	Christman, 1990
	Paternal attachment (Paternal Caretaking Activities Questionnaire)	Fortier, 1988
Ratio	Heart rate	Thomas & Friedmann, 1990
	Length of time lived in the United States	Upvall, 1990
	Hemodynamic stability (blood pressure, thermodilution cardiac outputs)	Ley et al., 1990
	Number of years of nursing experience	Owen, 1989
	Number of children	Fortier, 1988

ety, measured by the State–Trait Anxiety Inventory, which yielded interval-level data. The trait portion of the scale was administered at baseline, and the state portion was administered both at baseline and after the intervention (the support group for the experimental subjects).

The analysis did not reveal any group differences in trait anxiety or in state anxiety at either point in time. However, anxiety was found to be related to several of the background variables. For example, relatives whose socioeconomic status was higher tended to have higher state anxiety scores than those of a lower socioeconomic status. Also, among those relatives in the experimental group, men were less anxious than women.

≡ *SUMMARY*

Measurement involves a set of rules according to which numerical values are assigned to objects to represent varying degrees of some attribute. Strictly speaking, we do not measure "things," but rather some abstract characteristic of things, such as height, weight, pain, and so on. The quantification aspect of measurement usually focuses on developing a numerical system to indicate how much of the critical attribute the object possesses. This quantification process is not performed haphazardly, but rather according to well-formulated rules. The researcher must strive to locate or develop measures that are *isomorphic* with reality; that is, there must be some correspondence between or equivalence of the actual attributes and the measurements of them.

Measurement offers the research scientist a number of benefits. Objectivity is enhanced through measurements, inasmuch as it permits observations to be independently verified by other researchers. Greater precision can be attained through measurement than through casual observation, making it easier for the researcher to differentiate among the varying degrees of an attribute possessed by objects. Measurement also constitutes an important channel of communication among scientists.

The kinds of rules that can be applied to the measurement of an attribute usually depend on the nature of the attribute. The four major levels of measurement are (1) nominal, (2) ordinal, (3) interval, and (4) ratio. *Nominal measurement* classifies characteristics of attributes into mutually exclusive and collectively exhaustive categories. Nominal measurements, which represent the lowest level of measurement, cannot be manipulated mathematically. *Ordinal measurement* involves the sorting of objects on the basis of their relative standing to each other on a specified attribute. Ordinal-level data yield rank orderings among objects. *Interval measurements* indicate not only the rank-ordering of objects on an attribute but also the amount of distance between each object. Distances between numerical values on the interval scale represent equivalent distances in the attribute being measured. *Ratio measurements,* which constitute the highest form of measurement, are distinguished from interval measurements by virtue of having a rational zero point. Because ratio scales have an absolute zero, all arithmetic operations are permissible. In general, researchers should strive to measure key variables (especially dependent variables) on as high a measurement scale as possible.

≡ *STUDY SUGGESTIONS*

1. What types of data collection procedure (i.e., observation, self-report, or physiological index) might a researcher use to measure the following concepts: fear of death, loneliness, body image, self-esteem, sensitivity to pain, motor coordination, ease of fluid intake, adherence to a nutritional regime, and nursing effectiveness?
2. For one or more of the concepts listed in study suggestion 1, develop rules for quantitatively measuring the variable.
3. Read a research report in a recent issue of *Nursing Research.* Were the levels of measurement used by the author the highest possible? If not, explain how the researcher could have attained higher levels of measurement than were used or defend the re-

searcher's use of a lower level of measurement.

4. For each of the following variables, specify the highest level of measurement that you feel would ordinarily be attainable: number of siblings; rank in class; color of urine specimen; time to first voiding for postoperative patients; faculty status (i.e., professor, assistant professor, or instructor); attitude toward abortion; exposure to genetic counseling; length of stay in hospital; diastolic blood pressure; hospital nursing positions; sleeping state; anxiety level.

5. Below are presented fictitious data for the length in centimeters of ten newborns. Convert this information to interval, ordinal, and nominal measurements.

   a. 45 cm
   b. 52 cm
   c. 61 cm
   d. 49 cm
   e. 60 cm
   f. 58 cm
   g. 63 cm
   h. 58 cm
   i. 53 cm
   j. 57 cm

≡ *SUGGESTED READINGS*

METHODOLOGICAL REFERENCES

Allen, M.J., & Yen, W.M. (1979). *Introduction to measurement theory.* Monterey, CA: Brooks-Cole.

Blalock, H.M., Jr. (1982). *Conceptualization and measurement in the social sciences.* Beverly Hill, CA: Sage.

Churchman, C.W., & Ratoosh, P. (Eds.). (1963). *Measurement: Definitions and theories.* New York: John Wiley and Sons.

Downs, F.S. (1989). A meterstone. *Nursing Research, 38,* 3.

Kaplan, A. (1971). Measurement in behavioral sciences. In B.J. Franklin & H.W. Osborne (Eds.), *Research methods: Issues and insights* (pp. 121–128). Belmont, CA: Wadsworth.

Kerlinger, F.N. (1986). *Foundations of behavioral research* (3rd ed.). New York: Rinehart & Winston. (Chapter 25)

Lazarsfeld, P.F., & Barton, A. (1971). Qualitative measurement in the social sciences. In B.J. Franklin & H.W. Osborne (Eds.), *Research methods: Issues and insights* (pp. 140–160). Belmont, CA: Wadsworth.

Nunnally, J.C. (1978). *Psychometric theory.* New York: McGraw-Hill.

Stevens, S.S. (1946). On the theory of scales of measurement. *Science, 103,* 677–680.

Thorndike, R.L. (Ed.). (1971). *Educational measurement* (2nd ed.). Washington: American Council on Education.

Thorndike, R.L., & Hagen, E. (1986). *Measurement and evaluation in psychology and education* (5th ed.). New York: John Wiley and Sons.

Waltz, C.F., Strickland, O.L., & Lenz, E.R. (1984). *Measurement in nursing research.* Philadelphia: F.A. Davis.

SUBSTANTIVE REFERENCES

Christman, N.J. (1990). Uncertainty and adjustment during radiotherapy. *Nursing Research, 39,* 17–20.

Fortier, J.C. (1988). The relationship of vaginal and cesarean births to father–infant attachment. *Journal of Obstetric, Gynecologic, and Neonatal Nursing, 17,* 128–134.

Halm, M.A. (1990). Effects of support groups on anxiety of family members during critical illness. *Heart and Lung, 19,* 62–71.

Ley, S.J., Miller, K., Skov, P., & Preisig, P. (1990). Crystalloid versus colloid therapy after cardiac surgery. *Heart and Lung, 19,* 31–40.

Miller, Sr. P., Wikoff, R., McMahon, M., Garrett, M.J., & Ringel, K. (1990). Marital functioning after cardiac surgery. *Heart and Lung, 19,* 55–61.

Owen, B.D. (1989). The magnitude of low-back pain problem in nursing. *Western Journal of Nursing Research, 11,* 234–242.

Schraeder, B.D., Heverly, M.A., & Rappaport, J. (1990). Temperament, behavior problems and learning skills in very low birth weight preschoolers. *Research in Nursing and Health, 13,* 27–34.

Thomas, S.A., & Friedmann, E. (1990). Type A behavior and cardiovascular responses during verbalization in cardiac patients. *Nursing Research, 39,* 48–53.

Upvall, M.J. (1990). A model of uprooting for international students. *Western Journal of Nursing Research, 12,* 95–107.

Part V

The Analysis of Research Data

20
Quantitative Analysis: Descriptive Statistics

Statistical methods are techniques for rendering quantitative information meaningful and intelligible. Without the aid of statistics, the quantitative data collected in a research project would be little more than a chaotic mass of numbers. Statistical procedures enable the researcher to reduce, summarize, organize, evaluate, interpret, and communicate numerical information.

A knowledge of basic statistical methods is indispensable for those who want to keep abreast of research developments in their field. Many individuals are intimidated by statistics because they feel they are "no good in math," but strong mathematical talent is not required to use or understand statistical analysis. To apply and interpret statistics, one needs only basic arithmetic skills and logical thinking ability. In the remainder of this chapter and in Chapters 21 and 22, there will be no emphasis on the theoretical rationale or mathematical derivation of statistical operations. In fact, even computation will be underplayed because this is not a statistics text and also because statistics are seldom calculated by hand in this era of computers and calculators. The emphasis will be on how to use statistics appropriately in different research situations and how to understand what they mean once they have been applied.

Statistics usually are classified as either descriptive or inferential. *Descriptive statistics* are used to describe and synthesize data. Averages and percentages are examples of descriptive statistics. Actually, when such indices are calculated on data from a population, they are referred to as *parameters*. A descriptive index from a sample is called a *statistic*. Most scientific questions are about parameters, but researchers usually calculate statistics to estimate those parameters. When researchers use statistics to make inferences or draw conclusions about a population, then *infer-*

Table 20-1. *AIDS Knowledge Test Scores*

22	27	25	19	24	25	23	29	24	20
26	16	20	26	17	22	24	18	26	28
15	24	23	22	21	24	20	25	18	27
24	23	16	25	30	29	27	21	23	24
26	18	30	21	17	25	22	24	29	28
20	25	26	24	23	19	27	28	25	26

ential statistics are required. This chapter focuses on descriptive statistical procedures.

≡ FREQUENCY DISTRIBUTIONS

Raw data that are neither analyzed nor organized are overwhelming. It is not even possible to discern general trends until some order or structure is imposed on the data. Consider the 60 numbers presented in Table 20-1. Let us assume that these numbers represent the scores of 60 nurses on a 30-item test to measure knowledge about acquired immunodeficiency syndrome (AIDS). Visual inspection of the numbers in this table is not too helpful in understanding how the nurses performed. The data are too numerous to make much sense of them in this form.

A set of data can be completely described in terms of three characteristics: (1) the shape of the distribution of scores, (2) central tendency, and (3) variability. Central tendency and variability are dealt with in subsequent sections.

Constructing Frequency Distributions

Frequency distributions represent a method of imposing some order on a mass of numerical data. A *frequency distribution* is a systematic arrangement of numerical values from the lowest to the highest, together with a count of the number of times each value was obtained. The fictitious test scores of the 60 nurses are presented as a frequency distribution in Table 20-2. It should be apparent that this organized arrangement makes it convenient to see at a glance how the nurses performed. We can see what the highest and lowest scores were, where the bulk of scores tended to cluster, and what the most common score was.

Table 20-2. *Frequency Distribution of Test Scores*

SCORE (X)	TALLIES	FREQUENCY (f)	PERCENTAGE (%)
15	I	1	1.7
16	I I	2	3.3
17	I I	2	3.3
18	I I I	3	5.0
19	I I	2	3.3
20	I I I I	4	6.7
21	I I I	3	5.0
22	I I I I	4	6.7
23	⊞	5	8.3
24	⊞ I I I I	9	15.0
25	⊞ I I	7	11.7
26	⊞ I	6	10.0
27	I I I I	4	6.7
28	I I I	3	5.0
29	I I I	3	5.0
30	I I	2	3.3
		$n = 60 = \Sigma f$	$\Sigma\% = 100\%$

None of this was easily discernible before the data were organized.

The construction of a frequency distribution is very simple. It consists basically of two parts: (1) the classes of observations or measurements (the Xs) and (2) the frequency or count of the observations falling in each class (the fs). The observations are listed in numerical order in one column and the corresponding frequencies are listed in another. Table 20-2 shows the intermediary step in which the observations were actually tallied by the familiar method of four vertical bars and then a slash for the fifth observation. The only requirement for a frequency distribution is that the classes of observation must be mutually exclusive and collectively exhaustive. The sum of the numbers appearing in the frequency column must be equal to the size of the sample. In less verbal terms, $\Sigma f = n$, which translates as the sum of (signified by the Greek letter sigma, Σ) the frequencies (f) equals the sample size (n).

It is often useful to display not only the frequency counts for different values but also the

percentages of the total, as shown in the fourth column of Table 20-2. The percentages are calculated by the simple formula: $\% = (f \div n) \times 100$. Just as the sum of all frequencies should equal n, the sum of all percentages should equal 100.

Rather than listing frequencies in tabular form, many researchers prefer to display their data graphically. Graphs have the advantage of being able to communicate a lot of information almost instantaneously. The most widely used types of graphs are *histograms* and *frequency polygons*. These two types are actually similar forms of presenting the same data.

Both histograms and frequency polygons are constructed in much the same fashion. First, score classes are placed on a horizontal dimension, with the lowest value on the left, ascending to the highest value on the right. Next, the vertical dimension is used to designate the frequency count or, alternatively, percentages. The numbering of the vertical axis usually begins with zero. Using these dimensions as a base, a histogram is constructed by drawing bars above the score

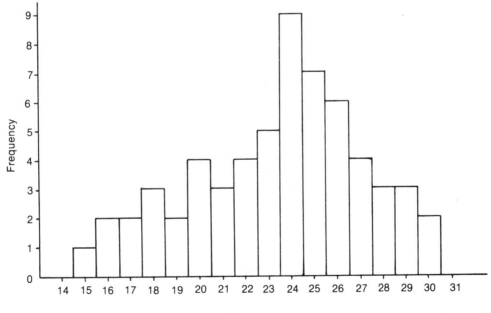

Figure 20-1. *Histogram of test scores.*

classes to the height corresponding to the frequency for that score class. An example is presented in Figure 20-1, using the same fictitious data on nurses' AIDS knowledge test scores.

Instead of vertical bars, the frequency polygon uses dots connected by straight lines to show frequencies for score classes. A dot corresponding to the frequency is placed above each score, as shown in Figure 20-2. It is conventional to connect the figure to the base (zero line) at the score below the minimum value obtained and above the maximum value obtained. In this particular example, however, the graph is terminated at 30 and brought down to the base at that point with a dotted line because a score of 31 was not possible.

Shapes of Distributions

A distribution of numerical values can assume an almost infinite number of shapes or forms. However, there are general aspects of the shape that can be described verbally. A distribution is said to be *symmetrical* in shape if, when folded over, the two halves of the distribution would be superimposed on one another. In other words, symmetrical distributions consist of two halves that are mirror images of one another. All of the distributions shown in Figure 20-3 are symmetrical. With real data sets, the distributions are rarely as perfectly symmetrical as shown in this figure. However, minor discrepancies are often ignored in trying to briefly characterize the shape of a distribution.

Asymmetrical distributions usually are described as being *skewed*. In skewed distributions, the peak is "off center" and one tail is longer than the other. Distributions that are skewed are usually described in terms of the direction of the skew. When the longer tail is pointing toward the right, the distribution is said to be *positively skewed*. Figure 20-4 (A) depicts a positively skewed distribution. If, on the other hand, the tail points to the left, the skew is described as negative. A *negatively skewed* distribution is illustrated in Figure 20-4 (B). An example of an actual attribute that is positively skewed is personal income.

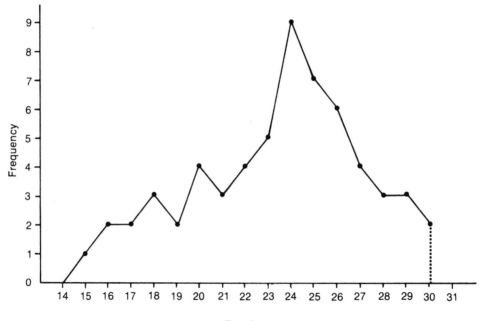

Figure 20-2. *Frequency polygon of test scores.*

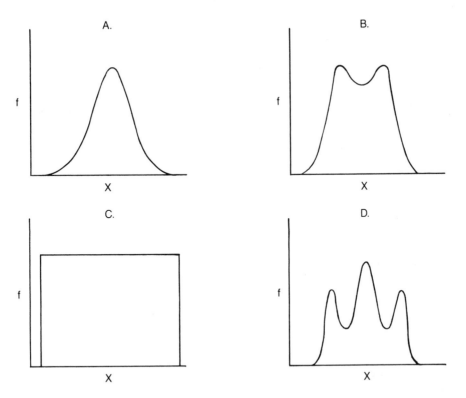

Figure 20-3. *Examples of symmetrical distributions.*

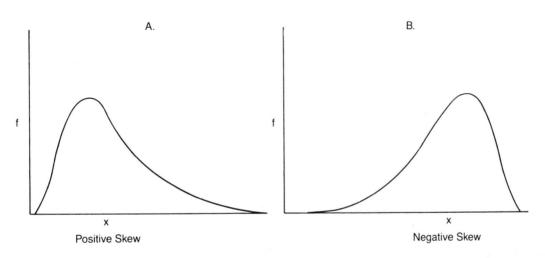

Figure 20-4. *Examples of skewed distributions.*

The bulk of people have low to moderate incomes, with relatively few people in very high income brackets at the tail of the distribution. An example of a negatively skewed attribute is age at death. Here, the bulk of people are at the upper end of the distribution, with relatively few people dying at an early age.

A second aspect of a distribution's shape is its modality. A *unimodal* distribution is one that has only one peak or high point (i.e., a value with high frequency), whereas a *multimodal* distribution has two or more peaks (i.e., two or more values of high frequency). The most common type of multimodal distribution is one with two peaks, which is called *bimodal*. Figure 20-3 (*A*) is unimodal, as are both graphs in Figure 20-4. Multimodal distributions are illustrated in Figure 20-3 (*B*) and (*D*). Symmetry and modality are completely independent aspects of a distribution. Knowledge of skewness does not tell you anything about how many peaks the distribution has.

Some distributions are encountered so frequently that special labels are used to designate them. Of particular interest in statistical analysis is the distribution known as the *normal curve* (sometimes called a *bell-shaped curve*). A normal curve is one that is symmetrical, unimodal, and not too peaked, as illustrated by the distribution in Figure 20-3 (*A*). Many physical and psychologic attributes of humans have been found to approximate a normal distribution. Examples include height, intelligence, age at menarche, and grip strength. As we will see in Chapter 21, the normal curve plays a central role in inferential statistics.

≡ *CENTRAL TENDENCY*

Frequency distributions are an important means of imposing order on a set of raw data and of clarifying group patterns. For many purposes, however, a group pattern is of less interest to a researcher than an overall summary of a group's characteristics. The researcher usually asks such questions as, What is the average oxygen consumption of myocardial infarction patients during bathing? What is the average blood pressure reading of hypertensive patients during relaxation therapy? How much information does the average pregnant teenager have about nutrition? Such questions seek a single number that best represents a whole distribution of measures. Because an index of "typicalness" is more likely to be representative if it comes from the center of a distribution than if it comes from either extreme, such indices are referred to as measures of *central tendency*. To lay people the term "average" is normally used to designate central tendency. Researchers seldom use this term because it is too ambiguous, inasmuch as there are three commonly used kinds of averages, or indices of central tendency: (1) the mode, (2) the median, and (3) the mean. Each can be used as an index to represent a whole set of measurements.

The Mode

The *mode* is that numerical value in a distribution that occurs most frequently. The mode is the simplest to determine of the three measures of central tendency. Actually, the mode is not computed, but rather is determined through inspection of a frequency distribution. In the following distribution of numbers, one can readily determine that the mode is 53:

50   51   51   52   53   53   53   53   54   55   56

The score of 53 was obtained four times, a higher frequency than for any other number. In the knowledge about AIDS example presented earlier, the mode of the AIDS knowledge test scores is 24 (Table 20-2). The mode, in other words, identifies the most "popular" score. (In multimodal distributions, of course, there is more than one score value that has high frequencies.) The mode is seldom used in research reports as the only index of central tendency. Modes are a quick and easy method of determining an "average" at a glance but are unsuitable for further computation and also are rather unstable. By unstable, we mean that modes tend to fluctuate widely from one sample drawn from a population to another sample drawn from the same population. The mode is infrequently used, except for describing "typical" values on nominal-level measures. For instance, researchers often characterize their samples by providing modal information on nominal-level demographic variables, as in the following example: "The typical subject was a white female, unmarried, living in an urban area, and with no prior history of sexually transmitted diseases."

The Median

The *median* is that point on a numerical scale above which and below which 50% of the cases fall. As an example, consider the following set of values:

$$2 \quad 2 \quad 3 \quad 3 \quad 4 \quad 5 \quad 6 \quad 7 \quad 8 \quad 9$$

The value that divides the cases exactly in half is 4.5, which is the median for this set of numbers. The point that has 50% of the cases above and below it is halfway between 4 and 5. An important characteristic of the median is that it does not take into account the quantitative values of individual scores. The median is an index of average *position* in a distribution of numbers. The median is insensitive to extreme values. Let us take the previous example to illustrate this point, making only one small change:

$$2 \quad 2 \quad 3 \quad 3 \quad 4 \quad 5 \quad 6 \quad 7 \quad 8 \quad 99$$

Despite the fact that the last value has been increased from 9 to 99, the median remains unchanged at 4.5. Because of this property, the median is often the preferred index of central tendency when the distribution is skewed and when one is interested in finding a "typical" value in measures on an ordinal scale or higher.

The Mean

The *mean* is the point on the score scale that is equal to the sum of the scores divided by the total number of scores. The mean is the index of central tendency that is usually referred to as an average. The computational formula for a mean—which everyone knows, but whose symbols need to be learned—is

$$\bar{X} = \frac{\Sigma X}{n}$$ where $\bar{X}$ = the mean
Σ = the sum of
X = each individual raw score
n = the number of cases

The researcher should become familiar with these symbols because they are commonly used to report results in the research literature.

Let us apply the above formula to calculate the mean weight of eight subjects whose individual weights are as follows:

$$85 \quad 109 \quad 120 \quad 135 \quad 158 \quad 177 \quad 181 \quad 195$$

$$\bar{X} = \frac{\begin{array}{c} 85 + 109 + 120 + 135 \\ + \ 158 + 177 + 181 + 195 \end{array}}{8}$$

$$= 145$$

Unlike the median, the mean is affected by the value of each and every score. If we were to exchange the 195-pound subject in this example for a subject weighing 275 pounds, the mean would increase from 145 to 155. A substitution of this kind would leave the median unchanged.

The mean is unquestionably the most widely used measure of central tendency. Many of the important tests of statistical significance, addressed in Chapter 21, are based on the mean. When researchers work with interval-level or ratio-level measurements, the mean rather than the median or mode is almost always the statistic reported.

Comparison of the Mode, Median, and Mean

Of the three indices of central tendency, the mean is the most stable. If repeated samples were drawn from a given population, the means would vary or fluctuate less than the modes or medians. Because of its stability, the mean is the most reliable estimate of the central tendency of the population.

The arithmetic mean is the most appropriate index in situations in which the concern is for totals or combined performance of a group. If a school of nursing were comparing two graduating classes in terms of scores on the national licensure examination, then the calculation of two means would be in order. Sometimes, however, the primary concern is learning what a "typical" value is, in which case a median might be preferred. In efforts to understand the economic well-being of United States citizens, for example, we would get a distorted impression of the financial status of the typical individual by considering the mean. The mean in this case would be inflated by the wealth of a small minority. The median, on the other hand, would reflect more realistically how the "average" person fared financially.

When a distribution of scores is symmetrical and unimodal, the three indices of central tendency coincide. In skewed distributions, the values of the mode, median, and mean differ. The mean is always pulled in the direction of the long tail, as shown in Figure 20-5. It is only in skewed distributions, therefore, that one must consider which index to use. When the distribution is

asymmetrical, it might be preferable to simply report all three values than to select a single index, because all three indices contain some information.

≡ VARIABILITY

Although measures of central tendency are of immense importance in descriptions of data, averages do not give a total picture of a distribution. Two sets of data with identical means could be different from one another in several respects. For one thing, two distributions with the same mean could be very different in shape: they could be skewed in opposite directions, for example. The characteristic of concern in this section is how spread out or dispersed the data are. The variability of two distributions could be quite different, even when the means are identical.

The concept of *variability* is concerned with the degree to which the subjects in a sample are similar to one another with respect to the critical attribute. Consider the two distributions in Figure 20-6, which represent the hypothetical Scholastic Aptitude Test (SAT) scores of freshmen students from two schools of nursing. Both distributions have an average of 500, but the patterns of scores

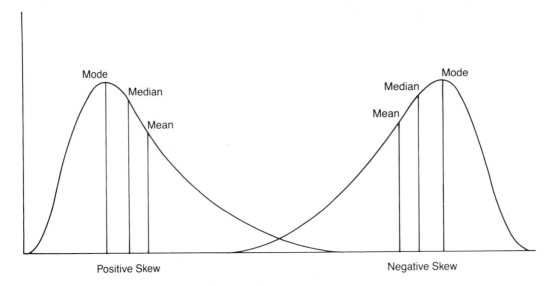

Figure 20-5. Relationships of central tendency indices in skewed distributions.

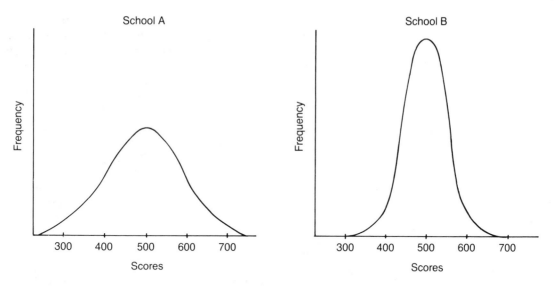

Figure 20-6. *Two distributions of different variability.*

are clearly different. In School A, there is a wide range of obtained scores: from scores below 300 to some above 700. This school has many students who performed among the best, but also has many students who were well below average. In School B, on the other hand, there are few students at either extreme. School A is said to be more *heterogeneous* than School B, and School B may be described as more *homogeneous* than School A.

To describe a distribution adequately, there is clearly a need for a measure of variability that expresses the extent to which scores deviate from one another. Several such indices have been developed, the most common of which are the range, semiquartile range, and standard deviation.

The Range

The *range* is simply the highest score minus the lowest score in a given distribution. In the examples shown in Figure 20-6, the range for School A is approximately 500 (750 − 250), and the range for School B is approximately 300 (650 − 350). The range indicates the distance on the score scale between the lowest and highest values.

The chief virtue of the range is the ease with which it can be computed. As an index of variability, the shortcomings of the range outweigh this modest advantage. The range, being based on only two scores, is a highly unstable index. From sample to sample drawn from the same population, the range tends to fluctuate considerably. Another difficulty with the range is that it ignores completely variations in scores between the two extremes. In School B of Figure 20-6, suppose that one "deviant" student obtained a score of 250 and another obtained a score of 750. The range of both schools would then be 500, despite obvious differences in the heterogeneity of scores. For these reasons, the range is used largely as a gross descriptive index and is typically reported in conjunction with, not instead of, other measures of variability.

Semiquartile Range*

A previous section described the median as the point below which 50% of the cases fall. It is computationally possible to determine the point

---

* Some statistical texts use the term semiquartile range, while others refer to this statistic as the semi-interquartile range or the quartile deviation.

below which any percentage of the scores fall. For example, an admissions committee for a school of nursing might establish a minimum standard at the 40th percentile on the SAT for its entrants. The *semiquartile range* is calculated on the basis of quartiles within a distribution. The upper quartile (Q^3) is the point below which 75% of the cases fall, and the lower quartile (Q^1) is the point below which 25% of the scores lie.[†] The semiquartile range is half the distance between Q^1 and Q^3, or

$$SQR = \frac{Q_3 - Q_1}{2}$$

The semiquartile range indicates half the range of scores within which the middle 50% of scores lie. Because this index is a measure based on middle cases rather than extreme scores, it is considerably more stable than the range. In the case of the two nursing schools in Figure 20-6, School A would have an semiquartile range in the vicinity of 125, and the semiquartile range of School B would be approximately 75. The addition of one deviant case at either extreme for School B would leave the semiquartile range virtually untouched.

Standard Deviation

The most widely used measure of variability is the standard deviation (SD). Like the mean, the standard deviation considers every score in a distribution.

What is needed in a variability index is some way of capturing the degree to which scores deviate from one another. This concept of deviation is represented in both the range and the semiquartile range by the presence of a minus sign, which produces an index of deviation, or difference, between two score points. The standard deviation is similarly based on score differences. In fact, the first step in calculating a standard deviation is to compute deviation scores for each subject. A *devi-*

[†] The computational formulas for percentiles are not presented here. Most standard statistics texts contain this information.

ation score (usually symbolized with a small *x*) is the difference between an individual score and the mean. If a person weighed 150 pounds and the sample mean were 140, then the person's deviation score would be +10. Symbolically, the formula for a deviation score is

$$x = X - \overline{X}.$$

Because what one is essentially looking for in an index of variability is a kind of "average" deviation, one might think that a good variability index could be arrived at by summing the deviation scores and then dividing by the number of cases. This gets us close to a good solution, but the difficulty is that the sum of a set of deviation scores is always zero. Table 20-3 presents an example of deviation scores computed for nine numbers. As shown in the second column, the sum of the *x*s is equal to zero. The deviations above the mean always balance exactly those deviations below the mean.

The standard deviation overcomes this problem by squaring each deviation score before summing. After dividing by the number of cases, one takes the square root to bring the index back to the original units. The formula for the standard deviation[‡] is

$$SD = \sqrt{\frac{\Sigma x^2}{n}}$$

The standard deviation has been completely worked out in the example in Table 20-3. First, a deviation score is calculated for each of the nine raw scores by subtracting the mean ($\overline{X} = 7$) from them. The third column shows that each deviation score is squared, thereby converting all

[‡] Some statistical texts indicate that the formula for an unbiased estimate of the population SD is

$$SD = \sqrt{\frac{\Sigma x^2}{n - 1}}$$

Knapp (1970) clarifies when n or $n - 1$ should be used in the denominator. He indicates that n is appropriate when the researcher is interested in *describing* variation in sample data.

Table 20-3. *Computation of a Standard Deviation*

X	$x = X - \overline{X}$	$x^2 = (X - \overline{X})^2$
4	−3	9
5	−2	4
6	−1	1
7	0	0
7	0	0
7	0	0
8	1	1
9	2	4
10	3	9

$$\Sigma X = 63 \qquad \Sigma x = 0 \qquad \Sigma x^2 = 28$$
$$\Sigma X/n = \overline{X}$$
$$= 63/9 = 7$$

$$SD = \sqrt{\frac{28}{9}} = \sqrt{3.11} = 1.76$$

values to positive numbers. The squared deviation scores are summed ($x^2 = 28$), divided by 9 (n), and a square root taken to yield an SD of 1.76.

Most researchers routinely report the standard deviation of a data set along with the mean. Sometimes, however, one will find a reference to an index of variability known as the variance. The *variance*[§] is simply the value of the standard deviation before a square root has been taken. In other words,

$$Var = \frac{\Sigma x^2}{n} = SD^2$$

In the above example, the variance is $(1.76)^2$, or 3.11. The variance is less widely reported because it is an index that is not the same unit of measurement as the original data. The variance, however, is an important component in many inferential statistical tests that will be encountered later. In any event, once a variance is obtained, it is a simple step to get a standard deviation, and vice versa.

§ Various symbols are used for the variance and standard deviation. The most common are $\sigma^2(\sigma)$ or s^2 (s), respectively.

A standard deviation is typically more difficult for students to interpret than other statistics such as the mean or range. In our previous example, we calculated an SD of 1.76. One might well ask, 1.76 *what?* What does the number mean? We will try to answer these questions from several vantage points. First, as we already know, the standard deviation is an index of the variability of scores in a data set. If two distributions had a mean of 25.0, but one had an SD of 7.0 and the other had an SD of 3.0, then we would immediately know that the second sample was more homogeneous.

A convenient way to conceptualize the standard deviation is to think of it as an average of the deviations from the mean. The mean tells us the single best point for summarizing an entire distribution, whereas a standard deviation tells us how much, on the average, the scores deviate from that mean. A standard deviation might thus be interpreted as an indication of our degree of error when we use a mean to describe an entire data set.

The standard deviation can also be used in interpreting individual scores from within a distribution. Suppose we had a set of weight measures from a sample whose mean weight was 125 and whose SD was ten. We can think of the standard deviation as actually providing a "standard" of variability. Weights greater than 1 SD away from the mean (i.e., greater than 135 or less than 115) are greater than the average variability for that distribution. Weights less than 1 SD from the mean, by consequence, are less than the average variability for that sample.

When the distribution of scores is normal, it is possible to say even more about the standard deviation. A normal curve, it will be recalled, is a symmetric, unimodal distribution. There are approximately 3 SDs above and below the mean with normally distributed data. To illustrate some further characteristics, suppose that we had a normal distribution of scores whose mean was 50 and whose SD was 10. Such a distribution is shown in Figure 20-7. In a normal distribution such as this, a fixed percentage of cases fall within certain distances from the mean. Sixty-eight per-

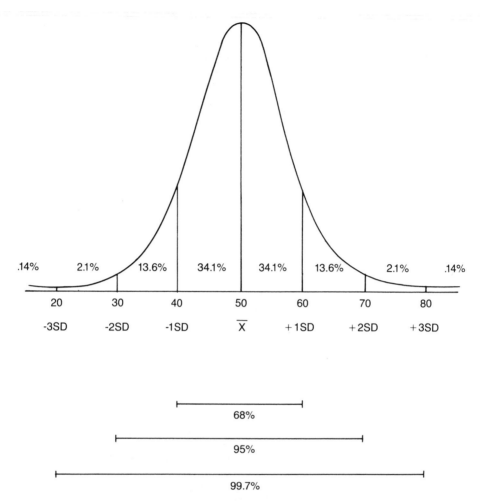

Figure 20-7. *Standard deviations in a normal distribution.*

cent of all cases fall within 1 SD of the mean (34% above and 34% below the mean). In this example, nearly seven out of every ten scores fall between 40 and 60. Ninety-five percent of the scores in a normal distribution fall within 2 SDs from the mean. Only a handful of cases—about 2% at each extreme—lie more than 2 SDs from the mean. Using this figure, we can see that a person who obtained a score of 70 got a higher score than about 98% of the sample.

In sum, the standard deviation is a useful index of variability that can be used to describe an important characteristic of a distribution and that also can be used to interpret the score or perfor-

mance of an individual *vis-à-vis* others in the sample. Like the mean, the standard deviation is a stable estimate of a population parameter and also is used extensively in more advanced statistical procedures. The standard deviation is the preferred measure of a distribution's variability.

≡ LEVELS OF MEASUREMENT AND DESCRIPTIVE STATISTICS

The kinds of statistics discussed thus far cannot be indiscriminantly applied to a set of data without considering the measurement characteristics of the scores. In Chapter 19, it was pointed out that there are four levels of measurement: nominal, ordinal, interval, and ratio. The level of measurement plays a role in determining the appropriate descriptive statistic for a variable.

In general, the higher the level of measurement, the greater the flexibility one has in choosing a descriptive statistic. Variables measured on an interval or ratio scale can use any of the three indices of central tendency, although it usually will be preferable to use the mean. However, for nominal-level data, it would make little sense to compute a mean. If we coded marital status as "1" for single, "2" for married, and "3" for other, a mean marital status of 1.73 would be nonsensical. It would, however, be reasonable to determine the modal response for nominal data.

Table 20-4 presents a rough guide of the statistics appropriate with different levels of measurement. It is always possible to choose a statistic from a lower level, but not from a higher one. One could use the range as an index of variability for data on a person's pulse rate (ratio level), but it would not be meaningful to calculate a standard deviation for a measure of ethnicity (nominal level). Generally, it is inadvisable to select a statistic that is suitable to a lower level of data, but circumstances may warrant it, as in the case of using a median with a severely skewed distribution.

≡ *BIVARIATE DESCRIPTIVE STATISTICS: CONTINGENCY TABLES AND CORRELATION*

The discussion has so far focused on a description of single variables. The mean, mode, standard deviation, and so forth are all used in describing data for one variable at a time. We have been examining what is referred to as *univariate* (one-variable) statistics. As indicated throughout this text, research usually is concerned with relationships between variables. What is needed then is some method of describing such relationships. In this section, we look at *bivariate* (two-variable) descriptive statistics.

Contingency Tables

A *contingency table* is essentially a two-dimensional frequency distribution in which the frequencies of two variables are cross-tabulated. Suppose we had data on subjects' sex and responses to a question on whether they were nonsmokers, light smokers, or heavy smokers. We might be interested in learning if there is a tendency for members of one sex to smoke more heavily than members of the opposite sex. Some fictitious data on these two variables are presented in Table 20-5. It is difficult to make sense of these data in their present form. To describe the data, we need a method of organizing this mass of numbers. The best way to do so in a manner that highlights the research question is to construct a contingency table.

A contingency table for the data in Table 20-5 is presented in Table 20-6. Six "cells" are created by placing one variable (sex) along the vertical dimension and the other variable (smoking status) along the horizontal dimension. The system of bars and crosshatches can then be used to tabulate the number of subjects belonging in each cell. The first subject, who has a code of "1" for sex and "1" for smoking status, would be marked in the upper left-hand cell, and so on.

Table 20-4. *Guide to Use of Descriptive Statistics*

	LEVEL OF MEASUREMENT		
Type of Statistic	*Nominal*	*Ordinal*	*Interval or Ratio*
Measure of Central Tendency	Mode	Median	Mean
Measure of Variability	Range	Semiquartile range	Standard deviation/variance

Table 20-5. *Fictitious Data on Sex/Smoking Relationship*

SUBJECT SEX*	SMOKING STATUS†	SUBJECT SEX	SMOKING STATUS	SUBJECT SEX	SMOKING STATUS
1	1	2	2	2	1
2	3	2	3	1	1
2	1	1	1	2	2
1	2	2	2	1	2
1	1	1	2	1	1
2	2	1	1	2	2
2	1	1	3	2	3
2	3	1	2	2	3
1	1	2	2	2	2
2	3	2	1	1	2
1	2	1	3	1	1
1	3	2	3	2	1
1	1	1	1	1	2
2	3	1	3	2	2
2	1	1	2		

* 1 = female; 2 = male.
† 1 = nonsmoker; 2 = light smoker; 3 = heavy smoker.

After all subjects have been "assigned" to the appropriate cells, the frequencies can be tabulated and percentages computed. This simple procedure allows us to see at a glance that, in this particular sample, women were more likely to be nonsmokers and less likely to be heavy smokers than males. Contingency tables, or *cross-tabulations* as they are sometimes called, are easy to construct and have the ability to communicate a lot of information. The use of contingency tables usually is restricted to nominal data or to ordinal data that have few levels or ranks. In the sex/ smoker relationship example, sex is a nominal measure and smoking status is an ordinal measure. We will encounter contingency tables again in the discussion on inferential statistics in Chapter 21.

Correlation

The most common method of describing the relationship between two measures is through correlation procedures. The computation of a correlation coefficient is normally per-

Table 20-6. *Contingency Table for Sex/Smoker Relationship*

SUBJECT SEX	NONSMOKER (1)		LIGHT SMOKER (2)		HEAVY SMOKER (3)		TOTAL
Female (1)	⳥⳥ (45% of females)	10	⳥ ⏐⏐⏐ (36% of females)	8	⏐⏐⏐⏐ (18% of females)	4	22 (50% of sample)
Male (2)	⳥ ⏐ (27% of males)	6	⳥ ⏐⏐⏐ (36% of males)	8	⳥ ⏐⏐⏐ (36% of males)	8	22 (50% of sample)
TOTAL	(36% of sample)	16	(36% of sample)	16	(27% of sample)	12	44 (100% of sample)

formed when two variables are measured on either the ordinal, interval, or ratio scale. Correlation coefficients were briefly described in Chapter 18, and this section extends that discussion.

The correlation question asks, To what extent are two variables related to each other? For example, to what extent are height and weight related? To what degree are anxiety test scores and blood pressure measures related? These questions can be answered graphically or, more commonly, by the calculation of an index that describes the magnitude of the relationship.

The graphic representation of a correlation between two variables is called a *scatter plot* or *scatter diagram*. To construct a scatter plot, one first sets up a scale for the two variables constructed at right angles, making a rectangular coordinate graph. The range of values for one variable (*X*) is scaled off along the horizontal axis, while the same is done for the second variable (*Y*) along the vertical axis. Such a graph is presented in Figure 20-8. To locate the position for Subject A, one goes two units to the right along the X-axis,

and one unit up on the Y-axis. The same procedure is followed for all subjects, resulting in the scatter plot shown. The letters shown on the plot in this figure have been included to help identify each point. Normally only the "dots" appear on the diagram.

From a scatter plot it is possible to determine both the direction and approximate magnitude of a correlation. The direction of the slope of points indicates the direction of the correlation. It may be recalled from Chapter 18 that correlations can be either positive or negative in direction. A *positive correlation* is obtained when high values on one variable are associated with high values on the second variable. If the slope of points begins at the lower-left corner and extends to the upper-right corner, then the relationship is positive. In the current example, we would say that *X* and *Y* are positively related. Inspection of the values shows that, indeed, people who have a high score on variable *X* also tend to have a high score on variable *Y*, and low scorers on *X* tend to score low on *Y*.

A *negative* (or *inverse*) *relationship* is one in

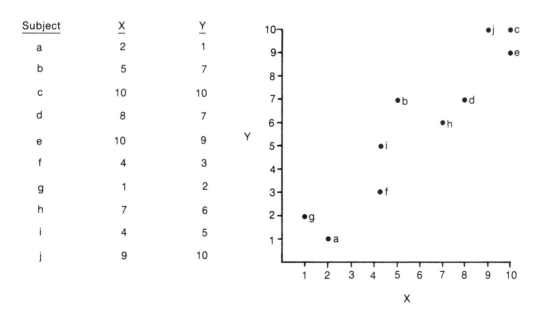

Figure 20-8. *Construction of a scatter plot.*

which high values on one variable are related to low values on the other. On a scatter plot, negative relationships are depicted by points that slope from the upper-left corner to the lower-right corner. A negative correlation is shown in Figure 20-9 (A) and (D).

Relationships are described as "perfect" when it is possible to know precisely a person's score on one variable by knowing his or her score on the other. For instance, if all people who were 6′2″ tall weighed 180 pounds, and all people who were 6′1″ tall weighed 175 pounds, and so on, then we could say that weight and height were perfectly, positively related. In such a situation, one would only need to be informed of a person's height to know his or her weight, or vice versa. On a scatter plot, a perfect relationship is represented by a sloped straight line, as shown in Figure 20-9 (C). When a relationship is not per-

fect, as is usually the case, one can interpret the degree of correlation from a scatter plot by seeing how closely the points cluster around a straight line. The more closely packed the points are about a diagonal slope, the higher the correlation. When the points are scattered all over the graph, the relationship is very low or nonexistent. Various degrees and directions of relationships are presented in Figure 20-9 (A–F).

Usually it is more convenient and more succinct to express the direction and magnitude of a linear relationship by means of a numerical index that is called a correlation coefficient. A *correlation coefficient* is an index whose values range from −1.0 for a perfect negative correlation, through zero for no relationship, to +1.0 for a perfect positive correlation. All correlations that fall between 0.0 and −1.0 are negative, and all correlations that fall between 0.0 and +1.0 are

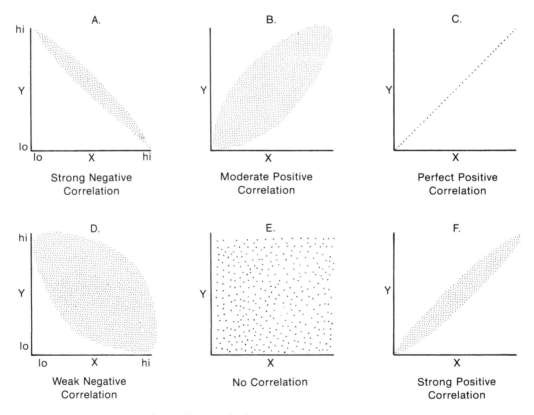

Figure 20-9. *Various relationships graphed on scatter plots.*

positive. The higher the absolute value of the coefficient (i.e., the value disregarding the sign), the stronger the relationship. A correlation of −.80, for instance, is stronger than a correlation of +.20.

The most commonly used correlation index is the product-moment correlation coefficient, also referred to as *Pearson's r*. This coefficient is computed when the variables being correlated have been measured on either an interval or ratio scale. The calculation of the *r* statistic is rather laborious and seldom performed by hand.*

Perfect correlations (+1.00 and −1.00) are extremely rare in research with humans. It is difficult to offer guidelines on what should be interpreted as strong or weak relationships. This determination depends, to a great extent, on the nature of the variables. If we were to measure patients' body temperatures both orally and rectally, a correlation of .70 between the two measurements would be considered low. For most variables of a social or psychologic nature, however, an *r* of .70 is quite high; correlations between variables of a psychosocial nature are typically in the .10 to .40 range.

≡ *THE COMPUTER AND DESCRIPTIVE STATISTICS*

In the previous sections, we introduced the basic concepts of univariate and bivariate statistics that are used to organize, summarize, and describe data. In this section, we work through a fictitious

---

* For those who may wish to understand how a correlation coefficient is computed, we offer the following formula:

$$r_{xy} = \frac{\Sigma(X - \overline{X})(Y - \overline{Y})}{\sqrt{[\Sigma(X - \overline{X})^2][\Sigma(Y - \overline{Y})^2]}}$$

where r_{xy} = the correlation coefficient for variables X and Y

$\quad$ X = an individual score for variable X

$\quad$ $\overline{X}$ = the mean score for variable X

$\quad$ Y = an individual score for variable Y

$\quad$ $\overline{Y}$ = the mean score for variable Y

$\quad$ Σ = the sum of

example of a study and illustrate these concepts through the use of computer printouts. The intent of this section is both to make the concepts less abstract by illustrating them with some data and to familiarize the reader with printout from a standard computer program (SPSS[x]). Information regarding the use of such programs is described in greater detail in Chapter 25.

Suppose that a nurse researcher were interested in improving the childbirth outcomes among a group of young, low-income pregnant women. A program of intensive health care, nutritional counseling, and contraceptive counseling is developed, and an experiment is designed to test the effect of the program: half of a sample of pregnant women, assigned randomly, will receive the special treatment, and the other half will be assigned to a group receiving routine care. The two outcomes that the researcher is primarily interested in are the birthweight of the infant and whether or not the young woman becomes pregnant again within 18 months of delivery. Some fictitious data for this example are presented in Table 20-7.

Figure 20-10 presents a frequency distribution printout for the birthweight variable. Under the term "VALUE," each birthweight in the sample is listed in ascending order. In the next column, "FREQUENCY," the number of occurrences of each birthweight is indicated. Thus, there was one 76-ounce baby, two 89-ounce babies, and so on. The next column, "PERCENT," indicates the percentage of birthweights in each class: 3.3% of the babies weighed 76 ounces at birth, 6.7% weighed 89 ounces, and so on. The next column, "VALID PERCENT," shows the percentage in each category after removing any missing data. In this example, birthweights were obtained for all 30 cases, but if one piece of data had been missing, the adjusted frequency for the 76-ounce baby would have been 3.4% (1 ÷ 29 rather than 30). The last column, "CUM PERCENT," adds the percentage for a given birthweight value to the percentage for all preceding values. Thus, we can tell by looking at the row for 99 ounces that, cumulatively, 33.3% of the babies weighed *under* 100 ounces in this example.

The bottom of this printout provides a number of the descriptive statistics discussed in this chapter. The MEAN is equal to 104.7, whereas the MEDIAN is 102.5, and the MODE is 99. This suggests that the distribution is somewhat skewed. The RANGE is 52, which is equal to the MAXIMUM of 128 minus the MINIMUM of 76. The SD (STD DEV) is 10.955, and the VARIANCE is 120.010 (10.955²).

In addition to tabular information, such as that shown in Figure 20-10, many programs can produce graphic materials. Figure 20-11 presents a histogram for the variable of a mother's age. In this case, all of the values for age are shown on the vertical axis, and the frequency on the horizontal axis. The histogram shows at a glance that the modal age is 19 ($f = 7$) and that this variable is negatively skewed (i.e., there are fewer younger girls). Descriptive statistics shown at the bottom of the printout indicate that the mean age for this group was 18.167, with an SD of 2.086.

If we were interested in comparing the repeat-pregnancy experience of the two groups of young women (experimental versus control), we would instruct the computer to cross-tabulate the two variables, as shown in the contingency table

Table 20-7. *Fictitious Data on Low-Income Pregnant Young Women*

GROUP (1 = EXPERIMENTAL; 2 = CONTROL)	WEIGHT OF INFANT (IN OZ)	REPEAT PREGNANCY WITHIN 18 MONTHS (1 = YES; 0 = NO)	AGE OF MOTHER
1	107	1	17
1	101	0	14
1	119	0	21
1	128	1	20
1	89	0	15
1	99	0	19
1	111	0	19
1	117	1	18
1	102	1	17
1	120	0	20
1	76	0	13
1	116	0	18
1	100	1	16
1	115	0	18
1	113	0	21
2	111	1	19
2	108	0	21
2	95	0	19
2	99	0	17
2	103	1	19
2	94	0	15
2	101	1	17
2	114	0	21
2	97	0	20
2	99	1	18
2	113	0	18
2	89	0	19
2	98	0	20
2	102	0	17
2	105	0	19

WEIGHT   BIRTHWEIGHT OF BABY

VALUE LABEL	VALUE	FREQUENCY	PERCENT	VALID PERCENT	CUM PERCENT
	76	1	3.3	3.3	3.3
	89	2	6.7	6.7	10.0
	94	1	3.3	3.3	13.3
	95	1	3.3	3.3	16.7
	97	1	3.3	3.3	20.0
	98	1	3.3	3.3	23.3
	99	3	10.0	10.0	33.3
	100	1	3.3	3.3	36.7
	101	2	6.7	6.7	43.3
	102	2	6.7	6.7	50.0
	103	1	3.3	3.3	53.3
	105	1	3.3	3.3	56.7
	107	1	3.3	3.3	60.0
	108	1	3.3	3.3	63.3
	111	2	6.7	6.7	70.0
	113	2	6.7	6.7	76.7
	114	1	3.3	3.3	80.0
	115	1	3.3	3.3	83.3
	116	1	3.3	3.3	86.7
	117	1	3.3	3.3	90.0
	119	1	3.3	3.3	93.3
	120	1	3.3	3.3	96.7
	128	1	3.3	3.3	100.0
	TOTAL	30	100.0	100.0	

MEAN	104.700	STD ERR	2.000	MEDIAN	102.500
MODE	99.000	STD DEV	10.955	VARIANCE	120.010
KURTOSIS	.473	S E KURT	.833	SKEWNESS	-0.254
S E SKEW	.427	RANGE	52.000	MINIMUM	76.000
MAXIMUM	128.000	SUM	3141.000		

VALID CASES   30   MISSING CASES   0

Figure 20-10. *SPSS^x computer printout: frequency distribution.*

in Figure 20-12. This cross-tabulation resulted in four cells: (1) experimental subjects with no repeat pregnancy (upper-left cell); (2) control subjects with no repeat pregnancy (upper-right cell); (3) experimental subjects with a repeat pregnancy (lower-left cell); and (4) control subjects with a repeat pregnancy (lower-right cell). Each cell contains four pieces of information, which we will explain for the first cell. The first number is the number of subjects in that cell. Ten experimental subjects did not have a repeat pregnancy within 18 months of their delivery. The next number is the *row* percentage: 47.6% of the

women who did not become pregnant again were in the experimental group (10 ÷ 21). The next number represents the *column* percentage: 66.7% of the experimentals did not become pregnant (10 ÷ 15). The last number is the *overall* percentage of women in that cell (10 ÷ 30 = 33.3%). This order need not be memorized. It is shown in the upper-left corner of the table:

COUNT
ROW PCT
COL PCT
TOT PCT

```
       COUNT       VALUE      ONE SYMBOL EQUALS APPROXIMATELY    .20 OCCURRENCES

         1        13.00   ****
         1        14.00   ****
         2        15.00   **********
         1        16.00   ****
         5        17.00   ***************************
         5        18.00   ***************************
         7        19.00   *************************************************
         4        20.00   *******************
         4        21.00   *******************
                          I.........I.........I.........I.........I.........I
                          0         2         4         6         8         10
                                       HISTOGRAM FREQUENCY


   MEAN         18.167      STD ERR       .381      MEDIAN        18.500
   MODE         19.000      STD DEV      2.086      VARIANCE       4.351
   KURTOSIS       .143      S E KURT      .833      SKEWNESS      -0.701
   S E SKEW       .427      RANGE        8.000      MINIMUM       13.000
   MAXIMUM      21.000      SUM        545.000


   VALID CASES     30       MISSING CASES      0
```

Figure 20-11. *SPSS[x] computer printout: histogram.*

```
- - - - - - - - - - - - - - - - - - -    C R O S S T A B U L A T I O N   O F
    REPEAT                                                BY   GROUP
- - - - - - - - - - - - - - - - - - - - - - - - - - - - - - - - - - - - - -

                     GROUP
             COUNT   |
             ROW PCT |EXPERIME CONTROL      ROW
             COL PCT |NTAL                  TOTAL
             TOT PCT |       1|        2|
   REPEAT.           --------+--------+--------+
                   0 |     10 |     11 |     21
    NO REPEAT PREG   |   47.6 |   52.4 |   70.0
                     |   66.7 |   73.3 |
                     |   33.3 |   36.7 |
                     +--------+--------+
                   1 |      5 |      4 |      9
    REPEAT PREG      |   55.6 |   44.4 |   30.0
                     |   33.3 |   26.7 |
                     |   16.7 |   13.3 |
                     +--------+--------+
             COLUMN         15       15       30
             TOTAL        50.0     50.0    100.0
```

Figure 20-12. *SPSS[x] computer printout: crosstabulation.*

Thus, Figure 20-12 indicates that a somewhat higher percentage of experimentals (33.3%) than controls (26.7%) experienced a repeat pregnancy. The row totals on the far right indicate that, overall, 30.0% of the sample (N = 9) had a subsequent pregnancy. The column total at the bottom indicates that, overall, 50% of the subjects were in the experimental group and 50% were in the control group.

≡ *RESEARCH EXAMPLES*

Table 20-8 presents some examples of descriptive statistics (measures of central tendency and variability) that have been presented in six nursing studies. One research example is discussed in greater detail below.

> Gross and colleagues (1989) explored the factors that are predictive of maternal confidence during toddlerhood among mothers of children born preterm (PT) and full term (FT). Information on the mothers' background was obtained in a questionnaire and information on the children's characteristics at birth was obtained from hospital records. Maternal confidence, the dependent variable, was measured by the Toddler-Care Questionnaire (TCQ), a 37-item Likert-type scale that yielded interval-level data.
>
> A wide variety of descriptive statistics were used to report study findings and sample characteristics. For example, the PT infants' mean birthweight was 2,004 grams (SD = 565), and that of the FT infants was 3,503 grams (SD = 423). This indicates that the PT infants weighed substantially less at birth and were more heterogeneous with respect to birthweight than FT infants. The mothers' mean age at the time of the study was similar in the two groups: 30.7 (SD = 4) in the PT group and 31.3 (SD = 3.7) in the FT group, with a range of 22 to 40 in both groups. Percentages were also used to describe the sample. For example, 26% of the PT children had

Table 20-8. *Examples of Descriptive Statistics Used in Nursing Research Reports*

VARIABLE	*CENTRAL TENDENCY INDEX*	*VARIABILITY INDEX*	*REFERENCE*
Uncertainty in illness (MUIS scale)	Mean: 1173.3	SD: 435.4 Range: 211–2,570	Braden, 1990
Total number of questions asked during clinic visit	Mean: 6.3 Median: 4 Modes: 0, 2	SD: 7.4 Range: 0–27	Barsevick & Johnson, 1990
Depression (Center for Epidemiological Studies Depression Scale, CES-D)	Mean: 8.7 Median: 6.0	SD: 8.9 Range: 0–46	Scalzi, 1990
Age of head of household eligible for Medicaid	Mean: 30.8 Median: 29	SD: 8.8	Selby et al., 1990
Number of stresses reported by hemodialysis patients	Mean: 16.4	SD: 7.2 Range: 2–32	Gurklis & Menke, 1988
Pulmonary artery wedge pressure at peak-inspiration	Mean: 25.9	SD: 8.9 Range: 12–42	Levine-Silverman & Johnson, 1990

handicaps or major health problems compared with 4% of the FT children. Group membership (PT versus FT) was cross-tabulated with various demographic variables, such as maternal education and ethnicity. These cross-tabulations revealed that the groups were fairly similar, except for a substantially higher percentage of white mothers in the FT group (96%) than in the PT group (77%).

Scores on the TCQ were found to be the same for both FT mothers ($\overline{X}$ = 3.96, SD = .45) and PT mothers ($\overline{X}$ = 3.96, SD = .50). Correlations between the TCQ and background variables revealed that maternal confidence was modestly related to the child's birth order among those in the PT group (r = .41), but negligibly related among the mothers in the FT group (r = .11). By contrast, mothers' age was positively related to maternal confidence in the FT group (r = .36), but essentially unrelated in the PT group (r = −.04). For both groups, the best predictor of maternal confidence was prior child care experience, with a correlation coefficient of .45.

☰ SUMMARY

Descriptive statistics enable the researcher to reduce, summarize, and describe quantitative data obtained from empirical observations and measurements. Raw data that have not been organized or analyzed are difficult, if not impossible, to interpret and communicate to others. A *frequency distribution* is one of the easiest methods of imposing some order on a mass of numbers. In a frequency distribution, numerical values are ordered from the lowest to the highest with a count of the number of times each value was obtained. *Histograms* and *frequency polygons* are two common methods of displaying frequency information graphically.

A set of data may be completely described in terms of the shape of the distribution, central tendency, and variability. The most important attributes of the distribution's shape are its symmetry and modality. A distribution is *symmetrical* if its two halves are mirror images of each other. A

skewed distribution, by contrast, is asymmetrical, with one "tail" longer than the other. The modality of a distribution refers to the number of peaks present: a *unimodal* distribution has one peak and a *multimodal* distribution has more than one peak.

Measures of *central tendency* are indices, expressed as a single number, that represent the "average" or typical value of a set of scores. The *mode* is the numerical value that occurs most frequently in the distribution (or with greater frequency than other scores in its vicinity). The *median* is that point on a numerical scale above which and below which 50% of the cases fall. The *mean* is the arithmetic average of all the scores in the distribution. In general, the mean is the preferred measure of central tendency because of its stability and its usefulness in further statistical manipulations.

Variability refers to the spread or dispersion of the data. Measures of variability include the range, the semiquartile range, and the standard deviation. The *range* is the distance between the highest and lowest score values. The *semiquartile range* indicates one half of the range of scores within which the middle 50% of scores lie. The most commonly used measure of variability is the *standard deviation.* This index is calculated by first computing *deviation scores,* which represent the degree to which the scores of each person deviate from the mean. The standard deviation is designed to indicate how much, on average, the scores deviate from the mean. A related index, *the variance,* is equal to the standard deviation squared.

Bivariate descriptive statistics describe the degree and magnitude of relationships between two variables. A *contingency table* is a two-dimensional frequency distribution in which the frequencies of two variables are cross-tabulated. When the scores have been measured on an ordinal, interval, or ratio scale, it is more common to describe the relationship between two variables with correlational procedures. A *correlation coefficient* can be calculated to express in numerical terms the direction and magnitude of a linear relationship. The values of the correlation coefficient range from −1.00 for a perfect negative correlation, through 0.0 for no relationship, to +1.00 for a perfect positive correlation. The most frequently used correlation coefficient is the product-moment correlation coefficient, also referred to as *Pearson's r*. The graphic representation of a relationship between two variables is called a *scatter plot* or scatter diagram.

≡ STUDY SUGGESTION

1. Construct a frequency distribution for the following set of scores obtained from a scale to measure attitudes toward primary nursing:

   32 20 33 22 16 19 25 26 25 18 22 30 24 26 27 23 28
   26 21 24 31 29 25 28 22 27 26 30 17 24

2. Construct a frequency polygon or histogram with the data from above. Describe the resulting distribution of scores in terms of symmetry and modality. How closely does the distribution approach a normal distribution?

3. What are the mean, median, and mode for the following set of data?

   13 12 9 15 7 10 16 8 6 11

   Compute the range and standard deviation.

4. Two hospitals are interested in comparing the tenure rates of their nursing staff. Hospital A finds that the current staff has been employed for a mean of 4.3 years, with an SD of 1.5. Hospital B, on the other hand, finds that the nurses have worked there for a mean of 6.4 years, with an SD of 4.2 years. Discuss what these results signify.

5. Suppose a researcher has conducted a study concerning lactose intolerance in children. The data reveal that 22 boys and 16 girls have lactose intolerance, out of a sample of 60 children of each sex. Construct a contingency table and calculate the percentages for each cell in the table. Discuss the meaning of these statistics.

6. A researcher has collected data on pulse rate and scores on a final exam for 10 students and would like to know if there is a relationship between the two measures. Compute Pearson's *r* for these data:

Pulse rate: 84 72 82 68 96 64 92 88 76 74
Test scores: 92 84 88 72 68 74 72 90 82 86

≡ SUGGESTED READINGS

METHODOLOGICAL REFERENCES

Blalock, H.M., Jr. (1979). *Social statistics* (2nd ed.). New York: McGraw-Hill.

Games, P.A., & Klare, G.R. (1967). *Elementary statistics: Data analysis for the behavioral sciences.* New York: McGraw-Hill.

Glass, G.V., & Stanley, J.C. (1984). *Statistical methods in education and psychology* (2nd ed.). Englewood Cliffs, NJ: Prentice-Hall.

Knapp, R.G. (1984). *Basic statistics for nurses* (2nd ed.). New York: John Wiley and Sons.

Knapp, T.R. (1970). N vs. N − 1. *American Educational Research Journal, 7,* 625−626.

McNemar, Q. (1969). *Psychological statistics* (4th ed.). New York: John Wiley and Sons.

Runyon, R.P., & Haber, A. (1984). *Fundamentals of behavioral statistics* (5th ed.). Reading, MA: Addison-Wesley.

Sokal, R.R., & Rohlf, F.J. (1981). *Biometry: The principles and practice of statistics in biological research* (2nd ed.). San Francisco: W.H. Freeman.

Spence, J.T., et al. (1983). *Elementary statistics* (4th ed.). New York: Appleton-Century-Crofts.

SUBSTANTIVE REFERENCES*

Aberman, S., & Kirchhoff, K.T. (1985). Infant-feeding practices: Mothers' decision making. *Journal of Obstetric, Gynecologic, and Neonatal Nursing, 14,* 394−398. [Percentages, cross-tabulations]

Barsevick, A.M., & Johnson, J.E. (1990). Preference for information and involvement, informational seeking and emotional responses of women undergoing colposcopy. *Research in Nursing and Health, 13,* 1−7. [Means, medians, modes, SDs, ranges, percentages, correlation coefficients]

*A comment in brackets after each citation designates the descriptive statistics of interest.

Braden, C.J. (1990). A test of the self-help model: Learned response to chronic illness experience. *Nursing Research, 39,* 42–47. [Means, SDs, ranges, skewness]

Brubaker, B.H. (1988). An attributional analysis of weight outcomes. *Nursing Research, 37,* 282–287. [Means, SDs, percentages]

Engstrom, J.L., & Chen, E.H. (1984). Prediction of birthweight by the use of extrauterine measurements during labor. *Research in Nursing and Health, 7,* 314–323. [Means, medians, SDs, ranges]

Gross, D., Rocissano, L., & Roncoli, M. (1989). Maternal confidence during toddlerhood: Comparing preterm and fullterm groups. *Research in Nursing and Health, 12,* 1–9. [Means, SDs, ranges, percentages, cross-tabulations, correlation coefficients]

Gurklis, J.A., & Menke, E.M. (1988). Identification of stressors and use of coping methods in chronic hemodialysis patients. *Nursing Research, 37,* 236–239. [Means, SDs, ranges, correlation coefficients]

Levine-Silverman, S., & Johnson, J. (1990). Pulmonary artery pressure measurements. *Western Journal of Nursing Research, 12,* 488–496. [Percentages, means, SDs, ranges]

Metheny, N., Williams, P., Wiersema, L., Wehrle, M.A., Eisenberg, P., & McSweeney, M. (1989). Effectiveness of pH measurements in predicting feeding tube placement. *Nursing Research, 38,* 280–285. [Means, SDs, percentages]

Robb, S.S. (1985). Urinary incontinence verification in elderly men. *Nursing Research, 34,* 278–282. [Means, SDs, percentages, cross-tabulations]

Scalzi, C.C. (1990). Role stress in top-level nurse executives. *Western Journal of Nursing Research, 12,* 85–94. [Means, medians, SDs, ranges, percentages, correlation coefficients]

Selby, M.L., Riportilla-Muller, R., Sorensen, J.R. Quade, D., Sappenfield, M.M., Potter, H.B., & Farel, A.M. (1990). Public health nursing interventions to improve the use of a health service. *Public Health Nursing, 7,* 3–12. [Means, medians, SDs]

Updike, P.A., Accurso, F.J., & Jones, R.H. (1985). Physiologic circadian rhythmicity in preterm infants. *Nursing Research, 34,* 16–163. [Means, SDs]

21
Inferential Statistics

Descriptive statistics such as means, standard deviations (SDs), and correlation coefficients are useful for summarizing univariate and bivariate sets of data. Usually, however, the researcher needs to do more than simply describe data obtained from a sample. Normally, subjects selected to participate in a research project are only a sample of individuals drawn from a population with certain characteristics. *Inferential statistics* provide a means for drawing conclusions about a population, given the data actually obtained for the sample. Inferential statistical reasoning would help us with such questions as, "What do I know about the average Apgar score of premature babies [the population] after having learned that a sample of 50 premature babies had a mean Apgar score of 7.5?" or "What can I conclude about the differential need for health education among women over age 25 [the population] after having found in a sample of 500 women that 50% of college-educated women but only 20% of high school-educated women practiced breast self-examination?" With the assistance of inferential statistics, researchers make judgments about or generalize to a large class of individuals based on information from a limited number of subjects.

Generally, the purpose of testing or measuring a sample is to gather data that allow us to make statements about the characteristics of a population. One estimates the parameters of a population from the statistics or attributes of the sample. These estimates are based on laws of probability, and, as we shall see, probabilistic estimates involve a certain degree of error. The difference between estimates based on inferential statistics and estimates arrived at through the ordinary thinking process is that the statistical method provides a framework for making judgments in a systematic, objective fashion. Different re-

429

searchers working with identical data would be likely to come to the same conclusion after applying inferential statistical procedures.

☰ *SAMPLING DISTRIBUTIONS*

If a sample is to be used as a basis for making estimates of population characteristics, then it is clearly advisable to obtain as representative a sample as possible. As we saw in Chapter 13, random samples (i.e., probability samples) are the most effective means of securing representative samples. Inferential statistical procedures are based on the assumption of random sampling from populations.

Even when random sampling is used, however, it cannot be expected that the sample characteristics will be identical to those of the population. Suppose we had a population of 10,000 freshmen nursing students who had taken the Scholastic Aptitude Test (SAT). Let us say, for the sake of this example, that the mean SAT score for this population is 500 and the SD is 100. Now, suppose that we do not know these parameters but that we must estimate them by using the scores from a random sample of 25 students. Should we expect to find a mean of exactly 500 and an SD of 100 for this sample? It would be extremely unlikely to obtain the exact population value. Let us say instead that we calculated a mean of 505. If a completely new sample of 25 students were drawn and another mean computed, we might obtain a value such as 497. The tendency for the statistics to fluctuate from one sample to another is known as *sampling error.*

A researcher actually works with only *one* sample on which statistics are computed and inferences made. However, to understand inferential statistics, we must perform a small mental exercise. With the population of 10,000 nursing students, consider drawing a sample of 25 individuals, calculating a mean and an SD, replacing the 25 students, and drawing a new sample. Each mean computed in this fashion will be considered a separate piece of data. If we draw 5000 such samples, we will have 5000 means or data points, which could then be used to construct a

frequency polygon, such as the one shown in Figure 21-1. This kind of frequency distribution has a special name: it is called a sampling distribution of the mean. A *sampling distribution* is a theoretical rather than actual distribution because one does not in practice draw consecutive samples from a population and plot their means. The concept of a theoretical distribution of sample values is basic to inferential statistics.

Characteristics of Sampling Distributions

When an infinite number of samples are drawn from an infinite population, the sampling distribution of means from those samples has certain known characteristics. Our example of a population of 10,000 students, and 5000 samples with 25 students each, deals with finite quantities, but the numbers are large enough to approximate these characteristics.

Statisticians have been able to demonstrate that sampling distributions of means follow a normal curve. Furthermore, the mean of a sampling distribution consisting of an infinite number of sample means is always equal to the population mean. In the current example, the mean of the sampling distribution is 500, the same value as the mean of the population.

In Chapter 20 we discussed the SD in terms of percentages of cases falling within a certain distance from the mean. When scores are normally distributed, 68% of the cases fall between +1 SD and −1 SD from the mean. Because a sampling distribution of means is normally distributed, we can make the same type of statement. The probability is 68 out of 100 that any randomly drawn sample mean lies within the range of values between +1 SD and −1 SD of the mean on the sampling distribution. The problem, then, is to determine the value of the SD of the sampling distribution.

Standard Error of the Mean

The SD of a theoretical distribution of sample means is called the *standard error of the mean* (SEM). The word "error" signifies that the

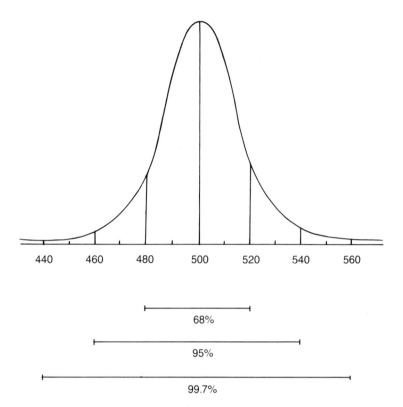

Figure 21-1. *Sampling distribution.*

various means composing the distribution contain some error in their estimates of the population mean. The *standard* error indicates the magnitude of a standard, or average, error. The smaller the standard error—that is, the less variable the sample means—the more accurate are those means as estimates of the population value.

Because one does not ever actually construct a sampling distribution, how can its SD be computed? Fortunately, there is a formula for estimating the standard error of the mean from the data from a single sample. It has been shown that the value of the standard error (symbolized as $s_{\bar{x}}$) has a systematic relationship to the standard deviation of the population and to the size of the samples drawn from it. The population SD is estimated by the sample SD to yield the following equation.

$$s_{\bar{x}} = \frac{SD}{\sqrt{n}}$$

where SD = the standard deviation of the sample
  n = sample size
  $s_{\bar{x}}$ = standard error of the mean

If we use this formula to calculate the standard error of the mean in our current example, we obtain

$$s_{\bar{x}} = \frac{100}{\sqrt{25}} = 20.0$$

The standard deviation of the sampling distribution is 20, as shown in Figure 21-1. This statistic is an estimate of how much sampling fluctuation or sampling error there would be from one sample mean to another.

We can now use these calculations to estimate the probability of drawing a sample with a certain mean. With a sample size of 25, the chances are about 95 out of 100 that the mean would fall between the values of 460 and 540.

Only five times out of 100 would the sample mean exceed 540 or be less than 460. In other words, only five times out of 100 would we be likely to draw a sample whose mean deviates from the population mean by more than 40 points.

From the formula for the standard error of the mean, it can be shown that to increase the accuracy of our estimate of the population mean, we need only increase the sample size. Suppose that instead of using a sample of 25 nursing students to estimate the average SAT score, we used a sample of 100 students. With this many students, the SEM would be

$$s_{\bar{x}} = \frac{100}{\sqrt{100}} = 10.0$$

In such a situation, the probability of obtaining a sample mean greater than 520 or less than 480 would be about 5 in 100. The chances of drawing a sample with a mean very different from that of the population is reduced as the sample size increases because large numbers promote the likelihood that extreme cases will cancel each other out.

≡ ESTIMATION VERSUS HYPOTHESIS TESTING

Statistical inference consists of two major types of techniques: (1) estimation of parameters versus (2) the testing of hypotheses. Of the two, hypothesis testing is more commonly encountered in research reports, but estimation plays an important role as well. Regardless of which approach is used, the overall goal remains the same: to use data from samples to draw conclusions about populations.

Estimation of Parameters

Estimation procedures are used when the researcher has no preestablished hypothesis about the value of a population characteristic and desires to determine that value. Suppose a new drug has been developed for people suffering from high blood pressure and a researcher administers the drug to a sample of patients. The researcher could use estimation procedures to estimate the average blood pressure of a population of people with high blood pressure (or the average reduction in blood pressure) after administration of the drug. Estimation is the method used when no *a priori* prediction can be made about the attributes of a population, as would probably be the case for the effects of a new drug.

Estimation can take one of two forms: (1) point estimation or (2) interval estimation. *Point estimation* involves the calculation of a single numerical value—a statistic—to estimate the unknown population parameter. To continue with the SAT population example, if we calculated the mean SAT score for a sample of 25 students and found that it was 510, then this number would represent the point estimation of the population mean.

The problem with point estimates is that they convey no information concerning the accuracy of the estimation. *Interval estimation* of a parameter is more useful because it indicates a range of values within which the parameter has a specified probability of lying. Interval estimates usually are referred to as *confidence intervals,* and the upper and lower limits of the range of values are called *confidence limits*.

The construction of a confidence interval around a sample mean establishes a range of values for a population parameter and also establishes a certain probability of being correct. In other words, we make the estimation with a certain degree of confidence. Although the degree of confidence one wishes to attain is somewhat arbitrary, researchers conventionally use either a 95% or a 99% confidence interval.

The calculation of the confidence limits involves the use of the SEM and the principles associated with the normal distribution. As shown in Figure 21-1, 95% of the scores in a normal distribution lie within about 2 SDs from the mean. The precise number of SDs is 1.96.

Returning to our example, let us say once again that the point estimation of the mean SAT score is 510, with an SD of 100. The SEM for a sample of 25 would be 20. We can now build a 95% confidence interval by using the following formula:

$$\text{Conf. } (\overline{X} \pm 1.96\ s_{\overline{x}}) = 95\%$$

That is, the confidence is 95% that the population mean lies between the values equal to 1.96 times the standard error, above and below the sample mean. In the example at hand, we would obtain the following:

$$\text{Conf. } (510 \pm (1.96) \times (20.0)) = 95\%$$
$$\text{Conf. } (510 \pm (39.2)) = 95\%$$
$$\text{Conf. } (470.8 \le \mu \le 549.2) = 95\%$$

The final statement may be read as follows: the confidence is 95% that the population mean (symbolized by the Greek letter mu[μ] by convention) is greater than or equal to 470.8 but less than or equal to 549.2. Another way to interpret the confidence interval concept is in terms of a probabilistic statement. One could say that out of 100 samples with an n of 25, 95 out of 100 such confidence intervals would contain the parameter (the population mean).

The confidence interval reflects the degree of risk the researcher is willing to take of being wrong. With a 95% confidence interval, the researcher accepts the probability that she or he will be wrong five times out of 100. A 99% confidence interval sets the risk at only 1% by allowing a wider range of possible values. The formula is as follows:

$$\text{Conf. } (\overline{X} \pm 2.58\ s_{\overline{x}}) = 99\%$$

The 2.58 reflects the fact that 99% of all cases in a normal distribution lie within ± 2.58 SD units from the mean. In the example, the 99% confidence interval would be:

$$\text{Conf. } (510 \pm (2.58) \times (20.0)) = 99\%$$
$$\text{Conf. } (510 \pm (51.6)) = 99\%$$
$$\text{Conf. } (458.4 \le \mu \le 561.6) = 99\%$$

In 99 out of 100 samples with 25 subjects, the confidence interval so constructed would contain the population mean. One accepts a re-duced risk of being wrong at the price of reduced specificity. In the case of the 95% interval, the range between the confidence limits was only about 80 points; here the range of possible values is more than 100 points. The risk of error that one is willing to accept depends on the nature of the problem. In research that could affect the well-being of humans, it is not unusual to use stringent 99.9% confidence intervals, but for many research projects, a 95% confidence interval is sufficient.

Hypothesis Testing

Statistical hypothesis testing is essentially a process of decision making. Suppose a nurse researcher hypothesized that cancer patients' participation in a stress management program would result in lower anxiety. The sample consists of 25 patients in a control group who do not participate in the stress management program, and 25 subjects in the experimental group who do. All 50 subjects are administered a self-report scale of anxiety. The researcher finds that the mean anxiety level for the experimental group is 15.8 and that for the control group is 17.5. Should the researcher conclude that the hypothesis has been supported? True, the group differences are in the predicted direction, but the results might simply be the result of sampling fluctuations. Statistical hypothesis testing allows researchers to make objective decisions concerning the results of their studies. Scientists need such a mechanism for helping them to decide which outcomes are likely to reflect only chance differences between groups and which are likely to reflect true population differences.

THE NULL HYPOTHESIS

The procedures used in testing hypotheses are based on rules of negative inference. This logic often seems somewhat awkward and peculiar to beginning researchers, so we will try to convey the concepts with a concrete illustration. In the stress management program example, a nurse researcher tested the effectiveness of a special program designed to reduce stress and anxiety in cancer patients. The researcher found that those participating in the program had lower mean anxiety scores than those not participating in the program. Two explanations for this outcome are that (1) the experimental treatment was successful in reducing patients' anxiety or (2) the differences resulted from chance factors (such as differences in the anxiety levels of the two groups even before any special treatment). The first explanation is the researcher's scientific hypothesis, but the second explanation is known as the null hypothesis. The *null hypothesis* is a statement that there is no actual relationship between variables and that any such observed relationship is only a function of chance, or sampling fluctuations. The need for a null hypothesis lies in the fact that statistical hypothesis testing is basically a process of rejection. It is impossible to demonstrate directly that the first explanation—the scientific hypothesis—is correct. However, it is possible to show that the null hypothesis has a high probability of being incorrect, and such evidence lends support to the scientific hypothesis. The rejection of the null hypothesis, then, is what the researcher seeks to accomplish through statistical tests.

The null hypothesis is sometimes stated as a formal proposition, using the following symbols:

$$H_0 : \mu_A = \mu_B$$

The null hypothesis (H_0) predicts that the population mean for method A (μ_A) is the same as the population mean for method B (μ_B) with regard to, in this case, anxiety scores. The *alternative,* or research, *hypothesis* may also be stated in similar terms:

$$H_A : \mu_A \neq \mu_B$$

Although null hypotheses are accepted or rejected on the basis of sample data, the hypothesis is made about population values. The real interest in testing hypotheses, as in all statistical inference, is to use samples to draw conclusions about relationships within the population.

TYPE I AND TYPE II ERRORS

The researcher's decision about whether to accept or reject the null hypothesis is based on a consideration of how probable it is that observed differences are the result of chance alone. Because information concerning the entire population is unavailable, it is not possible to flatly assert that the null hypothesis is or is not true. The researcher must be content with the knowledge that the hypothesis is either probably true or probably false. We make statistical inferences based on incomplete information, so that there is always a risk of error.

There are two types of errors that a researcher can commit: (1) the rejection of a true null hypothesis or (2) the acceptance of a false null hypothesis. The possible outcomes of a researcher's decision are summarized in Figure 21-2. When the investigator errs by concluding that the null hypothesis is false when it is in fact true, a Type I error is committed. For instance, if

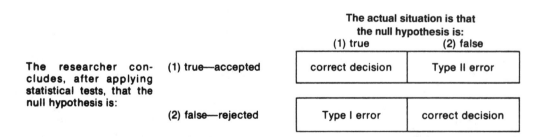

Figure 21-2. *Outcomes of statistical decision making.*

we concluded that the experimental treatment was more effective than the control treatment in alleviating patients' anxiety when in actuality the observed sample differences in anxiety scores resulted only from sampling fluctuations, then we would have made a Type I error. In the reverse situation, we might conclude that observed differences in average group anxiety levels were the result of chance, when in fact the experimental treatment did have an effect on anxiety. This situation of accepting a false null hypothesis constitutes a Type II error.

LEVEL OF SIGNIFICANCE

The researcher does not know when an error in statistical decision making has been committed. The truth or falseness of a null hypothesis could only be definitively ascertained by collecting information from the entire population, in which case there would be no need for statistical inference.

The degree of risk of a Type I error is controlled by the researcher. The selection of a level of significance determines the chance of making a Type I error. *Level of significance* is the phrase used to signify the probability of committing a Type I error. As in the case of confidence levels, the probability level can be established by the investigator.

The two most frequently used levels of significance (often referred to as α, or alpha) are .05 and .01. If we say we are using a .05 significance level, this means that we are accepting the risk that out of 100 samples, a true null hypothesis would be rejected five times. With a .01 significance level, the risk of a Type I error is *lower:* in only 1 sample out of 100 would we erroneously reject the null hypothesis. By convention, the minimum acceptable level for α in scientific research generally is .05. A stricter level may be desirable for statistical tests when the decision has important consequences for humans.

Naturally, researchers would like to reduce the risk of committing both types of error. Unfortunately, lowering the risk of committing a Type I error increases the risk of a Type II error. The stricter the criterion we use for rejecting a null hypothesis, the greater the probability that we will accept a false null hypothesis. There is a kind of trade-off that the researcher must consider in establishing criteria for statistical decision making. Procedures for addressing Type II errors are discussed in Chapter 22.

TESTS OF STATISTICAL SIGNIFICANCE

When a researcher uses quantitative analysis to test a hypothesis, the data collected for the study are used to compute a test statistic. For every test statistic there is a related theoretical distribution. Hypothesis testing uses theoretical distributions to establish "probable" and "improbable" values for test statistics, which are in turn used as a basis for accepting or rejecting the null hypothesis.

A simple example illustrates the process. Suppose a researcher wanted to test the hypothesis that the average SAT score for high school students who went on to a nursing program was higher than that for all high school students, whose mean score was 500. The null hypothesis is $H_0: \mu_{NURS} = 500$, and the alternate hypothesis is $H_A: \mu_{NURS} \neq 500$. That is, our null hypothesis is that the population mean for students who went on to a nursing program is equal to 500; the alternative hypothesis (which is the research hypothesis) is that the population mean is not equal to 500. To test this hypothesis, we draw a sample of 100 freshmen students in nursing programs. Let us say that the mean score for this sample of students turns out to be 525, with an SD of 100. Using statistical procedures, we can assess the likelihood that a mean score of 525 represents a chance fluctuation from the population mean of 500.

In hypothesis testing, one "assumes" that the null hypothesis is true and then gathers evidence to disprove it. Assuming a population mean of 500, a sampling distribution can be constructed with a mean of 500 and an SD equal to 10 ($s_{\bar{x}} = 100 \div \sqrt{100}$), as shown in Figure 21-3. Based on our knowledge of normal distribution characteristics, we can determine "probable" and "improbable"

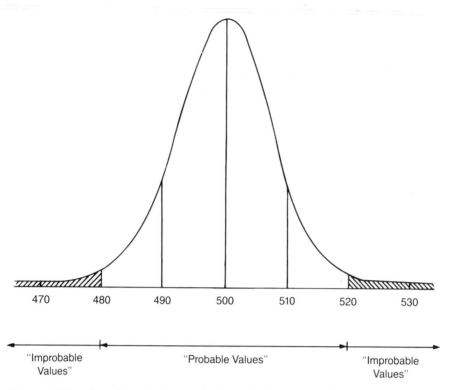

Figure 21-3. *Sampling distribution for hypothesis test example.*

values of sample means drawn from the nursing student population. If, as is assumed, the population mean is actually 500, then 95% of all sample means would fall between 480 and 520. The obtained sample mean of 525 is "improbable" given the null hypothesis, if we use as our criterion of "improbability" a significance level of .05. We would reject, therefore, the null hypothesis that the population mean for nursing students equals 500. We would not be justified in saying that we have "proved" the alternative hypothesis, because there is a 5% possibility of having made a Type I error.

Researchers reporting the results of hypothesis tests often say that their findings were *statistically significant.* This terminology has a very precise meaning. The word "significant" should not be given the familiar interpretation of "important" or "meaningful." In statistics, significant means that the obtained results are unlikely to have been the result of chance, at some specified level of probability. A nonsignificant outcome means that any difference between an obtained statistic and a hypothesized parameter could have been the result of a chance fluctuation.

The example used in this section was highly contrived; researchers rarely predict a specific value for a population mean. The use of theoretical distributions to determine "probable" and "improbable" values of a test statistic, however, is common to all tests of statistical significance.

ONE-TAILED AND TWO-TAILED TESTS

In most hypothesis-testing situations, researchers apply what is known as *two-tailed tests.* This means that both ends, or "tails," of the sampling distribution are used to determine the range of "improbable values." In Figure 21-3, for example, the critical region that contains 5% of

the area of the sampling distribution really involves 2.5% at one end of the distribution and
2.5% at the other. If the level of significance were
.01, then the critical regions would involve .5% of
the distribution at both tails.

However, when the research has a strong
basis for using a directional hypothesis (see
Chapter 8), it might be justifiable to use what is
referred to as a one-tailed test. For example, if a
nurse researcher instituted an outreach program
to improve the prenatal practices of low-income
rural women, then it might be hypothesized that
women in the experimental program would not
just be *different* from control women not exposed
to the intervention (in terms of outcomes such as
pregnancy complications, infant mortality, infant
birthweight, and so on). One would expect the
experimentals to have an advantage. It might
make little sense to use the tail of the distribution
that would signify *worse* outcomes among the
experimental than the control mothers. In a one-
tailed test, the critical region of improbable values
is entirely in one tail of the distribution—the tail

corresponding to the directionality of the hypothesis. Figure 21-4 illustrates that, in a one-tailed
test, the region of "improbable values" lies entirely at one end of the distribution. When a one-
tailed test is used, the critical area of .05 covers a
bigger region of the specified tail, and for this
reason, one-tailed tests are less conservative. This
means that it is easier to reject the null hypothesis
with a one-tailed test than with a two-tailed test.

The use of one-tailed tests has been the
subject of considerable controversy. Most researchers follow the convention of using a two-
tailed test, even if they have stated a directional
hypothesis. In reading research reports, one can
assume that a two-tailed test has been used, unless
the investigator specifically mentions a one-tailed
test. However, when there is a strong logical or
theoretical reason for using a directional hypothesis and for assuming that findings opposite to the
direction hypothesized are virtually impossible, a
one-tailed test may be warranted.

In the remainder of this chapter, the examples that are worked out use two-tailed tests. If a

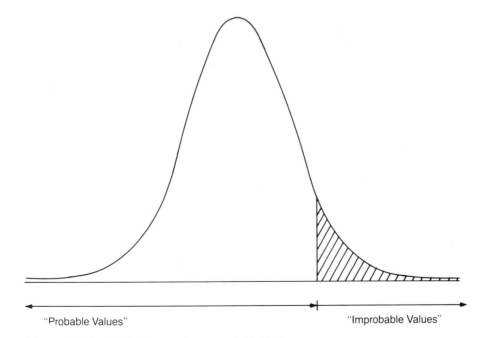

"Probable Values"   "Improbable Values"

Figure 21-4. *Critical range for a one-tailed test.*

computer is used to perform statistical analyses, then two-tailed hypothesis testing is almost always assumed.

PARAMETRIC AND NONPARAMETRIC TESTS

A distinction is often made between two classes of statistical tests. The bulk of the tests that we consider in this chapter—and also the majority of tests used by researchers—are called parametric tests. *Parametric tests* are characterized by three attributes: (1) they involve the estimation of at least one parameter; (2) they require measurements on at least an interval scale; and (3) they involve several other assumptions about the variables under consideration, such as the assumption that the variables are normally distributed in the population.

Nonparametric tests may be contrasted with parametric tests in terms of several of these characteristics. This second class of statistical tests is not based on the estimation of parameters. Nonparametric methods also involve less restrictive assumptions concerning the shape of the distribution of the critical variables than do parametric tests. For this reason, nonparametric tests are sometimes called *distribution-free* statistics. Finally, nonparametric tests are usually applied when the data have been measured on a nominal or an ordinal scale.

Statisticians disagree about the utility and virtues of most nonparametric tests. Purists insist that if the strict requirements of parametric tests are not met, then parametric procedures are inappropriate. Many statistical research studies have shown, however, that the violation of the assumptions for parametric tests usually fails to affect statistical decision making or the number of errors made. The more moderate position in this debate, and the one that we feel is reasonable, is that nonparametric tests are most useful when the data under consideration cannot in any manner be construed as interval-level measures or the distribution of data is markedly non-normal. Parametric tests are usually more powerful and offer more flexibility than nonparametric tests and are, for these reasons, generally preferred.

OVERVIEW OF HYPOTHESIS-TESTING PROCEDURES

In the pages that follow, various types of statistical procedures for testing research hypotheses are examined. The emphasis throughout is on explaining applications of statistical tests rather than on describing actual computations. One computational example is worked out to illustrate that numbers are not just "pulled out of a hat." However, calculators and computers have virtually eliminated the need for manual calculations, so that computational examples have been minimized. Researchers involved in statistical analyses are urged to pursue other references for a fuller appreciation of statistical methods. In this basic text on research methods, our primary concern is to alert researchers to the potential use (or misuse) of statistical tests for different purposes.

Although each of the statistical tests described in the remaining sections of this chapter has a particular application and can be used only with particular kinds of data, the overall process of testing hypotheses is basically the same. The six steps are essentially as follows:

1. *Determine the test statistic to be used.* Is a parametric test justified? What level of measurement was used for the measures? Is the distribution of data a reasonable approximation of a normal curve? (The summarization in Table 21-6 may help in the selection of an appropriate test.)
2. *Select the level of significance.* An α level of .05 will usually be acceptable. If a more stringent test is required, then α may be set at .01 or .001.
3. *Select a one-tailed or two-tailed test.* In most cases, a two-tailed test should be used to answer questions such as the following: Are the two groups different? Is there a relationship between the two variables? If the researcher has a firm basis for hypothesizing not only a

difference or a relationship, but also the *nature* of that difference or relationship, then a one-tailed test may be appropriate.

4. *Compute a test statistic.* Using the values from the collected data, calculate a test statistic using the appropriate computational formulas. Or, alternatively, have the computer calculate the statistic using a program designed for this purpose.

5. *Calculate the degrees of freedom* (symbolized as *df*). *Degrees of freedom* is a concept used throughout hypothesis testing to refer to the number of observations free to vary about a parameter. The concept is too complex for full elaboration here, but fortunately the computation (the formulas for the df vary from one test statistic to another) is extremely easy.

6. *Compare the test statistic to a tabled value.* Theoretical distributions have been developed for all test statistics. These theoretical distributions enable the researcher to discover whether obtained values are beyond the range of what is "probable" if the null hypothesis is true. That is, at some probability level specified by the researcher, the obtained value of the test statistic reflects a true relationship between variables (or a reliable estimate of a hypothesized population parameter) and not just a relationship or value that occurred in the sample by chance. The researcher examines a table appropriate for the test used, obtains the tabled value by entering the table at a point corresponding to the relevant degrees of freedom and level of significance, and compares the tabled value with the computed value of the statistic. If the absolute value of the test statistic is *larger* than the tabled value, then the results are statistically significant. If the computed value is smaller, then the results are nonsignificant.

When a computer program is used to test hypotheses, the researcher really only needs to follow the first step and then make the necessary commands to the computer. The computer will calculate the test statistic, the degrees of freedom, and the *actual* probability that the relationship being tested results from chance. For example, the computer may print that the probability (p) of an experimental group doing better on a measure of postoperative recovery than the control group on the basis of chance alone is .025. This means that fewer than three times out of 100 (or only 25 times out of 1000) would a difference between the two groups as large as the one obtained reflect haphazard sampling differences rather than differences resulting from an experimental intervention. This computed probability level can then be compared with the investigator's desired level of significance. If the significance level desired were .05, then the results would be said to be significant, because .025 is more stringent than .05. If .01 were the significance level, then the results would be nonsignificant (sometimes abbreviated NS). Any computed probability level greater than .05 (e.g., .20) indicates a nonsignificant relationship—that is, one that could have occurred on the basis of chance alone in more than five out of 100 samples.

In the sections that follow, a number of specific statistical tests and their applications are described. Examples of hypothesis tests using computerized computations are provided at the end of the chapter.

≡ *TESTING DIFFERENCES BETWEEN TWO GROUP MEANS*

A common research situation is the comparison of two groups of subjects on the dependent variable of interest. For instance, we might wish to compare an experimental and control group of patients on various physiologic measures such as heart rate, blood pressure, and tidal volume. Or, perhaps we would be interested in contrasting the average number of schools days missed because of illness among children who had been born preterm versus full term. This section describes methods for testing the statistical significance of differences between two group means.

The basic parametric procedure for testing differences in group means is the *t-test* (sometimes referred to as Student's *t*). A distinction must be drawn between the case in which the two groups are independent (such as an experimental and control group, or male versus female subjects) or dependent (as when a single group yields pretreatment and posttreatment scores). Procedures for handling independent samples are described below to illustrate the computation of the *t* statistic.

t-Tests for Independent Samples

Suppose that a researcher wanted to test the effect of special instruction on pregnant women's attitudes toward breast-feeding. Twenty primiparas from a prenatal education program compose the sample. Ten of these 20 women are randomly assigned to an experimental group, which will be exposed to special films and lectures on the beneficial effects of breast-feeding. The remaining ten women compose the control group, which will not receive special instruction on breast-feeding. At the end of the experiment, both groups are administered a scale measuring attitudes toward breast-feeding. The hypotheses being tested are

$$H_0 : \mu_A = \mu_B \qquad H_A : \mu_A \neq \mu_B$$

To test these hypotheses, the *t*-statistic must be computed. With independent samples such as in the current example, the formula is

$$t = \frac{\overline{X}_A - \overline{X}_B}{\sqrt{\dfrac{\Sigma_{x_A}^2 + \Sigma_{x_B}^2}{n_A + n_B - 2}\left(\dfrac{1}{n_A} + \dfrac{1}{n_B}\right)}}$$

This formula looks rather complex and intimidating, but it boils down to simple components that can be calculated with elementary arithmetic. Let us work through one example with data shown in Table 21-1.

The first column of numbers presents the scores of the experimental group on a measure of attitudes toward breast-feeding. The mean score for group A is 25.0. In column 4, similar scores are

Table 21-1. *Computation of the* t-*Statistic for Independent Samples*

EXPERIMENTAL GROUP A			CONTROL GROUP B			
(1)	(2)	(3)	(4)	(5)	(6)	
X_A	x_A	$x_A{}^2$	X_B	x_B	$x_B{}^2$	
30	5	25	23	4	16	$t = \dfrac{25 - 19}{\sqrt{\dfrac{242 + 154}{(10 + 10 - 2)}\left(\dfrac{1}{10} + \dfrac{1}{10}\right)}} =$
27	2	4	17	-2	4	
25	0	0	22	3	9	
20	-5	25	18	-1	1	
24	-1	1	20	1	1	
32	7	49	26	7	49	$t = \dfrac{6}{\sqrt{(22.0)(.2)}} =$
17	-8	64	16	-3	9	
18	-7	49	13	-6	36	
28	3	9	21	2	4	$t = \dfrac{6}{\sqrt{4.4}} =$
29	4	16	14	-5	25	
$\Sigma X_A = 250$		$\Sigma x_A^2 = 242$	$\Sigma X_B = 190$		$\Sigma x_B^2 = 154$	$t = \dfrac{6}{2.1} = 2.86$
$\overline{X}_A = 25.0$			$\overline{X}_B = 19.0$			

shown for the control group, whose mean is 19.0. The question is, Is this six-point difference significant? What is the probability that a difference of this size is the result of chance alone? The calculation of the *t*-statistic will enable such questions to be answered. In columns 2 and 5, deviation scores are obtained for each subject: 25.0 is subtracted from each score in Group A and 19.0 is subtracted from each score in Group B. Then, each deviation score is squared (columns 3 and 6), and the squared deviation scores are added. We now have all of the components for the formula presented above, as follows:

$\overline{X}_A = 25.0$ mean of Group A

$\overline{X}_B = 19.0$ mean of Group B

$\Sigma_{x_A}^2 = 242$ sum of Group A squared deviation scores

$\Sigma_{x_B}^2 = 154$ sum of Group B squared deviation scores

$n_A = 10$ number of subjects in Group A

$n_B = 10$ number of subjects in group B

When these numbers are used in the *t*-equation, the value of the *t*-statistic is computed to be 2.86, as shown in Table 21-1.

To ascertain whether this *t*-value is statistically significant, we need to consult a table that specifies the probability points associated with different *t*-values for the theoretical *t*-distributions. To make use of such a table, the researcher must have two pieces of information: (1) the α level sought—that is, the degree of risk of making a Type I error that one is willing to accept—and (2) the number of degrees of freedom available. For a *t*-test with independent samples, the formula for degrees of freedom is

$$df = n_A + n_B - 2$$

That is, the degrees of freedom is equal to the number of subjects in the two groups, minus 2. Thus, in the attitudes toward breast-feeding example, the degrees of freedom is equal to 18 [(10 + 10) − 2].

A table of *t*-values is presented in Table B-1, Appendix B. The left-hand column lists various

degrees of freedom, and the top row specifies different α values. If we use as our decision-making criterion a two-tailed probability (*p*) level of .05, we find that with 18 degrees of freedom, the tabled value of *t* is 2.10. This value establishes an upper limit to what is "probable," if the null hypothesis were true; values in excess of 2.10 would be considered "improbable." Thus, our calculated *t* of 2.86* is improbable (i.e., statistically significant). We are now in a position to say that the subjects in the experimental group scored significantly higher than those in the control group on the attitude toward breast-feeding scale. The probability that the mean difference of six points was the result of chance factors rather than the experimental intervention is less than 5 in 100 ($p < .05$). The null hypothesis is rejected, therefore, and the alternative hypothesis retained.

Paired t-Tests

In some studies, the researcher may obtain two measures from the same subjects or measures from paired sets of subjects (such as two siblings). Whenever two sets of scores on the dependent variable are not independent, then the procedures just described are inappropriate.

Suppose that we were interested in studying the effect of a special diet on the cholesterol level of adult males older than age 60. A sample of 50 men is randomly selected to participate in the study. The cholesterol levels are measured before the start of the investigation and measured again after two months on the special diet. The central concern here is the change in the cholesterol levels—the average difference in cholesterol values before and after the treatment. The hypotheses being submitted to a statistical test are

$$H_0 : \mu_x = \mu_Y \qquad H_A : \mu_x \neq \mu_Y$$

In these hypotheses, μ_X is the population

---

* The tabled *t*-value should be compared with the absolute value of the calculated *t*. Thus, if the calculated *t* value had been − 2.86, then the results would still be significant.

mean for pretreatment cholesterol levels, and μ_Y is that for posttreatment cholesterol levels.

As in the previous example, a t statistic would be computed from the pretest and posttest measures (using, however, a different formula).† The obtained t would be compared with the t values in Table B-1, Appendix B. For this particular type of t-test, the degrees of freedom equals the number of paired observations minus one ($df = n - 1$).

Other Two-Group Tests

In certain two-group situations the t-statistic might be inappropriate. If the researcher is working with ordinal-level data, or if the distribution is markedly non-normal, then a nonparametric test may be preferred. We mention a few such tests here without actually working out examples.

The *median test* involves the comparison of two independent groups on the basis of deviations from the median rather than the mean. In the median test, the scores for both samples are combined and the overall median calculated. Then the number of cases above and below this median is counted separately for each sample, resulting in a 2 × 2 contingency table; (above/below median) × (group A/group B). From such a contingency table, a chi-squared statistic (described in a subsequent section) can be computed to test the null hypothesis that the medians are the same for the two populations.

The *Mann-Whitney* U *test* is another nonparametric procedure for testing the difference between two independent samples when the de-

† The t-statistic for paired measures is computed according to the following equation:

$$t = \frac{\overline{D}_{x-y}}{\sqrt{\dfrac{\Sigma d^2}{n(n-1)}}}$$

where D_{x-y} = the difference between two paired scores
$\overline{D}_{x-y}$ = the mean difference between the paired scores
d = the deviation scores for the difference measure
Σd_2 = sum of the squared deviation scores
n = number of pairs

pendent variable is measured on an ordinal scale. The test is based on the assignment of ranks to the two groups of measures. The sum of the ranks for the two groups can be compared by calculating the U statistic. The Mann-Whitney U test tends to throw away less information than a median test and, therefore, is more powerful.

When ordinal-level data are paired rather than independent, either the sign test or the Wilcoxon signed-rank test can be used. The *sign test* is an extremely simple procedure, involving the assignment of a " + " or " − " to the differences between a pair of scores, depending on whether X is larger than Y, or vice versa. The *Wilcoxon test* involves taking the difference between paired scores and ranking the absolute difference.

Compared with t-tests, all of these nonparametric tests are computationally quite easy. Because they are generally less powerful, however, the ease of computation should not be used as the basis for choosing which statistic is most appropriate, especially if a computer is being used to analyze the data.

≡ TESTING DIFFERENCES BETWEEN THREE OR MORE GROUP MEANS

The procedure known as *analysis of variance* (ANOVA) is another commonly used statistical test. Like the t-test, ANOVA is a parametric procedure, used to test the significance of differences between means. However, ANOVA is not restricted to two-group situations: the means of three or more groups can be compared with ANOVA.

The statistic computed in an ANOVA is the *F-ratio* statistic. Because the statistic is based on more than two groups, it should not be too surprising that the computation of an F-ratio is somewhat more complex than that for a t-statistic. A brief overview of the logic of ANOVA might prove helpful.

Consider for the moment the raw scores shown in Table 21-1. The 20 scores—ten for each group—are not identical. The scores vary from one person to another. Some of that variability can be attributed to ingrained individual differences in feelings toward breast-feeding. Some of that variability could also result from measurement error (unreliability), and some of it could be the result of the subjects' mood on that day, and so forth. The research question is, Can a significant portion of the variability be attributed to the independent variable, which in this case is exposure or nonexposure to special instruction on breast-feeding?

ANOVA decomposes the total variability of a set of data into two components: (1) the variability resulting from the independent variable and (2) all other variability, such as individual differences, measurement unreliability, and so on. Variation *between* treatment groups is contrasted with variation *within* groups to yield an *F*-ratio. If the differences between groups receiving different treatments is large relative to fluctuations within groups, then it is possible to establish the probability that the treatment is related to, or resulted in, the group differences.

One-Way ANOVA

Suppose that we were interested in comparing the effectiveness of different therapies to help individuals stop smoking. One group of smokers will undergo behavior modification therapy, which is based on reinforcement theory (Group A). A second group will be treated by means of hypnosis (Group B). A third group will serve as a control group and, therefore, will receive no special treatment (Group C). The dependent variable in this experiment will be cigarette consumption during the week following completion of the therapies. Thirty subjects who smoke regularly and who wish to stop smoking are randomly assigned to one of the three conditions. The ANOVA will permit a test of the following hypotheses:

$$H_0 : \mu_A = \mu_B = \mu_C \qquad H_A : \mu_A \neq \mu_B \neq \mu_C$$

The null hypothesis asserts that the population means for posttreatment cigarette smoking will be the same for all three groups, and the

alternative (research) hypothesis predicts inequality of means. Table 21-2 presents some hypothetical data for such a study.

For each of the three groups, the raw score for each subject and the mean group score are shown. The mean number of posttreatment cigarettes consumed is 20, 25, and 33 for groups A, B, and C, respectively. These means are different but are they significantly different? Or, are these differences attributable to random fluctuations?

The underlying concepts and terms for a one-way ANOVA are briefly explained without working out the computations for this example. Again, the reader is urged to consult a statistics text for formulas and more detailed explanations. In calculating an *F*-statistic, the total variability within the data is broken down into two sources. The portion of the variance resulting from group membership (i.e., from exposure to different treatments) is determined by calculating a component known as the *sum of squares between groups,* or SS_B. This SS_B represents the sum of squared deviations of the individual group means from the overall mean for all the data. The SS_B term reflects the variability in individual scores attributable to group membership.

The second component is the *sum of squares within groups,* or SS_W. This is an index of the sum of the squared deviations of each individ-

Table 21-2. *Fictitious Data for a One-Way ANOVA*

GROUP A	GROUP B	GROUP C
28	22	33
0	31	44
17	26	29
20	30	40
35	34	33
19	37	25
24	0	22
0	19	43
41	24	29
16	27	32
$\Sigma X_A = 200$	$\Sigma X_B = 250$	$\Sigma X_C = 330$
$\bar{X}_A = 20$	$\bar{X}_B = 25$	$\bar{X}_C = 33$

ual score from its own group mean. The SS_W term indicates variability attributable to individual differences, measurement error, and so on.

It may be recalled from Chapter 20 that the formula for calculating a variance is $Var = \Sigma x^2 \div n - 1$. The two sums of squares described above are analogous to the numerator of this equation. The sums of squares represent sums of squared deviations from means. Therefore, to compute the variance within and the variance between groups, we must divide by a quantity analogous to $(n - 1)$. This quantity is the degrees of freedom associated with each sum of squares. For between groups, $df = G - 1$, which is the number of groups minus one. For within groups, $df = (n_A - 1) + (n_B - 1) + \ldots (n_G - 1)$. That is, degrees of freedom within is found by adding together the number of subjects less 1 for each group.

In an ANOVA context, the variance is conventionally referred to as the *mean square*. The formula for the mean square between groups and the mean square within groups is

$$MS_B = \frac{SS_B}{df_B} \quad MS_W = \frac{SS_W}{df_W}$$

The *F*-ratio is the ratio of these mean squares, or

$$F = \frac{MS_B}{MS_W}$$

All of these computations for the data in Table 21-2 are presented in the summary table shown in Table 21-3. As this table shows, the calculated *F*-statistic for our fictitious example is 3.84.

The last step is to compare the obtained *F*-statistic with the value from a theoretical *F*-distribution. Table B-2, Appendix B, contains the upper limits of "probable" values for distributions with varying degrees of freedom. The first part of the table lists these values for a significance level of .05, and the second and third parts list those for .01 and .001 significance levels. Let us say that for the current example we have chosen the .05 probability level. To enter the table, we find the column headed by our between-groups degrees of freedom (2), and go down this column until we reach the row corresponding to the within-groups degrees of freedom (27). The tabled value of *F* with 2 and 27 degrees of freedom is 3.35. Because our obtained *F*-value of 3.84 exceeds 3.35, we reject the null hypothesis that the population means are equal. The differences in the number of cigarettes smoked after treatment are beyond chance expectations. In fewer than five samples out of 100 would differences of this magnitude be obtained by chance alone. The data support the hypothesis that the therapies affect cigarette-smoking behaviors.

The ANOVA procedure does not allow us to say that each group differed significantly from all other groups. We cannot tell from these results if Treatment A was significantly more effective than Treatment B. Some researchers incorrectly use *t*-tests to compare the different pairs of means (A versus B, A versus C, B versus C) when this type of information is required. There are methods known as *multiple comparison procedures* that should be used in such situations. The function of these procedures is to isolate the comparisons between group means that are responsible for the rejection of the ANOVA null hypothesis. Multiple comparison methods are described in most intermediate statistical textbooks.

Table 21-3. *ANOVA Summary Table*

SOURCE OF VARIANCE	SS	df	Mean Square	F	p
Between groups	860.0	2	430.00	3.84	< .05
Within groups	3,022.0	27	111.93		
Total	3,882.0	29			

The techniques described in this section are suitable only in the case in which the samples are independent. When three or more measures are obtained from the same set of subjects, a repeated measures ANOVA is required. The treatment of repeated measures is beyond the scope of this book, but a full explanation and description of the necessary computations may be found in many statistical texts.

Multifactor ANOVA

The type of problem described above is known as a one-way ANOVA because it deals with the effect of one independent variable (the different therapies) on a dependent variable. Chapter 8 pointed out that hypotheses are sometimes complex and make predictions about the effect of two or more independent variables on a dependent variable. The analysis of data from such studies is often performed by means of a multifactor ANOVA.

In this section, we describe some of the principles underlying a two-way ANOVA. The actual computations, however, will not be worked out. Suppose that we were interested in determining whether the two smoking cessation therapies were equally effective in helping both men and women stop smoking, with no control group in the study. We could design an experiment using a randomized block design, with four groups: women and men would be randomly assigned, separately, to the two therapy conditions. After the experimental period, each subject would be required to report the number of cigarettes smoked. Some fictitious data for this problem are shown in Table 21-4.

With two independent variables, there is

Table 21-4. *Fictitious Data for a Two-Way (2 × 2) ANOVA*

Factor B—Sex	Factor A—Treatment			
	Behavior Modification (1)		**Hypnosis (2)**	
Female (1)	24 28 22 19 27 25 18 21 0 36	Group 1 $\overline{X} = 22$	27 0 45 19 22 23 18 20 12 14	Group 2 $\overline{X} = 20$	Females $\overline{X}_{B1} = 21$
Male (2)	10 21 17 0 33 16 18 13 15 17	Group 3 $\overline{X} = 16$	36 31 28 32 25 22 19 30 35 42	Group 4 $\overline{X} = 30$	Males $\overline{X}_{B2} = 23$
	Treatment 1	$\overline{X}_{A1} = 19$	Treatment 2	$\overline{X}_{A2} = 25$	$\overline{X}_G = 22$

more than one hypothesis to be tested. First, we are testing whether, for both sexes, the behavior modification therapy is more effective than hypnosis as a means of reducing smoking, or vice versa. Second, we are testing for sex differences in smoking behavior, irrespective of the therapeutic treatment. Third, we are examining the differential effect of the two treatments on males and females. This last hypothesis is the *interaction hypothesis.* Interaction is concerned with whether the effect of one independent variable is consistent for every level of a second independent variable. In other words, do the two therapies have the same effect on both sexes?

The data in Table 21-4 reveal that, overall, subjects in Treatment 1 smoked less than those in Treatment 2 (19 versus 25); that females smoked less than males (21 versus 23); and that males smoked less when exposed to Treatment 1 but females smoked less when exposed to Treatment 2. By performing a two-way ANOVA on these data, it would be possible to ascertain the statistical significance of these differences.

Multifactor ANOVA is an extremely important analytic technique. Human behaviors, conditions, and feelings are complex, and the ability to examine the combined effects of two or more independent variables permits this complexity to be incorporated into research designs. Multifactor ANOVA is not restricted to two-way schemes. Theoretically, any number of independent variables is possible, although in practice studies with more than three or four factors are rare because of the large number of subjects required and the complexity of the design.

Nonparametric "ANOVA"

Nonparametric tests do not, strictly speaking, analyze variance. There are, however, nonparametric procedures analogous to the parametric ANOVA for use with ordinal-level data or when a markedly nonnormal distribution renders parametric tests inadvisable. When the number of groups is greater than two and a one-way test for independent samples is desired, one may use a

statistic developed by statisticians named Kruskal and Wallis. The *Kruskal-Wallis test* is a generalized version of the Mann-Whitney *U* test, based on the assignment of ranks to the scores from the various groups. When the researcher is working with paired groups, or when several measures are obtained from a single sample, then the *Friedman test* for "analysis of variance" by ranks may be applied. These tests are described in Hays (1973) and Siegel (1956).

≡ TESTING DIFFERENCES IN PROPORTIONS

The Chi-square Test

The *chi-square* statistic is used when we have categories of data and hypotheses concerning the proportions of cases that fall into the various categories. In Chapter 20, we discussed the construction of contingency tables to describe the frequencies of cases falling in different classes. The chi-square (χ^2) statistic is applied to contingency tables to test the significance of different proportions.

Consider the following example. A researcher is interested in studying the effect of planned nursing instruction on patients' compliance with a self-medication regimen. An experimental group of 100 patients is instructed by nurses who are implementing a new instructional approach. A second (control) group of 100 patients is cared for by nurses who continue their usual mode of instruction. The hypothesis being tested is that a higher proportion of subjects in the experimental group will report self-medication compliance than will subjects in the control group.

The chi-square statistic is computed by comparing two sets of frequencies: (1) those observed in the collected data and (2) those that would be expected if there were no relationship between two variables. The expected frequencies are calculated on the basis of the observed total frequencies for the rows and columns of a contin-

Table 21-5. *Observed Frequencies for a Chi-Square Example*

GROUP	COMPLIANCE	NON-COMPLIANCE	TOTAL
Experimental	60	40	100
Control	30	70	100
Total	90	110	200

gency table. Observed frequencies for the example are shown in Table 21-5. As this table shows, 60% of the experimentals but only 30% of the controls reported self-medication compliance. The chi-square test will enable us to decide whether a difference in proportions of this magnitude is likely to reflect a real experimental effect or only chance fluctuations.

The chi-square statistic is computed* by summarizing differences between observed and expected frequencies for each cell. In this example, there are four cells, and thus χ^2 will be the sum of four numbers. More specifically, $\chi^2 = 18.18$ in the current case. As usual, we need to compare this test statistic with the value from a theoretical chi-square distribution. A table of chi-square values for various degrees of freedom and significance levels is provided in Table B-3, Appendix B. For the chi-square statistic, the degrees of freedom are equal to $(R - 1) \times (C - 1)$, or the number of rows minus 1 times the number of columns minus 1. In the current case, $df = 1 \times 1$, or 1. With 1 degree of freedom, the value that must

---

*The formula of a χ^2 statistic is

$$\chi^2 = \Sigma \frac{(f_o - f_E)^2}{f_E}$$ where f_o = observed frequency for a cell
f_E = expected frequency for a cell
Σ = sum of the $(f_o - f_E)^2/f_E$ ratios for all cells

$$f_E = \frac{f_R f_c}{N}$$ where f_R = observed frequency for the given row
f_c = observed frequency for the given column
N = total number of subjects

be exceeded to establish significance at the .05 level is 3.84. The obtained value of 18.18 is substantially larger than would be expected by chance. Thus, we can conclude that a significantly larger proportion of patients in the experimental group than in the control group complied with self-medication instructions.

Other Tests of Proportions

In certain situations, it may be inappropriate to calculate a chi-square statistic. When the total sample size is small (total N of 30 or under) or when there are cells with a value of 0, *Fisher's Exact Test* is usually used to test the significance of differences in proportions. Also, when the proportions being compared are derived from two dependent or paired groups (e.g., when a pretest–posttest design is used to compare changes in proportions on a nominal-level dichotomous variable), then the appropriate test is the *McNemar test.*

≡ *TESTING RELATIONSHIPS BETWEEN TWO VARIABLES*

Pearson's r

In Chapter 20, the computation and interpretation of the Pearson product-moment correlation coefficient were explained. Pearson's r is both a descriptive and inferential statistic. As a descriptive statistic, the correlation coefficient summarizes the magnitude and direction of a relationship between two variables. As an inferential statistic, r is used to test hypotheses concerning population correlations, which are ordinarily symbolized by the Greek letter rho, or ρ. The most commonly tested null hypothesis is that there is no relationship between two variables. Stated formally,

$$H_0 : \rho = 0 \qquad H_A : \rho \neq 0$$

For instance, suppose we were studying the

relationship between patients' self-reported level of stress (higher stress scores imply more stress) and the pH level of their saliva. With a sample of 50 subjects, we find that $r = -.29$. This value implies that there was a slight tendency for people who received higher stress scores to have lower pH levels than those with low stress scores. But we need to question whether this finding can be generalized to the population. Does the coefficient of $-.29$ reflect a random fluctuation, caused only by the particular group of subjects sampled, or is the relationship significant? The table of significant values in Table B-4, Appendix B, allows us to make the determination. Degrees of freedom for correlation coefficients are equal to the number of subjects minus 2, or $(n - 2)$. With $df = 48$, the critical value for r (for a .05 two-tailed test) lies between .2732 and .2875, or approximately .2803. Because the absolute value of the calculated r is .29, the null hypothesis can be rejected. Therefore, we may conclude that there is significant relationship between a person's self-reported level of stress and the acidity of his or her saliva.

Other Tests of Bivariate Relationships

Pearson's r is a parametric statistic. When the assumptions for a parametric test are violated, or when the data are inherently ordinal level, then the appropriate coefficient of correlation is either *Spearman's rho* or *Kendall's tau*. The values of these statistics range from -1.00 to $+1.00$ and their interpretation is similar to that of Pearson's r.

Measures of the magnitude of relationships can also be computed with nominal-level data. For example, the *phi coefficient* (ø) is an index describing the relationship between two dichotomous variables. *Cramer's V* is an index of relationship applied to contingency tables larger than 2×2. Both of these statistics are based on the chi-square statistic and yield values that range between 0 and 1, with higher values indicating a stronger association between variables.

OVERVIEW OF VARIOUS STATISTICAL TESTS

As we have seen in the preceding section, the selection and use of a statistical test depends on several factors. In some cases, nonparametric tests are more appropriate than parametric tests. For some research problems, a two-way ANOVA rather than a one-way ANOVA will be required. To aid researchers in selecting a test statistic or evaluating statistical procedures used by researchers in the literature, a chart summarizing the major features of several commonly used tests is presented in Table 21-6.

THE COMPUTER AND INFERENTIAL STATISTICS

As in Chapter 20, we have stressed the logic and uses of various statistics rather than their computational formulas and mathematical derivations.* Because the computer is increasingly called on to perform the computations for hypothesis testing, and because it is important to be able to make sense of the printed information produced by the computer, we conclude this chapter with examples of computer-produced information for two of the tests described in this chapter.

We return to the example described in Chapter 20. A researcher has designed an experiment to test the effect of a special prenatal program on a group of young, low-income women. The raw data for the 30 subjects in this example were presented in Table 20-7. Given these data, let us test some hypotheses.

Hypothesis One: t-Test

Let us suppose that our first research hypothesis is

---

* It is important to note that this introduction to inferential statistics has necessarily been superficial. We urge novice researchers to undertake further exploration of statistical principles.

The babies of the experimental subjects will have higher birthweights than the babies of the control subjects.

In this example, there are two independent groups of subjects for which average birthweights are being compared. Birthweight, the dependent variable, is measured on a ratio scale. Therefore, the *t*-test for independent samples is used to test our hypothesis. The null and alternative hypotheses can be stated as follows:

H₀: μ experimental = μ control
Hₐ: μ experimental ≠ μ control

Figure 21-5 presents the computer printout for the *t*-test. The left side of the figure presents some basic descriptive statistics for the birthweight variable, separately for the two groups. Thus, the mean birthweight of the babies in Group 1 (the experimental group) was 107.5 ounces, compared with 101.9 ounces for the babies in Group 2 (the control group). These data, then, are consistent with our research hypothesis—the average weight of the experimentals is higher than the average weight of the controls. But do the differences reflect the impact of the experimental intervention or do they merely represent random fluctuations? To answer this, we examine the results of the *t*-test, shown on the right side of the figure. The computer program calculated the value of *t* as 1.44. With 28 degrees of freedom [(15 + 15) − 2], this value is not significant. The two-tailed probability (*p* value) for this *t* statistic is .16. This means that in 16 samples out of 100, one could expect to find a difference in weights at least this large as a result of chance alone. Therefore, we cannot conclude that the special intervention was effective in improving the birthweights of the experimental groups.†

---

† The average difference in birth weights is fairly sizable and in the hypothesized direction. The researcher might wish to pursue this study by increasing the sample size or by controlling some other variables, such as the mother's age, through analysis of covariance (see Chapter 22).

Hypothesis Two: Pearson Correlation

The second research hypothesis might be stated as follows:

Older mothers will have babies of higher birthweight than younger mothers.

In this case, both birthweight and age are measured on the ratio scale. Referring to Table 21-6, we find that the appropriate test statistic is the Pearson product-moment correlation. The hypotheses subjected to the statistical test are

H₀: ρ birthweight/age = 0
Hₐ: ρ birthweight/age ≠ 0

The printout for the test of the hypothesis is presented in Figure 21-6. This printout shows a two-dimensional *correlation matrix,* in which each variable specified is indicated on both a row and a column. To read a correlation matrix, one finds the row for one of the variables and reads across until the row intersects with the column indicating the second variable.

The correlation matrix in Figure 21-6 shows, in row one, the correlation of weight with weight and of weight with age; and in row two, the correlation of age with weight and of age with age. The correlation of interest to us for testing the hypothesis is weight with age (or age with weight—the result is the same). At the intersection of these two variables, we find three numbers. The first is the actual correlation coefficient, and the second shows the number of cases. In our example, *r* = .5938 and *N* = 30. The correlation indicates a moderately strong positive relationship: the older the mother, the higher the baby's weight tends to be, as hypothesized. Again, the data are consistent with the research hypothesis, but does this reflect a true relationship or merely chance fluctuations in the data? The third number at the intersection of age and weight shows the probability that the correlation oc-

(Text continues on page 452)

Table 21-6. Summary of Statistical Tests

NAME OF PROCEDURE	TEST STATISTIC	Degrees of Freedom	PARAMETRIC (P) OR NON-PARAMETRIC (NP)	PURPOSE	Variable 1 (Independent)	Variable 2 (Dependent)
					LEVELS OF MEASUREMENT	
t-Test for independent samples	t	$n_{\text{Group A}} + n_{\text{Group B}} - 2$	P	To test the difference between the means of two independent groups	Nominal	Interval or ratio
t-Test for dependent (paired) samples	t	$n - 1$	P	To test the difference between the means of two related groups or sets of scores	Nominal	Interval or ratio
Median Test	χ^2	(Rows $- 1$) $\times$ (Columns $- 1$)	NP	To test the difference between the medians of two independent groups	Nominal	Ordinal
Mann-Whitney U Test	U (Z)	$n - 1$	NP	To test the difference in the ranks of scores of two independent groups	Nominal	Ordinal
Wilcoxon Signed-Rank Test	Z	$n - 2$	NP	To test the difference in the ranks of scores of two related groups or sets of scores	Nominal	Ordinal
ANOVA	F	Between: n of groups $- 1$ Within: n of subjects $- n$ of groups	P	To test the difference among the means of three or more independent groups, or of more than one independent variable	Nominal	Interval or ratio
Kruskal-Wallis Test	H (χ^2)	n of groups $- 1$	NP	To test the difference in the ranks of scores of three or more independent groups	Nominal	Ordinal

Test	Statistic	df	P/NP	Purpose	Data type	Data type
Friedman Test	χ^2	n of groups $-$ 1	NP	To test the difference in the ranks of scores for three or more related sets of scores	Nominal	Ordinal
Chi-square Test	χ^2	(Row $-$ 1) $\times$ (Columns $-$ 1)	NP	To test the difference in proportions in two or more groups	Nominal	Nominal
McNemar's Test	χ^2	1	NP	To test the differences in proportions for paired samples (2 $\times$ 2)	Nominal	Nominal
Fisher's Exact Test	†	†	NP	To test the difference in proportions in a 2 $\times$ 2 contingency table when $N < 30$	Nominal	Nominal
Pearson Product-Moment Correlation	r	$n - 2$	P	To test that a correlation is different from zero (i.e. that a relationship exists)	Interval or ratio	Interval or ratio
Spearman's rho	ρ	$n - 2$	NP	To test that a correlation is different from zero (i.e., that a relationship exists)	Ordinal	Ordinal
Kendall's tau	τ	$n - 2$	NP	To test that a correlation is different from zero (i.e., that a relationship exists)	Ordinal	Ordinal
Phi coefficient	ϕ	1*	NP	To examine the magnitude of a relationship between 2 dichotomous variables (2 $\times$ 2)	Nominal	Nominal
Cramer's V	V	(R $-$ 1)(C $-$ 1)*	NP	To examine the magnitude of a relationship between variables in a contingency table (not restricted to 2 $\times$ 2)	Nominal	Nominal

*The test that $\phi \neq 0$ (or $V \neq 0$) is provided by the χ^2 test.

†Fisher's Exact Test computes exact probabilities directly.

| GROUP 1 - GROUP   EQ   1. | | | | | | | |
| GROUP 2 - GROUP   EQ   .2. | | | | | | | |

| | | | | | | * POOLED VARIANCE ESTIMATE | | |
VARIABLE	NUMBER OF CASES	MEAN	STANDARD DEVIATION	STANDARD ERROR	*	T VALUE	DEGREES OF FREEDOM	2-TAIL PROB.
WEIGHT BIRTHWEIGHT OF BABY					*			
GROUP 1	15	107.5333	13.378	3.454	*			
GROUP 2	15	101.8667	7.239	1.869	*	1.44	28	.160

Figure 21-5. *SPSS^x computer printout:* t-test.

- - - - - - - - - - - - P E A R S O N   C O R R E L A T I O N   C O E F F I C I E N T S

	WEIGHT	AGE
WEIGHT	1.0000 (30) S= #####	.5938 (30) S= .000
AGE	.5938 (30) S= .000	1.0000 (30) S= #####

Figure 21-6. *SPSS^x computer printout: Pearson correlation coefficients.*

curred by chance: S (for significance level) = .000. The printout only shows significance (p) levels to the nearest thousandth. In this case, the actual p value might be .0004 or .000001, but we do not know the real value. We *do* know, however, that $p < .001$. In other words, a relationship this strong would be found by chance alone in fewer than 1 out of 1000 samples of 30 young mothers. Therefore, the research hypothesis is accepted.

≡ RESEARCH EXAMPLES

The inferential statistics discussed in this chapter have been used in thousands of nursing studies. Some examples illustrating the use of these statistics are presented in Table 21-7. One research example is described in greater detail below.

> Hodnett and Osborn (1989) conducted an evaluation to determine the physical and psychologic effects of continuous, one-to-one professional support to pregnant women on childbirth outcomes. Data were gathered through personal interviews and through the use of medical records data from 103 low-risk women. All women in the sample attended

one of two types of prenatal education program: Lamaze or "General." Lamaze emphasized breathing and relaxation techniques and General placed greater emphasis on information about hospital routines and newborn care.

Within each of the two types of education, women were randomly assigned to either an experimental or control group. The experimental intervention consisted of continuous intrapartum professional support by a familiar care-giver. The care-givers were eight self-employed birth attendants or "labor coaches."

Three psychologic variables—(1) anxiety, (2) control, and (3) commitment to unmedicated birth—were measured with established scales that yielded interval-level measures. Data that were extracted from the subjects' medical records included use of intrapartum pain relief medication; incidence of intrapartum obstetric interventions (e.g., forceps or episiotomy); and labor length.

The analysis of data, only a portion of which is reported here, included many of the tests discussed in this chapter. Hodnett and Osborn found that experimental subjects were more likely than control subjects to labor and give birth without any analgesia or anesthesia. The chi-square value of 9.8 with 3 degrees of freedom was significant ($p < .02$). The experimental group was also significantly less likely than the control group (61% versus 85%) to have required an episiotomy ($\chi^2 = 6.44$, $p < .01$). However, another chi-square test revealed that the Cesarean section rate of 17% in the experimental group was not signifi-

cantly different from the rate of 18% in the control group.

A *t*-test indicated that the experimental and control groups were not significantly different in terms of length of time in labor. However, those subjects who had pharmacologic interventions (pain relief medication or oxytocics) were in labor longer than those without them (means of 17.1 hours versus 9.9 hours, respectively). The computed *t* value of

Table 21-7. *Examples of Inferential Statistics Used by Nurse Researchers*

STATISTICAL TEST	RESEARCH HYPOTHESIS	VALUE OF STATISTIC	p VALUE	REFERENCE
t-test, independent samples	Special cleaning before breast pumping will have an effect on lowering bacterial colony counts of cultured milk	$t = 2.55$	$< .05$	Costa, 1989
t-test, dependent samples	A male cancer awareness education program will improve men's knowledge of prostate cancer	*	$< .01$	Martin, 1990
Mann-Whitney *U* Test	The use of shoe covers results in less bacterial transfer to clean areas than use of street shoes	$Z = 4.80$	$< .001$	Copp et al., 1987
ANOVA	Resting diastolic and systolic blood pressure values differ among younger, middle-aged, and older people, for both men and women	$F = 15.4$ men $F = 15.1$ (women)	$< .01$ $< .001$	Storm et al., 1989
Kruskal-Wallis Test	Junior and senior nursing students and practicing nurses differ in their acquisition of information obtained for diagnostic reasoning	$H = 7.6$	$< .05$	Tanner et al., 1987
Chi-square Test	Compliance regarding a follow-up appointment among otitis media patients is higher for those receiving a special intervention than for controls	$\chi^2 = 16.2$	$< .01$	Jones et al., 1989
Pearson's *r*	There is a relationship between an elderly person's adoption of a healthy lifestyle and his or her			Speake et al., 1989
	• educational level	$r = .15$	$< .05$	
	• marital status	$r = -.05$	NS**	
	• past health	$r = .18$	$< .01$	

* The value of the test statistic was not reported in the article.
** NS = Not statistically significant.

5.69 was statistically significant at the .0001 level.

The four study groups—(1) experimental-Lamaze, (2) control-Lamaze, (3) experimental-General, (4) control-General—were compared in terms of postpartum scores on a measure of personal control, the Labor Agentry Scale. An ANOVA indicated that the groups were not significantly different in terms of experiences of control during labor. Pearson's correlation coefficients did indicate, however, that women who perceived a high degree of control during labor tended to be women who had lower levels of anxiety in the third trimester ($r = -.20, p < .05$) and who had more of a commitment to an unmedicated birth ($r = .27, p < .05$). Length of time in labor was not significantly related to the women's perceptions of control ($r = -.07$).

≡ SUMMARY

Inferential statistics provide a means for a researcher to make inferences about the characteristics of a population based on data obtained in a sample. The reason that we cannot make such inferences directly from the data is that sample statistics inevitably contain a certain degree of error as estimates of population parameters. Inferential statistics offer the researcher a framework for deciding whether the sampling error is too high to provide reliable population estimates.

The *sampling distribution* of the mean is a theoretical distribution of the means of many different samples drawn from the same population. When an infinite number of samples is drawn from a population, the sampling distribution of means follows a normal curve. Because of this characteristic, it is possible to indicate the probability that a specified sample value will be obtained. The *standard error of the mean* is the standard deviation of the theoretical sampling distribution of the mean. This index indicates the degree of average error in a sample mean as an estimate of the population mean. The smaller the standard error of the mean, the more accurate are the estimates of the population value. Sampling distributions are the basis for inferential statistics.

Statistical inference consists of two major types of approaches: (1) estimating parameters and (2) testing hypotheses. When a researcher wants to discover the value of an unknown population characteristic, he or she may estimate the value by means of either point or interval estimation. *Point estimation* provides a single numerical value. *Interval estimation* provides the upper and lower limits of a range of values between which the population value is expected to fall, at some specified probability level. The researcher is able to establish the degree of confidence that the population value will lie within this range. Interval estimates are often referred to as *confidence intervals.*

The testing of hypotheses by statistical procedures enables researchers to make objective decisions concerning the results of their studies. The *null hypothesis* is a statement that no relationship exists between the variables and that any observed relationships are the result of chance or sampling fluctuations. The null hypothesis, rather than the research hypothesis, is used in hypothesis testing. Failure to reject the null hypothesis means that any observed differences may be attributable to chance fluctuations. Rejection of the null hypothesis lends support to the research hypothesis.

It is possible to fail to reject a null hypothesis when, in fact, it should be rejected. Such an error is referred to as a *Type II error.* If a null hypothesis is rejected when it should not be rejected, then the error is termed a *Type I error.* Researchers are able to control the risk of committing a Type I error by establishing levels of significance. A *level of significance* indicates the probability of making a Type I error. The two most commonly used levels of significance (designated as the α level) are .05 and .01. A significance level of .01 means that in only 1 out of 100 samples will the null hypothesis be rejected when, in fact, it should be retained.

Researchers report the results of hypothesis testing as being either statistically significant or nonsignificant. The phrase *statistically significant* means that the obtained results are not likely to be the result of chance fluctuations at the specified level of probability. Although most hypothesis testing involves *two-tailed tests* in which both ends of the sampling distribution are used to define the region of "improbable values," a *one-tailed test* may be appropriate if the researcher has a strong rationale for a directional hypothesis.

Statistical tests are classified as parametric and nonparametric. *Nonparametric tests* require less stringent assumptions than parametric tests and usually are used when the level of data is either nominal or ordinal or when normality of the distribution cannot be assumed. *Parametric tests* involve the estimation of at least one parameter, the use of data measured on an interval or ratio level, and assumptions concerning the variables under consideration. Parametric tests are usually more powerful than nonparametric tests and generally are preferred.

The most common parametric procedures are the *t*-test and *ANOVA,* both of which can be used to test the significance of the difference between groups means. The *t*-test can only be applied to two-group situations whereas the ANOVA procedure can handle three or more groups, as well as more than one independent variable. Nonparametric analogues of these parametric tests include the *median test, the Mann-Whitney U test,* the *sign test* and the *Wilcoxon signed-rank test* (two-group situations), and the *Kruskal-Wallis* and *Friedman tests* (three or more group situations). The nonparametric test that is used most frequently is the *chi-square test,* which is used in connection with hypotheses relating to differences in proportions. Statistical tests to measure the magnitude of bivariate relationships and test whether the relationship is significantly different from zero include Pearson's *r* for interval-level data, *Spearman's rho* and *Kendall's tau* for ordinal-level data, and the *phi coefficient* and *Cramer's V* for nominal-level data.

≡ *STUDY SUGGESTIONS*

1. A researcher has administered a Job Satisfaction Scale to a sample of 50 primary nurses and 50 team nurses. The mean score on this scale for each group was found to be 35.2 for the primary nurses and 33.6 for the team nurses. A *t*-statistic is computed and is found to be 1.89. Interpret this result, using the table for *t*-values in Appendix B.

2. Compute the chi-square statistic for the following contingency table:

	Number of Complications Following Surgery		
Group	*None*	*One*	*More Than One*
Experimental	38	72	54
Control	29	50	11

How many degrees of freedom are there? At the .05 level of significance, what may be concluded?

3. Answer the following:
   Given:
   a. three groups of nursing school students, with 50 in each group
   b. $p = .05$
   c. value of test statistic = 4.43
   d. mean scores on test to measure motivation to attend graduate school: 25.8, 29.3, and 23.4 for groups A, B, and C, respectively
   Specify:
   a. what test statistic was used
   b. how many degrees of freedom there are
   c. whether the test statistic is statistically significant
   d. what the test statistic means

4. What inferential statistic would you choose for the following sets of variables? Explain your answers. (Refer to Table 21-6.)
   a. Variable 1 represents the weights of 100 patients; variable 2 is the patients' resting heart rate.
   b. Variable 1 is the patients' marital status; variable 2 is the patient's level of preoperative stress.
   c. Variable 1 is whether an amputee has a leg removed above or below the knee;

variable 2 is whether or not the amputee has shown signs of aggressive behavior during rehabilitation.

≡ *SUGGESTED READINGS*

METHODOLOGICAL REFERENCES

Abraham, I.L., Nadzam, D.M., & Fitzpatrick, J.J. (1989). *Statistics and quantitative methods in nursing.* Philadelphia: W.B. Saunders.

Armstrong, G. (1981). Parametric statistics and ordinal data: A pervasive misconception. *Nursing Research, 30,* 60–62.

Brogan, D.R. (1981). Choosing an appropriate statistical test of significance for a nursing research hypothesis or question. *Western Journal of Nursing Research, 3,* 337–363.

Glass, G.V., & Stanley, J.C. (1984). *Statistical methods in education and psychology* (2nd ed.). Englewood Cliffs, NJ: Prentice-Hall.

Hays, W.L. (1973). *Statistics for the social sciences* (2nd ed.). New York: Holt, Rinehart & Winston.

Hoel, P.G. (1983). *Elementary statistics* (4th ed.). New York: John Wiley and Sons.

Holm, K., & Christman, N.J. (1985). Post hoc tests following analysis of variance. *Research in Nursing and Health, 8,* 207–210.

Knapp, R.G. (1984). *Basic statistics for nurses* (2nd ed.). New York: John Wiley and Sons.

Liebetrau, A.M. (1983). *Measures of association.* Beverly Hills, CA: Sage.

Marks, R.G. (1982). *Analyzing research data: The basics of biomedical research methodology.* Belmont, CA: Life Long Learning.

Milton, J.S., & Tsokos, J.O. (1983). *Statistical methods in the biological and health sciences.* New York: McGraw-Hill.

Munro, B.H., Visintainer, M.A., & Page, E.B. (1986). *Statistical methods for health-care research.* Philadelphia: J.B. Lippincott.

Reynolds, H.T. (1984). *Analysis of nominal data.* Beverly Hills, CA: Sage.

Siegel, S. (1956). *Nonparametric statistics for the behavioral sciences.* New York: McGraw-Hill.

Triola, M. (1989). *Elementary statistics* (4th ed.). Menlo Park, CA: Addison-Wesley.

Welkowitz, J., Ewen, R.B., & Cohen, J. (1982). *Introductory statistics for the behavioral sciences* (3rd ed.). New York: Academic Press.

Winer, B.J. (1971). *Statistical principles in experimental design* (2nd ed.). New York: McGraw-Hill.

Young, R.K., & Veldman, D.J. (1981). *Introductory statistics for the behavioral sciences* (4th ed.). New York: Holt, Rinehart & Winston.

SUBSTANTIVE REFERENCES[*]

Aaronson, L.S., & MacNee, C.L. (1989). The relationship between weight gain and nutrition in pregnancy. *Nursing Research, 38,* 223–227. [t-tests, ANOVA, Pearson's r]

Brooten, D., Gennaro, S., Brown, L.P., Butts, P., Gibbons, A.L., Bakewell-Sachs, S., & Kumar, S.P. (1988). Anxiety, depression, and hostility in mothers of preterm infants. *Nursing Research, 37,* 213–216. [Paired t-tests]

Cahill, C.A. (1989). Beta-endorphin levels during pregnancy and labor: A role in pain modulation? *Nursing Research, 38,* 200–203. [t-tests]

Copp, G., Slezak, L., Dudley, N., & Mailhot, C.B. (1987). Footwear practices and operating room contamination. *Nursing Research, 36,* 366–369. [Mann-Whitney U test, Kruskal-Wallis test]

Costa, K.M. (1989). A comparison of colony counts of breast milk using two methods of breast cleansing. *Journal of Obstetric, Gynecologic, and Neonatal Nursing, 18,* 231–236. [t-tests]

Damrosch, S.P. (1981). How nursing students' reactions to rape victims are affected by a perceived act of carelessness. *Nursing Research, 30,* 168–170. [Two-way ANOVA]

Glanz, D., Ganong, L., & Coleman, M. (1989). Client gender, diagnosis, and family structure. *Western Journal of Nursing Research, 11,* 726–735. [ANOVA]

Hodnett, E.D., & Osborn, R.W. (1989). Effects of continuous intrapartum professional support on childbirth outcomes. *Research in Nursing and Health, 12,* 289–297. [t-tests, ANOVA, chi-square tests, Pearson's r]

Jalowiec, A., & Powers, M.J. (1983). Stress and coping in hypertensive and emergency room patients. *Nursing Research, 30,* 10–15. [t-tests, Pearson's r, Spearman's rho]

Jones, S.L., Jones, P.K., & Katz, J. (1989). A nursing intervention to increase compliance in otitis media patients. *Applied Nursing Research, 2,* 68–73. [chi-square tests]

[*]A comment in brackets after each citation designates the statistical test of interest.

Korniewicz, D.M., Laughton, B.E., Butz, A., & Larson, E. (1989). Integrity of vinyl and latex procedure gloves. *Nursing Research, 38,* 144–146. [chi-square tests, Fisher's Exact Test]

Martin, J.P. (1990). Male cancer awareness: Impact of an employee education program. *Oncology Nursing Forum, 17,* 59–64. [paired *t*-tests]

McCloskey, J.C., & McCain, B. (1988). Nurse performance: Strengths and weaknesses. *Nursing Research, 37,* 308–313. [Spearman's rho]

Mercer, R.T. (1986). The relationship of developmental variables to maternal behavior. *Research in Nursing and Health, 9,* 25–33. [*t*-tests, ANOVA, multiple comparison procedures, Pearson's *r*]

Reed, P.G. (1986). Religiousness among terminally ill and healthy adults. *Research in Nursing and Health, 9,* 35–41. [One-tailed *t*-test, chi-square tests, Pearson's *r*]

Speake, D.L., Cowart, M.E., & Pellet, K. (1989). Health perceptions and lifestyles of the elderly. *Research in Nursing and Health, 12,* 93–100. [Pearson's *r*]

Storm, D.S., Metzger, B.L., & Therrien, B. (1989). Effects of age on autonomic cardiovascular responsiveness in healthy men and women. *Nursing Research, 38,* 326–330. [*t*-tests, ANOVA, Pearson's *r*]

Tanner, C.A., Padrick, K.P., Westfall, U.E., & Putzier, D. (1987). Diagnostic reasoning strategies of nurses and nursing students. *Nursing Research, 36,* 358–363. [ANOVA, Kruskal-Wallis Test, chi-square tests, Pearson's *r*]

Tulman, L.J. (1985). Mothers' and unrelated persons' initial handling of newborn infants. *Nursing Research, 34,* 205–209. [Mann-Whitney *U* Test, Friedman two-way ANOVA]

Youngblut, J.M., Loveland-Cherry, C.J., & Horan, M. (1990). Factors related to maternal employment status following the premature birth of an infant. *Nursing Research, 39,* 237–240. [ANOVA, chi-square test, Pearson's *r*]

Ziemer, M.M. (1983). Effects of information on post-surgical coping. *Nursing Research, 32,* 282–287. [*t*-tests, ANOVA, chi-square tests, Pearson's *r*)

22
Advanced Statistical Procedures

The phenomena of interest to nurse researchers are generally complex. Patients' preoperative anxieties, a nurses's effectiveness in caring for people, the self-concept of a person with severe thermal injuries, the fears of cancer patients, or the abrupt elevation of a patient's body temperature are phenomena that have multiple facets and multiple determinants. Scientists, in attempting to explain, predict, and control the phenomena that interest them, have come increasingly to the recognition that a two-variable study is often inadequate for such purposes. The classical approach to data analysis and research design, which consists of studying the effect of a single independent variable on a single dependent variable, increasingly is being replaced by more sophisticated *multivariate** procedures. Whether one structures a study to be multivariate or not, the fact remains that most nursing phenomena are essentially and unalterably multivariate in nature. The modern researcher who is unfamiliar with multivariate techniques is at a serious disadvantage both as a designer of research studies and as a consumer of research reports.

Unlike the statistical methods reviewed in Chapters 20 and 21, multivariate statistics are computationally formidable. However, the widespread availability of computers has made complex manual calculations obsolete. Therefore, we make no attempt to provide formulas for the multivariate statistical procedures described here. The purpose of this chapter is to provide a general understanding of how, when, and why multivariate statistics are used rather than to explain their mathematical basis. References are available

---

* We use the term "multivariate" in this chapter to refer generally to analyses dealing with at least three variables. Some statisticians reserve the term for problems involving more than one dependent variable.

at the end of this chapter for those desiring to increase this understanding.

≡ *MULTIPLE REGRESSION/ CORRELATION*

Multiple regression analysis is a method used for understanding the effects of two or more independent variables on a dependent variable. The terms multiple correlation and multiple regression will be used almost interchangeably in reference to this technique, given the strong bond between correlation and regression. To comprehend the nature of this bond, we first explain simple regression—that is, bivariate regression—before turning to multiple regression.

Simple Linear Regression

Regression analysis is basically performed with the intention of making predictions about phenomena. In the health-care field, as in many other fields, the ability to make accurate predictions has important implications for the quality of services rendered. For example, whenever a costly or scarce resource such as home visitation by nurses is to be allocated, then it is important to be able to predict who will most benefit from that resource.

In simple regression, one variable (*X*) is used to predict a second variable (*Y*). For instance, we could use simple regression to predict weight from height, blood pressure from age, nursing school achievement from Scholastic Aptitude Test (SAT) scores, or stress from noise levels. An important feature of regression is that the higher the correlation between the two variables, the more accurate the prediction. If the correlation between diastolic and systolic blood pressure were perfect (i.e., if $r = 1.00$), then one would only need to measure one to be able to know the value of the other. Because most variables of interest to researchers are not perfectly correlated, most predictions made through regression analysis are imperfect.

A simple regression equation is a formula for making predictions about the numerical values of one variable based on the scores or values of another variable. The basic linear regression equation is

$$Y' = a + bX$$

where Y' is a predicted value of variable Y, a is the intercept constant, b is the regression coefficient, or slope of the line, and X is the score on variable X. Regression analysis solves for a and b, so that for values of X, predictions about Y can be made. Those readers with recollection of high school algebra may remember that the above equation is the algebraic equation for a straight line. *Linear regression* is essentially a method for determining a straight line to fit the data in such a way that deviations from the line are minimized.

An illustration may help to clarify some of these points. Two sets of scores for five subjects are shown in columns 1 and 2 of Table 22-1.

Application of the formula for Pearson's r reveals that the scores are strongly related, $r = .90$. What we wish to do is develop a way of predicting Y scores for a *new* group of subjects from whom we will only have information on the variable X. To do this, we must use the five sets of scores to solve for a and b in the regression equation.

The formulas for these two components are as follows:

$$b = \frac{\Sigma xy}{\Sigma x^2} \qquad a = \overline{Y} - b\overline{X}$$

where b = regression coefficient
a = intercept constant
$\overline{Y}$ = mean of variable Y
$\overline{X}$ = mean of variable X
x = deviation scores from $\overline{X}$
y = deviation scores from $\overline{Y}$

The calculations required for the various elements of these equations are worked out for the current example in columns 3 through 7 of Table 22-1. As shown at the bottom of the table, the solution to the regression equation is $Y' = 1.5 + .9X$. What does one do with this information?

Suppose for the moment that the X scores in column 1 were the only data available for the five subjects and that we wanted to predict their scores for variable Y. For the first subject with an $X = 1$, we would predict that $Y' = 1.5 + (.9)(1)$, or 2.4. Column 8 shows similar computations for each X value. These numbers show that Y' does not exactly equal the actual values obtained for Y. Most of the errors of prediction (e) are quite small, as shown in column 9. The errors of prediction result from the fact that the correlation between X and Y is not perfect. Only when $r = 1.00$ or -1.00 does $Y' = Y$. The regression equation solves for a and b in such a way as to minimize such errors. Or, more precisely, the solution minimizes the sums of squares of the prediction errors, which is why standard regression analysis is said to use a *least-squares principle* (standard regression is sometimes referred to as *ordinary least squares,* or *OLS regression*). In column 10 of Table 22-1, the error terms—usually referred to as the *residuals*—have been squared and summed to yield a value of 7.6. Any values of a and b other than those obtained above would have yielded a larger sum of the squared residuals.

The solution to this regression analysis ex-ample is displayed graphically in Figure 22-1. The actual X and Y values from the table are plotted on the graph with circles. The line running through these points is the representation of the regression solution. The intercept (a) is the point at which the line crosses the Y axis, which in this case is 1.5. The slope (b) is the angle of the line, relative to the X and Y axes. With $b = .90$, the line slopes in such a fashion that for every 4 units on the X axis, we must go up 3.6 units (.9 × 4) on the Y axis. The line, then, embodies the whole regression equation. To find a predicted value for Y, we could go to the point on the X axis for an obtained X score, find the point on the regression line vertically above the score, and read the predicted Y value horizontally from the Y axis. For example, with an X score of 5, we would predict a Y' of 6, as shown by the star designating that point on the figure.

The connection between correlation and regression can be made more evident by pointing out an important aspect of a correlation coefficient. The correlation coefficient, it may be recalled, is an index of the degree to which variables are related. Relationships, from a statistical point of view, are concerned with how variations in one

Table 22-1. *Computations for Simple Linear Regression*

(1) X	(2) Y	(3) x	(4) x^2	(5) y	(6) y^2	(7) xy	(8) Y'	(9) e	(10) e^2
1	2	−4	16	−4	16	16	2.4	− .4	.16
3	6	−2	4	0	0	0	4.2	1.8	3.24
5	4	0	0	−2	4	0	6.0	−2.0	4.00
7	8	2	4	2	4	4	7.8	.2	.04
9	10	4	16	4	16	16	9.6	.4	.16
$\Sigma X = 25$	$\Sigma Y = 30$		40		40	36		0.0	7.60
$\overline{X} = 5$	$\overline{Y} = 6$								$\Sigma e^2 = 7.60$

$$r = .90$$
$$b = \frac{\Sigma xy}{\Sigma x^2} = \frac{36}{40} = .90$$
$$a = \overline{Y} - b\overline{X} = 6 - (.9)(5.0) = 1.5$$
$$Y' = a + bX$$
$$Y' = 1.5 + .9X$$

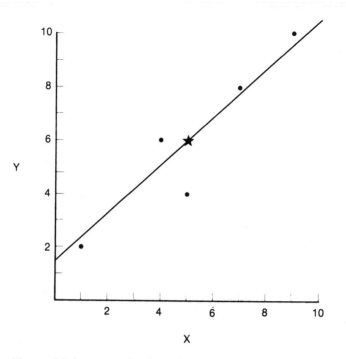

Figure 22-1. *Example of simple linear regression.*

score are associated with variations in another score. The r statistic enables us to specify how much variability can be "explained" or "accounted for" by two correlated variables. The square of r (r^2) tells us the proportion of the variance in Y that can be accounted for by X. In the previous example, $r = .90$, so $r^2 = .81$. This means that 81% of the variability in the Y scores can be understood in terms of the variability in the X scores. The remaining 19% constitutes variability resulting from some other source of influence.

Returning to the regression problem, it was found that the sum of the squared residuals (error terms) was 7.6. Column 6 of Table 22-1 also informs us that the sum of the squared deviations of the Y scores from the mean of Y (Σy^2) was 40. To demonstrate that the residuals constitute 19% of the unexplained variability in Y, we can compute the following ratio:

$$\frac{7.6}{40} = .19 = 1 - r^2$$

Although the computations are not shown, the sum of the squared deviations of the Y' scores from the mean of Y' ($\Sigma y'^2$) is equal to 32.4. As a proportion of the variability in the *actual Y* scores, this would equal

$$\frac{32.4}{40} = .81 = r^2$$

These calculations reinforce a point made earlier: the stronger the correlation the better the prediction. To put this another way, the stronger the correlation, the greater the percentage of variance explained.

Multiple Linear Regression

Because the correlation between two variables rarely is perfect, it is often desirable to try to improve one's ability to predict a Y score by including more than one X score as predictor variables. Suppose that we were interested in predicting graduate nursing students' grade point average (GPA). Because there are a limited number of students who can be accepted into graduate programs, there is naturally a concern for selecting those individuals who will have the greatest chance of success. Suppose from previous experience it had been found that those students who performed well on the verbal portion of the Graduate Record Examination (GRE) tended to obtain higher grades in graduate school than those with lower GRE scores. The correlation between the GRE verbal scores (GRE-V) and graduate grade point average has been calculated as .50. With only 25% ($.50^2$) of the variance of graduate grade point average accounted for, there will be many errors of prediction made: many admitted students will not perform as well as anticipated, and many rejected applicants would have made successful students. It may be possible, by using additional information about students, to make more accurate predictions. Multiple linear regression can assist us by developing a regression equation that provides the best prediction possible, given the correlations among several variables. The basic multiple regression equation is

$$Y' = a + b_1X_1 + b_2X_2 + \cdots b_kX_k$$

where Y' is the predicted value for variable Y, a is the intercept constant, k is the number of predictor (independent) variables, b_1 to b_k are the regression coefficients for the k variables, and X_1 to X_k are the scores on the k independent variables.

When the number of predictor variables exceeds two, the computations required to solve this equation are prohibitively laborious and complex. Therefore, we will restrict our discussion to hypothetical rather than worked-out examples. Our major interest is to facilitate the use and interpretation of multiple regression statistics.

In the example in which we wished to predict graduate nursing students' grade point average, suppose we decided that information on undergraduate grade point average (GPA-U) and

scores on the quantitative portion of the GRE (GRE-Q) should be added to the prediction equation. The resulting equation might be

$$Y' = .4 + .05\,(\text{GPA-U}) + \\ .003(\text{GRE-Q}) + .002\,(\text{GRE-V})$$

For instance, suppose an applicant had a GRE verbal score of 600, a GRE quantitative score of 550, and an undergraduate GPA of 3.2. The predicted graduate GPA would be

$$Y' = .4 + (.05)\,(3.2) + .003\,(550) + .002\,(600) = 3.41$$

We can assess the degree to which the addition of two independent variables improved our ability to predict graduate school performance through the use of the multiple correlation coefficient. In bivariate correlation, the index expressing the magnitude of a relationship is Pearson's r. When two or more independent variables are used, the index of correlation is the multiple correlation coefficient, symbolized as R. Unlike r, R does not have negative values. R varies only from 0.0 to 1.0, showing the *strength* of the relationship between several independent variables and a dependent variable but not *direction*. It would make no sense to indicate direction, because X_1 could be positively related to Y, and X_2 could be negatively related to Y. The R statistic, when squared, indicates the proportion of variance in Y accounted for by the combined simultaneous influence of the independent variables. Sometimes R^2 is referred to as the *coefficient of determination*.

The calculation of R^2 provides a direct means of evaluating the accuracy of the prediction equation. Let us say that with the three predictor variables used in the current example the value of $R = .71$. This means that 50% ($.71^2$) of the variability in graduate students' grades can be explained in terms of their verbal and quantitative GRE scores and their grades as undergraduates. The addition of two predictors doubled the variance accounted for by the single independent variable, from .25 to .50.

The multiple correlation coefficient cannot be less than the highest bivariate correlation between the dependent variable and one of the independent variables. Table 22-2 presents a correlation matrix that shows the Pearson correlation coefficients for all of the variables in this example, taken as pairs. It can be seen that all of the values on the diagonal are 1.00, resulting from the fact that every variable is "perfectly correlated" with itself. The independent variable that is correlated most strongly with graduate performance is undergraduate grade point average (GPA-U), $r = .60$. The value of R could not have been less than .60.

Another important point is that R tends to be larger when the independent variables have relatively low correlations among themselves. In the current case, the lowest correlation coefficient is between GRE-Q and GPA-U ($r = .40$) and the highest is between GRE-Q and GRE-V ($r = .70$). All correlations here are fairly substantial, a fact that helps to explain why R is not much higher than the r between the dependent variable and undergraduate grades alone (.71 compared with .60). This somewhat puzzling phenomenon can be explained in terms of redundancy of information among predictors. When correlations among the independent variables are high, they tend to add little predictive power to each other because they are redundant. When the correlations among the predictor variables are low, each variable has the ability to contribute something unique to the prediction of the dependent variable.

In Figure 22-2, a Venn diagram illustrates this concept. Each circle represents the total variability inherent in a variable. The circle on the left

Table 22-2. *Correlation Matrix*

	GPA-GRAD	GPA-U	GRE-Q	GRE-V
GPA-GRAD	1.00			
GPA-U	.60	1.00		
GRE-Q	.55	.40	1.00	
GRE-V	.50	.50	.70	1.00

GPA-GRAD, GPA for graduate students; GPA-U, GPA for undergraduate students; GRE-Q, GRE quantitative score; GRE-V, GRE verbal score.

(Y) is the dependent variable, graduate GPAs, whose values we are trying to predict. The overlap between this circle and the other circles represents the amount of variability that the variables have in common. If the overlap were complete—if the entire graduate GPA circle were covered by the other circles—then R would equal 1.00. As it is, only 50% of the circle is covered, because $R^2 = .50$. The hatched area on this figure designates the independent contribution of undergraduate GPA toward explaining graduate performance. This contribution amounts to 36% of Y's variance ($.60^2$). The remaining two independent variables do not contribute as much as one would anticipate by considering their bivariate correlation with graduate GPA (r for GRE-V = .50; r for GRE-Q = .55). In fact, their combined additional contribution is only 14% ($.50 - .36 = .14$), designated by the dotted area on the figure. The contribution is small because the two GRE scores have redundant information once the undergraduate grades are taken into account. The implication of this principle is that in selecting predictor variables, the researcher should choose independent variables that are strongly correlated with the dependent variable, but weakly correlated with each other.

A related point about multiple correlation is that, as more independent variables are added to the regression equation, the increment to R tends to decrease. It is rare to find many predictor variables that correlate well with a criterion measure and correlate only slightly with one another. Redundancy is difficult to avoid as more and more variables are added to the prediction equation. The inclusion of independent variables beyond the first four or five typically does little to improve the proportion of variance accounted for or the accuracy of prediction.

The dependent variable in multiple regression analysis, as in analysis of variance (ANOVA), should as a rule be measured on an interval or ratio scale. The independent variables, on the other hand, can either be continuous interval-level or ratio-level variables or dichotomous variables. A text such as that of Pedhazur (1982) should be consulted for information on how to

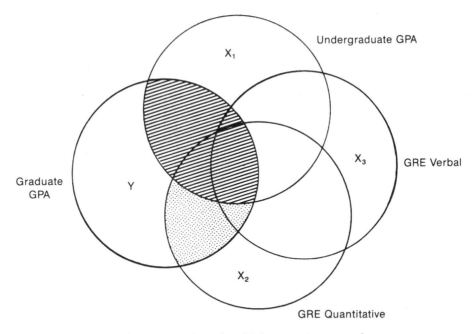

Figure 22-2. *Visual representation of multiple regression example.*

handle and interpret dichotomous "dummy" variables.

TESTS OF SIGNIFICANCE

In multiple correlation, as in bivariate correlation, researchers wishing to generalize their results must ask, Is the calculated R the result of chance fluctuations or is it statistically significant? To test the null hypothesis that the population multiple correlation coefficient is equal to zero, we can compute a statistic that can be compared with tabled values for the F distribution.

We stated in Chapter 21 that the general form for calculating an F-ratio is as follows:

$$F = \frac{SS_{\text{between}}/df_{\text{between}}}{SS_{\text{within}}/df_{\text{within}}}$$

In the case of multiple regression, the form is similar:

$$F = \frac{SS_{\text{due to regression}}/df_{\text{regression}}}{SS_{\text{of residuals}}/df_{\text{residuals}}}$$

In both cases the basic principle is the same: the variance resulting from the independent variables is contrasted with variance attributable to error or chance. To calculate the F-statistic for regression, we can use the following alternative formula:

$$F = \frac{R^2/k}{(1 - R^2)/(N - k - 1)}$$

where k equals the number of predictor variables and N equals the total sample size. In the example relating to the prediction of graduate GPAs, suppose that a multiple correlation coefficient of .71 (an R^2 of .50) had been calculated for a sample of 100 graduate students. The value of the F-statistic would be

$$F = \frac{.50/3}{.50/96} = 32.05$$

The tabled value of F with 3 and 96 degrees of freedom for a significance level of .01 is approximately 4.0. Thus, the probability that the R of .71

resulted from chance fluctuations is considerably less than .01.

Another question that researchers often seek to answer is, Does adding X_k to the regression equation significantly add to the prediction of Y over that which is possible with X_{k-1}? In other words, how effective is, say, a third predictor in increasing our ability to predict Y after two predictors have already been used? An F-statistic can also be computed for answering this question.

Let us number each independent variable in the example at hand, in order according to its correlation with Y: X_1 = GPA-U; X_2 = GRE-Q; and X_3 = GRE-V. We can then symbolize various correlation coefficients as follows: $R_{y.1}$ = the correlation of Y with GPA-U; $R_{y.12}$ = the correlation of Y with GPA-U *and* GRE-Q; and $R_{y.123}$ = the correlation of Y with all three predictors. The values of these Rs are as follows:

$$R_{y \cdot 1} = .60 \qquad R_{y \cdot 1}^2 = .36$$
$$R_{y \cdot 12} = .71 \qquad R_{y \cdot 12}^2 = .50$$
$$R_{y \cdot 123} = .71 \qquad R_{y \cdot 123}^2 = .50$$

These figures show at a glance that the verbal scores of the GRE made no independent contribution to the correlation coefficient. The value of $R_{y.12}$ is identical to the value of $R_{y.123}$. Figure 22-2 illustrates this point: if the circle for GRE-V were completely removed, then the area of the Y circle covered by X_1 and X_2 would remain the same.

We cannot tell at a glance, however, whether adding X_2 to X_1 *significantly* increases the prediction of Y. What we want to know, in effect, is whether or not X_2 would be likely to improve predictions in a new sample, or if its added predictive power in this particular sample resulted from chance. The general formula for the F-statistic for testing the significance of variables added to the regression equation is

$$F = \frac{(R_{y \cdot 12 \dots k_1}^2 - R_{y \cdot 12 \dots k_2}^2)/(k_1 - k_2)}{(1 - R_{y \cdot 12 \dots k_1}^2)/(N - k_1 - 1)}$$

where $R_{y.12 \dots k_1}^2$ is the squared multiple correlation coefficient for Y correlated with k_1 predictor variables (the larger number of predictors),

$R_{y.12 \dots k_2}^2$ is the squared R for Y correlated with k_2 predictor variables, and k_2 is the smaller of the two sets of predictors.

In the current example, the calculated *F-statistic* for testing whether the addition of GRE-Q scores results in significant improvement of prediction over GPA-U alone would be

$$F = \frac{(.50 - .36)/1}{.50/97} = 27.16$$

Consulting Table B-2 in the Appendix, we find that with df = 1 and 97 and a significance level of .01, the critical value is approximately 6.90. Therefore, the addition of GRE-Q to the regression equation significantly improved the accuracy of predictions of GPA-GRAD, beyond the .01 level of significance.

STEPWISE MULTIPLE REGRESSION

If the researcher had ten independent variables available for use in a regression equation, then the process of testing all possible combinations to determine which set of variables was significant, and yielded the highest R^2, would be exceedingly time consuming. *Stepwise multiple regression* is a method by which all potential predictors can be considered and through which the combination of variables providing the most predictive power can be chosen.

The computational aspects of stepwise multiple regression are too involved to discuss here, but some major features of this procedure can be pointed out. In stepwise multiple regression, predictors are stepped into the regression equation sequentially, in the order that produces the greatest increments to R^2. The first step involves the selection of the single best predictor of the dependent variable, which is the independent variable with the highest bivariate correlation coefficient with Y. The second variable to enter the regression equation is the one that produces the largest increase to R_2 when used simultaneously with the variable selected in the first step. The procedure continues until no additional predictor can significantly increase the value of R^2.

The basic principles of stepwise multiple regression are illustrated in Figure 22-3. The first variable to enter the regression, X_1, is correlated .60 with Y ($r^2 = .36$). No other predictor variable is correlated more strongly with the dependent variable. The variable X_1 accounts for the portion of the variability of Y represented by the hatched area in Step 1 of the figure. This hatched area is, in effect, removed from further consideration as far as subsequent predictors are concerned. This portion of Y's variability is "explained" or "accounted for." Therefore, the variable chosen in Step 2 is not necessarily the X variable with the second largest correlation with Y. The selected variable will be the predictor that explains the largest portion of what *remains* of Y's variability after X_1 has been taken into the account. Variable X_2, in turn, removes a second part of Y, so that the independent variable selected in Step 3 will be the variable that accounts for the most variability in Y after *both* X_1 and X_2 are removed.

RELATIVE CONTRIBUTION OF PREDICTORS

Scientists are concerned not only about the prediction of phenomena but about their explanation as well. Predictions can be made in the absence of understanding. For instance, in our graduate school example, we could predict performance moderately well without really understanding how the variables were functioning or what underlying factors were responsible for students' success. For practical applications, it may be sufficient to make accurate predictions, but scientists typically desire to understand the world around them and to make contributions to knowledge.

In multiple regression problems, one aspect of understanding the phenomenon under investigation is the determination of the relative importance of the independent variables. Unfortunately, the problem of determining the relative contributions of various independent variables in predicting a dependent variable is one of the thorniest issues in regression analysis. When the independent variables are correlated, as they usually are, there is no ideal way to untangle the effects of the variables in the equation.

It might appear that a solution could be found by comparing the contributions of the independent variables to R^2. In our graduate school example, undergraduate grades accounted for 36% of Y's variance, and GRE-Q explained an additional 14% of the variance. Should we conclude that undergraduate grades are about two

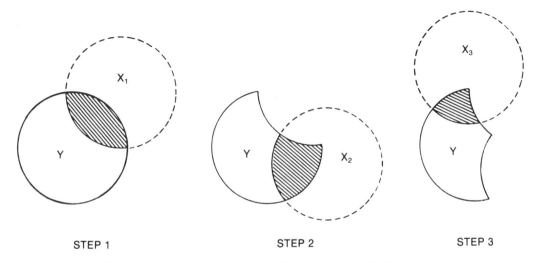

STEP 1   STEP 2   STEP 3

Figure 22-3. *Visual representation of stepwise multiple regression analysis.*

and one half times as important as GRE-Q scores in explaining graduate school grades? This conclusion would be inaccurate because the order of entry of variables in a regression equation affects their apparent contribution. If these two predictor variables were entered in reverse order, with GRE-Q first, then the R^2 would remain unchanged at .50; but GRE-Q's share would then be .30 ($.55^2$) and GPA-U's contribution would be .20 (.50 − .30). This circumstance results from the fact that whatever variance the independent variables share in common is attributed to the first variable entered in the regression analysis.

Another approach to assessing the relative importance of the predictors is to compare the regression coefficients. Earlier the regression equation was given as

$$Y' = a + b_1X_1 + b_2X_2 + \cdots b_kX_k$$

where b_1 to b_k are the regression coefficients. These b values are not directly comparable because they are in the units of raw scores, which differ from one X to another. X_1 might be in milliliters, X_2 in degrees Fahrenheit, and so forth. The use of *standard scores* (or *z scores*) eliminates this problem by transforming all variables to scores with a mean of zero and a standard deviation (SD) of one. The formula that accomplishes this standardization* is

$$z_x = \frac{X - \bar{X}}{SD_x}$$

In standard score form, the regression equation is

$$z_{Y'} = \beta_1 z_{x1} + \beta_2 z_{x2} + \cdots \beta_k z_{xk}$$

where $z_{Y'}$ is the predicted value of the standard score for Y, β_1 to β_k are the standardized regression weights for the k independent variables, and z_{x1} to z_{xk} are the standard scores for the k predictors.

---

* For a complete discussion of standard scores, an elementary statistical text should be consulted.

With all the βs (referred to as *beta* [β] *weights*) in the same measurement units, is it possible that their relative size could shed light on how much weight or importance to attach to the predictor variables? Many researchers have interpreted beta weights in this fashion, but there are problems in doing so. These regression coefficients will be the same no matter what the order of entry of the variables. The difficulty, however, is that regression weights are highly unstable. The values of beta tend to fluctuate considerably from sample to sample. Moreover, when a variable is added to or subtracted from the regression equation, the beta weights change. Because there is nothing absolute about the values of the regression coefficients, it is difficult to attach much theoretical importance to them.

Another method of disentangling relationships is path analysis. This procedure is a very important tool in the testing of theoretical expectations about relationships. Path analysis is described later in this chapter.

≡ ANALYSIS OF COVARIANCE

A significant portion of this chapter has been devoted to multiple regression analysis both because it is one of the most widely used multivariate techniques and because an understanding of it should facilitate comprehension of other related multivariate statistics. Analysis of covariance (ANCOVA) is a good example of a related procedure: it is a combination of analysis of variance and regression.

Analysis of covariance is used as a means of providing statistical control for one or more extraneous variables. This approach is especially appropriate in certain types of research situations. For example, when random assignment to treatment groups is not feasible, a quasi-experimental design is often adopted. The initial equivalency of the comparison groups in such studies is always questionable; therefore, the researcher must consider whether the obtained results were influenced by preexisting differences between the experimental and comparison groups. When experimental control such as the ability to randomize is lacking, ANCOVA offers the possibility of *post hoc* statistical control. Even in true experiments, ANCOVA can play a role in permitting a more precise estimate of group differences. This is because even when randomization procedures are used, there are typically slight differences between groups. Analysis of covariance can adjust for initial differences so that the final analysis will reflect more precisely the effect of an experimental intervention.

In both of these situations, the researcher is concerned with the possibility that the comparison groups differ in some respect at the beginning of the study. That is, the groups might differ with regard to an attribute or attributes that could affect the dependent variables and, hence, the outcome of the study. To use ANCOVA, a researcher must anticipate what those attributes are and must measure them at the outset of the study. For instance, suppose a researcher wanted to test the effectiveness of biofeedback therapy on patients' anxiety. An experimental group in one hospital is exposed to the treatment, and a comparison group of patients in another hospital is not. If the researcher wanted to be sure of the initial equivalence of the two groups, then the anxiety levels of all subjects could be measured both before and after the intervention. The initial anxiety score could be statistically controlled through ANCOVA. In such a situation, the posttest anxiety score is the dependent variable, experimental/comparison group status is the independent variable, and the pretest anxiety score is referred to as the covariate. *Covariates* can either be continuous variables (e.g., anxiety test scores) or dichotomous variables (male/female). However, the independent variables are categorical, that is, nominal-level variables.

The covariate or covariates should be selected with care. The variables chosen should be ones that the researcher strongly suspects are correlated with the dependent variable. A pretest measure is often selected as the controlled variable. A *pretest* is simply a measure of the same variable as the criterion variable, taken before a treatment is instituted. When pretests are not feasible, other related attributes can be controlled. For instance, if we were comparing the licensure exam scores for nursing students who had or had not attended schools using an integrated curriculum, there would be no possibility of a pretest, but other tests of academic aptitude or intelligence such as scores on the SAT could be used to control for initial differences in ability.

Analysis of covariance tests the significance of differences between group means after first adjusting the scores on the dependent variable to eliminate the effects of the covariate. The adjustment of scores utilizes regression procedures. In essence, the first step in ANCOVA is the same as the first step in a stepwise multiple regression analysis. The variability in the dependent measure that can be explained by the covariate is removed from further consideration. Analysis of variance is performed on what remains of Y's variability to see whether, once the covariate is controlled, significant differences between the groups remain. Figure 22-4 illustrates this two-step process. Pursuing the example just cited, Y might be scores on the licensure exam, the covariate X^* might be students' scores on the SAT, and the independent variable X might designate whether or not the students had attended schools using the integrated curriculum.

Another example may help to further explore aspects of the ANCOVA procedure. Suppose that we wanted to test the effectiveness of three different types of diets on overweight individuals. Although the sample of 30 subjects is randomly assigned to one of the three treatment groups, an ANCOVA, using pretreatment weights, permits a more sensitive analysis of weight change than a simple ANOVA. Some hypothetical data for such a study are displayed in Table 22-3.

Two aspects of the weight scores in this table are immediately discernible. First, despite random assignment to the treatment groups, the initial group means are different. Subjects assigned to Diet B differ from those assigned to Diet C by an average of ten pounds (175 versus 185

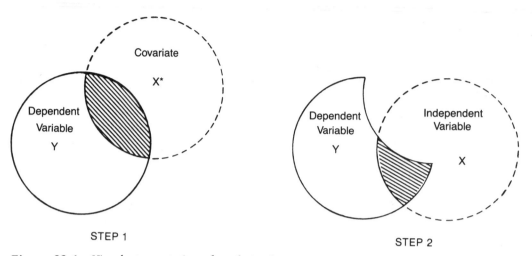

Figure 22-4. *Visual representation of analysis of covariance.*

pounds). This difference is not significant* but rather reflects chance sampling fluctuations. Second, the posttreatment means are similarly different by a maximum of only ten pounds. However,

---

* Calculations demonstrating nonsignificance are not shown. The calculated $F = .45$. With 2 and 27 degrees of freedom, $p > .05$.

the mean number of pounds *lost* ranged from ten pounds for Diets A and B to 25 pounds for Diet C.

An ordinary ANOVA for group differences in posttreatment means results in a nonsignificant F value. The ANOVA summary table is presented in part A of Table 22-4. Based on the ANOVA results, we would conclude that all three diets were equally effective in influencing weight loss.

Table 22-3. *Fictitious Data for ANCOVA Example*

DIET A (X_A)		DIET B (X_B)		DIET C (X_C)	
X_A^*	Y_A	X_B^*	Y_B	X_C^*	Y_C
195	185	205	200	175	160
180	170	150	140	210	165
160	150	145	135	150	130
215	200	210	190	185	170
155	145	185	185	205	180
205	195	160	150	190	165
175	165	190	175	160	135
180	170	165	150	165	140
140	135	180	165	180	160
195	185	160	160	230	195
1800	1700	1750	1650	1850	1600
$\overline{X}_A^* = 180$	$\overline{Y}_A = 170$	$\overline{X}_B^* = 175$	$\overline{Y}_B = 165$	$\overline{X}_C^* = 185$	$\overline{Y}_C = 160$

X, independent variable (diet); X^*, covariate (pretreatment weight); Y, dependent measure (posttreatment weight).

The second part of Table 22-4 presents the summary table for the ANCOVA. The first step of the analysis breaks the total variability of the post-treatments weights into two components: (1) that which can be accounted for by the covariate, which in this case is the pretreatment weights; and (2) residual variability. As the table shows, the covariate accounted for a significant amount of the variance, which is not surprising in light of the strong relationship between the pretreatment and posttreatment weights ($r = .91$). This merely indicates that people who started out especially heavy (or light), tended to stay that way, relative to others in the sample. In the second phase of the analysis, the residual variance is broken down to reflect the between-group and within-group contributions. With 2 and 26 degrees of freedom, the F of 17.54 is significant beyond the .01 level. The conclusion is that, after controlling for the initial weight of the subjects, there is a significant difference in weight loss resulting from exposure to different diets.

This fictitious example was deliberately contrived so that a result of "no difference" could be altered by the addition of a covariate to yield a significant difference. Most actual results are less dramatic than this example might suggest. Nonetheless, it is true that if the researcher can select meaningful covariates, then a more sensitive statistical test will always be made than if an ordinary ANOVA were performed. The increase in sensitivity results from the fact that the covariate reduces the error term (the within-group's variability), against which treatment effects are compared. In Part A of Table 22-4, it can be seen that the within-group's term is extremely large, thereby masking the contribution made by the experimental treatments.

Theoretically, it is possible to use any number of covariates. It is probably unwise to use more than five or six in practice, however. For one thing, the inclusion of more than five or six covariates is probably unnecessary because of the typically high degree of redundancy beyond the first few variables. Moreover, it may be to the researcher's disadvantage to add covariates that do not explain a statistically significant portion of the variability of a dependent variable. Each covariate "uses up" a degree of freedom, leaving the balance for the within-group's term. Fewer degrees of freedom means that a higher computed F is required for significance. For instance, with 2 and 26 degrees of freedom, an F of 5.53 is required for significance at the .01 level, but with 2 and 23 degrees of freedom (i.e., adding three covariates), an F of 5.66 is needed.

In sum, the analysis of covariance procedure is an extremely powerful and useful ana-

Table 22-4. *Comparison of ANOVA and ANCOVA Results*

SOURCE OF VARIATION	SUM OF SQUARES	df	MEAN SQUARE	F	p
A. Summary Table for ANOVA					
Between groups	500.0	2	250.0	55	> .05
Within groups	12,300.0	27	455.6		
Total	12,800.0	29			
B. Summary Table for ANCOVA					
Step 1 { Covariate	10,563.1	1	10,563.1	132.23	< .01
Residual	2236.9	28	79.9		
Total	12,800.0	29			
Step 2 { Between groups	1284.8	2	642.4	17.54	< .01
Within groups	952.1	26	36.6		
Total	2236.9	28			

lytic technique for controlling extraneous or confounding influences on dependent measures. Strictly speaking, analysis of covariance should not be used with intact groups because one of the underlying assumptions of ANCOVA is randomization. However, this assumption is frequently violated because no other alternative analysis works as effectively. Random assignment should always be done when possible but, in many situations in which randomization is not feasible, analysis of covariance could make an important contribution to the internal validity of a study.

≡ MULTIPLE CLASSIFICATION ANALYSIS

As shown in Part B of Table 22-4, an ANCOVA table provides information relating to significance testing. The table indicates that at least one of the three groups had a posttreatment weight that is significantly different from the overall grand mean, after adjusting for pretreatment weights. Sometimes it is extremely useful to examine *adjusted means*—that is, mean values on the dependent variable by group, after adjusting for covariates. It is possible to compute such adjusted means from information provided from regression analyses, as described in Pedhazur (1982). When several covariates are used to statistically control extraneous variables, however, manual computations become laborious.

Multiple classification analysis (MCA) is a versatile variant of multiple regression that will result in information about a dependent variable after adjustment for covariates, on one or more independent variables. MCA is versatile because it allows for dichotomous or continuous covariates, correlated independent variables or covariates, and nonlinear relationships between dependent and predictor variables (Andrews et al., 1973). In MCA, like ANCOVA, the independent variables are nominal-level. MCA can be performed on some standard statistical programs, such as SPSS^x (see Chapter 25).

Suppose a researcher wanted to examine whether there were differences in blood pressure among hypertensive pregnant women who had volunteered to participate in an educational program that encouraged ongoing self-monitoring of blood pressure during the pregnancy in comparison with pregnant women not participating in the program. The quasi-experiment was undertaken in two hospitals (Hospital A and B), both of which implemented the special program. The researcher collected information on preintervention blood pressure readings, as well as information on a number of background variables, such as number of prior pregnancies, number of years of schooling, and marital status. These four variables were used as the covariates in a multiple classification analysis.

Table 22-5 presents some hypothetical results. Overall, the mean posttreatment diastolic blood pressure (DBP) for the sample was 80 (grand mean). By adding or subtracting deviations from the grand mean we can determine group differences. The second column in the bottom half of Table 22-5 shows unadjusted group deviations, that is, the raw posttreatment group means without taking any of the covariates into account. Thus, without any covariate adjustments, women in the experimental group had a mean DBP of 75 (80 − 5) and those in the control group had a mean of 90 (80 + 10). However, some of the posttreatment differences between these two groups might reflect initial nonequivalences, rather than differences related to the program. The second column indicates that, after adjusting for four covariates *and* hospital, the women in the two groups still had rather sizable differences in mean postintervention DBPs. 76 for the experimentals (80 − 4) and 88 for the controls (80 + 8). ANCOVA would indicate whether this difference is significant. (In the SPSS^x program, ANCOVA and MCA can be performed simultaneously.) The R^2 at the bottom of the table indicates the proportion of variance in posttreatment DBP accounted for by all independent variables and covariates.

MCA provides a very useful method of displaying the results of complex analyses, especially to audiences that might be unfamiliar with sophisticated analytic techniques. Table 22-6 illustrates how the results from Table 22-5 could be presented in a report of research findings, after incorporating information on statistical testing from an ANCOVA. Tables such as this are generally easier to read and more meaningful than the numbers produced in an ANCOVA, such as shown in Table 22-4.

≡ *FACTOR ANALYSIS*

Factor analysis is a somewhat controversial multivariate procedure because it involves a higher degree of subjectivity than one ordinarily finds in a statistical technique. It is, nevertheless, a highly powerful and widely applied procedure and, therefore, merits attention. *Factor analysis* is related to multiple regression analysis in that both analyses develop equations that are linear combinations of the variables. The two procedures have little apparent resemblance, however, because

factor analysis does not deal with relationships between variables that the researcher classifies as dependent and independent variables.

The major purpose of factor analysis is to reduce a large set of variables into a smaller, more manageable set of measures. Factor analysis disentangles complex interrelationships among variables and identifies which variables "go together" as unified concepts. The underlying dimensions thus identified are called *factors*. As an example, consider a researcher who has prepared 100 Likert-type items aimed at measuring women's attitudes toward menopause. Suppose that the research goal was to compare the attitudes of premenopausal and postmenopausal women. If the researcher does not combine some of the items to form a scale, it would be necessary to calculate 100 chi-square statistics. The formation of a scale is preferable, but it involves adding together the scores from several individual items.

Table 22-5. *Example of Information From Multiple Classification Analysis*

Dependent variables	Postintervention diastolic blood pressure
Independent variable	Group (experimental/control)
	Hospital (A/B)
Covariates	Preintervention diastolic blood pressure
	Marital status (married/not married)
	Number of prior pregnancies
	Number of years of education

Grand Mean for Dependent Variable = 80

VARIABLE/CATEGORY	UNADJUSTED	ADJUSTED FOR INDEPENDENT VARIABLES AND COVARIATES
Group		
Experimental	−5	−4
Control	+10	+8
Hospital		
A	−10	−2
B	+5	+3
Multiple R = .866	Multiple R^2 = .750	

Table 22-6. *Example of Table Displaying MCA Results*

ADJUSTED GROUP MEANS FOR POSTTREATMENT DIASTOLIC BLOOD PRESSURE (DBP)

Group	Adjusted Mean*	p
Experimental	76.0	< .05
Control	88.0	
Hospital A	78.0	NS
Hospital B	83.0	

* The means presented have been statistically adjusted through multiple classification analysis for subjects' pretreatment DBP, parity, marital status, and educational level.

The problem is, which items are to be combined? Would it be meaningful to combine all 100 items? Probably not, because the 100 questions are not all asking exactly the same thing. There are various aspects, or various "themes" to a woman's attitude toward menopause. One aspect may relate to the problem of aging, and another aspect is concerned with a loss of the ability to reproduce. Other questions may touch on the general issue of sexuality, and yet others may concern the relief from monthly pain or bother. There are, in short, multiple dimensions to the issue of attitudes toward menopause, and these dimensions should serve as the basis for scale construction. The identification of these dimensions can be made *a priori* by the researcher, but the difficulty is that different researchers may read different concepts into the items. Factor analysis offers an empirical method of elucidating the underlying dimensionality of a large number of measures.

A factor, mathematically, is a linear combination of the variables in a data matrix. A data matrix contains the scores of N people on k different measures. For instance, a factor might be defined by the following equation:

$$F = b_1X_1 + b_2X_2 + b_3X_3 + \cdots b_kX_k$$

where F is a factor score, X_1 to X_k are original variables from the matrix, and b_1 to b_k are weights. The development of such an equation for a factor permits the reduction of the X_k scores to one (or perhaps several) factor scores.

Factor Extraction

Most factor analyses consist of two separate phases. The first step is to condense the variables in the data matrix into a smaller number of factors. Sometimes this first phase is referred to as the *factor extraction* phase. The factors usually are derived from the intercorrelations among the variables in the correlation matrix. The general goal is to seek clusters of highly interrelated variables within the matrix. There are various methods of performing the first step, each of which uses different criteria for assigning weights to the variables. Probably the most widely used method of factor extraction is called *principal components* (or principal factor or principal axes), but other methods that a researcher may come across are the image, alpha, centroid, maximum likelihood, and canonical techniques.

The result of the first step of the factor analysis is a *factor matrix* (sometimes labeled as the unrotated factor matrix), which contains coefficients or weights for each variable in the original data matrix on each extracted factor. Because unrotated factor matrices are difficult to interpret, we will postpone a detailed discussion of factor matrices until the second factor analysis phase is described. In the principal components method, weights for the first factor are defined such that the average squared weight is a maximum, thereby permitting a maximum amount of variance to be extracted by the first factor. The second factor, or linear combination, is formed in such a way that the highest possible amount of variance is again extracted from what *remains* after the first factor has been taken into account. The factors thus delineated represent independent sources of variation in the data matrix.

In extracting factors in this fashion, some criterion must be applied to delimit the number of factors or underlying dimensions. Factoring should continue until there is no further meaningful variance left. There are several criteria available from which the researcher can choose to specify when factoring should cease. It is partly the availability of so many different criteria or justifications for halting factor extraction that makes factor analysis a semisubjective process. Several of the most commonly used criteria can be described by illustrating information that is usually output from factor analysis programs. Table 22-7 presents hypothetical values for eigenvalues, percentages of variance accounted for, and cumulative percentages of variance accounted for, for ten factors. *Eigenvalues* are values equal to the sum of the squared weights for each factor. Many researchers establish as their cutoff point for factor extraction eigenvalues less than 1.00. In the example in the table, this would mean that the first five factors or dimensions would meet this criterion. Another cutoff rule that is adopted sometimes is a minimum of 5% of explained variance, in which case six factors would qualify for inclusion in our current example. Yet another criterion is based on a principle of discontinuity. According to this procedure, a sharp drop in the percentage of explained variance indicates the appropriate termination point. In Table 22-7, one might argue that there is considerable discontinuity between the third and fourth factors. The

general consensus seems to be that it is probably better to extract too many factors than too few.

Factor Rotation

The factor matrix produced in the first phase of factor analysis usually is rather difficult to interpret. For this reason, a second phase known as *factor rotation* is almost invariably performed on those factors that have met one or more of the criteria for inclusion. The concept of rotation is complex and can perhaps be best explained graphically. Figure 22-5 shows two coordinate systems, marked by axes A1 and A2, and B1 and B2. The primary axes (A1 and A2) represent Factors I and II, respectively, as they are defined before rotation. The points 1 through 6 represent six variables in this two-dimensional space. The weights associated with each variable can be determined in reference to the appropriate axis. For instance, before rotation, variable 1 is assigned a weight of .80 on Factor I and .85 on Factor II, and variable 6 has a weight of $-.45$ on Factor I and .90 on Factor II. The unrotated axes are designed to account for a maximum of variance but rarely provide a structure that has conceptual meaning. However, by rotating the axes in such a way that clusters of variables are distinctly associated with a factor, interpretability is enhanced. In the figure, B1 and B2 represent the rotated factors.

Table 22-7. *Summary of Factor Extraction Results*

FACTOR	EIGENVALUE	PERCENTAGE OF VARIANCE EXPLAINED	CUMULATIVE PERCENTAGE OF VARIANCE EXPLAINED
1	12.32	29.2	29.2
2	8.57	23.3	52.5
3	6.91	15.6	68.1
4	2.02	8.4	76.5
5	1.09	6.2	82.7
6	.98	5.8	88.5
7	.80	4.5	93.0
8	.62	3.1	96.1
9	.47	2.2	98.3
10	.25	1.7	100.0

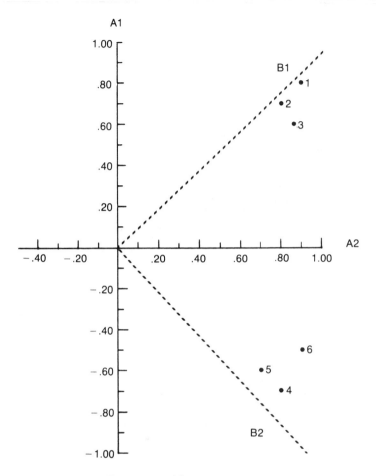

Figure 22-5. *Illustration of factor rotation.*

The rotation has been performed in such a way that variables 1, 2, and 3 would be assigned large weights on Factor I and small weights on Factor II, and the reverse would be true for variables 4, 5, and 6.

There are two general classes of rotation procedures from which a researcher must choose. Figure 22-5 illustrates *orthogonal rotation,* in which the factors are kept at right angles to one another. Orthogonal rotations maintain the independence of factors. That is, orthogonal factors are uncorrelated with one another. *Oblique rotations,* on the other hand, permit the rotated axes to depart from a 90° angle. In our figure, an oblique rotation would have put axis B1 between

variables 2 and 3 and axis B2 between variables 5 and 6. This placement of the axes strengthens the clustering of variables around an associated factor. The result is that oblique rotation produces correlated factors. Some researchers insist that orthogonal rotation leads to greater theoretical clarity; others claim that it is unrealistic. Those advocating oblique rotation point out that if the concepts *are* correlated, then the analysis should be permitted to reflect this fact. In practice, studies have revealed that similar conclusions are often reached by both rotational procedures.

The rotated factor matrix is what the researcher normally works with in interpreting the factor analysis. An example of such a matrix is displayed in Table 22-8 for discussion purposes. To make this discussion less abstract, let us say that the ten variables listed in the table are the first ten of the 100 items to measure attitudes toward menopause. The entries under each factor are the weights on that factor, which are called *factor loadings*. For orthogonally rotated factors, factor loadings can be readily interpreted. Like correlation coefficients, they range from -1.00 to $+1.00$. In fact, they can be interpreted in much the same way as a correlation coefficient. Factor loadings express the correlations between individual variables and factors (underlying dimensions). In this example, variable 1 is fairly highly correlated with Factor 1, .75. Therefore, it is possible to find which variables "belong" to a factor. For Factor I, variables 1, 3, 8, and 10 have fairly sizable loadings. Normally, a cutoff value of about .40 or .30 is used for such determinations. The researcher is now in a position to interpret the underlying dimensionality of the data. By inspecting items 1, 3, 8, and 10, it is usually possible to find some common theme that makes the variables go together. Perhaps these four questions have to do with the link between menopause and infertility and perhaps items 2, 5, and 6 (i.e., the items with high loadings on Factor II) are related to sexuality. The "naming" of factors is essentially a process of identifying theoretical constructs.

Factor Scores

In some cases in which the main purpose of factor analysis is to delineate the conceptual makeup of a set of measures, the analysis may end at this point. Frequently, however, the researcher will want to use the information obtained to develop *factor scores* for use in subsequent analyses. For instance, the factor analysis of the 100 menopause items might demonstrate that there are five principal dimensions or concepts being tapped. By reducing 100 variables to five variables, the analysis of differences between premenopausal and postmenopausal women using some procedure such as *t*-tests will be greatly simplified.

Several types of methods can be used to form factor scores. One procedure is to weight

Table 22-8. *Rotated Factor Matrix*

VARIABLE	FACTOR I	FACTOR II	FACTOR III
1	.75	.15	.23
2	−.02	.61	.18
3	−.59	−.11	.03
4	.05	.08	.48
5	.21	.79	.02
6	−.07	−.52	−.29
7	.08	.19	.80
8	.68	.12	−.01
9	−.04	.08	−.61
10	−.43	−.13	.06

the variables according to their factor loading on each factor. For example, a factor score for the first factor in Table 22-8 could be computed for each subject by the following formula:

$$F_1 = .75X_1 - .02X_2 - .59X_3$$
$$+ .05X_4 + .21X_5 - .07X_6 + .08X_7$$
$$+ .68X_8 - .04X_9 - .43X_{10} \ldots b_{100}X_{100}$$

where all of the X values* are the subject's scores on the 100 items. Some factor analysis computer programs have the capability of directly computing this type of factor score.

A second method of obtaining factor scores is to select certain variables to represent the factor and to combine them with unit weighting. This composite estimate method would produce a factor score on the first factor of our example in the following fashion:

$$F_1 = X_1 - X_3 + X_8 - X_{10} \pm \ldots$$

The variables here are those with high loadings on Factor I (the "$\pm \ldots$" indicates the inclusion of any of the other 90 variables with high loadings). This procedure is both computationally and conceptually simpler than the first approach, and both have been found to yield similar results.

---

* Standardized (z) scores are often used in lieu of raw scores in computing factor scores when the means and SDs of the variables differ substantially.

To illustrate the composite estimate approach more concretely, consider the rotated factor matrix in Table 22-8 and assume that factor scores were to be computed on the basis of this ten-item analysis, omitting for the sake of simplicity the remaining 90 items on the menopause scale. Suppose that two respondents had the following scores on these ten items:

Subject 1: 7, 1, 1, 5, 1, 6, 7, 6, 3, 2
Subject 2: 2, 5, 6, 3, 7, 3, 2, 3, 4, 4

Factor I has fairly high loadings on variables 1, 3, 8, and 10. Thus, the two subjects' factor scores on Factor 1 would be

$$7 - 1 + 6 - 2 = 10$$
$$2 - 6 + 3 - 4 = -5$$

The minus signs reflect the negative loadings on variables 3 and 10.* The same procedure would be performed for all three factors, yielding the following factor scores:

Subject 1: 10, −3, 9
Subject 2: −5, 9, 1

Factor scores would similarly be computed for all respondents, and these scores could then be used in the subsequent analyses as measures of different dimensions of attitudes toward menopause.

☰ OTHER LEAST-SQUARES MULTIVARIATE TECHNIQUES

In addition to analysis of covariance, several other multivariate techniques are closely related to least-squares multiple regression analysis. In this

---

* Researchers forming scale scores with Likert items often reverse the directionality of the scoring on negatively loaded items before forming the factor score to eliminate negative scores. Directionality of an item can be reversed by subtracting the raw score from the sum of 1 + the maximum item value. For example, in a 7-point scale, a score of 2 would be reversed to 6 [(1 + 7) − 2]. When such reversals have been done, all raw scores can be added in forming factor scores.

section, the methods known as discriminant function analysis, canonical correlation, and multivariate analysis of variance will be introduced. The introduction is brief and computations are entirely omitted, because these procedures are exceedingly complex. The intent of this review is to acquaint the reader with the types of research situations for which these methods are appropriate. Advanced statistical texts such as the ones listed in the references may be consulted for additional information.

Discriminant Analysis

In multiple regression, the dependent variable being predicted is normally a measure on either the interval or ratio scale of measurement. The regression equation makes predictions about scores that take on a large range of values. *Discriminant analysis,* in contrast, makes predictions about membership in categories or groups. The groups are identified by the researcher, and the purpose of the analysis is to distinguish the groups from one another on the basis of the independent variables available for prediction purposes. For instance, we may wish to develop a means of predicting membership in or affiliation with such groups as complying versus noncomplying cancer patients, graduating nursing students versus dropouts, or normal pregnancies versus those terminating in a miscarriage.

Discriminant analysis develops a regression equation—called a *discriminant function*—for a categorical dependent variable, with independent variables that are either categorical or continuous. The researcher begins with data from subjects whose group membership is known. The intent is to develop an equation that can be used to predict membership for new subjects for whom only measures of the independent variables are available. The discriminant function indicates to which group each subject will probably belong.

Discriminant analysis that is used to predict membership into only two groups (e.g., nursing school drop-out versus graduate) is relatively simple and can be interpreted in much the same fashion as a multiple regression. When there are more than two groups or categories, the calculations and interpretations are more complicated. With three or more groups, the number of discriminant functions is either the number of groups minus one or the number of independent variables, whichever is smaller. The first discriminant function is the linear combination of predictors that maximizes the ratio of between-group's variance to within-group's variance. The second function derived is the linear combination that maximizes this ratio, after the effect of the first function is removed. Because the independent variables are assigned different weights on the various functions, it is possible to develop theoretical interpretations based on the knowledge of which predictors are important in discriminating among different groups.

Discriminant analysis shares several features in common with multiple regression analysis, aside from the fact that prediction equations based on a linear combination of independent variables are developed. For one thing, it is possible to use a stepwise approach in entering predictors into the equation. Also, the analysis produces an index designating the proportion of variance in the dependent variable accounted for by the predictor variables. The index is known as *Wilks' lambda* (λ). Actually, λ indicates the proportion of variance *unaccounted for* by predictors, or $\lambda = 1 - R^2$.

In sum, discriminant analysis has potential for being quite useful to researchers, particularly those with practical problems of classification or diagnosis. An excellent and relatively simple guide to this procedure has been prepared by Tatsuoka (1970).

Canonical Correlation

Canonical correlation is the most general multivariate technique, of which other procedures are special cases. *Canonical correlation* analyzes the relationship between two or more independent variables and two or more dependent variables. Conceptually, one can think of this technique as an extension of multiple regression

to more than one dependent variable. Mathematically and interpretatively, the gap between multiple regression and canonical correlation is greater than this statement suggests.

Like other techniques described thus far in this chapter, canonical correlation uses the least-squares principle to partition and analyze variance. Basically, two linear composites are developed, one of which is associated with the dependent variables, the other of which is for the independent variables. The relationship between the two linear composites is expressed by the canonical correlation coefficient, R_C. As in the case of the coefficient of determination (R^2), R^2_C indicates the proportion of variance accounted for in the analysis. When there is more than one source or dimension of covariation in the two sets of variables, more than one canonical correlation can be found.

Examples of research utilizing canonical correlation are relatively rare. Perhaps the method is not well known, and it requires a higher degree of mathematical sophistication than is needed for most statistical techniques. Still, when a study involves multiple dependent and independent variables, canonical correlation may be the most suitable way to analyze the data.

Multivariate Analysis of Variance

Multivariate analysis of variance, sometimes abbreviated MANOVA, is the extension of analysis of variance procedures to more than one dependent variable. This procedure is used primarily to test the significance of differences between the means of two or more dependent variables, considered simultaneously. Like ordinary ANOVA, MANOVA was developed for use in experimental situations in which at least one independent variable has been manipulated. For instance, if we wanted to examine the effect of two methods of exercise (A_1 and A_2) and two lengths of exercise treatment (B_1 and B_2) on both diastolic and systolic blood pressure (Y_1 and Y_2), then a MANOVA would be appropriate. Researchers often analyze such data by performing two separate univariate

ANOVAs. Strictly speaking, this practice is incorrect. Separate ANOVAs imply that the dependent variables have been obtained independently of one another. In fact, the dependent measures have been obtained from the same subjects and are, therefore, correlated. Multivariate analysis of variance takes the intercorrelations of the dependent variables into account in computing the test statistics.

Links Among Multivariate Techniques

The analogy might be made that multiple regression is to canonical correlation what ANOVA is to MANOVA. This analogy, although correct, obscures a point that the astute reader has perhaps already suspected, and that is the close affinity between multiple regression and analysis of variance.

Pedhazur (1982) observed that ANOVA and multiple regression are virtually identical. Both techniques are concerned with analyzing the variability in a dependent measure and contrasting the proportion of the variability attributable to one or more independent variables with that attributable to unexplained sources of variation, or "error." Multiple regression and ANOVA use a somewhat different approach and use different symbols and terminology, but both analyses boil down to a final F-ratio. By tradition, experimental data are typically analyzed by ANOVA and *ex post facto* data are analyzed by regression procedures. Nevertheless, it should be realized that any data for which ANOVA is appropriate could also be analyzed by multiple regression, although the reverse is not true. In many cases, multiple regression is preferable because it can be used with a broader range of data and because it provides more information, such as a prediction equation and an index of association, R. However, with respect to the index of association issue, it should be noted that a formula can easily be applied to ANOVA results to derive the statistic known as *eta-squared* (η^2), which indicates the strength of association between variables and, like R^2, the proportion of variance in the dependent variable

explained by the independent variables. Eta-squared is simply the sum of squares between groups divided by the total sum of squares. The value of η^2 is computed routinely by most ANOVA computer programs.

≡ PATH ANALYSIS

Path analysis is a regression-based method for studying patterns of causation among a set of variables in *ex post facto* studies. As discussed in Chapter 10, path analysis usually begins with a theory or causal model that dictates the type of data to be collected. It is not a method for discovering causes; rather, it is a method applied to a prespecified model formulated on the basis of prior knowledge and theory.

Path analysis is a complex topic to which entire books have been devoted. Therefore, we briefly describe some of the key concepts without discussing actual analytic procedures. Path analytic reports often use a *path diagram* to display their results; we use such a diagram (Fig. 22-6) here to illustrate important concepts. This model postulates that patients' length of hospitalization (V4) is the result of their capacity for self-care (V3); this, in turn, is affected by nursing actions (V1) and the severity of their illness (V2).

In path analysis, a distinction is often made between exogenous and endogenous variables. An *exogenous variable* is a variable whose determinants lie outside the model. In Figure 22-6, nursing actions (V1) and illness severity (V2) are exogenous; no attempt is made in the model to elucidate what causes different nursing actions or different degrees of illness. An *endogenous variable*, by contrast, is one whose variation is determined by other variables in the model. In our example, self-care capacity (V3) and length of hospitalization (V4) are endogenous.

In path analysis, causal linkages are illustrated by arrows, drawn from the presumed causes to the presumed effects. In our illustration, severity of illness is hypothesized to affect length of hospitalization both directly (path p_{42}) and indirectly through the mediating variable self-

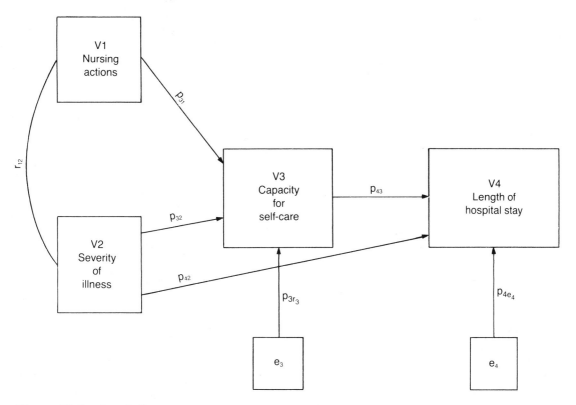

Figure 22-6. *A path diagram.*

care capacity (paths p_{32} and p_{43}). Correlated exogenous variables are indicated by curved lines, as shown by the curved line between nursing actions and illness severity.

Ideally, the model would totally explain the outcome of interest, which in this case is length of hospitalization. In practice, this almost never happens, because causal theories are rarely comprehensive when dealing with human phenomena. There are usually other determinants, which are generally referred to as *residual variables*. In Figure 22-6, there are two boxes labeled "e," which denote a composite of all determinants of self-care capacity and hospital stay that are not in the model. The residuals summarize our "ignorance" of other determinants of endogenous variables. If we can identify and measure additional causative forces and incorporate them into the overarching theory, then they should be in the model.

Figure 22-6 represents what is referred to as a *recursive model*. This means that the causal flow is unidirectional and without feedback loops. In other words, it is assumed that variable 2 is a cause of variable 3, and that variable 3 is *not* a cause of variable 2.

In Figure 22-6, causal paths are indicated by symbols denoting that a given variable (e.g., V3) is caused by another (e.g., V2), yielding a path labeled p_{32}. In research reports, the path symbols would be replaced by actual numbers developed by applying regression procedures. The numbers shown are called *path coefficients*, which are standardized partial regression slopes. For example, path p_{32} is equal to $\beta_{32.1}$—the beta weight between variables 2 and 3, holding variable 1 constant. Because path coefficients are in standard form, they indicate the proportion of a standard deviation difference in the caused variable that is directly attributable to a one SD difference in the specified causal variable. Thus, the path coefficients give us some indication of the relative importance of various determinants.

Path analysis involves estimation of the path coefficients through the use of *structural equations*. The structural equations for Figure 22-6 are as follows:

$$z_1 = e_1$$
$$z_2 = e_2$$
$$z_3 = p_{31} z_1 + p_{32} z_2 + e_3; \text{ and}$$
$$z_4 = p_{43} z_3 + p_{42} z_2 + e_4$$

These equations indicate that z_1 and z_2 (standard scores for variables 1 and 2) are determined by outside variables; that z_3 depends directly on z_1 and z_2 plus outside variables; and that z_4 depends directly on z_2, z_3, and outside variables. In our example, the structural equations could be solved to yield path coefficients by performing two multiple regressions: (1) by regressing variable 3 on variables 1 and 2 and (2) by regressing variable 4 on variables 2 and 3.

The model presented in Figure 22-6 may or may not be a reasonable construction of the hospitalization process. Path analysis involves a number of procedures for testing causal models and for determining effects. Pedhazur (1982) provides a good overview of path analytic techniques and the advanced student should refer to books such as that by Blalock (1972).

≡ *POWER ANALYSIS*

Many published (and even more unpublished) nursing studies result in nonsignificant findings—that is, one or more of the researcher's main hypotheses are not supported. Although standard statistical texts pay considerable attention to the problem of Type I errors, (wrongly rejecting a *true* null hypothesis), little attention has been paid to Type II errors (wrongly accepting a *false* null hypothesis). *Power analysis* represents a method for reducing the risk of Type II errors and for estimating their occurrence.

As indicated in Chapter 21, the probability of committing a Type I error is established by the investigator as the level of significance, or alpha (α). The probability of a Type II error is beta (β). The complement of $(1 - \beta)$ is the *probability of obtaining a significant result,* and is referred to as the *power* of a statistical test. It has been shown that many nursing studies have insufficient power (Polit & Sherman, 1990) and are therefore at high risk of committing a Type II error.

In performing a power analysis, there are four components, at least three of which must be known to or estimated by the researcher; power analysis solves for the fourth component. The four major factors are as follows:

1. *The significance criterion, α.* Other things being equal, the more stringent this criterion, the lower the power.
2. *The sample size, n.* As sample size increases, power increases.
3. *The population effect size, gamma (γ).* Gamma is a measure of how "wrong" the null hypothesis is, that is, how strong the effect of the independent variable is on the dependent variable in the population.
4. *Power, or $1 - \beta$.* This is the probability of rejecting the null hypothesis.

Researchers typically use power analysis for two purposes: (1) to solve for the sample size needed in a study to increase the likelihood of demonstrating significant results and (2) to determine the power of a statistical test. In this section, which is only a brief summary of power analysis, we focus on the first of these purposes.

To solve for an estimate of the needed sample size, the researcher must specify α, γ, and $1 - \beta$. Usually, the researcher establishes α, the risk of a Type I error, as (at most) .05; in some cases, a lower (stricter) criterion such as .01 may be required. Just as .05 has been adopted as the standard for the α criterion, a conventional standard for $1 - \beta$ is .80. With power equal to .80, there is a 20% risk of committing a Type II error. Although this risk may seem rather high, a stricter criterion would require sample sizes much larger than most nurse researchers could manage. The majority of nursing studies being conducted have a power well below .80, thus making it very difficult to avoid a Type II error.

With α and 1 − β specified, the only other piece of information needed to solve for *n* is γ, the population effect size. The *effect size* is an estimate of the magnitude of the relationship between the research variables. When relationships are strong, large samples are not needed to detect the effect at statistically significant levels. When the relationships are modest, then large sample sizes are needed to avoid Type II errors.

The value of γ is arrived at differently depending on the nature of the data and the statistical test to be performed. However, the principles for arriving at the estimate of γ are the same for all tests. The researcher needs to use available evidence to estimate the magnitude of the effect size. Sometimes this evidence comes from the researcher's own pilot study, a procedure that is highly recommended when the main study is likely to be costly. More often, the researcher uses evidence from other published studies on the same or a similar problem. That is, an effect size is calculated (through procedures that follow) based on other researchers' data.* When there are *no* data that could reasonably be construed as relevant, the researcher may be forced to use conventions based on whether the effect size is expected to be "small," "medium" or "large." In using these conventions, it is wise to be conservative because the majority of nursing studies have modest effect sizes.

The procedures for estimating effects and the relevant power tables vary from one statistical test to another. We provide formulas for four situations that are especially common in nursing research: (1) testing the difference between two group means (i.e., situations requiring a *t*-test);

(2) testing the difference between three or more group means (i.e., situations requiring an ANOVA); (3) testing the significance of a bivariate linear relationship (i.e., situations requiring Pearson's *r*); and (4) testing the significance of differences in proportions between two groups (i.e., situations requiring a chi-square test). Cohen (1977) and Jaccard and Becker (1990) discuss power analysis in the context of many other situations.*

Sample Size Estimates for Test of Difference Between Two Means

Suppose we were interested in testing the hypothesis that cranberry juice reduces the urinary *p*H of diet-controlled patients. In our study, we plan to randomly assign some subjects to a control condition (no cranberry juice) and others to an experimental condition in which they would be given 200 ml of cranberry juice with each meal for five days. How large a sample is needed for this study, given an α of .05 and power equal to .80?

To answer this question, we must first estimate γ. In a two-group situation in which the difference of means is of interest, the formula for the effect size is

$$\gamma = \frac{\mu^1 - \mu^2}{\sigma}$$

That is, γ is the difference between the population means, divided by the population SD. But how can the researcher know this information in advance? If we knew, for example, the mean urinary *p*H of all subjects who had or had not ingested cranberry juice, there might not be any point in doing the study. Nevertheless, as explained above, the researcher must *estimate* the population means and SD, based on whatever information is available. In our present example, suppose we found an earlier *ex post facto* study that compared the urinary *p*H of subjects who had

---

* Usually, a researcher will be able to find more than one piece of research from which the effect size can be estimated. In such a case, the estimate should be based on the study that yields the most stable and reliable results or whose design most closely approximates that of the new study. In some cases in which equally good (or equally bad) prior research is available, it may be desirable to combine information from multiple studies (through averaging or weighted averaging) to develop an effect size estimate.

* Computer software for performing power analyses is available for personal computers (Borenstein & Cohen, 1988).

or had not ingested cranberry juice in the previous 24 hours. The earlier and current studies are quite different. In the *ex post facto* study, the diets are uncontrolled; there may be selection biases in who drinks or does not drink cranberry juice, the length of ingestion is only one day, and so on. However, this study is a reasonable starting point. Suppose the results of the earlier study were as follows:

$$\bar{X}_1 \text{ (no cranberry juice)} = 5.70$$
$$\bar{X}_2 \text{ (cranberry juice)} \quad = 5.50$$
$$\sigma \text{ (pooled SD)} \quad\quad = .50$$

Thus, the value of γ would be .40:

$$\gamma = \frac{5.70 - 5.50}{.50} = .40$$

Table 22-9 presents approximate sample size requirements for various effect sizes and powers, and two values of α (for two-tailed tests), in a two-group mean-difference situation. In the upper half of the table for $\alpha = .05$, we find that the estimated n needed for an effect size of .40 and a power of .80 is 98 subjects per group. That is, assuming that the earlier study provided a roughly accurate estimate of the population effect size, the total number of subjects required in the new study would be about 200, with half assigned to the control group (no cranberry juice) and the other half assigned to the experimental group. A sample size much smaller than 200 would have a good chance of resulting in a Type II error.

If there is *no* prior relevant research (which is rarely the case), then the researcher can, as a last resort, estimate on the basis of readings or experience whether the expected effect is small, medium, or large. By a convention developed by Cohen (1977), the value of γ in a two-group test of mean differences is estimated at .20 for "small"

Table 22-9. *Approximate Sample Sizes* Necessary to Achieve Selected Levels of Power as a Function of Estimated Effect Size for Test of Difference of Two Means*

POWER	ESTIMATED EFFECT†									
	.10	.15	.20	.25	.30	.40	.50	.60	.70	.80
PART A: $\alpha = .05$										
.60	977	434	244	156	109	61	39	27	20	15
.70	1230	547	308	197	137	77	49	34	25	19
.80	1568	697	392	251	174	98	63	44	32	25
.90	2100	933	525	336	233	131	84	58	43	33
.95	2592	1152	648	415	288	162	104	72	53	41
.99	3680	1636	920	589	409	230	147	102	75	58
PART B: $\alpha = .01$										
.60	1602	712	400	256	178	100	64	44	33	25
.70	1922	854	481	308	214	120	77	53	39	30
.80	2339	1040	585	374	260	146	94	65	48	37
.90	2957	1324	745	477	331	186	119	83	61	47
.95	3562	1583	890	570	396	223	142	99	73	56
.99	4802	2137	1201	769	534	300	192	133	98	75

* Sample size requirements for *each* group; total sample size would be twice the number shown.

† Estimated effect (γ) is the estimated population mean group difference, divided by the estimated population SD, or:

$$\gamma = \frac{\mu_1 - \mu_2}{\sigma}$$

effects, .50 for "medium" effects, and .80 for "large" effects. With an α value of .05 and power of .80, the *total* sample size (number of subjects in both groups) for studies with expected small, medium, and large effects would be 784, 126, and 50, respectively. The majority of nursing studies cannot expect effect sizes in excess of .50, and those in the range of .20 to .40 are especially common. (In Polit and Sherman's [1990] analysis of effect sizes for studies appearing in *Nursing Research* and *Research in Nursing and Health* in 1989, the average effect size for *t*-test situations was .35). Cohen noted that in new areas of research inquiry, effect sizes are likely to be small. A medium effect should be estimated only when the effect is so substantial that it can be detected by the naked eye (i.e., without formal research procedures).

Sample Size Estimates for Test of Difference Between Three or More Means

Suppose we wanted to study the effectiveness of three different modes of stimulation—(1) auditory, (2) visual, and (3) tactile—on preterm infants' sensorimotor development. The dependent variable will be a standardized scale of infant development, such as the Denver Scale. With an α of .05 and power of .80, how many infants should be randomly assigned to the three groups?

There are alternative approaches to doing a power analysis in an ANOVA context, but the simplest approach is to calculate or estimate eta-squared, based on information from either other relevant studies or a pilot study. As noted earlier in this chapter, η^2 is the index indicating the proportion of variance explained in ANOVA, and is equal to the sum of squares between (SS_B) divided by the total sum of squares (SS_T). Eta-squared can be used directly as an estimate of the effect size.

In the modes of stimulation example, suppose we were able to find an earlier study that tested the same or a similar hypothesis and that

study yielded an η^2 of .05. Table 22-10 presents approximate sample size requirements for various ANOVA situations. Note that, for the sake of economy and practicality, this table presents much more limited information in terms of power (the power ranges between .70 and .95) and α (only .05) than was true for the two-group situation because of the increased complexity: here, the sample size requirements vary as a function of the number of groups in the study. The table presents sample size estimates only for the most common group sizes: 3, 4 and 5. Jaccard and Becker (1990) provide expanded tables for different alphas, powers, and group sizes.

Assuming that we desire a power of .80 and an α level of .05 in the hypothetical example, the number of subjects needed in each of the three stimulation groups would be 62 infants. If the experiment were undertaken with only 50 infants per group, there would be a 30% chance (power = .70) of finding nonsignificant results, even when the null hypothesis was false.

If no estimates of eta-squared can be developed on the basis of prior research, then the researcher would have to predict whether effects are likely to be small, medium, and large. For ANOVA-type situations, Cohen's conventional values of small, medium, and large effects would be values of η^2 equal to .01, .06, and .14, respectively. This would correspond to sample size requirements of approximately 319, 53, or 22 subjects *per group* (in a three-group study), assuming an α of .05 and power of .80.

Sample Size Estimates for Bivariate Correlation Tests

Suppose we wanted to study the effect of social support on primaparas' acceptance of the motherhood role. We plan to administer two scales to women who have had a normal vaginal delivery of full-term infants. One scale measures the amount of social support available to the mother in her family and community; the other scale measures the woman's positive and negative reactions to her new role. The hypothesis is that women who have more social support available to them will be more accepting of the role transition to motherhood. How many women should be included in the study, given an α of .05 and power of .80?

As in the previous cases, we need an estimate of γ. In this situation, we have two measures on an interval scale, and the relationship between them would be tested using Pearson's r. The estimated value of γ here is actually ρ, that is, the expected population correlation coefficient.

Suppose we found an earlier study that correlated a simple measure of social support (the number of people subjects felt they could "count on" in times of stress) with an observational measure of maternal warmth. Neither of these measures perfectly captures the variables in the new study, but they are conceptually close and, if no better information were available, they would provide a useful approximation. Suppose the completed study found $r = .18$, which we will use as our estimate of ρ, and hence of γ. Table 22-11

shows sample size requirements for various powers and effect sizes in situations in which Pearson's r is used. With an α of .05 and power of .80, the sample size needed in the study would lie between 197 (for an effect size of .20) and 349 (for an effect size of .15). Extrapolating for an effect size of .18, we would need a sample of approximately 250 subjects to achieve a power of .80 with an α of .05. With a sample this size, we would wrongly reject the null hypothesis only five times out of 100 and wrongly retain the null hypothesis 20 times out of a hundred. To increase the power to .95 (wrongly retaining the null hypothesis only five times out of 100), we would need a sample of about 400 women.

When prior estimates of effect size are unavailable, the conventional values of small, medium, and large effect sizes in a bivariate correlation situation are .10, .30, and .50, respectively. In Polit and Sherman's (1990) study, the average correlation found in nursing studies was in the vicinity of .20.

Table 22-10. *Approximate Sample Sizes* Necessary to Achieve Selected Levels of Power for $\alpha = .05$ as a Function of Estimated Population Values of Eta-Squared*

| POWER | \multicolumn{10}{c}{POPULATION ETA-SQUARED} |
	.01	.03	.05	.07	.10	.15	.20	.25	.30	.35
GROUPS = 3										
.70	255	84	50	35	24	16	11	9	7	6
.80	319	105	62	44	30	19	14	11	9	7
.90	417	137	81	57	39	25	18	14	11	9
.95	511	168	99	69	47	30	22	16	13	11
GROUPS = 4										
.70	219	72	43	30	21	13	10	8	6	5
.80	272	90	53	37	26	17	12	9	7	6
.90	351	115	68	48	33	21	15	12	9	8
.95	426	140	83	58	40	25	18	14	11	9
GROUPS = 5										
.70	193	64	38	27	18	12	9	7	6	5
.80	238	78	46	33	23	15	10	8	7	5
.90	306	101	59	42	29	18	13	10	8	7
.95	369	121	72	50	34	22	16	12	10	8

* The values are the number of subjects *per group*.

Sample Size Estimates for Testing Differences in Proportions

Estimating sample size requirements when differences in proportions between groups are being studied is more complex than in the previously described situations. For this reason, we present only a partial discussion of this topic here and recommend that other references such as Cohen (1977) or Jaccard and Becker (1990) be consulted. We restrict our coverage to 2 × 2 contingency tables.

Suppose we were interested in comparing the rates of breast-feeding in two groups of women: (1) those receiving a special intervention—home visits by nurses during the third trimester, in which the advantages of breast-feeding would be described—and (2) those in a control group not receiving any home visits. How many subjects should be randomly assigned to the two groups?

The effect size for this type of situation is not arrived at in a straightforward fashion. This is because the effect size is influenced not only by expected differences in proportions (e.g., 60% in one group versus 40% in another, a 20 percentage point difference) but also by the absolute values of the proportions. In other words, the effect size for 60% versus 40% is *not* the same as that for 30% versus 10%. In general, the effect size is *larger* (and consequently sample size needs are *smaller*) at the extremes than near the midpoint: a 20 percentage point difference is easier to detect when the two percentages are 10% and 30% (or 70% and 90%) than when they are near the middle, such as 40% and 60%.

The computation of the effect size index involves a complex transformation (the arcsine transformation) that we do not fully elaborate on here. Rather than present sample size estimates based on effect size, Table 22-12 presents the approximate sample size requirements for detecting differences in various proportions, assuming an α of .05 and a power of .80. To use this table, we would need to have estimates of the proportions for both groups. Then we would find the proportion for one group in the first column

Table 22-11. *Approximate Sample Sizes Necessary to Achieve Selected Levels of Power as a Function of Estimated Population Value of* ρ

POWER	POPULATION CORRELATION COEFFICIENT									
	.10	.15	.20	.25	.30	.40	.50	.60	.70	.80
PART A: α = .05										
.60	489	218	123	79	55	32	21	15	11	9
.70	616	274	155	99	69	39	26	18	14	11
.80	785	349	197	126	88	50	32	23	17	13
.90	1050	468	263	169	118	67	43	30	22	17
.95	1297	577	325	208	145	82	53	37	27	21
.99	1841	819	461	296	205	116	75	52	39	30
PART B: α = .01										
.60	802	357	201	129	90	51	33	23	17	14
.70	962	428	241	155	108	61	39	28	21	16
.80	1171	521	293	188	131	74	48	33	25	19
.90	1491	663	373	239	167	94	61	42	31	24
.95	1782	792	446	286	199	112	72	50	37	28
.99	2402	1068	601	385	267	151	97	67	50	39

and the proportion for the second group in the top row. The approximate sample size requirement *for each group* would be found at the intersection of the two appropriate proportions. Thus, in our example, if we had reason to expect (on the basis of a pilot study, say), that 20% of the control group mothers and 40% of the experimental group mothers would breast-feed their infants, then the sample size needed in the study (to keep the risk of a Type II error down to 20%) would be 80 subjects per group.

Because we have not presented information on the computationally complex effect size for the situation involving a 2 × 2 contingency table, we cannot conveniently identify Cohen's convention for small, medium, and large effects. We can, however, give *examples* of differences in proportions (i.e., the proportions in Group 1 versus Group 2) that conform to the conventions:

Small: .05 versus .10, .20 versus .29, .40 versus .50, .60 versus .70, .80 versus .87
Medium: .05 versus .21, .20 versus .43, .40 versus .65, .60 versus .82, .80 versus .96

Large: .05 versus .34, .20 versus .58, .40 versus .78, .60 versus .92, .80 versus .996

Thus, if the researcher expected a medium effect in which the proportion for Group 1 could be expected to be in the vicinity of .40, then the number of subjects in each of the two groups would need to be approximately 70 to 75. As in other situations, researchers are encouraged to avoid the use of the conventions, if possible, in favor of more precise estimates based on prior empirical evidence; when the use of the conventions is unavoidable, conservative estimates should be used to minimize the risk of finding nonsignificant results.

≡ OTHER STATISTICAL PROCEDURES

The statistical procedures described in this chapter and in Chapters 20 and 21 cover the vast majority of techniques for analyzing quantitative data used by nurse researchers today. However, the widespread use of computers and new develop-

Table 22-12. *Approximate Sample Sizes* Necessary to Achieve a Power of .80 for α = .05 for Estimated Population Difference Between Two Proportions*

GROUP II PROPORTIONS	GROUP I PROPORTIONS														
	.10	.15	.20	.25	.30	.35	.40	.45	.50	.55	.60	.70	.80	.90	1.00
.05	421	133	69	44	31	24	19	15	13	11	9	7	5	4	2
.10		689	196	97	59	41	30	23	18	15	12	9	6	5	3
.15			901	247	118	71	48	34	26	21	16	11	8	5	3
.20				1090	292	137	80	53	38	28	22	14	10	6	3
.25					1252	327	151	87	57	40	30	18	12	8	4
.30						1371	356	161	93	60	42	23	14	9	4
.35							1480	374	169	96	61	31	18	10	5
.40								1510	385	172	97	42	22	12	5
.45									1570	393	173	60	28	15	6
.50										1570	389	93	38	18	6
.55											1539	162	53	23	7
.60												356	80	30	8
.70													292	59	12
.80														195	18
.90															38

* The values are the number of subjects *per group*.

ments in statistical analysis have combined to give researchers more options for analyzing their data than were available in the past. Although a full exposition of other sophisticated statistical procedures is beyond the scope of this book, we briefly describe a few of these advanced techniques and provide references for readers interested in fuller discussions.

Life Table and Event History Analysis

Life table analysis is a procedure that is widely used by epidemiologists and medical researchers. It is used when the dependent variable represents the time interval between an initial event and a termination event. Life table analysis is often applied to situations in which mortality is the termination event—such as when the initial event is the onset of a disease, or the initiation of treatment for the disease, and death is the end event. Because of this fact, life table analysis is also referred to as *survival analysis*. Life table analysis involves the calculation of a survival score, which compares the survival time for one subject with that for all other subjects. When the researcher is interested in group comparisons—for example, comparing the survival function of subjects in a special treatment versus a control group—a statistic can be computed to test the null hypothesis that the groups are samples from the same survival distribution.

Life table analysis can be applied to many situations that are unrelated to mortality. For example, a life table analysis could be used to analyze such time-related phenomena as length of time in labor, length of time elapsed between release from a psychiatric hospital and reinstitutionalization, and duration of pain following surgery. Polit and her colleagues (1985) used life table analysis to study length of time between the termination of a first pregnancy and the onset of a second in a sample of economically disadvantaged teenagers. Further information about life table analysis may be found in Gross and Clark (1975), and Lee (1980).

More recently, extensions of life table analysis have been developed that allow researchers to examine the determinants of survival-type transitions in a multivariate framework. In these analyses, independent variables are used to model the risk (or hazard) of experiencing an event at a given point in time, given that one has not experienced the event before that time. The most common specification of the hazard is known as the *proportional hazards model.* These *event history* methodologies are likely to prove useful to nurse researchers in the 1990s. A relatively straightforward explanation and illustration of this technique is presented in Teachman (1982), and further discussion may be found in Allison (1984), Gross and Clark (1975), or Tuma and Hannan (1984).

Logistic Regression

Most of the analyses we have discussed thus far have been based on a single approach to estimating parameters, the least-squares approach. There are, however, alternative estimation procedures that are being used increasingly by researchers in certain situations. In particular, *maximum likelihood estimation* has gained in popularity and use in analyzing complex multivariate data. Although a full elaboration is beyond the scope of this text, we note that maximum likelihood estimators are ones that estimate the parameters most likely to have generated the observed measurements. For further discussions of maximum likelihood theory, the reader is urged to consult Hanushek and Jackson (1977).

Logistic regression (sometimes referred to as *logit analysis*) is a procedure that uses maximum likelihood estimation for analyzing relationships between multiple independent variables and categorical dependent variables. Logistic regression transforms the probability of an event occurring (e.g., that a woman will practice breast self-examination or not) into its odds—that is, into the ratio of one event's probability relative to the probability of a second event. As a result, probabilities that range between zero and one in actuality are transformed into continuous variables that range between zero and infinity. Because this range is still restricted, a further transformation is performed, namely calculating the logarithm of the odds. The range of this new variable (known as the *logit of the decision*) is now transformed from minus to plus infinity. Using the logit as a continuous dependent variable, maximum likelihood approaches are then used to estimate the coefficients of the independent variables. These techniques can also be used in the case of a dependent categorical variable that has more than two categories.

Logistic regression is often used in preference to discriminant function analysis for several reasons. First, as Cleary and Angel (1984) noted, logistic models are considered to be more theoretically appropriate than models based on the least-squares approach for exact model fitting. Second, logistic regression is concerned more with modeling the probability of an outcome rather than just with the prediction of group membership. Also, logistic regression enables the researcher to generate odds ratios that can be meaningfully interpreted and graphically displayed, and therefore may promote better understanding of the underlying relationships of the variables. Although logit analysis was avoided by researchers for many years because of the unavailability of convenient computer programs, that is no longer the case. We expect that logistic regression will be used increasingly by nurse researchers in the upcoming years.

Linear Structural Relation Analysis

Another statistical procedure that is based on maximum likelihood estimation is *linear structural relation analysis,* more commonly referred to as LISREL. LISREL is a versatile, but complex, approach used in the analysis of multivariate data. It is most frequently used as a method of testing causal models, much the same as path analysis, but it is also used as an approach to factor analysis.

One of the drawbacks of using ordinary least squares regression in doing path analysis is that the validity of the method is based on a set of very restrictive assumptions, most of which are virtually impossible to meet. First, it is assumed that the variables are measured without error. As we discussed in Chapter 18, most measures used by nurse researchers contain some degree of error. Second, it is assumed that any of the residuals (error terms) in the different regression equations are uncorrelated. However, because error terms often represent untapped sources of individual differences—differences that are not entirely random—this assumption is seldom tenable. Third, traditional path analysis assumes that the causal flow is unidirectional or recursive. In reality, causes and effects are often reciprocal or iterative.

LISREL avoids all of these problems. LISREL can be used for the analysis of models with multiple indicators,* reciprocal causation, measurement errors, and correlated residuals. Because of its versatility, LISREL is a highly complex procedure, and one whose computer program (LISREL VI) is not easy to learn. Readers interested in further information on LISREL are urged to consult texts by Sorbom and Joreskog (1981) or Kenny (1979).

≡ RESEARCH EXAMPLES

Table 22-13 illustrates some of the applications of multivariate statistics within nursing studies. The following study, which used multiple types of multivariate statistics, is described in greater detail.

> Muhlenkamp and her colleagues (1985) investigated nursing clinic clients' health beliefs, health values, and background characteristics in relation to health promotion activities. The subjects in the study were 175 clients of a nursing clinic who were administered instruments that measured health locus of control, health values, health-related elements of their

*LISREL generally involves the use of multiple indicators designed to tap complex latent (unobservable) variables, such as anxiety or motivation. Within LISREL, a measurement model is developed to specify the relations between unobserved and observed—that is latent and manifest—variables.

personal life style, and demographic variables such as marital status, religion, sex, education, income, and age.

The life style variables were measured with a 24-item Likert scale developed by the investigators—the Personal Lifestyle Questionnaire (PLQ). The Likert statements were designed to reflect health-related preferences and activities in six areas: (1) relaxation, (2) substance use, (3) health promotion, (4) safety, (5) nutrition, and (6) exercise. Responses to the PLQ were factor analyzed to determine its dimensionality. The factor analysis confirmed that six separate dimensions were being measured, supporting the calculation of six subscale scores. However, a total PLQ score was computed by adding the scores on all six subscales. The total score reflected the degree to which subjects engaged in an overall health-promoting life style.

The PLQ total score was used as a dependent variable in a multiple regression analysis designed to shed light on factors that could predict healthful life styles. Both demographic and attitudinal variables (such as the scores on the locus of control scale) were used as the predictor variables. Using stepwise multiple regression, five variables were found to be significantly related to the PLQ total score: (1) sex, (2) age, (3) education, (4) belief in chance as a determinant of health, and (5) self-rated health status. Education was found to be the best predictor—the better educated the subject, the higher his or her life style score. Overall, the five predictor variables accounted for only 16% of the variance in PLQ scores, suggesting that there were numerous unmeasured factors that led subjects to engage (or not engage) in a health-promoting life style.

Table 22-13. *Examples of Nursing Studies Using Multivariate Statistics*

RESEARCH PROBLEM	STATISTICAL PROCEDURE
Are prenatal and perinatal variables commonly found to predict breast-feeding duration also useful in predicting breast-feeding problems in the first week postpartum? (Kearney et al., 1990)	Multiple regression
With resting cardiovascular indices controlled, is there a difference—in terms of cardiovascular reactivity to a challenging situation—between preschool children classified as demonstrating Type A or Type B behavior? (Brown & Tanner, 1988)	ANCOVA
What are the dimensions of nurses' job satisfaction? (Mueller & McCloskey, 1990)	Factor analysis
Can adolescent female conduct disorders be predicted on the basis of such family characteristics as family income, family structure, and family routine adherence? (Keltner et al., 1990)	Discriminant function analysis
What is the relationship between sets of health, psychosocial and family variables on the one hand and various aspects of functional status following childbirth on the other? (Tulman et al., 1990)	Canonical correlation
What are the differences in sleep continuity, sleep architecture, sleep cycles, and rapid eye movement sleep measures between Alzheimer's, depressed, and healthy elderly individuals? (Hock et al., 1988)	MANOVA
Is the model of stress, appraisal, and coping developed by Lazarus and Folkman useful in explaining psychosocial health dysfunction in widows and widowers? (Gass & Chang, 1989)	Path analysis
Is the duration of breast-feeding among breast-feeding mothers related to the number of sources of support available? (Kaufman & Hall, 1989)	Life table analysis
Are maternal stressors and depressive symptoms in mothers related to behavior problems in young children? (Hall & Farel, 1988)	Logistic regression

≡ *SUMMARY*

The *multivariate* statistical procedures explored in this chapter are used to untangle complex relationships among three or more variables. One of the most versatile multivariate procedures is *multiple correlation/regression,* which is a statistical method for understanding the effects of two or more independent variables on a dependent variable. Regression analysis provides a mechanism for researchers to make predictions about phenomena. A simple regression equation is a formula for making predictions about the numerical values of one variable based on the values of a second variable. The researcher can often improve the precision of the predictions by including more than one predictor (independent) variable in the regression equation. The multiple correlation coefficient is symbolized by R. The multiple correlation coefficient, when squared (R^2), indicates the proportion of the variance of the dependent variable that is "explained" or "accounted for" by the combined influences of the independent variables. R^2 is sometimes referred to as the *coefficient of determination.* The versatility of multiple regression analysis is demonstrated by its various related analyses and special options. For example, in *stepwise multiple regression,* the researcher can identify from a pool of potential predictor variables those variables that in combination have the greatest predictive power.

Analysis of covariance is a procedure that permits the researcher to control extraneous or confounding influences on dependent variables. ANCOVA combines the principles of multiple regression and analysis of variance. The effect of one or more variable (called the *covariate*) is statistically controlled or removed before testing for group differences by way of traditional ANOVA procedures. ANCOVA is often used in *ex post facto* or quasi-experimental designs to control for potential pretreatment differences but can also be used in experimental designs to provide more precise estimates of experimental effects.

Multiple classification analysis (MCA) is a variant of regression that produces information about a dependent variable after adjusting for covariates. The information is usually provided in the form of values for the grand mean of the dependent variable and adjusted deviations from it.

Factor analysis is used to reduce a large set of variables into a smaller set of underlying dimensions, called *factors.* Mathematically, each factor represents a linear combination of the variables contained in a data matrix. The first phase of factor analysis, called *factor extraction,* identifies clusters of variables with a high degree of communality, or redundancy, and condenses the larger set of variables into a smaller number of factors. The second phase of factor analysis involves *factor rotation,* which enhances the interpretability of the factors by aligning variables more distinctly with a particular factor. The *factor loadings* shown in a rotated factor matrix can then be examined to identify and "name" the underlying dimensionality of the original set of variables and to compute *factor scores.*

Discriminant analysis is essentially a multiple regression analysis in which the dependent variable is categorical (i.e., nominal level of measurement). This procedure is useful for making predictions about membership in groups on the basis of two or more predictor variables. *Canonical correlation* is the most general of all the multivariate procedures: it analyzes the relationship between two or more independent *and* two or more dependent variables. Multivariate analysis of variance (MANOVA) is the extension of analysis of variance principles to cases in which there is more than one dependent variable. All of the procedures reviewed here are closely related methods that have as a common goal the identification, control, and prediction of variance.

Path analysis is a regression-based procedure for testing causal models. The researcher first prepares a *path diagram* that stipulates hypothesized causal linkages among variables. Using regression procedures applied to a series of *structural equations,* a series of *path coefficients* are developed. These path coefficients represent weights associated with a causal path in standard deviation units. The simplest form of a causal model is one that is *recursive,* that is, one in which causation is presumed to be unidirectional.

Power analysis refers to techniques for estimating either the likelihood of committing a Type II error or sample size requirements. Power analysis involves four components: (1) a desired significance level (α); (2) power ($1 - \beta$); (3) sample size, (n); and (4) an estimated *effect size* (γ). To calculate needed sample size, all three other components must be specified by the researcher. The most difficult part is estimating the effect size, but there is usually at least one existing study that can provide rough guidelines for the estimate. The application of power analysis would probably greatly reduce the number of nonsignificant findings reported in the nursing literature.

New statistical methodologies are likely to gain in popularity among nurse researchers in the 1990s. These include such techniques as *life table analysis, event history analysis, logistic regression,* and *LISREL.*

≡ *STUDY SUGGESTIONS*

1. Suppose that you were investigating job satisfaction among nurses. You have collected information on 12 variables concerning nurse

Factor	Eigenvalue	Percent of Variance	Cumulative Percentage
1	9.03	28.0	28.0
2	6.39	20.4	48.4
3	4.82	17.1	65.5
4	1.09	6.3	71.8
5	.98	5.8	77.6
6	.93	5.6	83.2
7	.87	4.9	88.1
8	.60	3.5	91.6
9	.52	2.8	94.4
10	.48	2.6	97.0
11	.30	1.8	98.8
12	.26	1.2	100.0

satisfaction. After submitting these variables to factor analysis, you obtain the following information (see table):

According to these data, how many dimensions underlie job satisfaction? On what did you base this decision?

2. Refer to Figure 22-1. What would the value of Y' be for the following X values: 8, 1, 3, 6?

3. A researcher has examined the relationship between preventive health care attitudes on the one hand and the person's educational level, age, and sex on the other. The multiple correlation coefficient is .62. Explain the meaning of this statistic. How much of the variation in attitudinal scores has been explained by the three predictors? How much is *unexplained*? What other variables might improve the power of the prediction?

4. Which multivariate statistical procedure(s) would you recommend using in the following situations:
   a. A researcher wants to test the effectiveness of a nursing intervention for reducing stress levels among surgical patients, using an experimental group of patients from one hospital and a control group from another hospital.
   b. A researcher wants to predict which students are at risk of venereal disease by using background information such as sex, socioeconomic status, religion, grades in sex education course, and attitudes toward sex.
   c. A researcher wants to test the effects of three different diets on blood sugar levels and blood pH.

5. Estimate the required total sample sizes for the following situations.
   a. Comparison of two group means: $\alpha = .01$; power $= .90$; $\gamma = .35$.
   b. Comparison of three group means: $\alpha = .05$; power $= .80$; $\eta^2 = .07$.
   c. Correlation of two variables: $\alpha = .01$; power $= .85$; $\rho = .27$.
   d. Comparison of two proportions: $\alpha = .05$; power $= .80$, $P_1 = .35$; $P_2 = .50$.

≡ SUGGESTED READINGS

METHODOLOGICAL REFERENCES

Aaronson, L.S. (1989). A cautionary note on the use of stepwise regression. *Nursing Research, 38,* 309–311.

Aaronson, L.S., Frey, M., & Boyd, C.J. (1988). Structural equation models and nursing research: Part II. *Nursing Research, 37,* 315–318.

Allison, P.D. (1984). *Event history analysis: Regression for longitudinal event data.* Beverly Hills, CA: Sage.

Anderson, S., et al., (1980). *Statistical methods for comparative studies.* New York: John Wiley and Sons.

Andrews, F.M., et al. (1973). *Multiple classification analysis.* Ann Arbor, MI: University of Michigan Institute for Social Research.

Bennett, S., & Bowers, D. (1978). *An introduction to multivariate techniques for the social and behavioral sciences.* New York: John Wiley and Sons.

Blalock, H.M., Jr. (1972). *Causal inferences in nonexperimental research.* New York: W.W. Norton.

Borenstein, M., & Cohen, J. (1988). *Statistical power analysis: A computer program.* Hillsdale, NJ: Erlbaum Associates.

Boyd, C.J., Frey, M.A., & Aaronson, L.S. (1988). Structural equation models and nursing research: Part I. *Nursing Research, 37,* 249–253.

Brown, B., Walker, H., Schimeck, M., & Wright, P. (1979). A life table analysis package for SPSS. *American Sociological Review, 33,* 225–227.

Cleary, P.D., & Angel, R. (1984). The analysis of relationships involving dichotomous dependent variables. *Journal of Health and Social Behavior, 25,* 334–348.

Cohen, J. (1977). *Statistical power analysis for the behavioral sciences.* New York: Academic Press.

Cohen, J., & Cohen, P. (1983). *Applied multiple regression: Correlation analysis for behavioral sciences* (2nd ed.). New York: Halsted Press.

Cox, D.R., & Oakes, D. (1984). *Analysis of survival data.* London: Chapman and Hall.

Dillon, W., & Goldstein, M. (1984). *Multivariate analysis: Methods and applications.* New York: John Wiley and Sons.

Draper, N., & Smith, H. (1981). *Applied regression analysis* (2nd ed.). New York: John Wiley and Sons.

Dwyer, J.H. (1983). *Statistical models for social and behavioral sciences.* New York: Oxford University Press.

Goodwin, L.D. (1984a). Increasing efficiency and precision of data analysis: Multivariate vs. univariate statistical techniques. *Nursing Research, 33,* 247–249.

Goodwin, L.D. (1984b). The use of power estimation in nursing research. *Nursing Research, 33,* 118–120.

Gross, A.J., & Clark, V. (1975). *Survival distributions: Reliability applications in the biomedical sciences.* New York: John Wiley and Sons.

Hanushek, E., & Jackson, J. (1977). *Statistical methods for social scientists.* New York: Academic Press.

Huitema, B.E. (1980). *The analysis of covariance and its alternatives.* New York: John Wiley and Sons.

Jaccard, J., & Becker, M.A. (1990). *Statistics for the behavioral sciences.* Belmont, CA: Wadsworth.

Kenny, D.A. (1979). *Correlation and causality.* New York: John Wiley and Sons.

Kerlinger, F.N. (1986). *Foundations of behavioral research* (3rd ed.) New York: Holt, Rinehart & Winston.

Kim, J., & Mueller, C. (1978). *Factor analysis: Statistical methods and practical issues.* Beverly Hills, CA: Sage.

Knapp, T.R., & Campbell-Heider, N. (1989). Numbers of observations and variables in multivariate analyses. *Western Journal of Nursing Research, 11,* 634–641.

Lee, E.T. (1980). *Statistical methods for survival data analysis.* Belmont, CA: Lifelong Learning.

Mason-Hawkes, J., & Holm, K. (1989). Causal modeling: A comparison of path analysis and LISREL. *Nursing Research, 38,* 312–314.

Maxwell, A.E. (1978). *Multivariate analysis in behavioral research: For medical and social science students* (2nd ed.). New York: Methuen.

Pedhazur, E.J. (1982). *Multiple regression in behavioral research* (2nd ed.). New York: Holt, Rinehart & Winston.

Polit, D.F., & Sherman, R. (1990). Statistical power in nursing research. *Nursing Research* (in press).

Rummel, R.J. (1970). *Applied factor analysis.* Evanston, IL: Northwestern University Press.

Sorbom, D., & Joreskog, K.E. (1981). The use of LISREL in sociological model building. In D.J. Jackson & E. Borgatta (Eds.), *Factor analysis and measurement in sociological research.* Beverly Hills, CA: Sage.

Schroeder, M.A. (1990). Diagnosing and dealing with multicollinearity. *Western Journal of Nursing Research, 12,* 175–187.

Tatsuoka, M. (1970). *Discriminant analysis: The study of group differences.* Champaign, IL: Institute for Personality and Ability Testing.

Tatsuoka, M. (1971). *Multivariate analysis: Techniques for educational and psychological research.* New York: John Wiley and Sons.

Teachman, J.D. (1982). Methodological issues in the analysis of family formation and dissolution. *Journal of Marriage and the Family, 44,* 1037–1053.

Tuma, N.B., & Hannan, M.T. (1984). *Social dynamics: Models and methods.* New York: Academic Press.

Verran, J.A., & Ferketich, S.L. (1984). Residual analysis for statistical assumptions of regression equation. *Western Journal of Nursing Research, 6,* 27–40.

Volicer, B.J. (1981). *Advanced statistical methods with nursing applications.* Bedford, MA: Merestat Press.

Weisberg, S. (1985). *Applied linear regression* (2nd ed.). New York: John Wiley and Sons.

Weissfeld, L.A., & Butler, P.M. (1988). Use of regression diagnostics in nursing studies. *Nursing Research, 37,* 119–122.

Welkowitz, J., Ewen, R.B., & Cohen, J. (1982). *Introductory statistics for the behavioral sciences* (3rd ed.). New York: Academic Press.

Wu, Y.B., & Slakter, M.J. (1989). Analysis of covariance in nursing research. *Nursing Research, 38,* 306–308.

SUBSTANTIVE REFERENCES*

Alexy, B. (1985). Goal setting and health risk reduction. *Nursing Research, 34,* 283–292. [ANCOVA]

Bowles, C. (1986). Measure of attitude toward menopause using the semantic differential model. *Nursing Research, 35,* 81–85. [Factor analysis, multiple regression]

Boyd, C. (1990). Testing a model of mother-daughter identification. *Western Journal of Nursing Research, 12,* 448–468. [LISREL]

Brown, M.S., & Tanner, C. (1988). Type A behavior and cardiovascular responsivity in preschoolers. *Nursing Research, 37,* 152–155. [ANCOVA]

Duffy, M.E. (1988). Determinants of health promotion in midlife women. *Nursing Research, 37,* 358–362. [Canonical correlation, multiple regression]

*A comment in brackets after each citation designates the multivariate statistical procedure of interest.

Froman, R.D., & Owen, S.V. (1990). Mothers' and nurses' perceptions of infant care skills. *Research in Nursing and Health, 13,* 247–253. [Multiple regression, MANOVA]

Gass, K.A., & Chang, A. (1989). Appraisals of bereavement, coping, resources, and psychosocial health dysfunction in widows and widowers. *Nursing Research, 38,* 31–36. [Path analysis]

Gortner, S.R., & Zyzanski, S.J. (1988). Values in the choice of treatment: Replication and refinement. *Nursing Research, 37,* 240–244. [Factor analysis]

Hall, L.A., & Farel, A.M. (1988). Maternal stresses and depressive symptoms: Correlates of behavior problems in young children. *Nursing Research, 37,* 156–161. [Logistic regression]

Hoch, C.C., Reynolds, C.F., & Houck, P.R. (1988). Sleep patterns in Alzheimer, depressed, and healthy elderly. *Western Journal of Nursing Research, 10,* 239–256. [ANCOVA, MANOVA]

Kaufman, K.J., & Hall, L.A. (1989). Influences of the social network on choice and duration of breastfeeding in mothers of preterm infants. *Research in Nursing and Health, 12,* 149–159. [Discriminant function analysis, life table analysis]

Kearney, M., Cronenwett, L., & Barrett, J.A. (1990). Breast-feeding problems in the first week postpartum. *Nursing Research, 39,* 90–95. [Multiple regression]

Keltner, B., Keltner, N.L., & Farren, E. (1990). Family routines and conduct disorders in adolescent girls. *Western Journal of Nursing Research, 12,* 161–174. [Discriminant function analysis]

Leidy, N.K. (1990). A structural model of stress, psychosocial resources, and symptomatic experience in chronic physical illness. *Nursing Research, 39,* 230–235. [Path analysis]

Melnyk, K. (1990). Barriers to care: Operationalizing the variable. *Nursing Research, 39,* 108–112. [LISREL factor analysis]

Metheny, N., Eisenberg, P., & McSweeney, M. (1988). Effect of feeding tube properties and three irrigants on clogging rates. *Nursing Research, 37,* 165–169. [MANOVA]

Mueller, C.W., & McCloskey, J.C. (1990). Nurses' job satisfaction: A proposed measure. *Nursing Research, 39,* 113–117. [Factor analysis]

Muhlenkamp, A., Brown A., Sands, D. (1985). Determinants of health promotion activities in nursing clinic clients. *Nursing Research, 34,* 327–332. [Factor analysis, multiple regression]

Murphy, S.A. (1984). Stress levels and health status of

victims of a natural disaster. *Research in Nursing and Health, 7,* 205–215. [Discriminant function analysis]

Polit, D.F., Kahn, J.R., & Stevens, D. (1985). *Final impacts from Project Redirection: A program for pregnant and parenting teens.* New York: Manpower Demonstration Research Corp. [Multiple regression, logistic regression, MCA, life table analysis]

Tulman, L., Fawcett, J., Groblewski, L., & Silverman, L. (1990). Changes in functional status after childbirth. *Nursing Research, 39,* 70–75. [Canonical correlation]

Williams, O.D., & Williams, A.R. (1989). Mild malnutrition and child development in the Philippines. *Western Journal of Nursing Research, 11,* 310–319. [Discriminant function analysis]

Yarcheski, A., & Mahon, N.E. (1989). A causal model of positive health practices: The relationship between approach and replication. *Nursing Research, 38,* 88–93. [LISREL]

23
The Analysis of Qualitative Data

As we saw in the chapters on data collection methods, data for nursing studies vary in their degree of structure. Some research questions and data collection strategies yield loosely structured, narrative materials, such as verbatim dialogue between an interviewer and a respondent, the field notes of a participant observer, or diaries used by historical researchers. These data are generally not amenable to the type of analyses we discussed in Chapters 20, 21, and 22. This chapter describes methods for analyzing such qualitative data. Before proceeding, we briefly discuss the arguments often made in favor of qualitative analysis.

≡ THE AIMS OF QUALITATIVE RESEARCH

Qualitative research has been described by Benoliel (1984) as "modes of systematic inquiry concerned with understanding human beings and the nature of their transactions with themselves and with their surroundings" (p. 3). Qualitative research is often described as holistic, that is, concerned with humans and their environment in all of their complexities. Qualitative research is often based on the premise that gaining knowledge about humans is impossible without describing human experience as it is lived and as it is defined by the actors themselves.

Qualitative research is often, though not always, allied with a phenomenological perspective. Phenomenological inquiries, because of an emphasis on the subjects' realities, require a minimum of researcher-imposed structure and a maximum of researcher involvement, as the researcher tries to comprehend those people whose experience is under study. Imposing structure on the research situation (e.g., by deciding in advance exactly what questions to ask and how to ask them) necessarily restricts the portion of the subjects' experiences that will be revealed.

A debate has emerged in recent years over whether qualitative or quantitative studies are better suited for advancing nursing science (e.g., Munhall, 1982; Webster et al., 1981), but there is a growing recognition that both approaches are needed (Bargagliotti, 1983; Downs, 1983; Goodwin & Goodwin, 1984; Gorenberg, 1983). The most balanced perspective seems to be that the degree of structure a researcher imposes should be based on the nature of the research question. For example, if the question under investigation is, "What are the processes by which infertile couples resolve their infertility?" then the investigator is really seeking to understand how men and women make sense of an experience that is complex, interpersonal, and dynamic. It would be possible to investigate this problem with structured instruments, but it is likely that the investigator would never really come to understand the *process* that is the focus of the inquiry.

On the other hand, if the research question is, "What is the effect of alternative topical gels applied during wound debridement on the patient's level of pain and extent of debridement accomplished?" it seems appropriate to seek specific, concrete data in a structured format. Both of these hypothetical questions have a place in nursing research, because both can contribute to the improvement of nursing practice.

Benoliel (1984) identified four broad areas in which unstructured, qualitative approaches appear most promising:

1. environmental influences on care-giving systems;
2. decision-making processes;
3. people's adaptation to critical life experiences, such as chronic illness or developmental changes; and
4. the nature of nurse–client social transactions in relation to stability and change

≡ APPLICATIONS OF QUALITATIVE ANALYSIS

Qualitative methods, as suggested in the previous section, are more appropriately applied to certain types of research problems than others. There is a fair amount of agreement that qualitative methods are less suitable than quantitative approaches for establishing cause-and-effect relationships, for rigorously testing research hypotheses, or for determining the opinions, attitudes, and practices of a large population. The unsuitability of qualitative methods for these purposes is based in part on the difficulties of analyzing qualitative data, as we discuss later. Another problem, however, is that qualitative research tends to yield vast amounts of narrative data—consequently, it is impractical for the researcher to use large, representative samples for obtaining the data. The extent to which the results can be generalized may therefore be called into question.

We must stress that these shortcomings of qualitative research are offset by some important advantages. Survey-type methods can never yield the rich and potentially insightful material that is generated using an unstructured approach. Among the important purposes of qualitative research are the following:

Description. When little is known about a group of people, an institution, or a social phenomenon of interest, in-depth interviewing or participant observation are good ways to learn about them. For example, suppose we wanted to learn about the experiences of deinstitutionalized mental patients. How do they cope with the transition to a new environment? What kinds of supports are available to them? What factors facilitate or impede improved mental health? For this type of study, a survey approach might be unfeasible or unprofitable.

Hypothesis generation. A researcher using qualitative techniques often has no explicit *a priori* hypotheses. The collection of in-depth information about some phenomenon might, however, lead to the formulation of hypotheses that could be tested more formally in subsequent research. For example, a researcher may be investigating by means of in-depth interviews the reasons for discontinued use of oral contraceptives among teenage girls. Open-ended discussion with a sample of girls might lead the researcher to observe that girls whose boyfriends have complained about the birth control pill's side effects on the girls (e.g., weight gain, moodiness, or headaches) appear to be substantially more likely to stop using the pill than girls whose boyfriends have not made such complaints. This hypothesis could be tested systematically in another study.

Theory development. Qualitative researchers often analyze their data with an eye toward developing an integrated explanatory scheme. The term *grounded theory* is frequently used in connection with a certain approach to analyzing qualitative data, as developed by two sociologists, Glaser and Strauss (1967). This approach involves the generation of theory on the basis of comparative analysis between or among groups within a substantive area, using methods of field research for data collection. The term "grounded theory" refers to the fact that a theorization does not spring from the investigator's preconceived hypotheses about a social situation, but rather is "discovered" by being *grounded* in the data.

Qualitative data can also serve a number of functions when combined with quantitative data. These purposes are discussed in Chapter 24.

≡ QUALITATIVE DATA: TO QUANTIFY OR NOT

One of the decisions a qualitative researcher must make is whether the narrative materials that compose the data will be quantified to some extent. After all, most quantitative measurement methods involve ascribing numbers to *qualities* of persons or objects—for example, their self-esteem, their degree of compliance, or their level of preoperative anxiety. In quantitative research, decisions about how to translate qualities of phenomena into numerical expression are generally made before data collection. However, researchers who collect qualitative materials often develop schemes for quantifying their narrative materials after the data have been gathered.

There are varying degrees to which qualitative materials can be quantified. At one extreme, the researcher can convert all of the narrative information to a numerical system and subject the data to quantitative analysis through statistical procedures. The technique known as content analysis, described in a later section of this chapter, often involves the complete quantification of narrative personal communications. At the other extreme, of course, all of the narrative materials can be left intact and can be analyzed through procedures that are described in the following section. In between are quantitative methods for introducing some checks and balances into qualitative analysis. For example, a procedure referred to as *quasi-statistics,* which resembles an accounting system more than a method of statistical analysis, is sometimes used in conjunction with qualitative analysis.

Qualitative materials can be quantified in a variety of ways. For example, suppose we asked patients to discuss, in their own words, the quality of nursing care they received during a long-term hospitalization. Suppose each patient's response was tape-recorded and then transcribed, yielding descriptions ranging from five to ten typewritten pages. How could the material be quantified? We could *count* the number of specific complaints mentioned; we could *count* the number of lines devoted to negative versus positive comments; we could *code* for the presence or absence of specific patient concerns, such as complaints about the time required for the nurse to respond to a call; or we could *rate* the description in terms of overall favorableness toward the care received. The researcher who wants to quantify qualitative material can be extremely creative and ingenious in developing a meaningful approach. The trick is to develop a system that is consistent with the aims of the research and faithful to the message conveyed in the qualitative materials.

Whether qualitative data *should* be quantified is a different issue. Some investigators argue that everything can be measured (quantified) and that quantitative analysis is the best way to determine objectively whether relationships between variables exist. This argument aside, it is often useful to quantify qualitative materials purely as a way of coping with the volume of data that is typically produced in qualitative research. Other researchers argue against any quantification, asserting that qualitative materials are richer than numbers and offer greater potential for understanding relationships and meanings. They also argue that because data collection and coding procedures are not immune to subjectivity, the use of numbers merely disguises potential bias and gives the illusion of objectivity. We are inclined to disagree with either extreme. We believe that an understanding of human behaviors, problems, and characteristics is best advanced by the judicious use of both qualitative and quantitative data. Sometimes, as we discuss in Chapter 24, that combination is appropriate in a single study.

≡ QUALITATIVE ANALYSIS PROCEDURES

The purpose of data analysis, regardless of the type of data one has, is to impose some order on a large body of information so that some general conclusions can be reached and communicated in a research report. This task is particularly challenging for the qualitative researcher for three major reasons. First, there are no systematic rules for analyzing and presenting qualitative data. It is at least partly because of this fact that qualitative methods have been described as "soft." The absence of systematic analytic procedures makes it difficult for the researcher engaged in qualitative analysis to present conclusions in such a way that their validity is patently clear. And, the absence of well-defined and universally accepted procedures makes replication difficult.

The second aspect of qualitative analysis that makes it challenging is the sheer amount of work that is required. The qualitative analyst must organize and make sense of pages and pages of narrative materials. In a qualitative study directed by one of the authors (Polit), the data consisted of transcribed, unstructured interviews with more than 100 women who had recently divorced. The transcriptions ranged from 40 to 80 pages in length, resulting in more than 6000 pages that had to be read, organized, integrated, and synthesized. It is this labor-intensive aspect of qualitative research, combined with the fact that samples must necessarily be rather small, that sometimes makes it difficult to obtain funding for qualitative studies; they are expensive but often are of limited generalizability.

The final challenge comes in reducing the data for reporting purposes. The major results of quantitative research can often be summarized in two or three tables. However, if one compresses qualitative data too much, the very point of maintaining the integrity of narrative materials during the analysis phase becomes lost. If one merely summarizes the conclusions reached without including numerous supporting excerpts directly from the narrative materials, then the richness of the original data disappears. As a consequence, it is extremely difficult to present the results of qualitative research in a format that is compatible with space limitations in professional journals. Most qualitative researchers find that the best medium for disseminating their results is books rather than journal articles.

Despite the fact that there are no universally accepted rules for the analysis of qualitative materials, numerous systems have evolved. It is beyond the scope of this book to describe all of the major systems in detail, but we present here some guidelines that should provide a basic understanding of the general process. We also describe the major features of two different strategies: (1) analytic induction and (2) grounded theory. However, we strongly encourage readers interested in performing qualitative analysis to consult several of the references listed at the end of this chapter.

Data Organization

Whether one is working with field notes from a participant observation study, transcriptions from unstructured interviews, historical documents, or some other qualitative material, a critical task is to carefully prepare for the analysis of data by imposing some structure on the mass of information. Some practical tips might prove helpful at this point.

First, as in quantitative studies, it is usually important to check that the data are all there, are of reasonably good quality, and are in a format that facilitates organization. You should confirm that the verbatim transcripts really *are* verbatim (some well-meaning typists are often tempted to "edit" or "clean up" dialogue). You should also ensure that all the field notes have been written up and that there are no glaring holes in the data. It is best to have all of the data typed or printed, double-spaced, and with wide margins so that notes and codes can be inserted into them. You should have at least one backup copy of all the data, but, depending on what system you use to index and analyze your data, you may need a total of three or four copies of the data.

The main task in organizing qualitative data is developing a method to index the materials. That is, the researcher must design a mechanism for gaining access to parts of the data, without having to read and re-read the set of data in its entirety. The traditional approach is to develop different types of files. One set of files, for example, would contain the master copy of the material and is ordinarily arranged in some administratively relevant manner, such as by chronological date or by subject identification number. The administrative files would ordinarily contain other types of cross-referenced materials, such as listings that link subject identification numbers with other types of information, such as dates and locations of data collection.

A second set of files usually is constructed on a conceptual/analytic basis. To develop such a file, the researcher must develop a coding scheme that relates to the major topics under investigation. An example of the topical coding scheme used in Polit's study of divorced women is presented in Box 23-1. Then, all of the data are reviewed for content and coded according to the topic that is being addressed. A file is subsequently developed for each of the various topics, and all of the materials relating to that topic are inserted into the file. In other words, the researcher "cuts up" a copy of the material by topic

---

BOX 23-1 EXAMPLE OF A CODING SCHEME FOR STUDY OF ADJUSTMENT TO DIVORCE

1. Divorce-related issues
   a. Adjustment to divorce
   b. Divorce-induced problems
   c. Advantages of divorce
2. General psychologic state
   a. Before divorce
   b. During divorce
   c. Current
3. Physical health
   a. Before divorce
   b. During divorce
   c. Current
4. Relationship with children
   a. General quality
   b. Communication
   c. Shared activities
   d. Structure of relationship
5. Parenting
   a. Discipline and child-rearing
   b. Feelings about parenthood
   c. Feelings about single parenthood
6. Friendships/social participation
   a. Dating and remarriage
   b. Friendships
   c. Social groups, leisure
   d. Social support
7. Employment/Education
   a. Employment experiences
   b. Educational experiences
   c. Job and career goals
   d. Educational goals
8. Workload
   a. Coping with workload
   b. Schedule
   c. Child care arrangements
9. Finances

area so that all of the content on a particular topic can be retrieved automatically.

This process of developing conceptual files is often more cumbersome and difficult than the preceding paragraph suggests, for several reasons. First, the researcher may discover in going through the data that the initial coding system was incomplete or otherwise inadequate. In some cases, this means going back and starting from scratch. For this reason, it is usually necessary to review a very large portion of the data before an adequate coding scheme can be developed. It is not unusual for some topics to emerge that were not initially conceptualized. When this happens, it is sometimes risky to assume that the topic failed to appear in materials that have already been coded. That is, a topic might not be identified as important until it has emerged three or four times in the data. In such a case, it would be necessary to reread all previously coded material to have a truly complete file on that topic.

Another problem stems from the fact that narrative materials are generally not linear. For example, paragraphs from transcribed interviews may contain elements relating to three or four different topics, in which case you would need as many copies of that paragraph as there are topics covered to place a copy in each of the topic files. (An example of a multitopic segment of an interview from the study of divorced women, with codes in the margin, is shown in Fig. 23-1.) Also, to understand the meaning of some statements about a topic, it may be necessary to include a lot of peripherally related material to provide a context, such as material preceding or following the directly relevant materials.

In setting up files based on a conceptual coding scheme, it is important to include pertinent administrative information on each item filed. For example, if your data consisted of transcribed interviews, each informant would ordinarily be assigned an identification number. Each master copy should bear the identification number, and each excerpt from the interview filed in the conceptual file should also include the appropriate identification number so that you could, if necessary, obtain additional information from the master copy.

In some cases, you would need to develop other types of files in addition to administrative

---

Subject 025
June 25, 1980
Page 32

Int: How did you feel right after the separation? Will you tell
           me a little more about that?

025:       Well, you know, when I look back...I mean I think anybody
           would have felt hopeless and helpless...because of, you
           know, emotionally...I think maybe it's a little easier if   2b
           you've got more security...more money. I was really stuck.
           I caught myself thinking..."Oh, if it wasn't for the   9
           kids..." I love them both dearly, but...I mean there have
           been times when I've said to myself--I think a lot of women
           go through this too--I really had thought of giving them   5c
           up. In the beginning I used to think, too, they'd be so
           much better off with somebody that could, you know...When I
           was really struggling--I was on welfare----I used to think,   1b.
           "My God, how am I going to educate them? What are they
           going to have? I can't make ends meet now." It's kinda
           projecting the unknown...fear of the unknown. I think you
           can get mixed up.

Figure 23-1. *Coded excerpt from an unstructured interview.*

and conceptual files. For example, if your data consisted of field notes from a participant observation study, you would ordinarily need to develop a method for indexing and retrieving methodological or personal notes.

Although many qualitative researchers have found that the development of a complex, multidimensional filing system is an indispensable preliminary task in preparation for the actual analysis, alternative methods have been used. For example, some people prefer to write abstracts of each interview or observation report on index cards, together with a listing of the coded categories and the relevant page numbers. An example, which used a special type of index card, is shown in Figure 23-2. These index cards have holes on all sides that can be used for easy retrieval of information on a given topic, or on analytic themes. That is, the researcher places notches in the holes corresponding to coded topical categories or concepts. Then, when information relating to a particular topic or theme is needed, all of the cards notched for that topic can easily be pulled from the deck of index cards. (In the example shown in Fig. 23-2, the notched holes correspond not to coded categories of content, but to themes developed in the analysis phase. Thematic analysis is described in the following section.) This method has at least three advantages. First, files with multiple copies of the data quickly become very bulky and cumbersome. Second, the abstract on the cards provides an immediate and useful overview of the entire observation or interview—an overview that is unavailable when one works directly from conceptual files. Third, the index cards can also be coded (with appropriate notches, if desired) for different characteristics of the subjects or observational settings. For example, basic demographic information about the respondents such as age, social class, marital status, and so on could be recorded for easy reference right on the card. On the other hand, when a

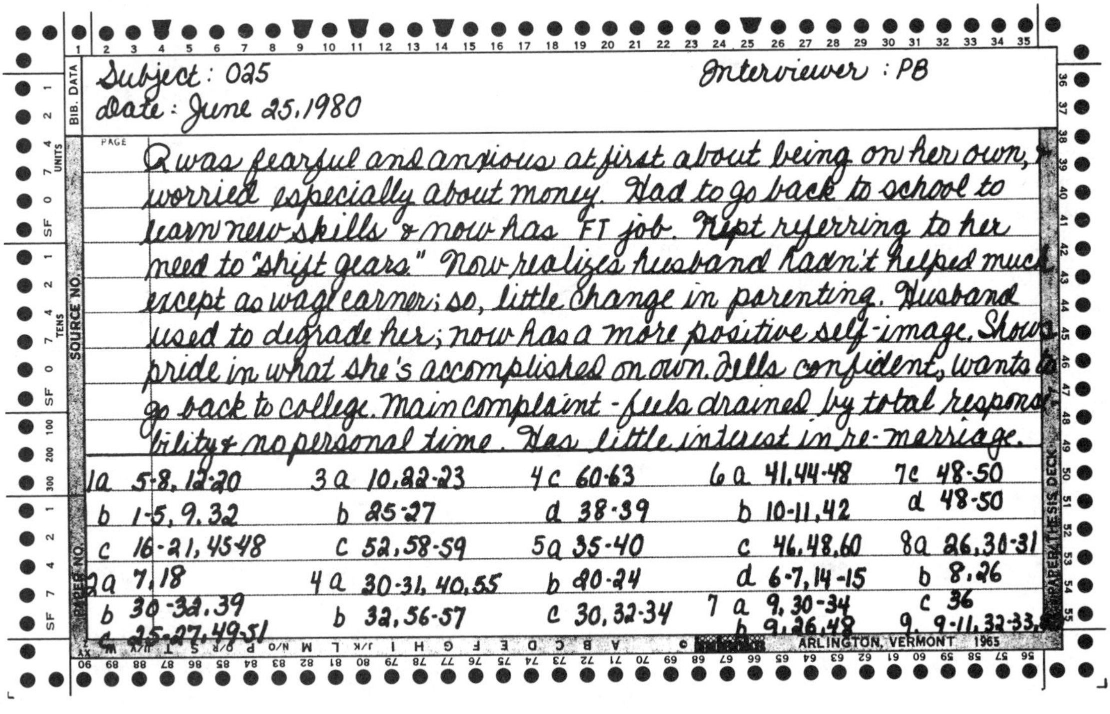

Subject: 025 Interviewer: PB
Date: June 25, 1980

R was fearful and anxious at first about being on her own, & worried especially about money. Had to go back to school to learn new skills & now has FT job. Kept referring to her need to "shift gears." Now realizes husband hadn't helped much except as wage earner; so, little change in parenting. Husband used to degrade her; now has a more positive self-image. Shows pride in what she's accomplished on own. Feels confident, wants to go back to college. Main complaint - feels drained by total responsibility & no personal time. Has little interest in re-marriage.

1a 5-8, 12-20	3a 10, 22-23	4c 60-63	6a 41, 44-48	7c 48-50
b 1-5, 9, 32	b 25-27	d 38-39	b 10-11, 42	d 48-50
c 16-21, 45-48	c 52, 58-59	5a 35-40	c 46, 48, 60	8a 26, 30-31
2a 7, 18	4a 30-31, 40, 55	b 20-24	d 6-7, 14-15	b 8, 26
b 30-32, 39	b 32, 56-57	c 30, 32-34	7a 9, 30-34	c 36
c 25-27, 49-51			b 9, 26, 48	9 9-11, 32-33

Figure 23-2. *Example of interview abstract with code and page summary.*

researcher is at the point of analysis, it is easier to go directly to the topical files than to start searching through the data with the index cards as a guide. In some cases, it might be worthwhile to combine these two approaches.

These traditional methods of organizing the data have a long and respected history, but they are becoming increasingly outmoded as a result of the widespread availability of personal computers (PCs) that can be used to perform the "filing" and indexing of qualitative material. Some systems involve numbering all paragraphs of the researcher's field notes or interviews, coding each paragraph for topical codes, and then entering the information into computer files. This is essentially an automated version of the manual indexing/retrieval systems described previously. However, increasingly sophisticated computer programs are being developed that permit the entire data file to be entered onto the computer, each portion of an interview or observation record coded and categorized, and then portions of the text corresponding to specified codes retrieved and printed (or shown on a screen) for analysis. The most prominent computer programs for qualitative data are known as Ethnograph, Superfile, TEXTAN, and LISPQUAL. When a study generates more qualitative data than can be conveniently handled on a microcomputer, it may be necessary to use a mainframe program such as QUAL (Morse & Morse, 1989).

Such computer programs are tremendous tools that can greatly facilitate the encoding and retrieval of complex qualitative materials. However, the careful researcher must be wary of two potential pitfalls: (1) too much elaboration in the coding scheme, which can occur simply because retrieval becomes so easy; and (2) atomism and context stripping, which can interfere with a meaningful analysis of the data.

Analytic Procedures

Although different approaches to qualitative data analysis have been advocated, there are some elements that are generally common to most approaches. We provide the following general guidelines, together with a description of one researcher's steps in performing a qualitative study.

The analysis of qualitative materials generally begins with a search for themes or recurring regularities. In some cases, the thematic analysis occurs in the field as the data are being collected. In other situations, the thematic analysis occurs after the data have been collected, during a reading (or re-reading) of the data set. Themes often develop within categories of data (i.e., within categories of the coding scheme used for indexing materials), but sometimes cut across them. For example, a theme that emerged repeatedly in Polit's study of divorced women was that, initially, the women's emotional well-being was so adversely affected by the divorce that they were unable to make plans for more than one day at a time. However, with the passage of time, many of these women became considerably more goal-oriented than they had ever been in their lives, developing long-range plans for their educational, occupational, and financial futures. This theme was one that cut across the coding categories (shown in Fig. 23-1) of "Adjustment to divorce" (1.a), "Current psychologic state" (2.c), and "Educational and employment goals" (7.c and d).

The search for themes involves not only the discovery of commonalities across subjects, but also a search for natural variation in the data. Themes that emerge from unstructured observations and interviews are never universal. The researcher must attend not only to what themes arise but also to how they are patterned. Does the theme apply only to certain subgroups? In certain types of communities or organizations? In certain contexts? At certain periods? What are the conditions that precede the observed phenomenon, and what are the apparent consequences of it? In other words, the qualitative analyst must be sensitive to *relationships* within the data.

The analyst's search for themes, regularities, and patterns in the data can sometimes be facilitated by charting devices that enable the researcher to summarize the evolution of behaviors, events, and processes. For example, for qualitative studies that focus on dynamic experiences—such as decision making—it is often useful to develop flow charts or time lines that highlight time sequences, major decision points and events, and factors affecting the decisions. An example of such a flow chart from a study of decision making among infertile couples is presented in Figure 23-3. The construction of such flow charts for all subjects would help to highlight certain regularities in the subjects' evolving behaviors.

A further step frequently taken involves the validation of the understandings that the thematic exploration has provided. In this phase, the concern is whether the themes inferred are an accurate representation of the perspectives of the people interviewed or observed. Several procedures can be used in this validation step. If there is more than one researcher working on the study, debriefing sessions in which the themes are reviewed and specific cases discussed can be highly productive. Multiple perspectives—what we referred to in Chapter 18 as investigator triangulation—cannot ensure the validity of the themes, but it can minimize any idiosyncratic biases. Using an iterative approach is almost always necessary. That is, the researcher derives themes from the narrative materials, goes back to the materials with the themes in mind to see if the materials really do fit, and then refines the themes as necessary. In some cases, it might also be appropriate to present the preliminary thematic analysis to some of the subjects/informants, who can be encouraged to offer suggestions that might support or contradict this analysis.

It is at this point that some researchers introduce what is referred to as "quasi-statistics." *Quasi-statistics* involve a tabulation of the frequency with which certain themes, relations, or insights are supported by the data. The frequencies cannot be interpreted in the same way as frequencies generated in survey studies, because of imprecision in the sampling of cases and enumeration of the themes. Nevertheless, as Becker (1970) pointed out,

Quasi-statistics may allow the investigator to dispose of certain troublesome null hypotheses. A simple frequency count of the number of times a given phenomenon appears may make untenable the null hypothesis that the phenomenon is infrequent. A comparison of the number of such instances with the number of negative cases—instances in which some alternative phenomenon that would not be predicted by his theory appears—may make possible a stronger conclusion, especially if the theory was developed early enough in the observational period to allow a systematic search for negative cases. Similarly, an inspection of the range of situations covered by the investigator's data may allow him to negate the hypothesis that his conclusion is restricted to only a few situations, time periods, or types of people in the organization or community. (p. 81)

In the final stage of analysis, the researcher strives to weave the thematic pieces together into an integrated whole. The various themes need to be interrelated in a manner that provides an overall structure (theory or model) to the entire body of data. The integration task is an extremely difficult one, because it demands creativity and intellectual rigor if it is to be successful. A strategy that sometimes helps in this task is to cross-tabulate dimensions that have emerged in the thematic analysis. For example, in the study of the emotional well-being of divorced women, one theme that emerged was the strong goal-orientation of many of the women. Another theme related to the women's interest in the possibility of remarriage. When these two dimensions were cross-tabulated, as shown in Figure 23-4, they revealed different mechanisms of women's coping with divorce. A further analysis revealed that the different coping mechanisms were linked with different psychologic outcomes and differential needs for intervention.

Qualitative researchers seldom discuss in any detail the ways in which they analyze their data. However, one researcher, who studied unmarried, pregnant women, described the stages of her analytic work (Macintyre, 1977). In the study, Macintyre used a computerized system for indexing (but not for actually analyzing) her mas-

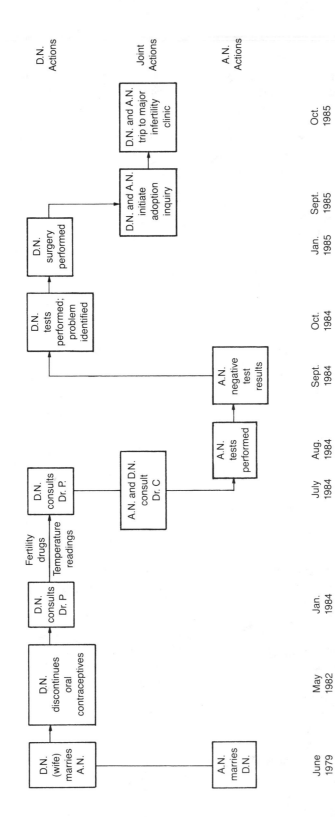

Figure 23-3. Example of a timeline for infertility study.

	Moderate to Strong Goal Orientation	Weak Goal Orientation
Actively seeks remarriage	Strong sense of self-efficacy and belief in own ability to control the future and build on past experiences; ability to cope tied in part to strong social suuport network; active in work and leisure pursuits.	Strong dependency needs; copes through "fantasies" of an ideal mate and home life; tends to use social supports as crutch; spends a lot of time worrying.
Open to marriage	Has made explicit efforts to forge a new life that sustains her self-esteem; would consider remarriage to mate willing to share in her personal growth; analytic, problem-solving approach to future decisions.	Focuses most of her energies on her children and derives major sense of self in mother role; would remarry primarily to benefit children; shows a sense of resignation.
Wary about/opposed to remarriage	Fiercely independent and determined not to revert to subservient wifely role; shown an almost martyr-like insistence on self-reliance and personal control.	Intensely bitter about divorce; uses denial and sustained self-righteousness as coping mechanisms, but has not yet adjusted to being divorced; engages in various compulsions (e.g., drinking); has isolationist tendencies.

Figure 23-4. *Example of a cross-tabulation of dimensions in a thematic analysis.*

sive narrative data. Her analysis involved seven different stages, which actually began before entering the field:

Stage 1. A list of research problems and concepts was prepared before entering the field. This stage continued as field work began. After the collection of some preliminary data, she developed the list of categories that could be used to index the data.

Stage 2. Coding occurred throughout the data collection period. Categories were constructed from statements and events so that comparisons could be made between the categories. New categories were added on the basis of new concepts emerging from the data.

Stage 3. After data collection and final coding of data, all of the data were re-read. Different types of materials (including interview transcripts, field notes, and documentary records) were brought together and linked in terms of conceptual themes and topics. From the various sources, the investigator prepared an account about each of her subjects.

Stage 4. This phase involved organizing for analysis. The investigator considered four organizational strategies: (1) use of detailed case studies; (2) comparison of what happened to the women at different points in time; (3) comparison of the accounts of the women themselves versus the professionals with whom they interacted; and (4) use of key concepts or themes that had emerged, such as "bargaining in encounters" and "moral character." (The compromise she reached was to organize by concept, but within a chronological order).

Stage 5. The indexing system she developed was used to locate data that were relevant for the major themes around which the analysis was organized.

Stage 6. The preliminary patterns and interrelationships were checked using quasi-statistical procedures. This approach was used to give credibility to major thematic categories, such as "moral career."

Stage 7. The relationships among the major topics were examined and incorporated into an overall model.

ANALYTIC INDUCTION

The general procedures and steps previously described provide a general outline of how qualitative researchers make sense of their data and distill from them their understandings of processes and behaviors operating in naturalistic settings. However, there are some variations in the goals and underlying philosophies of qualitative researchers that also lead to variations in how the analytic task is handled. One of the major strategies for analyzing qualitative data is referred to as *analytic induction,* an approach that was developed in the 1930s.

The analytic induction approach requires a careful scrutiny of all of the researcher's data, usually according to the following six steps:

1. Define the phenomenon to be studied and explained
2. Based on a review of the data, formulate a hypothetical explanation of the phenomenon, that is, develop an inductively derived hypothesis
3. Conduct an intensive analysis of individual cases to see whether the hypothesis fits particular cases
4. Search for negative cases that, if found, lead to a reformulation of the hypothesis *or* a redefinition of the phenomenon to exclude the particular case
5. Continue the examination of cases, redefinition of the phenomenon, and the reformulation of hypotheses until a universal pattern of relationships is established
6. Create a higher level of abstraction/conceptualization through comparison with other settings or groups

In practice, the use of analytic induction results in a procedure that alternates back and forth between tentative explanation and tentative

definition, each refining the other so that a sense of closure can be achieved when an integral relation between the two is established.

GROUNDED THEORY

A second major strategy is Glaser and Strauss's (1967) method of generating theories from data, using a procedure that they describe as the discovery of *grounded theory.* This approach is more than just a method of data analysis; it is an entire philosophy about how to conduct field research. For example, a study that truly follows Glaser and Strauss's precepts does not begin with a highly focused research problem; the problem itself emerges from the data.

One of the fundamental features of the grounded theory approach is that data collection and data analysis occur simultaneously. A procedure referred to as *constant comparison* is used to develop and refine theoretically relevant categories. The categories elicited from the data are constantly compared with data obtained earlier in the data collection so that commonalities and variations can be determined. As data collection proceeds, the inquiry becomes increasingly focused on emerging theoretical concerns.

In contrast to analytic induction, this approach requires "data saturation" rather than the consideration of all data. Glaser and Strauss identified the following four stages in the constant comparative method:

1. Establish categories based on similarity of content in incidents and dissimilarity of content with other categories, with the aim of elucidating the theoretical properties of each category.
2. Compare each incident within each category with the dimensions of the category for integration into a unified whole that reflects the relationships of the dimensions or properties of the category.
3. Examine categories and their properties for underlying uniformities that may reduce the number of categories. Look for theoretical saturation of content and add only new inci-

dents to categories when they explicate a new dimension.

4. Produce analytic memos to summarize the theoretical explanations; the memos provide the basis for the writing of publications and reports.

There are some obvious similarities between the grounded theory and analytic induction approach, but there are also some important differences. Of particular importance is their overall aims. Analytic induction is concerned with the testing of inductively derived hypotheses; it is purported to be a method for coming to terms with the problem of causal inference while remaining faithful to qualitative, naturalistic data. The grounded theory method is concerned with the generation of categories, properties, and hypotheses rather than testing them.

≡ CONTENT ANALYSIS

We are devoting a separate section of this chapter to *content analysis* because, although it is a method of handling narrative, qualitative material, it is a procedure that typically involves quantification. Although some researchers who do not quantify their data sometimes refer to their analytic work as a content analysis, the term in its classic sense refers to "a research technique for the objective, systematic, and quantitative description of the manifest content of communication" (Berelson, 1971, p. 18).

Content analysis is applied to people's written and oral communications. It can be used with such materials as diaries, letters, speeches, dialogues, reports, books, articles, and other linguistic expressions. The technique utilizes a number of controls designed to yield objective and systematic information. The researcher enhances objectivity by conducting the content analysis on the basis of explicitly formulated rules. The rules serve as guidelines to enable two or more people analyzing the same materials to obtain the same results. The analysis is rendered systematic by the inclusion or exclusion of materials according to consistently applied selection criteria.

Elements of Content Analysis

Holsti (1968) pointed out that communications comprise six basic elements: (1) a *source*—the sender; (2) an *encoding process* resulting in a message; (3) the *message;* (4) a transmitting *channel;* (5) a *detector*—the recipient of the message; and (6) a *decoding process.* The object of the analysis is the message, but content analysis can be used to answer questions concerning the remaining five elements. The questions one answers through content analysis are, Who said what? To whom? How? Why? With what effect? Table 23-1, adapted from Holsti (1968), links these questions to research problems and purposes.

The most common applications of content analysis have been directed toward the "what" question, that is, describing the characteristics of the content of the message. Several approaches can be used to analyze the attributes of a communication. These approaches share the feature of drawing some type of comparison. Usually a description is meaningless unless it is put into perspective through data comparisons. For instance, the fact that the dreams of ten patients' during hospitalization involved death and dying is in itself difficult to interpret. Holsti (1968) noted that the following types of comparisons are applicable to the "what" question: a comparison of messages from a single source over time, a comparison of messages from a single source in varying situations, a comparison of messages from a single source across audiences, a comparison of two or more concepts within a single message, and a comparison of messages from two or more different sources or types of sources.

Content Analysis Procedures

The methods used to analyze documents and communications overlap extensively with the procedures described earlier in this chapter, as well as with those used in observational studies. This is not too surprising in light of the fact that observational studies frequently deal with verbal behavior. Like the observational researcher, the investigator performing a content analysis must select the variables or concepts to be recorded and the *unit* of content that will be used. There are a variety of units for analyzing verbal expressions, not all of which will be of interest to nurse researchers. The smallest units, such as *letters* and *phonemes,* are unlikely to be useful to researchers in fields other than linguistics. Individual *words,* however, constitute an easy unit to work with and may be serviceable in a number of research applications. A *theme* is a more molar unit of analysis. A theme might be a phrase, sentence, or paragraph embodying ideas or making an assertion about some topic. Some examples of themes that might emerge in patients' accounts of a long-term illness experience include coping with pain, fear of death, loneliness, and loss of motivation for recovery. These are illustrations of themes organized around the content of a mes-

sage, but it is possible to detect stylistic themes such as different tones (proselytizing, admonishing, or informing); different grammatical structures; and so forth.

Another possible unit of analysis is the *item.* This unit refers to an entire message, document, or other production: a letter, editorial, diary entry, conference presentation, issue of a journal, and the like. The whole item can then be categorized in terms of one or more characteristics. For example, articles appearing in the journal *Nursing Research* can be classified according to whether the research problem was clinical in nature, and trends over time could then be analyzed. Finally, the unit may be a *space-and-time* measure. This type of unit consists of a physical measurement of content, such as the number of pages, number of words, number of speakers,

Table 23-1. *Content Analysis Questions, Problems, and Purposes*

QUESTIONS	RESEARCH PROBLEMS	PURPOSES
What?	To describe trends in communication content To relate attributes of the senders to the messages they produce To relate the message to the characteristics of situations	To describe characteristics of communication
How?	To analyze techniques of persuasion To analyze style	
To whom?	To relate the message to the characteristics of the recipients To describe patterns of communication	
Why?	To analyze psychologic traits of individuals To infer aspects of culture and cultural change	To make inferences as to the antecedents of communication (the encoding process)
Who?	To answer questions of disputed authorship To relate the message to the attributes of the sender	
With what effect?	To analyze the flow of information To assess responses to communication	To make inferences as to the effects of communication (the decoding process)

(Adapted from Table 1, Holsti, O.R. (1968). Content analysis. In G. Lindzey & E. Aronson (Eds.), *The handbook of social psychology,* (Vol. 2, 2nd ed., p. 604). Reading, MA: Addison-Wesley, with permission.)

amount of time spent in a discussion, and so forth. The units referred to here as "item" and "theme" are probably most useful for nurse researchers.

The next step in performing a content analysis is the development of a category system for classifying units of content. It is true that a category system is not always used by content analysis and may in some cases be unnecessary, but the use of such a system usually enhances the scientific validity of a content analysis study by making the operation more objective and systematic. A coding system enables the researcher to classify messages along relevant dimensions of content. For example, a nurse researcher may classify the descriptions of nursing programs issued in school catalogs in terms of the following variables: National League for Nursing accreditation, length of program, size of student body, student/teacher ratio, and state or private institution.

A variety of coding schemes are possible, even for a specific type of communication. The researcher may develop an original category system based on the idiosyncratic needs of the problem or theoretical framework. However, a criticism of content analyses is the absence of a generally useful and agreed-upon classification system for categorizing and comparing diverse materials. Because a number of systems have already been developed, the investigator might well use an existing scheme rather than generating a new one. Holsti's (1969, pp. 104–116) book provides many examples of category schemes and is a useful starting point for finding a system of classification. The careful training of coders assigned to do the job of categorization is essential to the success of content analysis studies.

Content analyses often apply a sampling plan in selecting materials to be analyzed. The sampling plan adopted depends on a number of considerations, the most salient being the extensiveness of the universe of content and the unit of analysis being used. If the unit of analysis is a word or theme, the researcher might use a systematic or random sampling procedure in which the *sampling unit* (not to be confused with the unit of analysis) might be pages or paragraphs in a document. That is, the investigator would select only some pages or paragraphs for examination, either on a systematic basis (e.g., every tenth page) or randomly with a table of random numbers.

The quantification of communication materials is normally linked with the category system. The most common form of quantifying materials is the enumeration of recorded occurrences in each category. A second approach is to simply create a binary index (yes–no) of whether the concepts covered in the coding scheme were present or absent in the materials. The ranking of materials according to prespecified criteria is a third possibility. Finally, rating scales can be used to assess various aspects of the communications.

Uses of Content Analysis

Content analysis can either be used alone or in conjunction with other data collection methods for a variety of applications in nursing research. Historical research, for example, deals almost exclusively with written documents and, therefore, is particularly amenable to content analysis. In psychiatric nursing, or for nurses working with handicapped people, linguistic productions can serve as a criterion for evaluating nursing interventions. Content analysis can be applied to pre-existing communications materials such as minutes of meetings, journal articles, and so forth or to messages produced specifically for a research project. For example, the nurses' notes in the records of patients with Alzheimer's disease could be examined for the dimensions of nursing care. The variable types that can be measured through content analysis include a broad range of social and psychologic concepts such as attitudes, emotional stability, motives, needs, expectations, stress, perceptions, values, creativity, and personality traits. This is not to say that content analysis is the *best* approach to measuring such variables. Content analysis suffers from several disadvantages such as the risk of subjectivity and the amount of tedious work involved. However, this technique may be expedient and efficient in its use of available materials, and there may be several research problems for which there are no data collection alternatives.

≡ RESEARCH EXAMPLES

The number of qualitative studies that have been published in nursing journals over the past decade has risen dramatically. Table 23-2 indicates some of the research problems that have been addressed through qualitative methods. Two additional examples are described in greater detail as follows.

Example Using Grounded Theory

Using the grounded theory approach, Forsyth and colleagues (1984) investigated the percep-

tions of hospitalized chronically ill patients concerning the effect of the illness on life style, needs during hospitalization, and attitudes toward health care. Data for the study were collected by interviewing patients and observing their interactions with nurses. The researchers tape-recorded both the interviews and observations and maintained a log of field notes. The tape recordings were fully transcribed for analysis. The initial interviews posed broad questions to the patients such as, "Can you tell me what this hospitalization has been like for you?" As conceptual categories of responses emerged from the interviews, additional questions were asked to help clarify the relationships among the properties of a category and among the categories themselves. For example, the researchers asked additional questions to clarify relationships between type of hospital setting and control of disease management.

Table 23-2. *Examples of Nursing Studies Involving Qualitative Analysis*

RESEARCH PROBLEM	NUMBER OF SUBJECTS	DATA SOURCE(S)
What is the meaning of inner strength as experienced in the personal lives of women? (Rose, 1990)	9	In-depth interviews
What are nurses' perceptions of the value of and the facilitators and inhibitors to nurse documentation in a hospital setting? (Tapp, 1990)	14	In-depth interviews
Among adolescents with cancer, what is their perception of how they helped themselves to achieve hopefulness? (Hinds & Martin, 1988)	58	In-depth interviews, observations
What are the experiences and needs of sleep apnea patients with tracheostomies? (Ashley, 1989)	12	In-depth interviews
What is the process of family caregiving for elderly family relatives with Alzheimer's dementia as experienced from the perspective of the caregiver? (Wilson, 1989)	20	In-depth interviews
What is it like to live the relentless drive to be ever thinner? (Santopinto, 1989)	2	Written narratives, in-depth interviews
What are the traditional health beliefs and practices of black women and how do these relate to their understanding of AIDs? (Flaskerud & Rush, 1989)	22	Focus group interviews
What is the process of adjustment experienced by individuals having a myocardial infarction? (Johnson & Morse, 1990)	14	In-depth interviews
What are the social and psychologic dimensions of childbearing among prisoners? (Shelton & Gill, 1989)	26	In-depth interviews, observations
What is the effect of a suicide death on family member survivors? (Van Dongen, 1990)	19	In-depth interviews

The researchers concurrently collected and analyzed the data from the interviews, observations, and field notes. They used the constant comparative method to determine the similarity of content in incidents before placing them into a category. The nature of the interviews changed as the study progressed in an effort to clarify relationships among dimensions of a category. Theoretical sampling was used to collect additional data.

Findings that emerged from the data indicated that the hospitalized, chronically ill patients developed strategies to cope with the illness and its unpredictability. The strategies permitted the patients to feel that they were "winning" in terms of controlling the progression of the disease. The specific strategies varied according to person and type of illness. When exacerbations of illness occurred, patients redesigned their strategies according to the lessened functional ability to maintain a positive self-image for their life style. Hospitalizations were viewed as a time for restabilization of their conditions in an effort to maintain a "winning position" over their illnesses. In terms of health-care professionals, the patients viewed physicians as a source of hope in symptom control. They viewed nurses as people who offered subtle support rather than as caregivers.

Example of Content Analysis

Swider and colleagues (1985) used content analysis to categorize the nursing actions that nursing students would take in resolving ethical dilemmas. The sample of 755 senior nursing students from 16 schools was divided into 146 groups. Each group was asked to list the nursing actions it would recommend taking in relation to a hypothetical ethical dilemma that could occur in nursing practice. The groups were instructed to assume that each nursing action they listed was unsuccessful in solving the problem and asked to continue listing actions until all reasonable decisions had been exhausted.

Based on a literature review, the researchers developed a coding scheme for categorizing the content of the proposed nursing actions. The three primary categories that evolved from the literature were (1) patient-centered, (2) physician-centered, and (3) bureaucratic-centered decisions.

Findings from the study indicated that 12% of the responses could not be classified into any of the three categories and were placed into a fourth category labeled "other." The groups made a total of 1163 nursing decisions. The number of decisions for each category were patient-centered, 9%; physician-centered, 19%; and bureaucratic-centered, 60%. The majority of first nursing actions were bureaucratically oriented. The last nursing decisions suggested by the nursing students spanned all four categories.

In the research study, the categories evolved from the literature and the researchers were able to classify successfully all but 12% of the responses. In addition to sorting the responses according to content, the researchers numerically quantified the number of responses for each category. The article failed to indicate whether more than one person independently sorted the responses into categories according to content.

≡ *SUMMARY*

Qualitative research typically involves the collection and analysis of loosely structured information regarding people in naturalistic settings. Qualitative nursing research has become an increasingly attractive method of inquiry, complementing more quantitative approaches in advancing nursing science.

Qualitative approaches are generally more holistic than quantitative approaches, and try to capture the totality of some aspect of human experience. Qualitative research is especially well suited to the following research purposes: description, hypothesis generation, and theory development. However, qualitative approaches are less suitable for establishing cause-and-effect relationships, for rigorously testing research hypotheses, and for determining the opinions, practices, and attitudes of a large population. Qualitative methods tend to yield in-depth insights into some phenomenon because data collection tends to be intensive. However, qualitative methods have been criticized because of the difficulty of analyzing in an objective and replicable fashion masses of narrative materials. Additional shortcomings of qualitative research are that it is extremely time consuming, usually restricted to relatively small samples, and difficult to adequately summarize in professional journals.

Although qualitative materials *can* be quantified and subsequently analyzed with statistical procedures, most qualitative researchers prefer to analyze their data through qualitative analysis. The first major step in analyzing qualitative data is to organize the materials according to some plan. One method of organization involves the development of an elaborate file system. In using this system, researchers generally develop a conceptual coding scheme and code all of the narrative materials (e.g., observational notes or transcripts of interviews); then a file is created for each of the topics covered in the coding scheme, so that the researcher can retrieve all of the information on one topic by going to a single file. The widespread availability of personal computers and appropriate software has lessened the burden of indexing, organizing, and retrieving qualitative materials.

The actual analysis of data begins with a search for *themes*. The search for themes involves not only the discovery of commonalities across subjects, but also of natural variation in the data. The next step generally involves a validation of the thematic analysis. Some researchers use a procedure known as *quasi-statistics,* which involves a tabulation of the frequency with which certain themes or relations are supported by the data. In a final step, the analyst tries to weave the thematic strands together into an integrated picture of the phenomenon under investigation.

Although this overview summarizes some of the major steps, there are a number of different philosophies underlying qualitative analysis. *Analytic induction* refers to an approach in which the researcher alternates back and forth between tentative definition of emerging hypotheses and tentative explanation, with each iteration making refinements. *Grounded theory* is a term used to describe field investigations, the purpose of which is to discover theoretical precepts grounded in the data. This approach makes use of a technique called *constant comparison*: Categories elicited from the data are constantly compared with data obtained earlier so that commonalities and variations can be determined. Both of these approaches have their intellectual roots in sociological inquiry.

Content analysis is a method for quantifying the content of narrative communications in a systematic and objective fashion. Communications include newspaper articles, diaries, speeches, and other verbal expressions. It is systematic in that data are methodically included or excluded according to predetermined criteria. Content analysis is most commonly used to describe the content of the message, although it may be used to answer questions concerning other elements of communication. A variety of units of analysis exist for verbal expressions. The most useful unit for nurse researchers are *themes,* which embody ideas or concepts, and *items,* which refer to the entire message. Once the researcher has chosen the unit of analysis, a classification system must be developed to permit the categorization of messages according to content. Coded data can then be analyzed using statistical or qualitative procedures.

≡ STUDY SUGGESTIONS

1. Suggest a research problem amenable to qualitative research. Explain why you think the problem is better suited to a qualitative than to a quantitative approach.

2. Read a qualitative nursing study (several are suggested in "Substantive References"). Do you think that if a different investigator had gone into the field to study the same problem, the conclusions would have been the same? How generalizable are the researcher's findings? What did the researcher learn that he or she would probably not have learned with a more structured and quantified approach?

3. As a class assignment, have each student ask

two people to describe their conception of preventive health care and what it means in their daily lives. Pool all of the narrative descriptions and develop a coding scheme to organize the reasons. What are the major themes that emerge?

4. What units of analysis would be appropriate for performing a content analysis of the following materials: letters from nurses stationed in Europe during World War II, the diary of an adolescent dying from leukemia, the minutes of meetings from a state nurses' association, and the articles appearing in the *American Journal of Nursing?*

≡ *SUGGESTED READINGS*

METHODOLOGICAL REFERENCES

Artinian, B.A. (1988). Qualitative modes of inquiry. *Western Journal of Nursing Research, 10,* 138–149.

Bargagliotti, L.A. (1983). The scientific method and phenomenology: Toward their peaceful coexistence in nursing. *Western Journal of Nursing Research, 5,* 409–411.

Becker, H.S. (1970). *Sociological work.* Chicago: Aldine.

Benoliel, J.Q. (1984). Advancing nursing science: Qualitative approaches. *Western Journal of Nursing Research, 6,* 1–8.

Berelson, B. (1971). *Content analysis in communication research.* New York: Free Press.

Chenitz, W.C., & Swanson, J.M. (1986). *From practice to grounded theory: Qualitative research in nursing.* Menlo Park, CA: Addison-Wesley.

Downs, F.S. (1983). One dark and stormy night. *Nursing Research, 32,* 259.

Evaneshko, V., & Kay, M.A. (1982). The ethnoscience research technique. *Western Journal of Nursing Research, 4,* 51–64.

Fielding, N.G., & Fielding, J.L. (1985). *Linking data.* Beverly Hills, CA: Sage.

Gephart, R.P., Jr. (1988). *Ethnostatistics: Qualitative foundations for quantitative research.* Newbury Park, CA: Sage.

Glaser, B.G., & Strauss, A.L. (1967). *The discovery of grounded theory: Strategies for qualitative research.* Chicago: Aldine.

Goodwin, L.D., & Goodwin, W.L. (1984). Qualitative vs. quantitative research or qualitative *and* quantitative research. *Nursing Research, 33,* 378–380.

Gorenberg, B. (1983). The research tradition of nursing: An emerging issue. *Nursing Research, 32,* 347–349.

Holsti, O.R. (1968). Content analysis. In G. Lindzey & E. Aronson (Eds.), *The handbook of social psychology* (Vol. 2, 2nd ed., pp. 596–692). Reading, MA: Addison-Wesley.

Holsti, O.R. (1969). *Content analysis for the social sciences and humanities.* Reading, MA: Addison-Wesley.

Klenow, D.J. (1981). Qualitative methodology: A neglected resource in nursing research. *Research in Nursing and Health, 4,* 281–292.

Knafl, K.A. (1988). Managing and analyzing qualitative data. *Western Journal of Nursing Research, 10,* 195–218.

Krippendorff, K. (1980). *Content analysis: An introduction to its methodology.* Beverly Hills, CA: Sage.

Leininger, M.M. (Ed.). (1985). *Qualitative research methods in nursing.* New York: Grune & Stratton.

McCain, G.C. (1988). Content analysis: A method for studying clinical nursing problems. *Applied Nursing Research, 1,* 146–147.

Miles, M.B., & Huberman, A.M. (1984). *Qualitative data analysis.* Beverly Hills, CA: Sage.

Morse, J.M., & Morse, R.M. (1989). QUAL: A mainframe program for qualitative data analysis. *Nursing Research, 38,* 188–189.

Munhall, P.L. (1982). Nursing philosophy and nursing research: In apposition or opposition? *Nursing Research, 31,* 176–177.

Oiler, C. (1982). The phenomenological approach in nursing research. *Nursing Research, 31,* 178–181.

Parse, R.R., Coyne, A.B., & Smith, M.J. (1985). *Nursing research: qualitative methods.* Bowie, MD: Brady.

Pfaffenberger, B. (1988). *Microcomputer applications in qualitative research.* Newbury Park, CA: Sage.

Simms, L.M. (1981). The grounded theory approach in nursing research. *Nursing Research, 30,* 356–359.

Stern, P.M. (1985). Using grounded theory method in nursing research. In M.M. Leininger (Ed.), *Qualitative research methods in nursing.* New York: Grune & Stratton.

Webster, G., Jacox, A., & Baldwin, B. (1981). Nursing theory and the ghost of the received view. In H. Grace & B. McCloskey (Eds.), *Contemporary issues in nursing.* Boston: Blackwell Scientific Publications.

SUBSTANTIVE REFERENCES

Ashley, M.J. (1989). Concerns of sleep apnea patients with tracheostomies. *Western Journal of Nursing Research, 11,* 600–608.

DeVellis, B.M., Adams, J.L., & DeVellis, R.F. (1984). Effects of information on patient stereotyping. *Research in Nursing and Health, 7,* 237–244.

DeVito, A. (1990). Dyspnea during hospitalizations for acute phase of illness as recalled by patients with chronic obstructive pulmonary disease. *Heart and Lung, 19,* 186–191.

Flaskerud, J.H., & Rush, C.E. (1989). AIDS and traditional health beliefs and practices of black women. *Nursing Research, 38,* 210–215.

Forsyth, G.L., Delaney, K.D., & Gresham, M.L. (1984). Vying for a winning position: Management style of the chronically ill. *Research in Nursing and Health, 7,* 181–188.

Hinds, P.S., & Martin, J. (1988). Hopefulness and the self-sustaining process in adolescents with cancer. *Nursing Research, 38,* 336–339.

Johnson, J.L., & Morse, J.M. (1990). Regaining control: The process of adjustment after myocardial infarction. *Heart and Lung, 19,* 126–135.

Jordan, P.L. (1990). Laboring for relevance: Expectant and new fatherhood. *Nursing Research, 39,* 11–16.

Knafl, K.A. (1985). How families manage a pediatric hospitalization. *Western Journal of Nursing Research, 7,* 151–176.

Macintyre, S. (1977). *Single and pregnant.* London: Croom Helm.

Miller, Sr. P., McMahon, M., Garrett, M.J., & Ringel, K. (1989). A content analysis of life adjustments post infarction. *Western Journal of Nursing Research, 11,* 559–567.

Nusbaum, J.G., & Chenitz, W.C. (1990). A grounded theory study of the informed consent process for pharmacologic research. *Western Journal of Nursing Research, 12,* 215–228.

Patterson, E.T., & Hale, E.S. (1985). Making sure: Integrating menstrual care practices into activities of daily living. *Advances in Nursing Science, 7,* 18–31.

Ritchie, J.A., Caty, S., & Ellerton, M.L. (1984). Concerns of acutely ill, chronically ill, and healthy preschool children. *Research in Nursing and Health, 7,* 265–274.

Rose, J.F. (1990). Psychologic health of women: A phenomenologic study of women's inner strength. *Advances in Nursing Science, 12,* 56–70.

Santopinto, M.D.A. (1989). The relentless drive to be ever thinner. *Nursing Science Quarterly, 2,* 29–36.

Schuster, E.A., Kruger, S.F., & Hebenstreit, J.J. (1985). A theory of protection: Parents as sex educators. *Advances in Nursing Science, 7,* 70–77.

Shelton, B.J., & Gill, D. (1989). Childbearing in prison: A behavioral analysis. *Journal of Obstetric, Gynecologic, and Neonatal Nursing, 18,* 301–307.

Swider, S.M., McElmurry, B.J., & Yarling, R.R. (1985). Ethical decision making in a bureaucratic context by senior nursing students. *Nursing Research, 34,* 108–112.

Tapp, R.A. (1990). Inhibitors and facilitators to documentation of nursing practice. *Western Journal of Nursing Research, 12,* 229–240.

Van Dongen, C.J. (1990). Agonizing questioning: Experiences of survivors of suicide victims. *Nursing Research, 39,* 224–229.

Walker, C.L. (1988). Stress and coping in siblings of childhood cancer patients. *Nursing Research, 37,* 208–212.

Wilson, H.S. (1989). Family caregiving for a relative with Alzheimer's dementia: Coping with negative choices. *Nursing Research, 38,* 94–98.

24
Integration of Qualitative and Quantitative Analysis

Until recently, nursing research was dominated by quantitatively oriented studies. However, consistent with the overall expansion of nursing research inquiry, qualitative studies gained considerable ground during the 1980s. An emerging trend, and one that we believe will gain momentum in the years to come, is the integration of qualitative and quantitative data within single studies or coordinated clusters of studies. This chapter discusses the reasons for such integration and strategies for accomplishing it.

≡ *RATIONALE FOR INTEGRATION*

The dichotomy between quantitative and qualitative data analysis represents the key epistemological and methodological distinction within the social and behavioral sciences. Some argue, and are likely to continue to argue, that qualitative and quantitative research are based on fundamentally incompatible paradigms. Thus, there undoubtedly are people who will disagree with the fundamental premise of this chapter, namely that many areas of inquiry can be enriched through the judicious blending of qualitative and quantitative data. It would be imprudent to argue that all (or even most) research problems could be enhanced by such integration or that all (or most) researchers should strive to collect and integrate both types of data. However, we believe that there are many noteworthy advantages of combining various types of data in a single investigation, and that these advantages will come to be increasingly recognized by nurse researchers in the years ahead. Some of the major advantages are reviewed in the following sections.

Complementarity

One argument in support of blending qualitative and quantitative data in a single project is that they are complementary; they represent words and numbers, the two fundamental languages of human communication. Webster's* defines *complementary* as "mutually supplying each other's lack," and this characterizes the two methodological strategies rather well. As we have noted repeatedly in this text, researchers address their problems with methods and measures that are invariably fallible. By integrating different methods and modes of analysis, the weaknesses of a single approach may be diminished or overcome.

Quantitative data derived from relatively large or representative samples have many strengths. Quantitative studies are often strong in terms of generalizability, precision, control over extraneous variables, and reliability of measurement. However, a major problem with quantitative research is that its validity is sometimes called into question. By introducing tight controls, quantitative studies may fail to capture the full context of a situation. Moreover, by reducing complex human experiences, behavior, and characteristics to numbers, such analyses sometimes suffer from superficiality. Another issue is that the use of tightly structured questions or observational instruments may lead to biases in capturing constructs under study. All of these weaknesses are aspects of the study's ability to yield valid and meaningful answers to the research questions.

Qualitative research, by contrast, has strengths and weaknesses that are diametrically opposite. The strength of qualitative research lies in its flexibility and its potential to yield insights into the true nature of complex phenomena through a wealth of in-depth information. However, such insights are not gratuitous. Because qualitative research is almost always based on small and unrepresentative samples and is often engaged in by a solitary researcher or small team of researchers using data collection and analytic

procedures that rely on subjective judgments, qualitative research may suffer in terms of reliability and generalizability.

This discussion suggests that *neither of the two styles of research can fully deliver on its promise to establish the "truth" about phenomena of interest to nurse researchers.* However, the strengths and weaknesses of quantitative and qualitative data are complementary. Haase and Myers (1988) also noted the complementarity of the assumptions underlying the two approaches. Combined judiciously in a single study, qualitative and quantitative data can "supply each other's lack." By using multiple methods, the researcher can allow each method to do what it does best, with the possibility of avoiding the limitations of a single approach. In essence, this argument in favor of integration represents an extension of the argument for methodological triangulation discussed in Chapter 18.

Enhanced Theoretical Insights

Most theories do not have paradigmatic or methodological boundaries. As discussed in Chapter 7, the major nursing theories embrace four broad concepts: (1) person, (2) environment, (3) health, and (4) nursing. There is nothing inherent in these concepts that demands (or excludes) a qualitative or quantitative orientation.

The world in which we live is complex and multidimensional, as are most of the theories we have developed to make sense of it. Qualitative and quantitative research constitute alternative ways of viewing and interpreting the world. These alternatives are not necessarily correct or incorrect; rather, they reflect and reveal different aspects of reality. To be maximally useful, nursing research should strive to understand these multiple aspects. We believe that the blending of quantitative and qualitative data in a single analysis can lead to insights on these multiple aspects that might be unattainable without such integration. Denzin (1989), who has been a staunch advocate of methodological triangulation, captured this notion eloquently:

*By permission. From Webster's Ninth New Collegiate Dictionary © 1985 by G. & C. Merriam Company, publishers of the Merriam-Webster ® Dictionaries.

Each method implies a different line of action toward reality—and hence each will reveal different aspects of it, much as a kaleidoscope, depending on the angle at which it is held, will reveal different colors and configurations of objects to the viewer. Methods are like the kaleidoscope: depending on how they are approached, held, and acted toward, different observations will be revealed. This is not to imply that reality has the shifting qualities of the colored prism, but that it too is an object that moves and that will not permit one interpretation to be stamped upon it. (p. 235)

Incrementality

It is sometimes argued that different approaches are especially appropriate for different phases in the evolution of a theory or problem area. In particular, it has been said that qualitative methods are well-suited to exploratory or hypothesis-generating research early in the development of a research problem area, and quantitative methods are needed as the problem area matures for the purposes of verification.

It is certainly true that in-depth qualitative research can be highly productive in revealing theoretically relevant aspects of a phenomenon and suggesting lines for further inquiry. It is also true that statistical analysis provides a useful framework for the testing of hypotheses. However, the fact remains that the evolution of a theory or problem area is rarely linear and unidirectional. The need for exploration and in-depth insights is rarely confined to the beginning of an area research inquiry, and subjective impressions may need to be checked for accuracy early and continuously.

Thus, progress in a developing area tends to be incremental, and to rely on multiple feedback loops. It therefore could be productive to build a loop into the design of a single study, thereby potentially speeding the progress toward understanding. This point is illustrated by inquiry in the area of work-related stress and coping. Bargagliotti and Trygstad (1987) described two separate studies of job stress among nurses, one using quantitative procedures and the other using qual-

itative procedures. The quantitative study identified discrete events as sources of stress, and the qualitative study revealed stress-related processes over time. The discrepant findings, because they were derived from different samples of nurses working in different settings, could not be easily integrated and reconciled. The investigators noted, "Comparison of findings from the two studies suggests that the questions raised by the findings in each study might have been more fully addressed by using a combined quantitative/qualitative methodology" (p. 172).

Enhanced Validity

Another advantage of combining quantitative and qualitative data lies in the potential for enhancements to the validity of the study findings. When a researcher's hypothesis or model is supported by multiple and complementary types of data, the researcher can be much more confident about the validity of the results. Scientists are basically skeptics, constantly seeking evidence to validate their theories and models. Evidence derived from different approaches can be especially persuasive. As Brewer and Hunter (1989) noted, "Although each type of method is relatively stronger than the others in certain respects, none of the methods is so perfect even in its area of greatest strength that it cannot benefit from corroboration by other methods' findings" (p. 51).

In Chapters 12 and 18, we discussed various types of validity problems—such problems as rival hypotheses to explain the data, difficulties of generalizing beyond the study circumstances, and measures that fail to really capture the constructs under investigation. The use of a single approach leaves the study vulnerable to at least one (and often more) of these problems. The integration of qualitative and quantitative data can provide better opportunities for testing alternative interpretations of the data, for examining the extent to which the context helped to shape the results, and for arriving at convergence in tapping a construct. For example, Hinds (1989), in her study of adolescents' change in hopefulness as they progressed through a program for substance abuse, used qualitative findings as a means of validating her quantitative findings. As Hinds noted, "Using both methods together results in an increased ability to rule out rival explanations of observed change and reduces skepticism of change-related findings" (p. 442).

Creating New Frontiers

Inevitably, researchers will sometimes find that qualitative and quantitative data are inconsistent with each other. This lack of congruity—when it happens in the context of a single investigation—can actually lead to insights that can push a line of inquiry farther than would otherwise have been possible.

When separate investigations yield inconsistent results, the differences are difficult to reconcile and interpret, because they may reflect differences in subjects and circumstances, rather than theoretically meaningful distinctions that merit further study. In a single study, any discrepancies that emerge can be tackled "head on." By probing into the reasons for any observed incongruities, the researchers can help to rethink the constructs under investigation and possibly to redirect the research process. The incongruent findings, in other words, can be used as a springboard for the investigation of the reasons for the discrepancies and for a thoughtful analysis of both the methodological and theoretical underpinnings of the study.

☰ APPLICATIONS OF INTEGRATED ANALYSES

Researchers make decisions about the types of data to collect and analyze based on the specific objectives of their investigation. In this section, we illustrate how the integration of qualitative and quantitative data can be used in addressing a variety of research goals.

Instrumentation

One of the most frequent uses of an integrated approach in nursing research involves the development of instruments. When a researcher becomes aware of the need for a new measuring tool, where do the items come from? The item pool is sometimes generated by the researcher based on theory, his or her clinical experience, readings in the field, or prior research. However, when a construct is new, these mechanisms may be inadequate to capture the full complexity and dimensionality of the construct. No matter how rich the researcher's experience or knowledge base, the fact remains that this base is highly personal and inevitably biased by the researcher's values and world view.

In recognition of this situation, many nurse researchers have begun to use data obtained from qualitative inquiries as the basis for generating items for quantitative instruments that are subsequently subjected to rigorous psychometric assessment. For example, Stokes and Gordon (1988), in developing the Stokes/Gordon Stress Scale for the elderly, conducted in-depth interviews with a sample of people aged 65 or older. The first part of the interview consisted of open-ended questions that asked respondents to describe events and situations perceived as stressful since turning 65, and the second part of the interview probed more deeply into specific areas of stress. Interviewing continued until saturation was achieved, that is, until an analysis of the data revealed redundancy in the stressors mentioned. The responses yielded 102 distinctive stressors that formed the basis of the new scale. This approach essentially represents a mechanism for building content validity into the instrument from its inception.

Qualitative data have also been used as a means of assessing the validity of a quantitative instrument at later stages in the development process. For example, Burckhardt and her colleagues (1989) undertook a psychometric assessment of the Flanagan Quality of Life Scale (QOLS). Their study involved the administration of the QOLS and other quantitative scales, as well as several open-ended questions such as, "What does quality of life mean to you?" and "What kinds of things are important to your quality of life?" A thematic analysis of the responses to these questions provided support for most of the dimensions of QOLS, but also revealed that one theme that emerged quite strongly in the qualitative analysis (the theme of independence) was not represented by the QOLS items.

These examples illustrate the important role that the integration of qualitative and quantitative data can play in enhancing the measurement of constructs important to nurse researchers.

Illustration

Qualitative data are sometimes combined with quantitative data to illustrate the meaning of descriptions or relationships. Such illustrations help to clarify important concepts, and serve further as a method of corroborating the understandings gleaned from the statistical analysis. In this sense, these illustrations often help to illuminate the analyses and give guidance to the interpretation of results.

As an example, suppose a researcher were studying stress and coping behavior among recently divorced women. The quantitative data might indicate that 80% of the sample had experienced severe distress in the postseparation period, and that 30% had sought professional assistance for that stress. These facts are interesting and may suggest the need for some type of early intervention, but the following excerpt illustrating a report of stress (from Polit's study of divorce) adds a perspective that the numbers alone could not provide:

> I've had a lot of emotional problems since my husband left. I can't foresee the future, and I don't want to because I don't think I could keep my sanity if I knew what was ahead. Sometimes when I wake up in the morning I just lie there staring at the ceiling, thinking about everything I've been through; and I'll think, "What am I here for? What's the use of going on? Will anything in my life ever go right for me?"

Qualitative materials can be used to illustrate specific statistical findings, or can also be used to provide more global and dynamic views of the phenomena under study, often in the form of illustrative case studies. For example, Polit and her colleagues (1987), in their study of the sexual and contraceptive behavior of teenagers who had been abused as children, used quantitative data to statistically model the risk of a premarital pregnancy in this high-risk sample. In addition, their report included several case studies illustrating the emotional and social problems these teenagers faced, and the evolution and resolution of these problems over time. The case studies were based on interviews with the teenagers, their parents or foster parents, and their social workers, as well as on information available in their case records.

Understanding Relationships and Causal Processes

Quantitative methods often demonstrate that variables are systematically related to one another, but they often fail to provide insights about *why* the variables are related. This situation is especially likely to occur with *ex post facto* research.

Typically, the discussion section of research reports is devoted to an interpretation of the findings. In quantitatively oriented studies, the interpretations are often speculative, representing the researcher's best guess (a guess that may, of course, be built on solid theory or prior research) about what the findings mean. In essence, the interpretations represent a new set of hypotheses that could be tested in another study. When a study integrates both qualitative and quantitative data, however, the researcher may be in a much stronger position to derive meaning immediately from the statistical findings. Suppose, for example, that we found that single men and women had significantly poorer health (based on a variety of quantitative indices) than married people. What is the meaning of this relationship? Are single people less healthy because they lack an important source of social support? Or are single people less financially able to obtain adequate health care? Or are single people less healthy to begin with, and do their health problems make them less "marriageable"? Qualitative methods might yield some understanding about the mechanisms underlying this relationship.

A study by Dennis (1987) provides a good illustration of this application of blended data collection methods. The purpose of her study was to identify activities that give patients a sense of control during their hospitalization. The data were collected by means of a psychosocial self-report scale (the Health Opinion Survey), a 45-item Q sort, and an open-ended post–Q-sort interview. The items for the Q sort (which themselves were based, in part, on open-ended interviews with patients and nurses), were designed to determine the relative importance patients attached to controlling hospital events. A factor analysis of the Q-sort items revealed that a major dimension involved what Dennis labeled "decisional control," i.e., the desire to be involved actively in decision making relating to these events. The qualitative analyses indicated that patients low on this factor tended to be people who thought that those decisions were the physician's prerogative, and that they would only complicate or impede the process if they participated in it.

Quantitative analyses can also help to clarify and give shape to findings obtained in qualitative analyses. For example, a thematic analysis of interviews with infertile couples could reveal various aspects of the emotional consequences of infertility and shed light on the meaning of those consequences to individuals; the administration of a standardized scale (such as the CES-D Depression Scale) to the same subjects could indicate more precisely the distribution of depressive symptoms and their magnitude among the infertile couples. A study by Duffy (1986) illustrates this approach. Her basically qualitative study of primary prevention behaviors in single mothers involved the use of health diaries and in-depth interviews. The investigators supplemented the qualitative data by asking respondents to complete a card sort of primary prevention behaviors and barriers to their practice, which yielded a profile of the frequency of certain behaviors, and provided a context for interpreting the qualitative data.

The integration of qualitative and quantitative materials for the purpose of enhancing the interpretability of study results is essentially a mechanism of substantive validation. In some studies, it may be useful to use multiple data sources as a methodological check. For example, if a researcher is concerned with biases that could result from attrition in a longitudinal survey, it might be profitable to undertake a small number of in-depth interviews with nonrespondents (if feasible) to evaluate the direction and magnitude of such biases.

Theory Building, Testing, and Refinement

The most ambitious application of an integrated approach is in the area of theory development. As we have pointed out repeatedly, a theory is never proven nor confirmed, but rather is supported to a greater or lesser extent. A theory gains acceptance as it escapes disconfirmation. The use of multiple methods provides greater opportunity for potential disconfirmation of the theory. If the theory can survive these assaults, then it can provide a substantially stronger context for the organization of our clinical and intellectual work. Brewer and Hunter (1989), in their discussion of the role of multimethod research in theory development, made the following observation:

> Theory building and theory testing clearly require variety. In building theories, the more varied the empirical generalizations to be explained, the easier it will be to discriminate between the many possible theories that might explain any one of the generalizations. And in testing theories, the more varied the predictions, the more sharply the ensuing research will discriminate among competing theories. (p. 36)

≡ STRATEGIES FOR INTEGRATION

The ways in which a researcher might chose to integrate qualitative and quantitative methods in a single study are almost limitless—or rather, are limited only by the ingenuity of the investigator. Therefore, it is impossible to develop a catalog of integration strategies. However, some of the following scenarios are apt to be especially common.

Embedding Qualitative Approaches Within a Survey

By far the most common form of data collection method currently used by nurse researchers is structured self-reports, either in the form of a structured interview/questionnaire or the administration of social–psychologic scales. Once the researcher has gained the cooperation of the sample for the structured portion of a study, he or she is in an ideal position to move into a second in-depth stage with a subset of the initial respondents. The second stage might involve such approaches as in-depth or focus-group interviews, unstructured observations in a naturalistic environment such as a hospital or nursing home, or the use of health diaries.

From a practical point of view, it would be efficient to have the two forms of data collection occurring simultaneously. For example, the researcher could administer social–psychologic scales and an in-depth interview on the same day for a subset of the entire sample. In some studies, this procedure is likely to work quite well. However, a two-stage approach has two distinct advantages. First, if the second stage data collection can be postponed until after the quantitative data have been collected and analyzed, then the researcher will have greater opportunity to probe deeply into the reasons for any obtained results. This is especially likely to be beneficial if the quantitative analyses did not confirm the researcher's hypotheses or if there were any inconsistencies in the results. The second-stage respondents, in other words, can be used as informants to help the researcher interpret the outcomes.

A second reason for using a two-stage approach is that the researcher can use information from the first stage to select a useful sample for the second. One strategy might be to use a stratified design so that the subset participating in the second stage will be roughly comparable with that in the larger sample. Alternatively, the researcher might want to use information from the

first round to "hand-pick" respondents with certain characteristics—for example, respondents who are most knowledgeable about the phenomena under investigation, or ones who represent "typical" cases, or ones who are at opposite extremes with regard to the key constructs.

Shirley Murphy's longitudinal study of the consequences and processes relating to a natural disaster (the eruption of Mt. St. Helens in southwestern Washington state in 1980) provides an example of multimethod research in which qualitative interviews were embedded within a larger survey (Murphy, 1989). In the study, the bulk of the data were collected by way of structured self-report instruments administered to three groups of individuals: (1) a bereaved group (individuals who experienced the loss of a family member or close friend); (2) a property loss group (individuals who experienced serious damage or destruction to their homes); and (3) a matched "no disaster loss" group for comparison purposes. Complex multivariate analyses of the quantitative data were undertaken to test alternative theories regarding disaster-related effects. In addition, in-depth interviews were conducted with stratified subsets of the study group participants to obtain richer information regarding disaster-induced stress, coping strategies, and processes of recovery.

Embedding Quantitative Measures Into Field Work

Field research, more than other types of research, has a long history of using multiple methods of data collection. Generally, the methods used in field studies are ones that yield data amenable to qualitative analysis, such as field notes from participant observation, unstructured interviews, and narrative documents such as diaries and letters. However, field researchers can in some cases profit from the collection of more structured information from a larger or more representative sample than is possible in collecting the qualitative data. The secondary data might be in the form of structured self-reports by way of a survey, or formal quantifiable records. For example, if the researcher's field work focused on family violence, police and hospital records could be used to gather systematic data amenable to statistical analysis.

As field work progresses, researchers typically gain considerable insight into the communities, organizations, or social groups under study. With this knowledge, the researcher can generate hypotheses that can be subjected to more systematic scrutiny through structured data collection methods. Alternatively, the quantitative portion of the study could be used to gather descriptive information about the characteristics of the community or group, so that the qualitative findings could be understood in a broader context. In either case, having already gained entree into the community and the trust and cooperation of its members, the field researcher may be in an ideal position to pursue a survey or a record-extraction activity.

A study by Browner (1987) provides an example of a field study that included the use of quantitative measures. Browner's qualitative study focused on the relationship between work stress, social support, and health in ancillary nursing staff employed in a state psychiatric institution. The hypothesis was that staff who were integrated into supportive work-based social networks would be in better health than those who were not. Although the bulk of data were collected through participant observation, quantitative information on health was obtained through the use of the 195-item Cornell Medical Index.

Qualitative and Quantitative Data in Experimental Research

Because experimental research involves highly controlled designs and the testing of causal hypotheses, it is easy to get the impression that only quantitative data are appropriate. However, qualitative data can greatly enrich studies that use an experimental or quasi-experimental design. Through in-depth, unstructured approaches, the researcher can better understand qualitative differences between groups, including differences in the reactions of subjects to the experimental conditions, and experiences and processes underlying experimental effects.

The use of qualitative data collection methods may be especially useful when the researcher is evaluating complex interventions. When an experimental treatment is simple and straightforward—for example, a new drug—it might be relatively easy to interpret the results. Any posttreatment group differences (assuming that sufficient controls have been instituted) can be attributed to the intervention. However, many nursing interventions are not so straightforward. They may involve new ways of interacting with patients or new approaches to organizing the delivery of care. Sometimes the intervention is multidimensional, involving several different components. At the end of the experiment, even when hypothesized results are obtained, people may ask, What *is* it that really caused the group differences? (If there were no group differences, then the important question would be, *Why* was the intervention unsuccessful?) In-depth qualitative interviews with subjects could help to address these questions. In other words, qualitative data may help researchers to address the "*black box*" question—understanding what it is about the complex intervention that is driving any observed effects. This knowledge can be helpful for theoretical purposes, and can also help to streamline an intervention and make it more efficient and cost-effective.

Another reason for gathering qualitative data in evaluations of complex interventions is that there is often a need to understand exactly what the intervention was like in practice and how people reacted to it. Unstructured observations and interviews with people with different perspectives (e.g., nurses, physicians, hospital administrators, patients, or patients' family members) are especially well-suited for such process evaluations.

A study by one of the authors (Polit et al., 1988) provides an example of using both qualitative and quantitative data collection/analysis in a quasi-experimental study. The study was a multifaceted evaluation of a comprehensive program for poor teenage mothers, implemented in several sites nationwide. The intervention, known as Project Redirection, included educational, health, parenting, and social services for participating young mothers and their children. Data were collected over a 5-year period, and included structured interviews with young mothers in the experimental and comparison groups, the administration of several social–psychologic tests to the mothers and their young children, and structured observations of the home environment. The evaluation also involved in-depth ethnographic interviews with the mothers and significant others (e.g., boyfriends or relatives) and unstructured observations of program operations.

☰ *OBSTACLES TO INTEGRATION*

Throughout this chapter, we have stressed the advantages of blending qualitative and quantitative data in a single investigation. We believe that the potential for advancing nursing science through such integration is great, and is as yet relatively untapped. We also believe that integration efforts such as those proposed are inevitable because, at the level of the problem, almost all research questions are inherently multimethod.

Nevertheless, we recognize that there are various obstacles that may constrain the gathering of qualitative and quantitative data in a single investigation. Among the most salient are the following:

- *Epistemological biases.* Qualitative and quantitative researchers often operate with a different set of assumptions about the world and ways of learning about it. For those with a hard-line view, these assumptions may be seen as mutually and inevitably irreconcilable. According to a survey of nurses with doctorates, however, extreme biases of this type are atypical among nurse researchers (Damrosch & Strasser, 1988).
- *Costs.* A major obstacle facing researchers who would like to gather qualitative and quantitative data is that such integrated re-

search is usually expensive. Agencies that sponsor research activities may need to be "educated" about the contribution that integrated data collection efforts can make. In addition to the many substantive advantages that integration offers, it can also be argued that blending qualitative and quantitative data in a single study is actually less costly and more efficient than two discrete research projects on the same topic.
- *Researcher training.* Most researchers obtain graduate-level training that stresses either qualitative or (more typically) quantitative research methods. According to a survey by Damrosch and Strasser (1988), only about one third of doctorally prepared academic nurses have training in both qualitative and quantitative methods. Thus, investigator skills may pose an obstacle to integration. However, there is nothing about the integration model that suggests that all phases of the investigation must be done by a single researcher. Collaboration among researchers might, indeed, be an important byproduct of the decision to use an integrated approach. Such collaboration provides opportunities for both methodological and investigator triangulation.
- *Publication biases.* Some journals have a distinct preference for studies that are qualitative, and others lean toward quantitative studies. Because of this fact, researchers might be concerned that they would need to write up the qualitative and quantitative results separately, thereby foregoing many of the advantages of an integrated analysis. However, publication biases are much less evident today than they were a decade ago. All of the major nursing journals devoted to research publish qualitative and quantitative studies, and are increasingly publishing reports of integrated analyses.

In conclusion, although it is recognized that there are various obstacles to integrated analyses, we believe that the simultaneous use of qualitative and quantitative data to address problems of interest to the nursing profession represents a powerful methodological strategy. We are confident that nurse researchers will develop mechanisms for dealing with the obstacles.

≡ RESEARCH EXAMPLES

We have provided examples of studies using integrated analyses throughout this chapter in an effort to demonstrate the advantages of such an approach, as well as to illustrate different applications to which such integration has been put. Table 24-1 identifies some additional studies in which qualitative and quantitative data were blended, and one additional example is described in greater detail as follows.

> Hinds and Young (1987) conducted a study designed to assess the effects of standardized self-care instruction by community health nurses together with a follow-up nursing contact on the wellness outcomes of adults partici-

pating in a wellness program. Within the theoretical framework of the study, wellness was conceived of as a multidimensional, dynamic phenomenon, and hence was well-suited to a study involving both qualitative and quantitative measures.

Data were gathered by means of structured questionnaires, an observational measure, archival records, field notes, and structured interviews. The questionnaires consisted primarily of two Likert scales: (1) the Wellness Appraisal Scale and (2) the Health Goals Progress Scale. The observational measure was a structured measure of client's morale: the Behavior-Morale Scale (BMS). Clinic records included ratings of the participants' health habits and risks, as well as narrative descriptions of the participants' wellness goals. Field notes were maintained to document the investigators' impressions of participant reactions and spontaneous comments made by participants. Finally, at the last three data collection points (1 week, 3 weeks, and 6 months after the clinic visit), structured interviews were administered to gather data on the

Table 24-1. *Examples of Studies That Have Combined Qualitative and Quantitative Data*

RESEARCH PROBLEM	DATA COLLECTION METHODS
What are the defining characteristics for the nursing diagnoses *fear* and *anxiety?* (Taylor-Loughran et al., 1989)	Records, narrative written descriptions
How is a child's psychosocial identity developed within the context of the family? (Sohier, 1988)	Structured questionnaires, records, social-psychological scales, in-depth interviews, participant observation, ethnographic diaries
What are the effects of hearing loss on older women? (Magilvy, 1985)	Social-psychologic scales, in-depth interviews
What importance do mothers give to issues in the first 3 months of infants' lives and how is importance related to perceived need for action and maternal experience? (Pridham et al., 1987)	Daily diaries, rating scales
Do adults with chronic disease manifest a different pattern of health behavior than adults without diagnosed disease? (Laffrey, 1990)	Structural questionnaire and scales; semistructured interview

participants' perceived level of wellness and satisfaction with it.

The analysis carefully integrated findings from the qualitative and quantitative data. For example, using a multivariate analysis of covariance, the investigator explored changes over time on morale (BMS scores) among the follow-up groups. When no statistically significant differences were found, the investigator turned to the field notes. In these notes, the investigator had observed a high level of homogeneity of morale among the participants, which helped to explain the nonsignificant BMS findings. In other aspects of the analyses, the investigator used data from multiple sources to corroborate findings and validate the wellness construct as multidimensional and nonstatic. The researcher's summary of the strengths of her study nicely describes many of the advantages of an integrated approach:

The triangulated approach, thus, (a) tested the study hypotheses, (b) validated study findings, (c) explained divergent findings, (d) provided theoretical integrations, and (e) gave information to rule out a rival explanation. The convergence between methods served to increase confidence in the adequacy of how the construct of wellness was made operational. (p. 198)

≡ *SUMMARY*

The judicious blending of qualitative and quantitative data collection and analysis in a single project offers many advantages. The most obvious advantage is that the two methods have complementary strengths and weaknesses and offer the possibility of "mutually supplying each other's lack." Second, an integrated approach can lead to theoretical and substantive insights into the multidimensional nature of reality that might otherwise be unattainable. Third, integration can provide feedback loops that augment the incremental gains in knowledge that a single-method study could achieve. Fourth, the potential for confirmation of the study hypotheses through multiple and complementary types of data can strengthen the researcher's confidence in the val-

idity of the findings. Fifth, when the multiple methods yield inconsistent findings, a careful scrutiny of the discrepancies could push the line of inquiry farther than might otherwise have been possible. Although nurse researchers have not frequently adopted an integrated approach in their investigations, it seems likely that, in recognition of these advantages, the blending of methods in a single project will become more prevalent as we move toward the twenty-first century.

The integration of qualitative and quantitative data can be used in many applications. In nursing, one of the most frequent uses of multimethod research has been in the area of instrument development. Qualitative data are also used in some studies to illustrate the meaning of quantified descriptions or relationships. Integrated analyses are also used in efforts to interpret and give shape to relationships and causal processes. Finally, the most ambitious application of an integrated approach is in the area of theory development.

Researchers can implement an integrated approach in a variety of ways, but three strategies are especially likely to be common. The first is to embed qualitative methods (such as in-depth interviews or unstructured observations) within a survey. The second is to add structured data collection (such as a survey or a systematic analysis of records data) into field work. The third is to collect both types of data within the context of an experimental or quasi-experimental design. In some studies, the simultaneous collection and analysis of qualitative and quantitative data might address the objectives of integration, but in many studies a multistage approach is likely to yield more insights.

Despite the advantages of blending both types of data in a single study, there are several obstacles to doing so. These obstacles include epistemological biases, high costs, inadequate researcher training, and publication biases. However, these obstacles are not insurmountable; the potential contribution that integration would afford nursing science makes the effort to surmount them a worthwhile investment.

≡ *STUDY SUGGESTIONS*

1. Suppose you were interested in studying the psychologic consequences of a miscarriage. Suggest ways in which qualitative and quantitative data could be gathered for such a study.

2. Read an article in a recent issue of a nursing research journal in which the researcher collected only quantitative data. Suggest some possibilities for how qualitative data might have enhanced the validity or interpretability of the findings.

3. Read one of the studies cited in "Substantive References" at the end of this chapter. To what extent were the qualitative and quantitative analyses integrated? Describe how the absence of either the quantitative or qualitative portions of the study might have affected the study quality and the study conclusions.

≡ *SUGGESTED READINGS*

METHODOLOGICAL REFERENCES

Brewer, J., & Hunter, A. (1989). *Multimethod research: A synthesis of styles.* Newbury Park, CA: Sage.

Bryman, A. (1988). *Quantity and quality in social research.* London: Unwin Hyman.

Damrosch, S.P., & Strasser, J.A. (1988). A survey of doctorally prepared academic nurses on qualitative and quantitative research issues. *Nursing Research, 37,* 176–180.

Denzin, N.K. (1989). *The research act* (3rd ed.). Englewood Cliffs, NJ: Prentice-Hall.

Duffy, M. (1967). Methodological triangulation: A vehicle for merging quantitative and qualitative research methods. *Image, 19,* 130–133.

Haase, J.E., & Myers, S.T. (1988) Reconciling paradigm assumptions of qualitative and quantitative research. *Western Journal of Nursing Research, 10,* 128–137.

Jicks, T.D. (1979). Mixing qualitative and quantitative methods: Triangulation in action. *Administrative Science Quarterly, 24,* 602–611.

Mitchell, E.S. (1986). Multiple triangulation: A methodology for nursing science. *Advances in Nursing Science, 8,* 18–26.

Murphy, S.A. (1989). Multiple triangulation: Applications in a program of nursing research. *Nursing Research, 38,* 294–298.

Myers, S.T., & Haase, J.E. (1989). Guidelines for integration of quantitative and qualitative approaches. *Nursing Research, 38,* 299–301.

Seiber, S.D. (1973). Integrating field work and survey methods. *American Journal of Sociology, 78,* 1335–1359.

Tilden, V.P., Nelson, C.A., & May, B.A. (1990). Use of qualitative methods to enhance content validity. *Nursing Research, 39,* 172–175.

Tripp-Reimer, T. (1985). Combining qualitative and quantitative methodologies. In M. Leininger (Ed.), *Qualitative research methods in nursing.* New York: Grune & Stratton.

SUBSTANTIVE REFERENCES

Bargagliotti, L.A., & Trygstad, L.N. (1987). Differences in stress and coping findings: A reflection of social realities or methodologies. *Nursing Research, 36,* 170–173.

Browner, C.H. (1987). Job stress and health: The role of social support at work. *Research in Nursing and Health, 10,* 93–100.

Burckhardt, C.S., Woods, S.L., Schultz, A.A., & Ziebarth, D.M. (1989). Quality of life of adults with chronic illness: A psychometric study. *Research in Nursing and Health, 12,* 347–354.

Corcoran-Perry, S., & Graves, J. (1990). Supplemental-information-seeking behavior of cardiovascular nurses. *Research in Nursing and Health, 13,* 119–127.

Dennis, K.E. (1987). Dimensions of client control. *Nursing Research, 36,* 151–156.

Duffy, M.E. (1986). Primary prevention behaviors: The female-headed, one-parent family. *Research in Nursing and Health, 9,* 115–122.

Hinds, P.S. (1989). Method triangulation to index change in clinical phenomena. *Western Journal of Nursing Research, 11,* 440–447.

Hinds, P.S., & Young, K.J. (1987). A triangulation of methods and paradigms to study nurse-given wellness care. *Nursing Research, 36,* 195–198.

Laffrey, S.C. (1990). An exploration of adult health behaviors. *Western Journal of Nursing Research, 12,* 434–447.

La Montagne, L.L., & Pawlak, R. (1990). Stress and coping of parents in a pediatric intensive care unit. *Heart and Lung, 19,* 416–421.

Magilvy, J.K. (1985). Experiencing hearing loss in later life: A comparison of deaf and hearing-impaired older women. *Research in Nursing and Health, 8,* 347–353.

Murphy, S.A. (1986). Perceptions of stress, coping, and recovery one and three years after a natural disaster. *Mental Health Nursing, 8,* 63–77.

Murphy, S.A. (1987). Self-efficacy and social support: Mediators of stress on mental health following a natural disaster. *Western Journal of Nursing Research, 9,* 58–73.

Murphy, S.A. (1989). An explanatory model of recovery from disaster loss. *Research in Nursing and Health, 12,* 67–76.

Polit, D.F., Quint, J.C., & Riccio, J.A. (1988). *The challenge of serving teenage mothers: Lessons from Project Redirection.* New York: Manpower Demonstration Research Corp.

Polit, D.F., White, C.M., & Morton, T. (1987). *Family planning needs of the child welfare population.* Saratoga Springs, NY: Humanalysis, Inc.

Pridham, K.F., Chang, A.S., & Hansen, M. (1987). Mothers' problem-solving skill and use of help with infant-related issues. *Research in Nursing and Health, 10,* 263–275.

Sohier, R. (1988). Multiple triangulation and contemporary nursing research. *Western Journal of Nursing Research, 10,* 732–742.

Stokes, S.A., & Gordon, S.E. (1988). Development of an instrument to measure stress in the older adult. *Nursing Research, 37,* 16–19.

Taylor-Loughran, A.E., O'Brien, M.E., LaChapelle, R., & Rangel, S. (1989). Defining characteristics of the nursing diagnoses *fear* and *anxiety:* A validation study. *Applied Nursing Research, 2,* 178–186.

25
Computers and Scientific Research

High-speed electronic computers have evolved and expanded at a tremendous rate since their development in the 1940s. Few aspects of American society have remained untouched by the impact of computers: bills are sent out, weather is predicted, literature sources are retrieved, classroom schedules are determined, production machines are controlled, medical records are maintained, and diagnoses are made—all with the assistance of computers. With the advent of personal computers, computers have, indeed, become ubiquitous and their role in nursing and health care has vastly expanded.

The use of computers in scientific research, as one might suspect, is substantial and inevitably growing. Computers have, in fact, revolutionized research by making possible the kinds of operations that could not have been attempted with human labor alone. Computers are now used by researchers throughout the research process—to conduct bibliographic searches, to collect and store data of all types, to maintain administrative research records, to analyze data, and to prepare proposals and research reports. Although there are numerous applications of computer technology in scientific investigations, the discussion here focuses primarily on the use of computers to analyze data obtained during the course of a research project.

The purpose of this chapter is to introduce the reader to some of the basic principles of computer operations. Although computers are electronically complex machines, the basic logic of computers is not difficult to comprehend. One of the most striking features of modern computer technology is that computer users do not need to understand in detail how a computer works to benefit from its labor-saving computations. Computers have become accessible to broader and broader classes of users. It is hoped that an acquaintance with some of the basic characteristics of computers will be sufficient to demonstrate that computer analysis is within the reach of all readers of this book.

POWERS AND LIMITATIONS OF COMPUTERS

Computers are machines of tremendous power. Without any doubt, they are indispensable to modern scientists because of the characteristics we describe in this chapter. Computers are not, however, on the verge of making human intelligence obsolete. Respect for the potency of computers must be balanced by a recognition of their limitations.

Computer Capabilities

The most noteworthy characteristic of computers is unquestionably their remarkable speed. The fact that computers are fast probably is familiar to everyone, but it is difficult to grasp how incredibly speedy computers actually are. The most sophisticated computers can perform elementary arithmetic calculations such as addition and subtraction in billionths of a second. In other words, in a single second, computers are capable of executing tens of millions of operations. A large computer can perform more arithmetic in one second than a human could perform working 40-hour weeks for several years. The speediness of computers, therefore, removes the drudgery and delays of doing computations manually and can increase researcher productivity.

Not only are computers fast but they also are accurate. Highly complex calculations can be performed without error. By contrast, human "calculators" are fallible. The person who spends an hour calculating a statistic such as a correlation coefficient would probably have to spend at least as much time checking for computational errors. A computer could perform the same calculation, error-free, in a fraction of a second.* An additional advantage of computers is that they are dependably accurate. They can work hour after hour without making a mistake.

The memory capacity of large computers is impressive. The memory of a computer can store immense files of symbols to which it can gain access in a fraction of a second. Some memory devices can store millions of digits. What is even more impressive is that the information stored in memory is not permanent but can be erased and replaced with new information. In other words, the memory can be used over and over again to solve new problems.

Another noteworthy aspect of computers is their flexibility. Most computers have been built for a variety of purposes. A university computer, for instance, does the payroll, produces income tax forms, keeps track of scholarship monies, bills students, produces grade reports, analyzes data from faculty research, and so forth.

Finally, although computers do break down, they behave for the most part as our faithful servants. They do exactly what they are told to do, day in and day out, no matter how boring or repetitive the task might be.

Computer Limitations

One of the most conspicuous limitations of computers is their utter and complete stupidity. Computers are sometimes referred to as "giant brains," but computers have absolutely no innate intelligence. They do only those operations that they are told to do by humans. The computer's inability to think can result in many frustrating experiences for its users. Unlike humans, a computer is unable to make even the simplest of inferences. Consider the following equation: 1 + 1, = ?. The extraneous comma placed before the

---

* The accuracy of a computer is limited to numbers of a certain size, owing to limitations in the computer's memory. Usually numbers can be accurate to 16 significant digits (e.g., 0.000000000000001), which is sufficiently accurate for virtually all nursing research applications.

equal sign would probably not interfere with a 6-year-old's ability to come up with the answer "2." Yet most computers could not solve this equation. The computer would be incapable of inferring that the extraneous comma should be ignored. Actually, although this aspect of computers usually taxes the patience of computer users, it is often an advantage. In the above equation, perhaps the comma should actually have been a zero. In such a situation, it is preferable for the computer to alert the user to an error than to perform a faulty computation.

Computer time for the analysis of complex data sets can be quite costly, although computer costs have decreased dramatically over the past 10 years. For example, although costs vary markedly from one installation to another, it is not unusual for computer time on a large computer to cost $10 per minute. Of course, the computer could perform an enormous quantity of operations in one minute. Thus, although computer costs may be high, they are really a bargain in comparison with the costs of human labor.

Another limitation of computers is the detail with which instructions must be described. When a human is confronted with the task $2 + 2 = ?$, the solution is (at the conscious level at least) straightforward and simple. A computer normally requires several instructions to process such computations. Every logical and arithmetic operation must be "explained" to the computer in detail, a feature that makes most tasks seem more complex than they would to humans. Fortunately, the average researcher does not have to worry about such matters. The detailed instructions are developed by experts who have taken pains to simplify the use of computers.

≡ *TYPES OF COMPUTERS*

There are four major types of computers: (1) microcomputers, (2) minicomputers, (3) mainframes, and (4) supercomputers. These four types vary with respect to speed, memory capacity, cost, size, and direct accessibility to researchers. For the most part, nurse researchers are most likely to use either mainframes or microcomputers.

Most universities, hospitals, and other large institutions own what is referred to as a *mainframe computer,* which is a large multi-user system that usually can be accessed from multiple locations. Mainframes typically have huge memory capacities and operate at very high rates of speed. Figure 25-1 presents a picture of the main components of such a mainframe computer. Specialized mainframes that are needed to perform highly complex operations (such as the management of a space launch) are sometimes referred to as *supercomputers.*

Minicomputers are moderate-sized computers that operate at intermediate speeds. Such computers have most frequently been used for midsized applications, such as the storage and analysis of laboratory data. However, minicomputers are becoming less common with the advent of fairly powerful microcomputers.

Microcomputers or *personal computers (PCs)* are becoming increasingly popular both in institutions and in private homes and offices. PCs are slower and have less memory than mainframes, and are generally restricted to just one user (or a handful of users) who can use the machine at any given time. Yet PCs are inexpensive and generally easy to use and are becoming especially useful for certain applications, such as word processing and the analysis of small data sets. Figure 25-2 shows an example of a PC.

≡ *OVERVIEW OF COMPUTER COMPONENTS*

A computer system is an elaborate complex consisting of numerous components that perform specialized functions. The components of a computer system can be classified as either hardware or software. *Hardware* refers to the physical equipment that stores, processes, and controls information. *Software* refers to the instructions

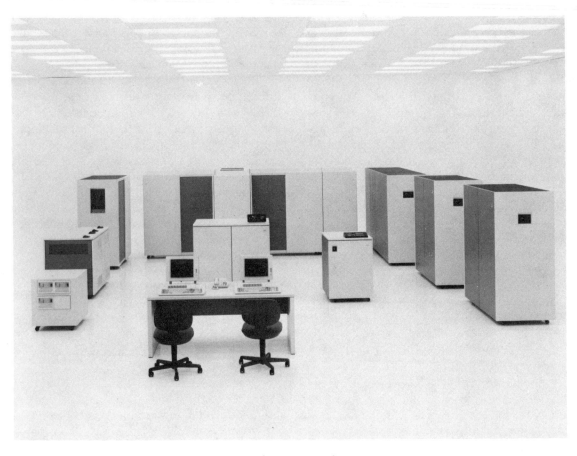

Figure 25-1.   *Computer hardware. (Courtesy of International Business Machines Corporation.)*

and procedures required to operate the computer. In this section, the major aspects of both hardware and software are reviewed.

Computer Hardware

A schematic diagram of computer hardware is presented in Figure 25-3. Essentially, the computer consists of five types of components. Information is fed into the computer through some type of *input device*. The information read in through an input device comprises data, on the one hand, and instructions concerning how the data are to be processed, on the other. After the computer has performed its necessary calculations,

the resulting information comes out through an *output device*. In a mainframe environment, input/output (sometimes abbreviated I/O) devices are generally the only parts of the machine with which a researcher comes in direct physical contact. Because it is more important for a researcher to become familiar with I/O devices than with other components of a computer, a separate section has been devoted to them.

The information that is read into the computer is stored in a device called *memory*. The computer memory comprises a series of cells, which may be likened to a set of pigeon holes or post office boxes. Each cell of memory can store either an instruction or a numerical value. The

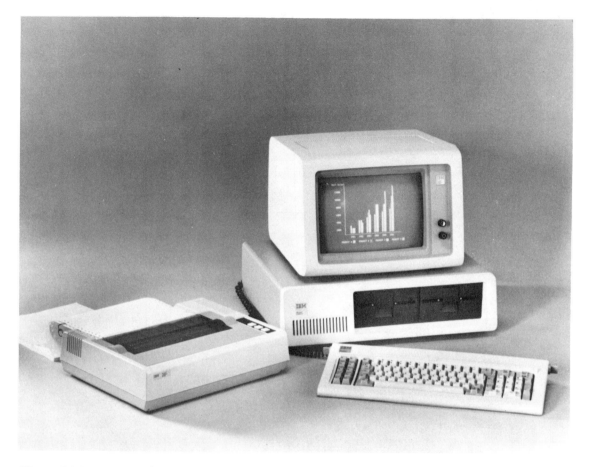

Figure 25-2. *A personal computer. (Courtesy of International Business Machines Corporation.)*

cells are organized into a series and assigned a number so that any piece of information stored in memory can be located by its "address." The memory unit of a computer is designed to store large amounts of information and to allow rapid access to any specific portion of that information. The capacity of computer's memory typically is measured in *kilobytes* (K) or *megabytes* (MB). A *byte* is a single character, such as a number, letter, or specialized symbol such as a " + " sign. One kilobyte equals 1000 bytes, and a megabyte equals 1 million bytes. Microcomputers generally have between 64K to 800K of memory.

From the memory, the instructions are sent to the *control unit.* This component coordinates the functions of the other components. The control unit interprets the instructions, determines the sequence of operations of the computer, and controls the movements of information from one component to another.

The *arithmetic/logic unit* is the component in which arithmetic operations are accomplished. The control unit and arithmetic/logic unit are together referred to as the *central processing unit* (CPU), which is where all of the decisions and calculations are performed.

All four types of computers consist of these same five basic components.

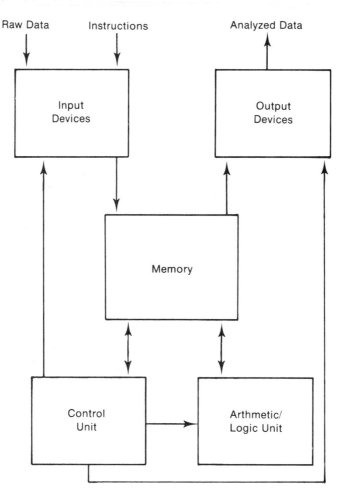

Figure 25-3. *Scheme of computer components and interrelationships.*

Computer Software

The software components of a computer include the instructions for performing operations and the documentation for those instructions. A set of instructions is referred to as a *program*. The ability of a computer to solve problems depends on computer programs, which specify clearly and precisely what operations the machine is to perform and how to perform them.

To give the computer a set of commands, people must be able to communicate with the machine. Computers, unfortunately, do not "speak" or understand natural languages such as English.

Direct machine language that a computer *can* comprehend is extremely complex and accessible to only programming experts. Happily, various *programming languages* have been developed that are reasonably easy to learn and that are structured in a manner comfortable to human communicators. The instructions to the computer can be written in a programming language, and then another program called a *compiler* translates the instructions into an equivalent machine language program that the computer can comprehend and execute.

Various programming languages are available to computer users. Many of these languages have been developed for a specific type of application. The language most commonly used in scientific applications is FORTRAN, which is an acronym for FORmula TRANslation. The language known as PL/1 (Programming Language 1) is becoming increasingly popular in the scientific community. It includes many features of FORTRAN, but has additional new features and capabilities that make it attractive for use with scientific and social scientific problems. One of the simplest languages for beginning programmers to learn is BASIC (Beginners All-purpose Symbolic Instruction Code). PASCAL is a relatively new language that is especially popular in introducing programming to students.

Most researchers can make ample use of computers without ever having to learn a computer language. This is because there are standard programs available for most types of statistical analysis. It would be inefficient to have every researcher write a program to compute an average or percentage, when a single program could be used by thousands of individuals.

Despite the fact that most readers will never need to master a programming language, a brief and simplified example of a BASIC program might help to demystify the process of computer functioning. Suppose that we had information concerning the weights of 100 subjects and that we wanted to know the mean weight of the sample. We could obtain the mean by using a program with eight statements as follows:

```
10 LET N = 0
20 LET S = 0
30 INPUT X
40 LET S = S + X
50 LET N = N + 1
60 IF N <100 THEN GO TO 30
70 LET M = S/N
80 PRINT M
```

In this program, the numbers 10, 20 . . . 80 are merely labels to help identify different commands. The symbol S is used to represent the sum of the subjects' weights, N represents the number of subjects, X stands for an individual datum (the weight of a subject), and M is the mean weight of the sample. The first two statements set the initial values of N and S to zero, as one would normally do when using a pocket calculator. Statement 30 tells the computer to read in the weight (X) of the first subject. The sum is incremented by the value of X in line 40. If the first person weighed 120 pounds, then S at this point would be equal to 120 pounds. In line 50, the value of N is increased by 1 to keep track of the number of subjects whose weights have been added to the sum. The first time through, N would be set equal to 1. In line 60, the computer is instructed to make a decision. If the number of cases processed is less than 100, then the computer is instructed to return to statement 30, where another case is read in. Once again, the weight would be added to the sum and the number counter would be increased. The cyclical process would continue until all 100 cases had been read into the computer. When N was equal to 100, the computer would proceed to execute statement 70, which calculates the mean (M) by dividing the sum by the number of cases. Finally, the computer would output the desired information by printing the average weight of the sample.

This short example demonstrates that there is nothing mysterious about instructing a computer to perform computational operations, although most computer tasks are considerably more complex than the task used here as an illustration. A great deal of skill and effort normally are required to develop efficient and sophisticated programs, but the logical processes underlying programming are much the same from one application to another.

The increasing availability of software packages to perform a variety of analytic jobs has made it possible for large numbers of nonprogrammers to profit from the advantages that computers offer. Knowledge of a programming language is definitely an asset to researchers. There are several operations that a packaged program does not perform, and researchers may also find that some specialized computation is required for their data. Nevertheless, for the typical researcher, ignorance of a computer language is not an adequate reason to avoid computer analysis.

≡ *INPUT AND OUTPUT DEVICES*

Both data and programs must be transmitted to the computer through some input medium. Similarly, the computer communicates back to the user through an output medium. Usually, researchers interact with the computer through I/O devices without having to worry too much about what happens inside the computer itself. Because researchers do operate and work with I/O devices, it is appropriate to describe them more fully than other hardware components.

Input Media and Devices

Input devices convert alphabetical and numerical characters to a form amenable to storage in the computer's memory. A variety of input devices exist, and most computer installations have more than one type of device available for use.

One input medium is the *punch card,* an illustration of which is presented in Figure 25-4. These cards have become virtually obsolete, but are discussed here because data are often entered onto other devices in card-image format. Punch cards contain 80 columns for storing a line of information, with each column representing a single character.

The most widely used method of input today is through direct communication devices. These devices transmit information to the CPU by way of electronic impulses and permit the user to communicate directly with the computer without the use of cards or other input devices. Direct communication devices take the form of a terminal or a keyboard onto which the user types the relevant information. The keyboard is connected to a display screen or monitor—the *cathode ray tube* (CRT). CRTs have screens that are typically 80 columns wide, corresponding to the width of a punch card. Other input devices include *optical scanners* and other optical devices for the direct input of specially prepared materials such as bar codes.

Several other kinds of input media are used in the analysis of scientific data that serve both as methods of inputting information into the computer and as *external storage devices.* In mainframe settings, the two most common devices for input and storage are magnetic tapes and magnetic disks. In the case of *magnetic tapes,* information is stored on reels similar to the reels for a tape recorder. Magnetic tape can break or become unreadable, but it is a much more durable input medium than punch cards. Information is often put onto tape by a transfer from input from a terminal. The input device through which tape information is passed on to the computer is called a *tape drive.*

Magnetic disks are flat spinning objects, analogous to a record, with magnetizable surfaces. Information is stored on disks on concentric tracks. Disks are a more dependable medium for storing information than either punch cards or magnetic tapes. Information typed into a terminal is typically stored on disks. Like magnetic tapes, disks have the advantage that they can be erased and reused.

Several types of storage/input media are available for use with PCs. Many have a built-in hard disk, analogous to the disks used by mainframes. However, most PCs use *floppy disks* as a means of putting information into the computer. Floppy disks or diskettes are small (usually 3″ or 5¼″ in diameter), flexible circular objects that resemble a 45-rpm record, protected by a paper cover. Floppies can be erased and reused many times. New I/O and external storage devices are constantly under development. One of the most noteworthy advances in recent years is the *CD-ROM* (compact disk, read-only memory). CD-ROM represents a microcomputer application of the technology responsible for the highly popular audio compact disks. A single CD-ROM can hold more than 550MB of information, the equivalent of 1500 floppy disks. CD-ROM can make data as easily accessible to the microcomputer as files on a floppy or hard disk.

Output Media and Devices

Output devices transfer the problem solutions from the computer's memory to a form that

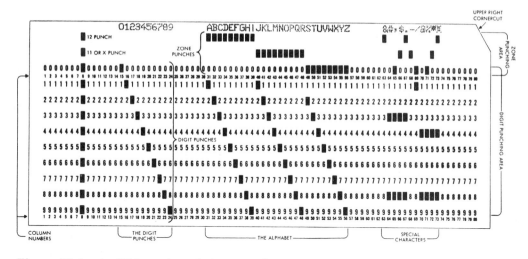

Figure 25-4. *An IBM punch card. Courtesy of International Business Machines Corporation.*

is understandable to humans. The most common output medium is a permanent readable record of the results of the analysis, referred to as a *hardcopy,* from a printer. A wide variety of printers are now available for both mainframe and microcomputers. The *line printer* is typically a principal output device for mainframe computers. These printers create an entire line of print at once and can print more than 1000 lines per minute. Printers connected to microcomputers include both impact printers (which print through the physical striking of paper, much like typewriters) and nonimpact printers, such as ink-jet and laser-jet printers. *Plotters* are another output device that can be used for producing printed graphs and diagrams. The copy produced by printers and plotters is usually called the *printout* or *printed output.*

Various visual display devices are often used to output information in direct communications systems. Examples include CRTs and special graphics terminals. Another output device that is less frequently used is the microfilm recorder, which enables output to be photographed for storage on microfilm.

In some cases, a researcher wants the results of one part of an analysis stored on a me-dium that the computer can then read for subsequent analyses. In such cases, information can be transferred to such external storage devices as tapes, disks, floppy disks, or CD-ROMs for later use. Such external storage devices are available for both mainframe and microcomputers.

≡ MODES OF COMMUNICATING WITH A COMPUTER

Researchers can communicate with a computer in one of several modes. For many mainframe applications, instructions to the computer are processed in the batch processing mode. *Batch processing* refers to a method in which a batch of programs is assembled for execution during the same machine run. The data and instructions regarding the analysis of the data are entered into the computer (sometimes through more than one input device if the data are being stored on an external storage device) and the program is processed without any further intervention. The researcher must normally wait some time before getting the output from a batch processing job. The delay between the input of the job and the availability of the output, which is referred to as the *turnaround time,* may be several minutes or several hours.

Some computer systems and software packages offer users the capability of interacting directly with the computer, in what is called the *interactive mode.* When direct communication devices such as terminals or consoles are used, a researcher may be able to type in information and receive feedback essentially immediately, either on a CRT display or on a typed copy. Microcomputers operate in an interactive mode. On large computer systems, direct communication between the computer and numerous users concurrently is made possible by a concept known as time sharing. *Time sharing* is a method of operation by means of which several different programs are interleaved, giving the users the impression that the jobs are being processed simultaneously. Time sharing usually operates on a "round robin" system. The computer spends a small amount of time (perhaps only one hundredth of a second) on each program, passing onto the next user. Because an entire cycle takes only seconds, it appears to all users as though they are getting instantaneous, personal service. The slowness of the keyboard and the rapidity of the CPU have combined to make time sharing feasible. The major advantages of the interactive mode are convenience, ease of use, and immediate feedback. In using an interactive mode, the researcher can communicate with the computer in a conversational way: to enter a program or commands, to enter data, to receive and answer questions from the computer, and to select a course of action to be followed. Because interactive terminals are connected to the computer by telephone lines, the terminals need not be in the same building or even the same city as the computer.

Programs written in the batch mode can often be executed on an interactive terminal. The researcher can, from a terminal, instruct the computer to load the program and data from some input storage device (e.g., from a disk file) and then direct the computer to execute the program without further interaction.

≡ AVAILABLE PROGRAMS FOR DATA ANALYSIS

A great boon to researchers unfamiliar with a programming language, as well as to those with programming skills, is the widespread availability of ready-made programs for the analysis of research data. The computer centers at universities are particularly likely to have a variety of software packages available to their users. Most computer centers have a professional staff that is accessible for consultation concerning the computer's library of programs. Sophisticated programs for performing statistical analysis are available for both mainframe and microcomputer. As discussed in Chapter 23, various programs also are available for the analysis of qualitative data.

Many mainframe computer facilities have a variety of simple, easy-to-use statistical programs in their general library. Often there are a large number of such "canned" programs that can be run from an interactive terminal. The use of these programs requires no expertise at all on the part of the researcher. For example, a researcher could obtain some basic descriptive statistics about a set of data by a simple instruction, such as RUN TALLY. The terminal would ask questions that would then guide the researcher in providing the necessary information to the computer.

These simple library programs are excellent heuristic devices when a user is first learning to work with a computer. When a researcher has a large number of cases, a large number of variables, or desires a sophisticated statistical procedure, however, a more complex statistical software package will usually be required.

Major Software Packages

The most widely used statistical software packages for use on mainframe computers include the Statistical Package for the Social Sciences, or SPSS^x (SPSS, Inc., 1987); Statistical Analysis System, or SAS (SAS Institute, 1985); and the Biomedical Computer Programs—P Series or BMD-P (Dixon, 1988). Each of these packages contains programs to handle a broad variety of statistical analyses. The reference section at the end of this chapter identifies the major statistical capabilities currently available for each of these packages. Because these packages are updated, refined, and expanded frequently, readers are advised to check with personnel at their computer facility for any modifications to the description and listings provided in this chapter.

SPSS^x

SPSS^X

SPSS^x was developed by researchers at the University of Chicago and National Opinion Research Center to assist researchers in the analysis of social science data. Like its earlier versions, the current SPSS^x package represents a highly flexible program with a syntax that is not technically oriented. For people with limited statistical and computer backgrounds, SPSS^x is relatively easy to learn. Among its many strong features, SPSS^x provides excellent capabilities for labeling variables and includes all of the most commonly used parametric and nonparametric statistical procedures, and many less frequently used ones, including survival analysis. SPSS is also available in a microcomputer version, SPSS/PC⁺.

SAS

SAS

SAS is a computer package that was developed at North Carolina State University, Raleigh, for use in research. It has evolved into a widely used and very flexible package. It is generally considered to be somewhat more sophisticated, from a statistical point of view, than SPSS. Like SPSS, the syntax of SAS is fairly easy to learn, even for those without a strong statistical or computer background. One disadvantage of SAS, in comparison with SPSS, is that SAS uses a more cumbersome approach for the labeling of variables (e.g., labeling the variable GENDER) and for categories within variables (e.g., MALE/FEMALE). However, SAS uses a less rigid format in syntax than SPSS and contains a more complete set of sophisticated statistical procedures. Like SPSS, SAS is also available in a PC version.

BMD-P

BMD-P

The programs referred to as Biomedical Programs were originally developed in the 1960s at the Health Sciences Computer Facility of the University of California, Los Angeles. The package has been vastly improved and simplified since its original development, and the current P series (BMD-P) is now widely used. The BMD-P package contains a large variety of elementary and advanced statistical procedures, and uses a highly flexible syntax. One major way in which BMD-P differs from SPSS and SAS is that the particular BMD-P program to be accessed must be indicated at the outset. Thus, only one program can be used for any given computer run (although the program may contain numerous statistical methods as options). In SPSS and SAS, the various statistical procedures are all incorporated as separate steps or subprograms. BMD-P also has a counterpart available for microcomputers.

Using a Packaged Program

Researchers using packaged programs do not need to know a programming language, but they still must be able to communicate to the computer some basic information about what their variables are and how the data are to be analyzed. This is accomplished by means of certain commands that are unique to each software package. To illustrate the kinds of commands the researcher would need to know, an example of a set-up for an analysis using the SPSS^x software is presented.

Suppose that we wanted to analyze the data that we used as an example in Chapters 20 and 21 concerning an intervention for low-income pregnant young women. The data for 30 subjects are shown in Table 20-7. The four variables, it may be recalled, are as follows: (1) group—experimental versus control; (2) weight of the infant; (3) repeat pregnancy; and (4) the mother's age. These data would most likely be entered into the computer directly by way of a terminal, with a separate record (in this case, a separate line of information) for each subject. Thus, the data would be entered onto 30 lines, with each line containing information on these four variables.

On each record or line, the information for the research variables would have to be entered according to some plan. Suppose, for example, the data were to be entered as follows: an identification number would be assigned and entered in columns 1 and 2; a designation of group status would be entered in column 3; the infant's birthweight (in ounces) would be entered in columns 4 through 6; whether the mother had a repeat pregnancy would be entered in column 7; and the

mother's age would be entered in columns 8 and 9. (Chapter 26 explains how such decisions are made.)

To use SPSS[x] to analyze the data, we must tell the computer how we have set up our data, just as we had to communicate this information to you in the preceding paragraph. Figure 25-5 presents the SPSS[x] instructions and the data that would be entered into the computer. The first line (DATA LIST) tells the computer that we are about to define the variables that are in the data file. The next line contains all of the variable definition and variable location information. The first entry on

```
DATA LIST
   /1  ID 1-2   GROUP 3   WEIGHT 4-6   REPEAT 7   MOMSAGE 8-9
FREQUENCIES   VARIABLES=WEIGHT,REPEAT,MOMSAGE/
   STATISTICS=ALL
BEGIN DATA
011107117
021101014
031119021
041128120
051089015
061099019
071111019
081117118
091102117
101120020
111076013
121116018
131100116
141115018
151113021
162111119
172108021
182095019
192099017
202103119
212094015
222101117
232114021
242097020
252099118
262113018
272089019
282098020
292102017
302105019
END DATA
FINISH
```

Figure 25-5. *Instructions for an SPSS[x] program.*

the line (/1) tells the computer that, in this case, all of the information for a given subject is contained on a single line. (If we had collected information on 50 variables per subject, we might well have needed two or three 80-column lines per subject, in which case the second line would have begun with /2.) Next, each variable is specified by a name, followed by the designation of the columns in which data for that variable will appear. In SPSS^x, variable names can be up to eight alphanumeric characters. In this example, we have called our variables ID, GROUP, WEIGHT, REPEAT, and MOMSAGE. Then, to the right of each variable name, we have designated the appropriate column numbers. For example, the data for mothers' age (MOMSAGE) is in columns 8 and 9.

The next two records, taken together, instruct the computer what statistical analysis to perform. These instructions will produce, for the variables WEIGHT, REPEAT, and MOMSAGE, a frequency count of every value obtained, together with many basic descriptive statistics, such as the mean, median, and standard deviation. The printout produced by this program for the WEIGHT variable was presented in Figure 20-10. If we wanted more complex statistics, such as those described in Chapters 21 and 22, we would need only to replace the FREQUENCIES/STATISTICS instructions with other instructions.

Finally, the command BEGIN DATA tells the computer to begin reading the data records, which follow immediately. There are 30 records here, because there were 30 subjects. The command following the data records (END DATA) tells the computer that all of the data have been read in, and the final command (FINISH) informs the computer that there are no further instructions for that particular run.

Hopefully, this simple example has made it clear that a researcher need not be a computer whiz or statistical expert to make use of a computer. SPSS^x has many features that were not described here, but these features are not difficult to understand either. Similarly, other packaged programs have commands that must be learned by users but that are designed to be easy to learn by people with limited computer skills.

≡ LOGGING ON TO A COMPUTER

Each mainframe computer installation has developed its own idiosyncratic procedures by which users gain access to computer facilities. If you are a first-time user of a system, you will need to learn exactly what steps must be taken to make use of the equipment. You may obtain such information from your instructors or from one of the many computer assistants who are generally available to guide you.

Generally, regardless of what your input mechanisms are, you will need to provide the computer with some administrative information that allows the computer to determine whether you should have access to it. If you are using an interactive terminal, the computer will request a user identification (ID) and a password, which allows you to *log on,* or gain access, to the computer. If you do not have this information, you will not be permitted to use the facilities.

Mainframe computers often have several options for interacting with the system and creating files. Two common options in university settings are TSO (Time Sharing Option) and CMS (Conversational Monitoring System). You will need to learn which monitoring system is available at your installation and how to gain access to it. You will also need to learn what statistical software packages are available.

PCs generally do not have as many security precautions, so an identification number may not be required. Most software for PCs is designed to be easy to learn to use through printed manuals and direct instructions from the computer. Easy-to-use programs are called "user friendly."

≡ SUMMARY

The advantages of computers to researchers include their speed, accuracy, and flexibility. On the other hand, computers require considerable attention to detail on the part of users, because computers have no capacity to "think."

Large, multi-user computer systems are often referred to as *mainframe computers* or, for certain applications, *supercomputers.* Midsized computers (*minicomputers*) are increasingly being replaced by powerful *microcomputers,* also known as *personal computers* or *PCs.* The components of a computer system are broadly categorized as either hardware or software. *Hardware* refers to the physical equipment that stores, processes, and controls information. *Software* refers to the instructions and procedures required to operate the computer.

The five essential components of computer hardware are the (1) *input device,* (2) *memory,* (3) *control unit,* (4) *arithmetic/logic unit,* and (5) *output device.* The control unit and the arithmetic/logic unit are collectively called the *central processing unit (CPU).* The input device is the means by which the researcher feeds information into the computer. The memory is the device that stores the information that is fed into the computer. The control unit coordinates the functions of the other components. The arithmetic/logic unit performs the arithmetic or logic operations requested. Finally, the output device produces the resulting information.

The most commonly used input device for mainframes and PCs is direct communication by means of a terminal or keyboard. Other input media that also serve as *external storage devices* include *magnetic tapes, magnetic disks, floppy disks,* and *CD-ROM.* The most commonly used output media are the paper *printout* (which is a permanent, readable record of the results of the analysis) and displays on CRTs and plotters.

A *program* is a set of instructions informing the computer what to do. *Programming languages* make it possible for humans to communicate with computers. FORTRAN, PL/1, and BASIC are examples of programming languages. Many packaged software programs exist for the researcher who is not greatly skilled in a programming language.

Researchers are able to communicate with computers in several ways. *Batch processing* refers to a process in which a batch of programs is assembled for execution during the same computer run. Generally, there is a delay between feeding the information into the computer and the output phase. The delay is referred to as *turnaround time. Interactive mode* permits direct communication between the researcher and the computer through the use of a terminal or console. Almost immediate feedback of information is possible when the interactive mode is used. *Time sharing* is a method in which several programs are processed "simultaneously" by the computer, which spends a small amount of time on each program in a "round robin" fashion.

Researchers generally do not need to learn programming to analyze their data by computer because of the widespread availability of sophisticated statistical packages. The most widely used packages, for both mainframes and PCs, are SPSS[x], SAS, and BMD-P.

≡ *STUDY SUGGESTIONS*

1. Can you solve the following equation:
$$10 - 3 = ?$$
Do you think a computer could? Why or why not?

2. Look at statement 40 in the BASIC program illustrated in this chapter (40 LET S = S + X). In which hardware component would this instruction actually be processed?

3. If you have access to a computer, find out how many cells or words of memory are available in your computer.

4. Visit a computer center. Check what types of I/O devices the computer has. Does the computer have a time sharing system? If possible, learn how to operate a terminal. Ask someone what software packages are available for doing statistical analyses.

5. Suppose you had data from 50 subjects on the following four variables: (1) age; (2) sex (coded 1 for females, 2 for males); (3) number of cigarettes smoked per day; and (4) number of days absent from work in the past year. Write out SPSS[x] instructions that would produce a frequency listing for these four variables. (Note: if necessary, first determine in which columns the data would be entered.)

☰ *SUGGESTED READINGS*

GENERAL REFERENCES

Ball, M.J., & Hannah, K.J. (1984). *Using computers in nursing.* Reston, VA: Reston Publishing.

Barcikowski, R.S. (Ed.). (1983). *Computer packages and research design, with annotations of input and output from the BMD-P, SAS, and SPSS[x] statistical packages.* New York: University of America Press.

Bronzino, J.D. (1982). *Computer applications for patient care.* Menlo Park, CA: Addison-Wesley.

Brownell, B.A. (1985). *Using microcomputers: A guidebook for writers, teachers, and researchers in the social sciences.* Beverly Hills, CA: Sage.

Capron, H.L., & Williams, B.K. (1984). *Computers and data processing* (2nd ed.). Menlo Park, CA: Benjamin/Cummings.

Chang, B.L. (1985). Computer use and nursing research. *Western Journal of Nursing Research, 7,* 142–144.

Cox, H., Harsanyi, B., & Dean, L. (1988). *Computers and nursing: Applications to practice, education and research.* Norwalk, CT: Appleton & Lange.

Grobe, S.J. (1984). *Computer primer and resource guide for nurses.* Philadelphia: J.B. Lippincott.

Jacobsen, B.S., Tulman, L., Lowery, B.J., & Garson, C. (1988). Experiencing the research process by using statistical software on microcomputers. *Nursing Research, 37,* 56–59.

Moore, R.W. (1978). *Introduction to the use of computer packages for statistical analyses.* Englewood Cliffs, NJ: Prentice-Hall.

Morse, J.M., & Morse, R.M. (1989). QUAL: A mainframe program for qualitative data analysis. *Nursing Research, 38,* 188–189.

Nicoll, L.H. (1987). The microcomputer: An alternative for data analysis. *Nursing Research, 36,* 320–323.

Saba, V.K., & McCormick, K.A. (1986). *Essentials of computers for nurses.* Philadelphia: J.B. Lippincott.

Schrodt, P.A. (1984). *Microcomputer methods for social scientists.* Beverly Hills, CA: Sage.

Stern, R., & Stern, N. (1983). *Computers in society.* Englewood Cliffs, NJ: Prentice-Hall.

Sweeney, M.A. (1985). *The nurse's guide to computers.* New York: Macmillan.

Turley, J.P. (1989). Transferring data files between microcomputer statistical packages. *Nursing Research, 38,* 315–317.

Walker, M.B., & Schwartz, C.M. (1984). *What every nurse should know about computers.* Philadelphia: J.B. Lippincott.

Webster, D.C. (1988). Personal computers and qualitative data analysis. *Western Journal of Nursing Research, 10,* 219–221.

REFERENCES ON SOFTWARE PACKAGES

Dixon, W.J. (Ed.) (1988). *Biomedical computer programs.* Berkeley, CA: University of California Press. [See also BMD-P (1986), *BMD-P statistical software PC user's guide.* Berkeley, CA: U of C Press. Major programs include summary statistics; correlations; analysis of variance (ANOVA); analysis of covariance (ANCOVA); multiple regression analysis; cluster analysis; factor analysis; canonical correlation; and discriminant analysis.]

SAS Institute. (1985). *SAS user's guide.* Cary, NC: SAS Institute. [See also SAS Institute. (1985). *SAS-STAT guide for personal computers.* Cary, NC: SAS Institute. This package includes all basic descriptive and inferential statistics, plus additional programs for cluster analysis, Guttman scalogram analysis, multiple regression, factor analysis, discriminant function analysis, canonical correlation, logit/probit analysis, and spectral analysis.]

SPSS, Inc. (1987). *SPSS[x] user's guide.* New York: McGraw-Hill. [See also SPSS, Inc. (1986). *SPSS/PC+ for the IBM PC/XT/AT.* Chicago, IL: Author. Major programs include descriptive statistics, frequency distributions, contingency tables and related measures of association, bivariate correlation and scatter diagrams, partial correlation, multiple regression analysis, *t*-tests, ANOVA, ANCOVA, multivariate ANOVA, discriminant analysis, factor analysis, canonical analysis, survival analysis, loglinear analysis, reliability analysis, and various nonparametric procedures.]

26
Preparation for Statistical Analysis

After a researcher gathers quantitative data in the course of a research investigation, there are typically a variety of tasks that must be undertaken before testing the research hypotheses. These tasks include editing and preparing the data for analysis by the computer, evaluating data quality, and undertaking data manipulations needed for the analyses. This chapter provides an overview of these preparatory steps.

≡ *CODING*

If a computer is to be used to perform statistical analyses—and this is almost always the case—the information must be converted to a form amenable to such analyses. Computers cannot process verbatim responses to open-ended questions. It is similarly difficult for a computer to read and analyze information with verbal labels such as male or female, agree or disagree. *Coding* is the process by which basic research information is transformed into symbols compatible with computer analysis. It is possible to code information using alphabetical symbols. For example, the code for females could be F and the code for males could be M. However, we strongly urge that a completely numerical coding scheme be developed because some packaged programs cannot handle alphabetical coding.

Inherently Quantitative Variables

Although the majority of data collected in the course of a project will need to be coded, there are certain variables whose measures are directly amenable to computer analysis because they are inherently quantitative. Variables such as age, weight, body temperature, and diastolic blood pressure do not normally require coding. Sometimes the researcher may ask for information of this type in a way that does call for the development of a coding plan. If a researcher asks respondents to indicate whether they are younger than 30, between the ages of 31 and 49, or older than 50, then the responses would have to be coded before being entered into a computer file. When the responses to questions such as age, height, income level, and so forth are given in their full, natural form, then the researcher should *not* reduce the information to coded categories for data entry purposes.

Information that is "naturally" quantitative thus may need no coding whatsoever, but the researcher should inspect and edit the data before having them entered. It is important that all of the responses be of the same form and precision. For instance, in entering a person's height, the researcher would need to decide whether to use feet and inches or to convert the information entirely to inches. Whichever method is adopted, it must be used consistently for all subjects. There must also be consistency in the method of handling information reported with different degrees of precision.

Precategorized Data

Much of the data from questionnaires, interviews, observation schedules, and psychologic scales can be coded easily through precategorization. Closed-ended questions that provide for response alternatives can easily be preassigned a numerical code, as in the following example:

From what type of program did you receive your basic nursing preparation?
1. Diploma school
2. Associate degree program
3. Baccalaureate degree program

Thus, if a nurse received his or her nursing preparation from a diploma school, the response to this question would be coded "1."

In many cases the codes will be arbitrary, as in the case of a variable such as gender. Whether a female is coded 1 or 2 will have no bearing on the

subsequent analysis as long as females are consistently assigned one code and males another. Other variables will appear to have a more obvious coding scheme, as in the following example:

How often do you suffer from insomnia?
1. almost never
2. once or twice a year
3. three to eleven times a year
4. at least once a month but not weekly
5. once a week or more

Sometimes respondents may have the option of checking off more than one answer in reply to a single question, as in the following illustration:

To which of the following journals do you subscribe?
( ) American Journal of Nursing
( ) Nursing Forum
( ) Nursing Outlook
( ) Nursing Research

With questions of this type, it is incorrect to adopt a 1-2-3-4 code because subjects may check several, or none, of the responses. The most appropriate procedure for questions such as this one is to treat each journal on the list as a separate question. In other words, the researcher would code the responses as though the item were four separate questions asking, "Do you subscribe to the American Journal of Nursing? Do you subscribe to Nursing Forum? . . . " A check mark beside a journal would be treated as though the reply were "yes." In effect, the question would be turned into four dichotomous variables, with one code (perhaps "1") signifying a "yes" response and another code (perhaps "2") signifying a "no" response.

Uncategorized Data

Qualitative data from open-ended questions, unstructured observations, and other narrative forms usually are not readily amenable to direct computer analysis. When this type of information is to be analyzed by the computer, it is necessary to categorize and code it. Sometimes it is possible for the researcher to develop a coding scheme in advance of data collection. For instance, a question might ask, "What is your occupation?" If the researcher knew the sample characteristics, he or she could probably predict such major categories as "Professional," "Managerial," "Clerical," and so forth.

Usually, however, unstructured formats for data collection are adopted specifically because it is difficult to anticipate the kind of information that will be obtained. In such a situation, it is necessary to code responses after all the data are collected if a computer is to be used to analyze the information, through procedures analogous to a content analysis. The researcher typically begins by scanning a sizable portion of the data to get a feel for the nature of the content. The researcher can then proceed to develop a scheme to categorize the material. The categorization scheme should be designed to reflect both the researcher's theoretical and analytic goals as well as the substance of the information. The amount of detail in the categorization scheme can vary considerably, but the researcher should keep in mind that too much detail is better than too little detail. In developing a coding scheme for unstructured information, the only "rule" is that the coding categories should be both mutually exclusive and collectively exhaustive.

Precise instructions should always be developed for the coders, and documented in a coding manual. Coders, like observers and interviewers, must be properly trained. Intercoder reliability checks are strongly recommended.

Coding Missing Data

A code should be designated for every question or variable for every subject, even if in some cases no response or information is available. Missing data can be of various types. A person responding to an interview question may be undecided, refuse to answer, or say "Don't know." An observer coding behavior may get distracted during a 10-second sampling frame, may be undecided about an appropriate categorization, or may observe behavior not listed on the observation schedule. In some cases, it may be important to distinguish between various types of missing data by specifying separate codes, and in other cases a single code may suffice. This decision must be made with the conceptual aims of the research in mind. A person who replied "Don't know" to a question seeking to understand the public's familiarity with health maintenance organizations should probably be distinguished from the person who refused to answer the question.

Insofar as possible, it is desirable to code missing data in the same manner for all variables. If a "no response" is coded as a 4 on variable 1, a 6 on variable 2, a 5 on variable 3, and so forth, there is a greater risk of error than if a uniform code is adopted. The choice of what number to use as the missing data code is fairly arbitrary, but the number must be one that has not been assigned to an actual piece of information. Many researchers follow the convention of coding missing data as 9, because this value is normally out of the range of codes for true information. Others use blanks, zeros, or negative values to indicate missing information.

Some software packages require a specific handling of missing information. For example, the Statistical Analysis System uses periods (.) for missing values. Therefore, the researcher should decide what software will be used for data analysis before finalizing coding decisions.

☰ ENTERING CODED DATA

For most types of computer analysis, the coded data are transferred onto a disk file through a terminal or keyboard. Coded data are transferred to a computer file in accordance with a predesignated plan. The next section discusses the considerations in designing and implementing such a plan.

Preparing Data for Data Entry

In many cases, data files are set up to store 80 columns of information, analogous to an 80-column punch card. In this section, we illustrate data preparation activities based on an 80-column scheme, but it is sometimes possible to use alternative schemes, depending on the software being used.

The researcher should plan in advance of the actual data entry the layout of information within the 80 columns. It is usually preferable to adopt what is known as a *fixed format,* which places the values for any specific variable in the same column for every case. Some packaged programs also permit data to be entered in a *free format,* in which there is no necessary correspondence between the variables entered in any particular column from one case to the next, although the variables are always in the same order. We recommend using a fixed format because many programs require it and checking for errors is easier.

With fixed format the researcher must specify in which columns all of the data are to be entered. Many variables will require no more than one column. If a variable has a code whose maximum value is one digit, then the variable can be assigned to a single column. Examples include variables whose responses are agree/disagree and yes/no/maybe. Other variables, such as age, weight, and blood pressure measures, must occupy more than one column. Anytime the maximum value of a variable exceeds 9, the researcher must be sure to reserve two (or more, if the number is larger than 99) columns. The space allocated to a particular variable is referred to as a *field.*

The researcher must be careful in dealing with a variable whose values may be of different widths. For example, if we were recording a person's weight, we would need only two digits for people weighing under 100 pounds, but three digits for those weighing 100 pounds or more. Because the maximum value would be three digits long, then three columns on the card would be required for all subjects. To record the weight of a 95-pound person, we would have to occupy the full three columns, so it would be necessary to enter 095. This procedure is known as *right-justifying* the data. Whenever a number smaller than the corresponding field is entered in fixed format, the number should be entered as far to the right as possible in the designated field. In the example, if columns 11, 12, and 13 were reserved for the weight measurement, 95 should be entered in columns 12 and 13. If, instead, 95 were entered in columns 11 and 12, then the value would be read as 950.

In designing the layout for the data, the researcher should allocate space for recording an identification number. Each individual case (i.e., the information from a single questionnaire, test, observation, and so forth) should be assigned a unique identifying number, and this number should be entered along with the actual data. This procedure permits the investigator to go back to the original source if there are any difficulties with the data file. The numbering is completely arbitrary and is used only as a label.

Usually, a consecutive numbering scheme is used, running from number 1 to the number of actual cases. The identification number normally is entered in the first columns of the record. If there are fewer than 100 subjects, then the first two columns are used, starting with subjects 01, 02, and so on. As in the case of other variables, the field width is determined by the maximum value of the identification number.

The researcher will often find that a single 80-column format is insufficient for recording all of the information obtained from a single case. There is no restriction on the number of records (lines) that may be used for a given case or subject. In fact, it is quite common to require multiple lines to enter all of the data for each subject. When multiple records are needed, the identification number for a particular case is often entered onto all records for that case. The researcher often enters a number identifying the order of the records within a case. That is, the first record of a case would be identified with a "1," the second card with a "2," and so forth. The record sequence number is often entered either immediately after the identification (ID) number, or in column 80.

A number of procedures are available to facilitate the actual data entry process. The first is to transfer codes from the original source (such as a questionnaire) onto a specially prepared coding sheet. These sheets, which are available commercially, are ruled off into a grid with 80 columns and 20 to 40 rows. The columns correspond to the columns in a data file, and each row represents a single record. The researcher can use these sheets to write numbers representing the desired codes in the appropriate columns.

A second procedure is to use a margin on the original source to write the appropriate numerical codes for the data entry person to follow. This *edge-coding* scheme may lead to fewer errors than the use of code sheets because the coder does not have to worry about losing his or her place in going back and forth between the original source and the code sheets. However, edge coding can also create problems because the coder inadvertently might fail to code a variable. Data entry from edge-coded materials usually proceeds more slowly than from coding sheets because the person entering must stop to turn pages and must pay attention to whether or not the data are being entered in the correct columns.

Other procedures exist for transferring data to computer files. Sometimes it is possible to enter data directly from an original source without edge coding if the source has been designed properly. Optical scanning sheets can, in some cases, be used to avoid manual data entry altogether.

Data Entry and Verification

The data entry operation can begin after the layout scheme has been developed and the codes have been specified for each variable. Data entry is a tedious and exacting task that is usually subject to numerous errors. Therefore, it is necessary to verify or check the entries to correct the mistakes that are inevitably made. Several verification procedures exist. The first is to visually compare the numbers printed on a printout of the data file with the codes on either the original source or the coding sheets. A second possibility is to enter all of the data twice and to compare the two sets of records. The comparison can be done either visually or with the assistance of the computer. Finally,

there are special verifying programs that are designed to perform comparisons during direct data entry. The use of such verification is recommended as the best method for eliminating data entry inaccuracies.

Data Cleaning

Even after the records are verified, the data usually contain a few errors. These errors could be the result of data entry mistakes but could also arise from coding or reporting problems. Data are not ready for analysis until they have been cleaned. Data cleaning involves two types of checks. The first is a check for *outliers* or wild codes. One procedure involves using a computer printout of the frequency counts associated with every value for every variable, and checking for undefined code values. The variable gender might have the following three defined code values: 1 for female, 2 for male, and 9 for not reported. If it were discovered that a code of 5 were entered in the column designated for the gender variable, then it would be clear that an error had been made. The computer could be instructed to list the ID number of the culpable record, and the error could be corrected by checking the appropriate code on the original source. Another procedure is to use a program for data entry that automatically performs range checks.

Editing of this type, of course, will never reveal mistakes that look "respectable" or plausible. If the gender of a male is entered incorrectly as a 1, then the mistake may never be detected. Because errors can have a profound effect on the analysis and interpretation of data, it is naturally quite important to perform the coding, entering, verifying, and cleaning with great care.

The second data-cleaning procedure involves performing *consistency checks,* which focus on internal data consistencies. In this task, the researcher looks for data entry or coding errors by testing whether data in one part of a record are compatible with data in another part. For example, one question in a questionnaire might ask respondents their current marital status and another might ask how many times they had been married. If the data were internally consistent, then the subjects who responded "Single, never married" to the first question should have a zero entered in the field for the second. As another example, if the respondent's sex were entered with the code for male and there was an entry of "2" for the variable "number of pregnancies," then one of those two fields would contain an error. The researcher should identify a number of such opportunities for checking the consistency of entered data.

Once the data have been cleaned to the researcher's satisfaction, a backup copy of the data file should be made immediately as a protection against loss or damage. The duplicate copy can be stored in a safe place, using any external storage medium such as magnetic tape, disk, or diskette.

Documentation

The decisions that a researcher makes concerning coding, field width, placement of data in columns, and so on should be documented in full. Documentation is essential for the proper handling of any data set. The researcher's own memory should not be trusted to store all of the required information. Several weeks after coding, the researcher may no longer remember if males were coded 1 and females 2, or vice versa. Moreover, colleagues may wish to borrow the data set to perform a secondary analysis. Whether one anticipates a secondary analysis or not, documentation should be sufficiently thorough so that a person unfamiliar with the original research project could use the data.

A major portion of the documentation involves the preparation of a codebook. A *codebook* is essentially a listing of each variable, the column(s) in which the variable has been entered, and the codes associated with the various aspects or attributes of the variable. The codebook is often prepared before coding so that it can be used as a guide by coders. In the next section, we present an example of a codebook. If the data are stored on a magnetic tape file, information concerning access to that file should also be prepared.

A Hypothetical Example of Coding/Cleaning

The concepts and recommendations presented thus far in this chapter can be best understood by reference to a detailed example. Figure 26-1 presents a questionnaire that was contrived to illustrate many of the points made in the preceding sections. This hypothetical instrument should not be taken as an example of good questionnaire design. The intent was to include a variety of item types to demonstrate how different coding problems could be handled.

On the left-hand margin of the questionnaire are the numerical codes to be transferred to a computer file. The first code—001—represents the ID number assigned to the respondent who completed the questionnaire. The three-digit number implies that at least 100 (but fewer than 1000) respondents participated in the study. Following the ID number are the codes corresponding to the subject's responses. In the second part of question 2, the missing values code of 9 signifies that the subject skipped over the question. With regard to question 5, each individual symptom is treated for data analysis purposes as a separate question, with a check of "X" being coded as "1" and no check coded as "2." Note that the subject's height, reported in question 10, has been converted into inches.

The data entry person using edge-coded questionnaires such as this would simply follow the numbers in the left margin, entering them in consecutive columns. To illustrate an alternative to edge coding, the same data have been transferred to the coding sheet presented in Figure 26-2. As this figure shows, the code sheets specify precisely the column in which each numerical code is to be entered. The total number of columns required to store the information from this fictitious questionnaire is 31. If there were 150 respondents, then there would be 150 records, all with information in the first 31 columns.

The example presented here involves a sim-

001	This questionnaire is part of a study on health-related habits and attitudes. We hope you will help us by answering the following questions.

1. Overall, how would you describe your health in comparison with that of others your age?

2
( ) above average health
(x) average health
( ) below average health

2. Have you been hospitalized within the past two years?

2
( ) yes ⎯⎯⎯⎯⎯⎯⎯⎯⎯⎯⎯⎯⎯↓
(x) no

If yes: how many times have you been hospitalized?
9
( ) once
( ) two times
( ) more than two times

3. Do you smoke cigarettes?

1
(x) yes ⎯⎯⎯⎯⎯⎯⎯⎯⎯⎯⎯↓
( ) no

If yes, how many cigarettes do you usually smoke per day?
1
(x) 1 pack or less
( ) between one and two packs
( ) two packs or more

4. How often do you drink alcoholic beverages?

4
( ) never   (x) 2 or 3 times a month
( ) 10 times a year or less   ( ) about once a week
( ) about once a month   ( ) several times a week
                            ( ) nearly every day

5. Below is a list of some common somatic complaints. Please check off those symptoms which have bothered you within the past month or so.

1 (x) headache
2 ( ) indigestion
1 (x) constipation
2 ( ) diarrhea
2 ( ) insomnia
2 ( ) lower back pains
2 ( ) lack of appetite

6. Which of the following statements best describes your health care practices?

( ) I go for regular physical checkups as a preventive health care measure.
2 (x) I see a health care professional only when I have a specific complaint.
( ) I have to be extremely ill before I will see a health care professional.

7. Please indicate how important the following things are to you by placing an "X" under the appropriate column:

		Extremely important	Somewhat important	Not too important
1	Abundant leisure time	X		
3	A long life			X
2	Financial success and security		X	
1	Good family relationships	X		
2	Good health		X	
2	Lots of friends, popularity		X	

38 8. What is your present age? ___38___ years.
135 9. How much do you weigh? ___135___ pounds.
66 10. How tall are you? ___5___ feet, ___6___ inches.
1 11. What is your sex?
(x) female
( ) male

Figure 26-1. *Example of a questionnaire with edge coding.*

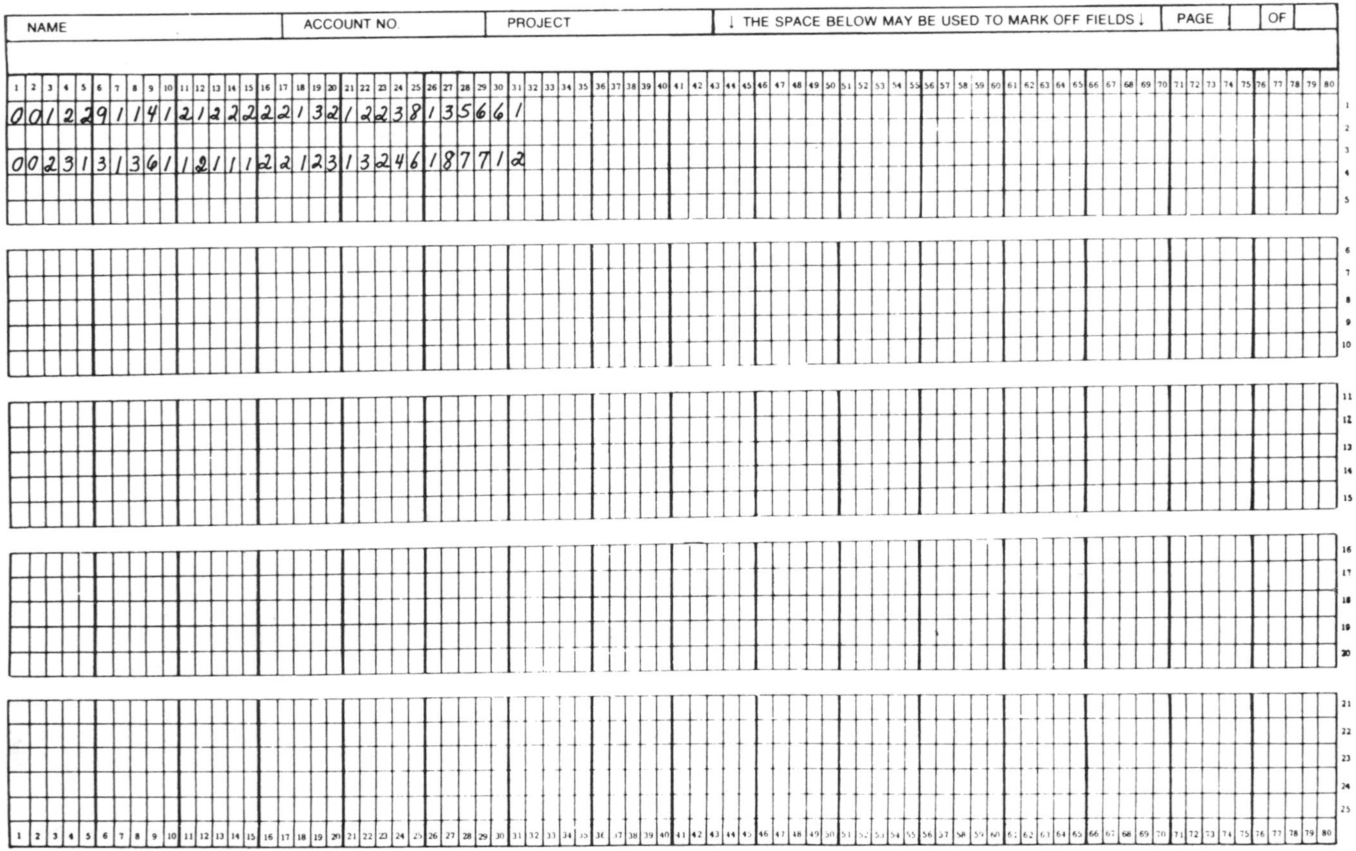

Figure 26-2. *Example of a coding sheet.*

ple and straightforward coding scheme. Because all the questions are closed-ended, there is little confusion or ambiguity concerning how to code the various responses. Even for uncomplicated data, it is a good practice to develop a codebook. The preparation of a codebook is not time consuming and represents a permanent record of the researcher's major data preparation decisions. An example of a codebook setup is shown in Figure 26-3, which includes the information for the first four questions of this example only.

The example can also be used to illustrate data cleaning. Figure 26-4 presents a computer listing of the frequency counts corresponding to all values entered for question 3, "Do you smoke cigarettes?" Of the 150 cases, 76 responses were entered as "1" or "yes" and 68 responses were entered as "2" or "no." Three respondents appar-

Card Column	Variable Description and Codes	Question Number
1-3	Respondent Identification Number (001 to 150)	
4	"Overall, how would you describe your health in comparison with that of others your age?" 1. above average health 2. average health 3. below average health 9. no response	1
5	"Have you been hospitalized within the past two years?" 1. yes 2. no 9. no response	2
6	"If yes: how many times have you been hospitalized?" 1. once 2. two times 3. more than two times 9. no response	2
7	"Do you smoke cigarettes?" 1. yes 2. no 9. no response	3
8	"If yes: how many cigarettes do you usually smoke per day?" 1. 1 pack or less 2. between one and two packs 3. two packs or more 9. no response	3
9	"How often do you drink alcoholic beverages?" 1. never 2. 10 times a year or less 3. about once a month 4. 2 to 3 times per month 5. about once a week 6. several times a week 7. nearly every day 9. no response	4

Figure 26-3. *Example of a section of a codebook.*

```
9-DEC-85    SPSS-X RELEASE 2.1 FOR VAX/VMS
15:31:09    BOSTON COLLEGE VAXCLUSTER          DEC VAX-11/780 VMS V4.1


SMOKE      DO YOU SMOKE CIGARETTES?
```

| | | | | VALID | CUM |
| | | | | VALID | CUM |
VALUE LABEL	VALUE	FREQUENCY	PERCENT	PERCENT	PERCENT
YES	1	76	50.7	51.7	51.7
NO	2	68	45.3	46.3	98.0
	3	2	1.3	1.4	99.3
	8	1	.7	.7	100.0
	9	3	2.0	MISSING	
	TOTAL	150	100.0	100.0	

```
MEAN        1.537    STD ERR      .062    MEDIAN      1.000
MODE        1.000    STD DEV      .752    VARIANCE     .565
KURTOSIS   36.298    S E KURT     .397    SKEWNESS    4.428
S E SKEW     .200    RANGE       7.000    MINIMUM     1.000
MAXIMUM     8.000    SUM       226.000


VALID CASES     147     MISSING CASES        3
```

Figure 26-4. *Hypothetical data for data cleaning example.*

ently failed to answer the question (entered as "9"). The printout tells us that, in two cases, a "3" was incorrectly entered for question 3, and in one case, an "8" was entered. This computer listing has informed us that there are errors on three records in column 7. We could now go through the data file—either manually, with a printout, or by the computer—to find the three records in question. The records would indicate the ID number of the questionnaires to be rechecked, and the necessary corrections could then be made.

≡ DATA TRANSFORMATIONS

Raw data entered directly onto a computer file often need to be modified or transformed before the hypotheses can be tested using statistical analysis. *Data transformations* can be of various types, and can easily be handled directly through instructions to the computer. We present several examples of such transformations in this section.

Sometimes response codes to certain items need to be completely reversed (i.e., high values becoming low, and vice versa, often for the purposes of combining items in scale construction).* Other transformations involve the construction of composite scales or indices, created by combining responses to several individual variables. The software packages described in Chapter 25 all have the ability to create totally new variables through arithmetic manipulations of variables in the original data set. For example, with the Statistical Package for the Social Sciences (SPSS^x) a 6-item Likert scale could be created with the following command:

COMPUTE SELFCARE = Q1 + Q2 +
(6 − Q3) + Q4 + (6 − Q5) + Q6

where the original values of items 1, 2, 4,

*For example, to reverse a 5-category Likert scale item, one would instruct the computer to set the value of the variable equal to 6 minus the original value. This would transform the value of 1 to 5, 2 to 4, and so on.

and 6, and the reversed values of items 3 and 5, would be combined to form a new variable labeled SELFCARE.

Other transformations involve recoded values. For example, in some analyses, an infant's original birthweight (entered on the computer files in grams) might be used as a dependent variable. In other analyses, however, the researcher might be interested in comparing the subsequent morbidity of low birthweight versus normal birthweight infants. In SPSS, a command such as the following could be used to recode the original variable (BWEIGHT) into a dichotomous variable with a code of 1 for a low birthweight infant and a code of 2 for a normal weight infant, based on whether the baby weighed less than 2500 g:

    RECODE BWEIGHT (LOWEST THRU 2500 = 1)
        (2501 THRU HIGHEST = 2)

Sometimes data transformations are necessary for the data to be meaningfully interpreted. For example, children's raw scores on a test may be uninterpretable unless the scores are standardized by age. In this situation, the researcher would need to transform the raw scores into standard scores (see Chapter 22) by using the means and standard deviations (SDs) for children of different ages. For example, the following SPSS commands would create standard scores with a mean of 0 and an SD of 1 for children in three different age groups, with different average scores and SDs:

    IF (CHILDAGE EQ 6) FEARSS =
        (FEAR − 15.0)/2.0
    IF (CHILDAGE EQ 7) FEARSS =
        (FEAR − 18.0)/2.5
    IF (CHILDAGE EQ 8) FEARSS =
        (FEAR − 20.5)/3.0

Thus, if a 6-year-old child's score on a scale named "FEAR" were 18.0, then the child's standardized score on this scale (FEARSS) would be 1.5 ($18 − 15 = 3$; $3 ÷ 2.0 = 1.5$); but if the child were 7 years old, a raw score of 18.0 would yield a standard score of 0 ($18 − 18 = 0$; $0 ÷ 2.5 = 0$).

Transformations are also undertaken to render data appropriate for certain statistical tests. For example, most parametric statistical tests assume that the distribution of values on a variable is normal. Parametric tests are fairly robust and can tolerate mild violations to the underlying assumptions. However, if a distribution is markedly non-normal, then a transformation may be needed to make the use of the powerful parametric procedures appropriate. A logarithmic transformation, for example, often tends to normalize the distribution. For example, in $SPSS^x$, the command that would be used to normalize the distribution of values on family income (which is often highly skewed) would be

COMPUTE INCLOG = LN(INCOME)

The new variable, INCLOG is actually the natural log of the original values on the INCOME variable; INCLOG would then be used in statistical tests in place of INCOME. Discussions of the use of transformations for changing the characteristics of a distribution may be found in Dixon and Massey (1969).

Whenever researchers create transformed or recoded variables, it is wise to check that the computer is performing the intended manipulation by examining a sample of values for the original and transformed variables. When transformed and recoded variables become an integral part of the researcher's data set, the researcher should remember to carefully document the transformations in the codebook.

≡ OTHER PREPARATORY ACTIVITIES

In addition to handling data transformations, researchers often undertake other activities before they can begin their main analyses. Although a comprehensive discussion of such activities is not possible in this introductory text, we do identify the following major activities and point readers toward useful references:

* *Handling missing data.* Researchers almost always find that their data set has missing

information on some variables for a subset of subjects. If the sample is large and the number of missing cases on a specific variable is small, then the missing data should not cause a problem. However, because many samples in nursing studies are small, missing data often cause considerable concern. A number of strategies have been used to deal with this situation: (1) deletion of the missing cases; (2) deletion of the variable with extensive missing cases; (3) substitution of the mean value on the variable for those cases with missing values; (4) estimation of the missing values using, for example, multiple regression; and (5) pairwise deletion of cases (e.g., the calculation of correlations based on all available data, with varying number of pairs for each coefficient). Each of these solutions has accompanying problems, so care should be taken in deciding how the missing data are to be handled. Procedures for dealing with missing data are discussed in Cohen and Cohen (1975) and Little and Rubin (1990).

- *Other assessments of data quality.* Other steps are often undertaken to assess the quality of data in the early stage of the analyses. For example, when psychosocial scales or composite indices are used, the researcher should generally assess the reliability of the measures (see Chapter 18). The distribution of data values for key variables also should be examined to determine any anomalies, such as limited variability, extreme skewness, or the presence of "ceiling" or "floor" effects (e.g., the use of a developmental test appropriate for 10-year-olds would yield a clustering of high scores for 12-year-olds, but a clustering of low scores for 8-year-olds). As described previously, the data may need to be transformed to meet the requirements for certain statistical tests.

- *Assessment of bias.* Before proceeding to the main analyses, researchers often undertake preliminary analyses designed to assess the direction and extent of any biases. For example, to determine whether a biased subset of the population volunteered to participate in a

study, the researcher may be able to compare the characteristics of those who did and did not volunteer. When a nonequivalent control group design is used (in a quasi-experimental or *ex post facto* study), the researcher should always check for selection biases by comparing the background characteristics of the groups. In longitudinal studies, it is always important to check for attrition biases, which involves a comparison of people who did and did not continue to participate in the study in later waves of data collection, based on characteristics of these two groups at the initial wave. In all of these cases, significant group differences are an indication of bias, and such biases must be taken into consideration in interpreting the results.[†]

≡ *PHASES IN THE ANALYSIS OF QUANTITATIVE DATA*

As the preceding discussion suggests, the processing of quantitative data normally proceeds through a number of different phases. The phases and the steps within the phases may vary from one project to another. For example, if a computer is not used, or if the data set is an extremely simple one, then the researcher may be able to proceed fairly quickly from the collection to the analysis of the data. Figure 26-5 summarizes what the flow of tasks might look like when a researcher uses a computer, and when the final analyses involve the use of complex multivariate statistical procedures. Progress in the analysis of data may not always be as linear as this figure suggests, however. For example, complications in the final phase may require some backtracking if a more fine-tuned analysis of data quality seems warranted.

[†] For certain types of bias, there are statistical procedures for correcting the bias, but these sophisticated two-stage regression techniques are beyond the scope of this book. Advanced students are advised to consult an econometrics text for a description of the *Heckman procedure* and other correction techniques.

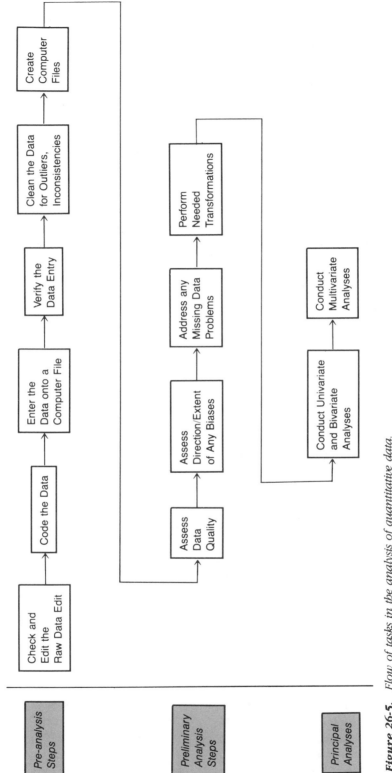

Figure 26-5. *Flow of tasks in the analysis of quantitative data.*

Pre-analysis Steps

Check and Edit the Raw Data Edit → Code the Data → Enter the Data onto a Computer File → Verify the Data Entry → Clean the Data for Outliers, Inconsistencies → Create Computer Files

Preliminary Analysis Steps

Assess Data Quality → Assess Direction/Extent of Any Biases → Address any Missing Data Problems → Perform Needed Transformations

Principal Analyses

Conduct Univariate and Bivariate Analyses → Conduct Multivariate Analyses

≡ SUMMARY

The focus of this chapter was on the preparation of data for statistical analysis. These preparatory activities include editing the data and preparing the data for entry onto computer files, evaluating data quality, and manipulating the data in various ways.

Information collected in a research project must be converted to machine-readable form if a computer is to be used. *Coding* is the procedure of transforming research data into symbols compatible with computer analysis. Preferably, the coding scheme adopted is completely numerical. If the data are inherently quantitative (such as a person's weight), or if a precategorization scheme was used to collect the data, then the coding task is straightforward. For uncategorized data, such as responses to open-ended questions, a coding system must be developed for analytic purposes. Special codes should be developed to signify missing data.

The researcher usually must plan in advance the layout of information on an 80-column record. In a *fixed-format* arrangement, which is commonly used for research data, each variable is entered onto the same column for every case. The width of the *field* (the space allocated to a particular variable) is determined by the maximum numerical value for that variable. The data should always be *right-justified,* or entered as far to the right as possible in the designated field. The researcher may transfer the codes from the original source onto specially prepared *coding sheets* or may use an *edge-coding* scheme, in which the numerical codes to be entered are written onto the margin of the original source. The researcher should document the decisions made concerning the coding, field placement, and the naming of variables. A fairly standard procedure is the preparation of a *codebook* that serves as a comprehensive, permanent record of the researcher's data processing decisions.

The next step is *data entry* onto an input medium, a task that is susceptible to a high error rate. Entered data, therefore, should be checked or *verified* for errors. Even after the data are veri-fied, they almost inevitably contain a few errors. Because of this fact, data should be *cleaned* before proceeding with any analyses. The cleaning process is primarily a check for *outliers* or numerical values that are not part of the coding scheme, and a check for internal consistency.

Raw data entered directly onto a computer file often need to be modified for analysis. *Data transformations* can be of many types, and are usually handled directly through commands to the computer. Examples of transformations include combining individual variables to form a composite scale, reversing the coding of a variable, recoding the values of a variable, obtaining standardized scores on a variable, and performing mathematical transformations for analytic purposes.

Finally, before the main analyses can proceed, the researcher usually has to undertake a number of steps to assess data quality and to maximize the value of the data. These steps include evaluating the extent of missing data and developing strategies to address missing data problems, evaluating the reliability of measures, examining the distribution of values on key variables for any anomalies, and analyzing the magnitude and direction of any biases.

≡ STUDY SUGGESTIONS

1. Prepare a codebook for the questionnaire (Nursing Research Subscriber Profile) presented on pages 64–65 of the 1984 volume (volume 33) of *Nursing Research.*
2. Complete the questionnaire referenced in study suggestion 1. Code your responses and transfer them to a coding sheet.
3. If you have access to a terminal, enter the data from the hypothetical example presented in this chapter. Enter the data from both the edge-coded questionnaire and the coding sheet. Compare the amount of time spent on each. Verify your data entry by checking for discrepancies on the two records.
4. What field width would you need for the following variables: marital status, annual income, body temperature, number of chil-

dren, white blood cell count, religious affiliation, days absent from work, Apgar score, time to first voiding, and pulse rate?

≡ *SUGGESTED READINGS*

Babbie, E.R. (1973). *Survey research methods.* Belmont, CA: Wadsworth. (Chapter 10).

Barhyte, D., & Bacon, L.D. (1985). Approaches to cleaning data sets. *Nursing Research, 34,* 62–65.

Cohen, J., & Cohen, P. (1975). *Applied multiple regression/correlation analysis for the behavioral sciences.* New York: John Wiley and Sons.

Dixon, W.J., & Massey, F.J. (1969). *Introduction to statistical analysis* (3rd ed.) New York: McGraw-Hill. (Chapter 16).

Harris, M.L. (1979). *Introduction to data processing* (2nd ed.). New York: John Wiley and Sons. (Chapters 1–3).

Jacobsen, B.S. (1981). Know thy data. *Nursing Research, 30,* 254–255.

Kim, J., & Curry, J. (1977). The treatment of missing data in multivariate analysis. In D.F. Alwin (Ed.), *Survey design and analysis.* Beverly Hills, CA: Sage.

Little, R.J.A., & Rubin, D.B. (1990). The analysis of social science data with missing values. In J. Fox & J.S. Long (Eds.), *Modern methods of data analysis.* Newbury Park, CA: Sage.

Marls, R.G. (1982). *Designing a research project: The basics of biomedical research methodology.* Belmont, CA: Life Long Learning.

Norusis, M.J. (1988). *The SPSS guide to data analysis.* Chicago, IL: SPSS, Inc.

Selltiz, C., Wrightsman, L.S., & Cook, S.W. (1976). *Research methods in social relations* (3rd ed.). New York: Holt, Rinehart & Winston. (Chapters 13 & 14).

Sorin, M.D. (1982). *Data entry without keypunching: Improved preparation for social data analysis.* Lexington, MA: Lexington Books.

Tabachnick, B.G., & Fidell, L.S. (1983). *Using multivariate statistics.* New York: Harper & Row. (Chapter 4).

Part VI

Communi-
cation
in the
Research
Process

27
Interpreting and Reporting Research Results

The final stages of a research project, like the beginning stages, are often more difficult than the intermediary steps of data collection and analysis. The interpretation and communication of the research results cannot be done mechanically by following methodological techniques that may at first seem cumbersome but that can be learned. To be sure, research skills are required for interpreting and reporting the findings of a study, but there is also a need for creativity, intellectual insights, logical reasoning, and theoretical grounding. These are not attributes that can be learned in a textbook. This chapter offers general guidelines for helping the researcher with the final steps in the scientific process, but it should be recognized that these guidelines tell only half the story of this challenging task.

≡ *INTERPRETATION OF RESULTS*

The analysis of research data provides what are referred to as the "results" of the study. These results need to be evaluated and interpreted by the researcher with due consideration to the overall aims of the project, its theoretical underpinnings, the specific hypotheses being tested, the existing body of related research knowledge, and the limitations of the adopted research methods.

The interpretive task primarily involves a consideration of five aspects of the study findings: (1) their accuracy, (2) their meaning, (3) their importance, (4) the extent to which they can be generalized, and (5) their implications. In this section, we review issues relating to each of these five aspects.

The Accuracy of the Results

One of the first tasks that the researcher faces in interpreting the results is assessing whether the findings are likely to be accurate. This assessment, in turn, requires a careful analysis of the study's methodological and conceptual limitations. Whether one's hypotheses are supported or not, the validity and meaning of the results depend on a full understanding of the study's shortcomings.

Such an assessment relies heavily on the researcher's critical thinking skills, as well as on an ability to be reasonably objective about one's own decisions. The researcher should carefully evaluate (using, for example, criteria such as those that we present in Chapter 28) all of the major methodological decisions made in planning and executing the study to determine whether alternative decisions might have yielded different results.

The assessment of accuracy, however, also depends on the ability of the researcher to assemble different types of evidence. One type of evidence is the body of prior research on the topic. The investigator should examine whether his or her results are consistent with those of other studies; if there are discrepancies, a careful analysis of the reasons for any differences should be undertaken.

Other types of evidence can often be developed through peripheral data analyses, some of which were discussed in Chapter 26. For example, the researcher needs to carefully assess the quality of the data collected, the reliability of measures used, and the presence or absence of any biases. Another highly recommended strategy in quantitative studies is the conduct of a power analysis. In Chapter 22, we described how power analysis is often used before a study is undertaken to estimate sample size requirements. However, the researcher who determines the actual power of his or her own analyses is in a good position to assess whether a Type II error has been committed. It is especially important to perform a power analysis when the results of the main hypothesis tests were not statistically significant.

A critical analysis of the research methods and conceptualization and an examination of various types of external and internal evidence will almost inevitably indicate some limitations. These limitations must be taken into account in interpreting the results.

The Meaning of the Results

In qualitative studies, interpretation and analysis occur virtually simultaneously. In quantitative studies, however, the results are in the form of test statistic values and probability levels. It is the researcher's role to imbue these results with meaning. In this section, we discuss the interpretation of various types of research outcomes within a hypothesis testing context. If the research was conceived on the basis of a theory or conceptual model, then it is important to relate the findings to that theoretical framework. That is, if a theoretical framework was truly the basis for the study, then it should also provide a basis for trying to understand the data.

INTERPRETING HYPOTHESIZED RESULTS

When the tests of statistical significance support the original research hypotheses, the task of interpreting the results is somewhat easier than when the hypotheses are challenged. In a sense, the interpretation has been partly accomplished beforehand in such a situation, because the researcher has already had to bring together prior research findings, a theoretical framework, and logical reasoning in the development of the hypotheses. This groundwork can then form the context within which more specific interpretations are made.

Naturally, researchers are gratified when the results of many hours of effort offer support for their predictions. There is a very decided preference on the part of individual researchers, advisers, and journal reviewers for studies whose hypotheses have been supported. This preference is understandable, but it is important not to let personal predilections interfere with the critical appraisal that is appropriate in all interpretive situations. A few cautionary suggestions should be kept in mind.

First, it is preferable to be somewhat conservative in drawing conclusions from the data. The intrusion of personal viewpoints and subjective judgments is inevitable in making sense of research results, but they must be held in check as much as possible. It is sometimes tempting to go far beyond the data in developing explanations for what the results mean, but conscientious scientists avoid doing so. A simple example might help to explain what is meant by "going beyond the data." Suppose a nurse researcher hypothesized that a relationship existed between a pregnant woman's level of anxiety about the labor and delivery experience and the number of children she has already borne. The data reveal that a negative relationship between anxiety levels and parity ($r = -.40$) does indeed exist. The researcher, therefore, concludes that increased experience with childbirth causes decreasing amounts of anxiety. Is this conclusion supported by the data? The conclusion appears to be logical but, in fact, there is nothing within the data that leads directly to this interpretation. An important, indeed critical, research precept is: *Correlation does not prove causation.* The finding that two variables are related offers no evidence suggesting which of the two variables—if either—caused the other. In the example, perhaps causality runs in the opposite direction, that is, that a woman's anxiety level influences how many children she bears. Or perhaps a third variable not examined in the study, such as the woman's social supports, "causes" or influences both anxiety and number of children.

Alternative explanations for the findings should always be considered. If these competing interpretations can be ruled out on the basis of the data or previous research findings, so much the better. However, every angle should be examined to see if one's pet explanation has been given adequate competition. Any evidence from the researcher's assessment of bias and data quality should be brought to bear at this point.

The support of research hypotheses with empirical evidence never constitutes proof of their veracity. Hypothesis testing, as we have seen, is probabilistic. There always remains a possibility that the obtained relationships resulted

from chance or from some artifact of the research methods.

Therefore, one must be tentative about both the results and the interpretations given to those results. In sum, even when the findings are in line with expectations, the researcher should exercise restraint in drawing conclusions and should give due consideration to any limitations identified in the assessment of the accuracy of the results.

INTERPRETING NONSIGNIFICANT RESULTS

Failure to reject a null hypothesis is particularly problematic from an interpretative point of view. The statistical procedures currently prevalent are geared toward disconfirmation of the null hypothesis. The failure to reject a null hypothesis could occur for one or more reasons, and the researcher does not usually know which of these reasons pertains. First, the null hypothesis could actually be true. The nonsignificant result, in this case, would accurately reflect the absence of a relationship among the research variables. On the other hand, the null hypothesis could be false, in which case a Type II error would have been committed.

The retention of a false null hypothesis can be attributed to several things, such as internal validity problems, the selection of a deviant sample, the use of a weak statistical procedure, or the use of too small a sample. Unless the researcher has special justification for attributing the nonsignificant findings to one of these factors, interpreting such results is a tricky business. However, we suspect that in the majority of cases, the failure to reject the null hypothesis is the consequence of insufficient power (usually reflecting too small a sample size). For this reason, the conduct of a power analysis can often come to the researcher's aid in interpretation when nonsignificant results are obtained.

In any event, there is never justification for interpreting a retained null hypothesis as proof of a *lack* of relationship among variables. *The safest interpretation is that nonsignificant findings represent a lack of evidence for either truth or falsity of the hypothesis.* Thus, one can see that if the researcher's actual research hypothesis states that no differences or no relationships will be observed, traditional hypothesis testing procedures will not permit the required inferences.

When no significant results are found, there is sometimes a tendency to be overcritical of one's research strategy and methods and undercritical of the theory or logical reasoning on which the hypotheses were based. This is understandable: it is easier to say "My ideas were sound, I just didn't use the right approach to demonstrate this" than to admit that one has reasoned incorrectly. It is important to look for and identify flaws in the research methods, but it is equally important to search for theoretical shortcomings. The result of such endeavors should be recommendations for how the methods or theory could be improved.

INTERPRETING UNHYPOTHESIZED SIGNIFICANT RESULTS

There probably is nothing more perplexing to a researcher than to obtain results opposite to those hypothesized. For instance, a nurse researcher might hypothesize that individualized patient teaching of breathing techniques is more effective than group instruction, but the results might reflect that the group method was better. Or a positive relationship might be predicted between a nurse's age and level of job satisfaction but a negative relationship might be found.

It should go without saying that it is unethical to alter the hypothesis after the results are in. Although some researchers may view such situations as awkward or embarrassing, there is really little basis for such feelings. The purpose of research is not to corroborate the scientist's notions, but to arrive at truth and enhance understanding. There is no such thing as a study whose results "came out the wrong way," if the "wrong way" is the truth.

In the case of unhypothesized significant findings, it is less likely, though not impossible, that the methods are flawed than that the reasoning or theory is incorrect. As always, the interpretation that the researcher gives to the findings should involve comparisons with other research,

a consideration of alternate theories, and a critical scrutiny of the data collection and analysis procedures. The final result of such an examination should be a tentative explanation for the unexpected findings, together with suggestions for how such explanations could be tested in other research projects.

INTERPRETING MIXED RESULTS

The interpretive process is often confounded by mixed results. The investigator may find some hypotheses supported by the data and others that cannot be supported. Or a hypothesis may be accepted when one measure of the dependent variable is used but rejected when using a separate measure of the same variable. Of all the situations mentioned, mixed results are probably the most prevalent.

When only some results run counter to a theoretical position or conceptual scheme, the research methods are probably the first aspect of the study deserving scrutiny. Differences in the validity and reliability of the various measures could account for such discrepancies, for example. On the other hand, mixed results could be indicative of how a theory needs to be qualified, or of how certain constructs within the theory need to be reconceptualized. Mixed results often present opportunities for making conceptual advances because close scrutiny and attempts to make sense of disparate pieces of evidence may lead to breakthroughs that otherwise might have been impossible. This point was elaborated on more fully in Chapter 24 on integrating qualitative and quantitative data.

In summary, the interpretation of research findings is a demanding task, but offers the possibility of unique intellectual rewards. The researcher must in essence play the role of a scientific detective, trying to make pieces of the puzzle fit together so that a coherent picture emerges.

The Importance of the Results

In quantitative studies, results in support of the researcher's hypotheses are described as being significant. A careful analysis of the results of a study involves an evaluation of whether, in addition to being statistically significant, they are important.

The fact that statistical significance was attained in testing the hypothesis does not necessarily mean that the results were of value to the nursing community and their clients. Statistical significance indicates that the results were unlikely to be a function of chance. This means that the observed group differences or observed relationships were probably real, but not necessarily important. With large samples, even modest relationships are statistically significant. For instance with a sample of 500, a correlation coefficient of .10 is significant at the .05 level, but a relationship of this magnitude might have little practical value. Researchers, therefore, must pay attention to the numerical values obtained in an analysis in addition to the significance level when assessing the implications of the findings.

The absence of statistically significant results does not mean that the results are unimportant—although because of the difficulty in interpreting nonsignificant results, the case is more complex. However, let us suppose that the study involved testing two alternative procedures for making a clinical assessment (e.g., body temperature). Suppose that a researcher retained the null hypothesis, that is, found no statistically significant differences between the two methods. If a power analysis revealed an extremely low probability of a Type II error (e.g., power = .99, a 1% risk of a Type II error), then the researcher might be justified in concluding that the two procedures yield equally accurate assessments. If one of these procedures was more efficient or less painful than the other, then the nonsignificant findings could indeed be clinically very important.

The Generalizability of the Results

Another aspect of the results that the researcher should carefully assess is their generalizability. Researchers are rarely interested in discovering relationships among variables for a specific group of people at a specific point in time. The aim of research is typically to reveal enduring relationships, the understanding of which can be used to improve the human condition. If a nursing intervention under investigation is found to be successful, others will want to adopt the procedure. Therefore, an important interpretive question is whether the intervention will "work" or whether the relationships will "hold" in other settings, with other people. Part of the interpretive process involves asking the question, "To what groups, environments, and conditions can the results of the study be applied?"

The Implications of the Results

Once the researcher has formed conclusions about the accuracy, meaning, importance, and generalizability of the results, he or she is in a good position to draw inferences about the implications of the results and to make recommendations for how best to use and build on the study findings. The researcher often considers the implications with respect to future research endeavors, theory development, and nursing practice.

The results of one study are often used as a springboard for additional research, and the investigator is typically in a very good position to recommend "next steps." Armed with a comprehensive understanding of the study's limitations and strengths, the researcher can pave the way for studies that avoid the same pitfalls or that capitalize on known strengths. Moreover, the researcher is in a good position to assess how a new study could move a topic area forward. Is a replication needed, and, if so, with what groups? If observed relationships are significant, what do we need to know next for the information to be maximally useful?

If the study was based on a theoretical framework or conceptual model, then the researcher should also consider the implications of the study results for the theory. If the analysis of the study methods leads the researcher to conclude that the study had many flaws, then it may be difficult to make any inferences about the validity of the theory. However, if the study was reasonably rigorous methodologically, then the results should be used to either document support for the theory, to suggest ways in which the theory ought to be modified, or to discredit the theory as a useful approach for studying the topic under investigation.

Finally, the researcher should carefully consider the implications of the findings for nursing practice and nursing education. How can client outcomes or the nursing process be improved, based on the findings of the study? Specific suggestions for implementing the results of the study in a real nursing context are extremely valuable in the utilization process, as we discuss in Chapter 28. Of course, if the study is seriously flawed it may be that the results are not usable within the nursing profession. But they will probably be useful, nevertheless, in designing an improved new study for the same research question.

≡ THE RESEARCH REPORT: CONTENT

No scientific project is ever complete until a research report has been prepared. The most brilliant piece of work is of little value to the scientific community unless that work is known. The task of preparing the final report may appear to be anticlimactic: after all, the researcher has satisfied his or her curiosity. Nevertheless, the reporting of results adds to knowledge on some issue and is a scientist's responsibility. It is also to the researcher's advantage to have research findings known by others, because proper credit should be given to the work that has been completed.

Research reports are prepared for different audiences and for different purposes. A thesis or dissertation not only communicates the research strategy and results but also serves as documentation of the student's thoroughness and ability to perform scholarly empirical work. Theses and dissertations, therefore, are rather lengthy documents. Journal articles, on the other hand, are typically short because they must compete with other reports for limited journal space and because they will be read by busy professionals. Oral reports and presentations at professional conferences are another mechanism for disseminating research results; they offer the possibility

of immediate two-way communications and are therefore highly useful.

Despite differences among various types of research reports, their general form and content are quite similar. The major distinction lies in the amount of detail reported and the emphasis given to different parts. In this section, we review the type of material that is covered in the four major sections of a research report: (1) introduction, (2) methods, (3) results, and (4) discussion. The distinctions among the various kinds of reports are described later in the chapter.

The Introduction

The purpose of the introductory section of a research report is to acquaint readers with the research problem, the significance of the problem for nursing and for a field of knowledge, and the context within which the problem was developed. The introduction sets the stage for a description of the study through the inclusion of a brief literature review, description of the conceptual framework, a presentation of the problem statement, hypotheses, and any underlying assumptions, and a discussion of the rationale for studying the problem.

Sometimes reports describe only the general purpose of an investigation. However, a precise and unambiguous problem statement, phrased in question form, is of immense value in communicating to the reader the major objectives of the study. If formal hypotheses have been developed, then they should also be identified in the introduction.

The researcher should explain enough of the background of the study to make clear the reasons that the problem was considered worth pursuing. The justification of a nursing research problem should ideally include both the practical and theoretical significance of the study. This ideal is not always feasible. Not all studies have a direct bearing on theoretical issues, nor should they all necessarily be expected to have such a bearing in a practicing profession such as nursing. With the current state of knowledge, no one should feel apologetic if a study can solve a practical problem but is not linked to a theory. Of course, studies that are framed within a theoretical context are most likely to make enduring contributions to knowledge about nursing and the nursing process. The introduction should make explicit such theoretical rationales when they exist.

The statement of the problem should also be accompanied by a summary of related research, so that the research may be seen in an appropriate context. The review of the literature helps to clarify the theoretical and practical foundations of the research problem. Chapter 6 describes in greater detail the write-up of the literature review section.

Finally, the introduction should incorporate definitions of the concepts under investigation. Sometimes complete operational definitions are reserved for the "Methods" section, but a reader should have a fairly good idea early in the report what the researcher had in mind with regard to such terms as "grief," "stress," "therapeutic touch," and so forth if they are the key concepts under study.

In sum, the introduction should prepare readers for the description of what was done and what was discovered. The introduction should answer the questions, "What did the researcher want to know?" "Why did he or she want to know it?" and "What is the likely significance of such a study?"

The Methods Section

The consumer needs to understand what the researcher did to address the problem identified in the introduction. The methods section should have as its goal a description of what was done to collect and analyze the data in sufficient detail such that another researcher could replicate the study if desired. In theses and final reports to funding agencies, this goal should always be satisfied. In journal articles, however, it is often necessary to condense the methods section. For example, it is typically impossible to include a complete questionnaire, interview schedule, or observation schedule. Nevertheless, the degree

of detail should be sufficiently adequate to permit a reader to evaluate the manner in which the research problem was solved.

The methods section is often subdivided into several parts. The reader needs to know, first of all, who the subjects participating in the study were. The description of the subjects normally includes the specification of the population from which the sample was drawn and the setting for the research. The method of sample selection, the rationale for the sampling design, and the sample size should be clearly delineated so that the reader can estimate the generalizability of the findings. It is advisable to describe the basic characteristics of the subjects, such as their age, sex, and other relevant attributes, and to indicate, if known, the degree to which these characteristics are representative of the population. For instance, if it is known that a sample of nurses tends to underrepresent those who have not received a Bachelor's or higher degree, then this fact should be pointed out.

The design of the study also needs to be described. The design is often given more detailed coverage in an experimental project than in a nonexperimental one. In an experiment, the researcher should indicate what variables were manipulated, how subjects were assigned to groups, the nature of the experimental intervention, and the specific design adopted. In longitudinal studies, the report should indicate the amount of time elapsed between waves of data collection. Regardless of study design, the report should offer a rationale for its use. Also, in most types of study, it is essential to identify what steps were taken to control the research situation in general and extraneous variables in particular.

A critical component of the methods section is the description of the instruments used to collect the data. In rare cases, this description may be accomplished in three or four sentences, such as when a standard physiologic measure has been utilized. More often, a detailed explanation of the instruments and a rationale for their use are required to communicate to the reader the manner in which the variables were operationalized. When it is not feasible to include the actual research instrument within the report, its form and content should be outlined in as much detail as possible. If the measuring devices were constructed specifically for the research project, then the report should describe how they were developed, the methods used for pretesting, revisions made as a result of pretesting, scoring procedures, and guidelines for interpretation. Any information relating to the validity and reliability of the instruments should also be mentioned.

A procedures section provides information about what steps were followed in actually collecting the data. In an experiment, how much time elapsed between the intervention and the measurement of the dependent variable? In an interview study, where were the interviews conducted and how long, on the average, did each one last? In an observational study, what was the role of the observer *vis-à-vis* the subjects? When questionnaires are used, how were they delivered to respondents and were follow-up procedures used to increase the response rate? Any unforeseen events occurring during the collection of data that could affect the findings should be described and assessed. Those reading a report must be in a position to evaluate the quality of the data obtained, and a description of research procedures assists in this evaluation.

A delineation of the analytic procedures is sometimes incorporated into the methods section and sometimes put with the results of the analyses. In qualitative studies, where there is less standardization than is true in analyzing quantitative data, analytic procedures are usually described in some detail. In quantitative studies, it is often sufficient to merely identify the statistical procedures used. It is unnecessary to give computational formulas or even references for commonly used statistics. For unusual procedures, or unusual applications of a common procedure, a technical reference justifying the approach should be noted.

Table 27-1 illustrates the content covered in the methods section of research reports, using excerpts from several studies published in nursing research journals.

The Results Section

The results section summarizes the results of the analyses. In qualitative studies, the researcher presents a summary of the thematic analysis and the integration of the narrative materials, often including direct quotes to illustrate important points. In quantitative studies, if both descriptive and inferential statistics have been used, then the descriptive statistics ordinarily come first. If both quantitative and qualitative analysis has been performed, the qualitative analyses are often placed later because of their ability to explain the meaning of statistical analyses. On the other hand, in some cases, quantitative results may serve a useful summation or confirmatory function and may be more meaningful after a presentation of qualitative results. The researcher must be careful to report all results as accurately and completely as possible, whether or not the hypotheses were supported. If there are too many analyses for inclusion in the report, then the criterion used to select analyses should be their relevance to the overall objectives of the study.

When the results of several statistical analyses are to be presented, it is frequently useful to summarize the findings in a table. Good tables, with precise headings and titles, are an important way to economize on space and to avoid dull, repetitious statements. Important findings can then be highlighted in the text. Beginning researchers are encouraged to carefully study tables presented in research journals to acquaint themselves with the format and content normally considered appropriate for reporting the kinds of analyses they have undertaken. Figures may also be used to summarize results. Figures that display the results in graphic form are used less as an economy than as a means of dramatizing important findings and relationships. Tables and figures should be numbered for easy reference.

Although we will discuss style in a later section, it is difficult to avoid the mention of style here. The write-up of statistical results is often a difficult task for beginning researchers, because they are unsure both about what should be said and about the style in which to say it. A few suggestions may prove helpful. By now, it is hopefully clear that research evidence does not constitute proof of anything, but the point bears repeating here. The research report should never claim that the data "proved," "verified," "confirmed," or "demonstrated" that the hypotheses were correct or incorrect. Hypotheses are "supported" or "unsupported," "accepted" or "rejected." It may seem a trivial point, but the presentation of results should be written in the past tense. For example, it is inappropriate to say, "Nurses who receive special training perform triage functions significantly better than those without training." In this sentence, "receive" and "perform" should

be changed to "received" and "performed." The present tense implies that the results are generalizable to all nurses, when in fact the statement pertains only to a particular sample whose behavior was observed in the past.

When the results of statistical tests are reported, three pieces of information are normally included: the value of the calculated statistic, the number of degrees of freedom, and the significance level. For instance, it might be stated, "A chi-square test revealed that patients who were exposed to the experimental intervention were significantly less likely to develop decubitus ulcers than patients in a control group ($\chi^2 = 8.23$, $df = 1$, $p < .01$)."

Table 27-1. *Excerpts From Methods Sections of Nursing Research Reports**

ASPECT DESCRIBED	EXCERPT
Research design	The study design was a randomized crossover trial, where one half of the nurses would carry out the present system of team nursing and the other half would use primary nursing; then after 5 months, the primary nurses would cross over to team nursing and the former team nurses would practice primary nursing. (McPhail et al., 1990)
Sampling plan	Participation was solicited through exercise classes and various community and church groups. 524 individuals consented to participate. 478 questionnaires were returned with the complete data necessary for inclusion in the study. This convenience sample of 478 consisted of 291 men and women, aged 18 to 74. (Volden et al., 1990)
Instrument	The Sickness Impact Profile (SIP) is a standardized, structured interview that was given in self-administered form to measure perceived health status. The questionnaire contains 136 items in 12 categories .... Bergner et al. (1981) reported high test-retest reliability ($r = .92$) and internal consistency (Cronbach's alpha = .94) of the SIP. Convergent and discriminant validity were evaluated using multitrait–multimethod technique. (Cornwell & Schmidt, 1990)
Data collection procedures	Data were collected by trained interviewers at seven points in time spanning the period following the birth of the infant until approximately two years later. Each couple was first interviewed in the hospital after the birth of their infant, and then was interviewed every 3 to 4 months for two years thereafter in the couple's home. (Rustia & Abbott, 1990)
Data analysis	The descriptions reported during the interviews were transcribed to memo form. As the data were received, a system of open coding was applied. Content analysis was applied by reviewing the descriptions and comparing the accounts of different subjects. Data were clustered and assigned to themes according to obvious fit. Additional subjects were interviewed and the process of coding and clustering data continued until the "point of saturation ...." (DeVito, 1990)

* These brief exerpts illustrate the content and style used to describe various aspects of a study's methods and do not reflect the investigators' entire description of the methods used in their studies.

To further acquaint readers with the write-up of quantitative results, Table 27-2 presents excerpts from the results sections of several studies published in nursing journals. The researcher who is writing a results section for the first time is also likely to profit from a careful examination of a full research report published in a professional journal, which could be used as a model.

The Discussion Section

A bare report of the findings is never sufficient to convey their full implications. The meaning that a researcher gives to the results plays a rightful and important role in the report. The discussion section is typically devoted to a consideration of the study's limitations, the interpretations of the results, and recommendations that incorporate the study's implications. In short, the discussion section is devoted to the issues covered in the first section ("Interpretation of Results") of this chapter.

The interpretation of the results, as discussed earlier, involves the "translation" of statistical findings into practical and conceptual meaning. The interpretative process is a global one, encompassing the investigator's knowledge of the results, the methods, the sample characteristics, related research findings, clinical dimensions, and theoretical issues. The researcher

Table 27-2. *Excerpts From Results Sections of Nursing Research Reports**

TYPE OF ANALYSIS	EXCERPT
Qualitative	The majority of subjects described a dilemma between documentation and doing something for the patients. Most believed that documentation is done at the expense of patient care time. One subject expressed a feeling that was often repeated: "The main inhibitor of documentation is feeling that it will detract from the amount of patient care that can be given and you feel like you're in a dilemma of either documenting or being in there with the patient and actually doing something." (Tapp, 1990)
t-tests	The patient satisfaction questionnaire was completed by 108 patients, with 53 patients receiving primary nursing and 55 patients receiving team nursing. . . . The mean score (SD) for primary nursing patients was 101.3 (12.4) and was 103.5 (12.2) for the team nursing patients, t (106) = 0.93, p = NS. (McPhail et al., 1990)
ANOVA	The fathers and their teenagers shared self-concept perceptions (M = 26.3 and 24.1, respectively), very much unlike the mothers' perceptions (M = 19.5) of their teenagers' self-concept following sibling death, F (2,37) = 11.90, p = .0001. The mothers had a much more favorable opinion of their teenagers' self-concept than the fathers or the teenagers themselves. (Hogan & Balk, 1990)
Pearson correlation	The correlation between supine and left lateral pulmonary artery wedge pressures was 0.888 and between supine and right-sided measurements was .877 (both significant at p = .000). (Groom et al., 1990)
Factor analysis	This (factor) analysis showed that 13 of the 15 items (on the HIV-Impact Questionnaire) belonged in three scales: (1) Precautions, (2) Worry and Policies, and (3) Job Change. (Wiley et al., 1990)
Logistic regression	Logistic regression revealed that female sex, preexisting peripheral vascular disease, and diabetes mellitus each demonstrated a significant (p < .05) and independent relation to lower limb ischemia in the presence of the two other factors. (Funk et al., 1989)

* These brief excerpts illustrate the content and style used to describe a portion of a study's results and do not reflect the investigators' entire description of the results of their analyses.

should justify his or her interpretations, explicitly stating why alternative explanations have been ruled out. If the findings conflict with those of earlier research investigations, then tentative explanations should be offered. A discussion of the generalizability of the study findings and an analysis of their importance should also be included.

Although the readers should be told enough about the methods of the study to identify its major weaknesses, report writers should point out the limitations themselves. The researcher is in the best position to detect and assess the impact of sampling deficiencies, design problems, instrument weaknesses, and so forth, and it is a professional responsibility to alert the reader to these difficulties. Moreover, if the writer shows that he or she is aware of the study's limitations, then the reader will know that these limitations were not ignored in the development of the interpretations.

The implications derived from a study are often speculative and, therefore, should be couched in tentative terms. For instance, the kind of language appropriate for a discussion of the interpretation is illustrated by the following sentence: "The results suggest that it may be possible to improve nurse–physician interaction by modifying the medical student's stereotype of the nurse as the physician's 'handmaiden'." The interpretation is, in essence, a hypothesis and as such can presumably be tested in another research project. The discussion section, therefore, should include recommendations for studies that would help to test this hypothesis, as well as suggestions for other research to answer questions raised by the findings.

Other Aspects of the Report

The materials covered in the four major sections are found in some form in virtually all research reports, although the organization might differ slightly. In addition to these major divisions, some other aspects of the report deserve mention.

Every research report should have a title. The phrases "Research Report" or "Report of a Nursing Research Investigation" are inadequate. The title should indicate to prospective readers the nature of the study. Insofar as possible, the dependent and independent variables should be named in the title. It is also desirable to indicate the population studied. However, the title should be brief (no more than about 15 words), so the writer must balance clarity with brevity. Some examples of titles include the following:

> The Effect of Advance Information on Pain Perception in Hospitalized Children
> Attitudes Toward Preventive Health Care in the Urban Working Class
> Educational Preparation: Its Effects on Role Conflict Among Nurses

If the title gets too unwieldy, its length can often be reduced by omitting unnecessary terms such as "A Study of . . . " or "An Investigation to Examine the Effects of . . . " and so forth. The title should communicate clearly and concisely the phenomena that were researched.

Research reports often include an abstract or a summary. *Abstracts* are brief descriptions of the problem, methods, and findings of the study, written so that a reader can assess whether the entire report should be read. Sometimes a report concludes with a brief summary, and the summary, in such cases, usually substitutes for the abstract. Abstracts and summaries are typically only 100 to 200 words in length. Finally, each report concludes with a list of cited references so that the reader can locate other relevant materials.

≡ THE STYLE OF A RESEARCH REPORT

Research reports are generally written in a distinctive style. Some stylistic guidelines were discussed previously in this chapter and in Chapter 6, but additional points are elaborated on in this section.

A scientific report is not an essay but rather a factual account of how and why a problem was studied and what results were obtained. The report should generally not include overtly subjective statements, emotionally laden statements, or exaggerations. When opinions are stated, they should be clearly identified as such, with proper attribution if the opinion was expressed by another writer. In keeping with the goal of objective reporting, personal pronouns such as "I" and "my" and "we" are often avoided, because the passive voice and impersonal pronouns do a better job of conveying impartiality. However, some journals are beginning to break with this tradition and are encouraging a greater balance between active and passive voice and first person and third person narration. If a direct presentation can be made without sacrificing objectivity, a more readable and lively product usually will result.

It is not easy to write simply and clearly, but these are important goals of scientific writing. The use of pretentious words or technical jargon does little to enhance the communicative value of the report, although colloquialisms should be avoided. Similarly, complex sentence constructions are not necessarily the best way to convey ideas. The style should be concise and straightforward. If writers can add elegance to their reports without interfering with clarity and accuracy, so much the better, but the product is not expected to be a literary achievement. Needless to say, this does not imply that grammatical and spelling accuracy should be sacrificed. The research report should reflect scholarship, not pedantry.

With regard to references and specific technical aspects of the manuscript, various styles have been developed. The writer may be able to select a specific style but often such considerations are imposed by journal editors and university regulations. Specialized manuals such as those of the University of Chicago Press (1982), the American Psychological Association (APA, 1983), and the American Medical Association (1989) are widely used. Four nursing research journals (*Nursing Research, Research in Nursing and Health, Western Journal of Nursing Research,* and *Applied Nursing Research*) use the reference style recommended by the APA, which is the reference style used in this book.

A common flaw in the reports of beginning

researchers is inadequate organization. The overall structure is relatively inflexible and, therefore, should pose no difficulties, but the organization within sections and subsections needs careful attention. Sequences should be in an orderly progression with appropriate transition. Themes or ideas should not be introduced too abruptly nor abandoned suddenly. Continuity and logical thematic development are critical to good communication.

First drafts of research reports are almost never perfect. The assistance of a colleague or an adviser can be invaluable in improving the quality of a scientific paper. Objective criticism can often be achieved by simply putting the report aside for a few days and then rereading it with a fresh outlook. As a final check, one might try to subject one's manuscript to an evaluation according to the guidelines presented in Chapter 28.

≡ TYPES OF RESEARCH REPORTS

Although the general form and structure of a research report are fairly consistent across different types of reports, certain requirements vary. This section describes the content, structure, and features of three major kinds of research reports: (1) theses and dissertations, (2) journal articles, and (3) papers for professional meetings. Reports for class projects are excluded not because they are unimportant but rather because they so closely resemble theses on a smaller scale. Final reports to agencies that have sponsored research are also not described. Most funding agencies issue guidelines for their reports and these guidelines can be secured from project officers. In most cases, reports to funding agencies require nearly as much detail and documentation as dissertations.

Theses and Dissertations

Most doctoral degrees are granted upon the successful completion of an empirical research project. Empirical theses are sometimes required of master's degree candidates as well. Theses and dissertations typically document completely the steps performed in carrying out the research investigation. Faculty members overseeing the project must be able to judge whether the student has understood the research problem both substantively and methodologically. The length of the majority of doctoral dissertations is between 150 and 250 typewritten double-spaced pages.

Most universities have a preferred format for their dissertations, but the following format is fairly typical:

Preliminary Pages
   Title Page
   Acknowledgment Page
   Table of Contents
   List of Tables
   List of Figures
Main Body
   Chapter I. Introduction
   Chapter II. Review of the Literature
   Chapter III. Methods
   Chapter IV. Results
   Chapter V. Discussion and Summary
Supplementary Pages
   Bibliography
   Appendix

The preliminary pages for a dissertation are much the same as those for a scholarly book. The title page indicates the title of the study, the author's name, the degree requirement being fulfilled, the name of the university awarding the degree, the date of submission of the report, and the signatures of the dissertation committee members. The acknowledgment page gives the writer the opportunity to express appreciation to those who contributed to the completion of the project. The table of contents outlines the major sections and subsections of the report, indicating on which page the reader will find those sections of interest. The lists of tables and figures identify by number, title, and page the tables and figures that appear in the text.

The main body of a dissertation incorporates those sections that were described earlier. The literature review often is so extensive for doctoral dissertations that a separate chapter may be devoted to it. When a short review is sufficient, the first two chapters may be combined. In some cases, a separate chapter may also be required to elaborate the study's conceptual framework.

The supplementary pages include a bibliography or list of references used to prepare the report, and one or more appendixes. An appendix contains information and materials relevant to the study that are either too lengthy or too unimportant to be incorporated into the body of the report. Data collection instruments, listings of special computer programs, detailed scoring instructions, cover letters, permission letters, listings of the raw data, and peripheral statistical tables are examples of the kinds of materials included in the appendix. Some universities also require the inclusion of a brief *curriculum vitae,* or autobiography, of the author.

Journal Articles

Progress in nursing research depends on researchers' efforts to share their work with others. Dissertations and final reports to funders are rarely read by more than a handful of individuals. They are too lengthy and too inaccessible for widespread use. Publication in a professional journal ensures broadest possible circulation of scientific findings. From a personal point of view, it is exciting and professionally advantageous to have one or more publications.

A journal article generally follows the same form as that for the main body of a thesis, but articles are much shorter. The purpose of an article is not to demonstrate research competence but rather to communicate the contribution that the study makes to knowledge. Because readers are particularly interested in the findings of a research project, a relatively large proportion of the journal report normally is devoted to the results and discussion sections. For the sake of economy of journal space, the typical research article is only approximately 10 to 25 typewritten double-spaced pages.

Several nursing journals accept research articles for publication. *Nursing Research,* which is currently published six times annually, is a major communication outlet for research in the field of nursing and has been published for four decades. Other nursing journals that focus primarily on empirical studies are *Advances in Nursing Science, Applied Nursing Research, Research in Nursing and Health,* and the *Western Journal of Nursing Research.* Nursing journals that are not devoted exclusively or even primarily to research but do accept research reports for publication include the *American Journal of Nursing; Heart and Lung; Nursing Forum; Nursing Outlook; Journal of Advanced Nursing; Journal of Obstetric, Gynecologic, and Neonatal Nursing; Oncology Nursing Forum; Psychiatric Nursing Forum; Public Health Nursing;* and the *Journal of Gerontological Nursing.* Many journals not directly focusing on nursing also publish articles by nurse authors, such as *The American Journal of Public Health, Journal of School Health, Perceptual and Motor Skills, Family Planning Perspectives,* and numerous others.

The prospective author should check through recent issues of journals under consideration for guidance concerning the journals' stylistic requirements and content coverage. Many publications make an explicit statement concerning the type of manuscripts they are seeking. Swanson and McCloskey (1986) have prepared a valuable report on publishing opportunities for nurses, which includes information on the circulation of the journal, number of copies of a manuscript required for submission, typical article word length, time needed to arrive at an editorial decision, and acceptance rate for 139 journals in nursing and related health fields.

Before submitting a paper to a journal, it is wise to let at least one person read and comment on it. Usually an independent reader is able to spot weaknesses more readily than the authors. When the manuscript is finally prepared for journal submission, the required number of copies should be sent to the editor with a brief cover letter indicating the mailing address of at least one author.* Generally, the receipt of the manuscript

is acknowledged immediately but the final decision concerning the paper's acceptance or rejection may require several months.

Many journals have a policy of independent, anonymous (sometimes referred to as "blind") *reviews* by two or more knowledgeable persons. By "anonymous," we mean that the reviewers do not know the identity of the authors of the article, and the authors do not learn the identity of the reviewers. Journals that have such a policy are sometimes described as *refereed journals* and are generally more prestigious than nonrefereed journals.

Accepted manuscripts almost invariably are revised somewhat, either by the authors at the editor's request or by the editorial staff of the journal. If the manuscript is not accepted, authors are usually sent copies of the reviewers' comments or a summary of the reasons for its rejection. This information can be used to revise a manuscript before submitting it to another journal. A rejection by one journal should not discourage researchers from sending the manuscript to another journal. The competition for journal space is quite keen and a rejection does not necessarily mean that a study is unworthy of publication. Although it is considered unethical to submit an article to two journals simultaneously, manuscripts may need to be reviewed by several journals before final acceptance.

Presentations at Professional Conferences

Numerous professional organizations sponsor annual national meetings at which research activities are presented, either through the reading of a research report or through visual display in a poster session. The American Nurses' Association is an example of an organization that holds meetings where nurses have an opportunity to share their knowledge with others interested in their research topic. Many local chapters of Sigma Theta Tau devote one or more of their annual activities to research reports. Examples of regional organizations that sponsor research conferences are the Western Society for Research in Nursing, the Southern Council on Collegiate Edu-

---

* By convention, the ordering of authors' names on a research report usually is alphabetical if authors have contributed equally, or in order of the importance of their contribution if otherwise. See Waltz et al., (1985) and Hanson (1988) for a discussion of author credits.

cation for Nursing, the Eastern Nursing Research Society of MARNA/NEON, and the Midwest Nursing Research Society. Other nursing organizations such as the Society for Research in Nursing Education, the American Association of Critical Care Nurses, the American Association of Neurosurgical Nurses, and the Congress of Nursing in Child Health sponsor research conferences. Professional organizations such as the Association for the Care of Children's Health, the American Anthropological Association, the American Public Health Association, and the Orthopsychiatry Society also have sessions that are of interest to nurses.

Presentation of research results at a conference has at least two advantages over journal publication. First, there is generally less time elapsed between the completion of a research project and its communication to others when a presentation is made at a meeting. Second, there is an opportunity for dialogue between the researcher and the audience at a professional conference. The listeners can request clarification on certain points and can suggest interesting modifications to the research paradigm. For this reason, a professional conference is a particularly good forum for presenting results to a clinical audience. At professional conferences, researchers also can take advantage of meeting and talking with others who are working on the same or similar problems in different parts of the country.

The mechanism for submitting a presentation to a conference is somewhat simpler than in the case of journal submission. The association sponsoring the conference ordinarily publishes a "Call for Papers" in its newsletter or journal about six to nine months before the meeting date. The notice indicates requirements and deadlines for submitting a paper. The journal *Nursing Research* publishes a "Call for Papers" section as one of its regular departments, and most universities and major health care agencies also receive and post "Call for Papers" notices. Usually, an abstract of 500 to 1000 words is submitted rather than a full paper. If the submission is accepted, the researcher is committed to appear at the conference to make a presentation.

Papers of empirical work presented at professional meetings follow much the same format as a journal article. The report is typically quite condensed, inasmuch as the time allotted for presentation ranges from 10 to 20 minutes. Therefore, only the most important aspects of the study can be included in the paper. A handy rule of thumb is that a page of double-spaced text requires 2½ to 3 minutes to read aloud. Presentations are usually more effective, however, if they are informal summaries of research than if they are read verbatim from a written text.

Researchers sometimes elect to present their findings in a poster session. In such a session, several researchers simultaneously present visual displays summarizing the highlights of the study, and conference attendees circulate around the room perusing these displays. In this fashion, those interested in a particular topic can devote considerable time to discussing the study with the researcher, and avoid those posters dealing with topics of lesser personal interest. Poster sessions are thus efficient and encourage one-on-one discussions. Lippman and Ponton (1989) and Ryan (1989) have presented some useful tips for poster sessions.

≡ SUMMARY

The interpretation of research findings basically represents the researcher's attempts to understand the research results. The interpretation typically involves five subtasks: (1) analyzing the accuracy of the results, (2) searching for the meaning underlying the results, (3) considering the importance of the findings, (4) analyzing the generalizability of the findings, and (5) assessing the implications of the study *vis-à-vis* future research, theory development, and nursing practice.

The research project is not complete until the results have been communicated in the form of a report. Despite some differences in the length, purposes, and audience of different types of research reports, the general form and content are similar. In general, the four major sections of a research report are the (1) introduction, (2) methods, (3) results, and (4) discussion.

The purpose of the introduction is to acquaint the readers with the research problem. This section includes the problem statement, the research hypothesis, a justification of the importance or value of the research, a summary of relevant related literature, the identification of a theoretical framework, and definitions of the concepts being studied. The methods section acquaints the reader with what the researcher did to solve the research problem. This section normally includes a description of the subjects, how they were selected, the instruments and procedures used to collect the data, and the techniques used to analyze the data. In the results section, the findings obtained from the analyses are summarized. Finally, the discussion section of a research report presents the researcher's interpretation of the results, a consideration of the study's limitations, and recommendations for future research and for utilization of the findings.

Scientific communications should be written as simply and clearly as possible. Emotionally laden statements and overtly subjective statements should be excluded from research reports. Various reference manuals exist to assist the researcher in selecting a consistent and acceptable style for noting references and handling other technical aspects of report writing. The style should be congruent with that of the university or journal to which the report is submitted.

The major types of research reports are theses and dissertations, reports to funding agencies, journal articles, and presentations at professional meetings. When space or time are at a premium—as in the case of journal articles and conference papers—detail should be kept to a minimum. In other types of reports, however, extensive documentation may be required.

≡ STUDY SUGGESTIONS

1. Write an abstract for an article appearing in a recent issue of the *Western Journal of Nurs-*

ing Research. Compare your abstract with that written by a classmate.

2. Read the article "Predictors of depression among wife caregivers" by Robinson in the November–December 1989 issue of *Nursing Research* in which mixed results were obtained. How did Robinson interpret the results? What are some other interpretations that could be made?

3. What are the similarities and differences of research reports that are written for journal publication and for presentation at a professional meeting?

4. Suppose that a researcher has found that women who experience severe cramps during menstruation are more likely than women who do not experience the discomforts of menstrual cramps to smoke cigarettes. Suggest two or three different ways that this finding might be interpreted.

≡ SUGGESTED READINGS

METHODOLOGICAL/STYLISTIC REFERENCES

American Medical Association. (1989). *American Medical Association manual of style* (8th ed.). Baltimore: Williams & Wilkins.

American Psychological Association. (1983). *Publication manual of the American Psychological Association* (3rd ed.). Washington, DC: Author.

Burns, N. (1989). Standards for qualitative research. *Nursing Science Quarterly, 2,* 44–52.

Fuller, E.O. (1983). Preparing an abstract of a nursing study. *Nursing Research, 32,* 316–317.

Gay, J.T., & Edgil, A.E. (1989). When your manuscript is rejected. *Nursing and Health Care, 10,* 459–461.

Hanson, S.M.H. (1988). Collaborative research and authorship credit: Beginning guidelines. *Nursing Research, 37,* 49–52.

Huth, E.J. (1982). *How to write and publish papers in the medical sciences.* Philadelphia: Institute for Scientific Information.

Jackle, M. (1989). Presenting research to nurses in clinical practice. *Applied Nursing Research, 2,* 191–193.

Johnson, S.H. (1982). Selecting a journal. *Nursing and Health Care, 3,* 258–263.

Juhl, N., & Norman, V.L. (1989). Writing an effective abstract. *Applied Nursing Research, 2,* 189–191.

Knafl, K.A., & Howard, M.T. (1984). Interpreting and reporting qualitative research. *Research in Nursing and Health, 7,* 17–24.

Kolin, P.C., & Kolin, J.L. (1980). *Professional writing for nurses in education, practice, and research.* St. Louis, MO: C.V. Mosby.

Lippman, D.T., & Ponton, K.S. (1989). Designing a research poster with impact. *Western Journal of Nursing Research, 11,* 477–485.

Markman, R.H., & Waddell, M.J. (1989). *Ten steps in writing the research paper* (4th ed.). Woodbury, NY: Barron's Educational Series.

McCloskey, J.C., & Swanson, E. (1982). Publication opportunities for nurses: A comparison of 100 journals. *Image, 14,* 50–56.

Mirin, S.K. (1981). *The nurse's guide to writing for publication.* Wakefield, MA: Nursing Resources.

Ryan, N.M. (1989). Developing and presenting a research poster. *Applied Nursing Research, 2,* 52–55.

Selby, M., Tornquist, E., & Finerty, E. (1989). How to present your research. *Nursing Outlook, 37,* 172–175.

Sexton, D.L. (1984). Presentation of research findings: The poster session. *Nursing Research, 33,* 374–377.

Smith, T.C. (1984). *Making successful presentations: A self-teaching guide.* New York: John Wiley and Sons.

Strunk, W., Jr., & White, E.B. (1979). *The elements of style* (3rd ed.). New York: Macmillan.

Swanson, E., & McCloskey, J. (1982). The manuscript review process of nursing journals. *Image, 14,* 72–76.

Swanson, E., & McCloskey, J. (1986). Publishing opportunities for nurses. *Nursing Outlook, 45,* 227–235.

Tornquist, E.M. (1986). *From proposal to publication: An informal guide to writing about nursing research.* Menlo Park, CA: Addison-Wesley.

Tornquist, E.M., Funk, S.G., & Champagne, M.T. (1989). Writing research reports for clinical audiences. *Western Journal of Nursing Research, 11,* 576–582.

University of Chicago Press. (1982). *The Chicago manual of style* (13th ed.). Chicago: Author.

Van Till, W. (1985). *Writing for professional publication* (2nd ed.). Boston: Allyn & Bacon.

Waltz, C.F., Nelson, B., & Chambers, S.B. (1985). Assigning publication credits. *Nursing Outlook, 33,* 233–238.

SUBSTANTIVE REFERENCES

Cornwell, C.J., & Schmidt, M.H. (1990). Perceived health status, self-esteem and body image in women with rheumatoid arthritis or systemic lupus erythematosus. *Research in Nursing and Health, 13,* 99–107.

DeVito, A.J. (1990). Dyspnea during hospitalization for acute phase of illness as recalled by patients with chronic obstructive pulmonary disease. *Heart and Lung, 19,* 186–191.

Funk, M., Gleason, J., & Foell, D. (1989). Lower limb ischemia related to use of the intraaortic balloon pump. *Heart and Lung, 18,* 542–552.

Groom, L., Frisch, S.R., & Elliott, M. (1990). Reproducibility and accuracy of pulmonary artery pressure measurement in supine and lateral position. *Heart and Lung, 19,* 147–151.

Hogan, N.S., & Balk, D.E. (1990). Adolescent reactions to sibling death: Perceptions of mothers, fathers, and teenagers. *Nursing Research, 39,* 103–106.

McPhail, A., Pikula, H., Roberts, J., Browne, G., & Harper, D. (1990). Primary nursing: A randomized crossover trial. *Western Journal of Nursing Research, 12,* 188–200.

Rustia, J., & Abbott, D.A. (1990). Predicting paternal role enactment. *Western Journal of Nursing Research, 12,* 145–160.

Tapp, R.A. (1990) Inhibitors and facilitators to documentation of nursing practice. *Western Journal of Nursing Research, 12,* 229–240.

Volden, C., Langemo, D., Adamson, M., & Oechsle, L. (1990). The relationship of age, gender, and exercise practice to measures of health, life-style, and self-esteem *Applied Nursing Research, 3,* 20–26.

Wiley, K., Heath, L., Acklin, M., Earl, A., & Barnard, B. (1990). Care of HIV-infected patients: Nurses' concerns, opinions, and precautions. *Applied Nursing Research, 3,* 27–33.

28
Evaluating Research Reports

Research in a practicing profession such as nursing contributes not only scholarly knowledge but also information concerning how that practice can be improved. Nursing research, then, has relevance for all nurses, not just the minority of nurses who actually engage in research projects. As professionals, nurses should possess skills with which to critically evaluate reports of research in their field. Hopefully, this text has provided a foundation for the development of such skills. In this chapter, more specific guidelines for the critical and intelligent review of research are presented.

≡ *THE RESEARCH CRITIQUE*

If nursing practice is to be based on a solid foundation of scientific knowledge, then the worth of studies appearing in the nursing literature must be critically appraised. Sometimes consumers have the mistaken belief that if a research report was accepted for publication, then it must be a good study. Unfortunately, this is not the case. Indeed, *most* research has limitations and weaknesses, and for this reason no single study can provide unchallengeable answers to research questions. Nevertheless, the scientific method continues to provide us with the best possible means of answering certain questions. Knowledge is accumulated not by an individual researcher conducting a single, isolated study, but rather through the conduct and evaluation of several studies addressing the same or similar research questions. Thus, consumers who can thoughtfully critique research reports also have a role to play in the advancement of scientific knowledge.

Critiquing Research Decisions

Although no single study is infallible, there is a tremendous range in the quality of studies—from nearly worthless to exemplary. The quality of the research is closely tied to the kinds of decisions the researcher makes in conceptualizing, designing, and executing the study, and in interpreting and communicating the study results. Each study tends to have its own peculiar flaws, because each researcher, in addressing the same or a similar research question, makes somewhat different decisions about how the study should be done. It is not uncommon for researchers who have made different research decisions to arrive at different answers to the same research question. It is precisely for this reason that consumers of research must be knowledgeable about the research process. As a consumer, you must be able to evaluate the decisions that investigators made so that you can determine how much faith should be put in their conclusions. The consumer must ask, "What other approaches could have been used to study this research problem?" and "If another approach had been used, would the results have been more reliable, believable, or replicable?" In other words, the consumer must evaluate the impact of the researcher's decisions on the study's ability to reveal the "Truth."

Much of this book has been designed to acquaint consumers with a range of methodological options for the conduct of research—options on how to control extraneous variables, on how to collect and analyze data, on how to select a study sample, on how to operationalize variables, and so on. Hopefully, an acquaintance with these options has provided you with the tools to challenge a researcher's decisions and to suggest alternative methods.

The Purpose of a Research Critique

Research reports are evaluated for a variety of purposes. Students are often asked to prepare a critique to demonstrate their mastery of methodological and analytic skills. Seasoned researchers are sometimes asked to write critiques of manuscripts to help journal editors make publication decisions, or to accompany the report as published commentaries.* Journal clubs in clinical or other settings may meet periodically to critique and discuss research studies. For all of these purposes, the goal is generally to develop a balanced evaluation of the study's contribution to knowledge.

A research critique is not just a review or summary of a study, but rather a careful, critical appraisal of the strengths and limitations of a piece of research. A written critique should serve as a guide to researchers and practitioners. With respect to the research community, the critique should inform them of the ways in which the study results have possibly been compromised, and should alert them to how to better go about addressing the research question. The critique should thus help to advance a particular area of knowledge. With respect to clinical nurses, the critique should help those who are practicing nursing to decide how the findings from the study can best be incorporated into their practice, if at all.

It should be recognized that the function of critical evaluations of scientific work is not to dogmatically hunt for and expose "mistakes." A good critique objectively identifies adequacies and inadequacies, virtues as well as faults. Sometimes the need for such balance is obscured by the terms "critique" and "critical appraisal," which connote unfavorable observations. The merits of a study are as important as its limitations in coming to conclusions about the worth of its findings. Therefore, the research critique should reflect a thoughtful, objective, and balanced consideration of the study's validity and significance. If the critique is not balanced, then it will be of little utility to the researcher who conducted the study because it might engender defensiveness, and the practitioner may erroneously get the impression that the study has no merit at all.

* The *Western Journal of Nursing Research*, for example, usually publishes a research report followed by one or two commentaries that include appraisals of the report.

BOX 28-1 GUIDELINES FOR THE CONDUCT OF A WRITTEN RESEARCH CRITIQUE

1. Be sure to comment on the study's strengths as well as its weaknesses. The critique should be a balanced consideration of the worth of the research. Each research report has at least *some* positive features—be sure to find them and note them.
2. Give specific examples of the study's weaknesses and strengths. Avoid vague generalities of praise and fault-finding.
3. Try to justify your criticisms. Offer a rationale for how a different approach would have solved a problem that the researcher failed to attend to.
4. Be as objective as possible. Try to avoid being overly critical of a study because you are not particularly interested in the topic or because you have a bias against a certain research approach (e.g., qualitative vs. quantitative).
5. Without sacrificing objectivity, be sensitive in handling negative comments. Try to put yourself in the shoes of the researcher receiving the critical appraisal. Try not to be condescending or sarcastic.
6. Suggest alternatives that the researcher (or future researchers) might want to consider. Don't just identify the problems in the research study—offer some recommended solutions, making sure that the recommendations are practical ones.
7. Evaluate all aspects of the study—its substantive, methodological, interpretive, ethical, and presentational dimensions.

Box 28-1 summarizes general guidelines to consider in preparing a written research critique. In the section that follows, we present some specific guidelines for evaluating various aspects of a research report.

≡ ELEMENTS OF A RESEARCH CRITIQUE

Each research report has several important dimensions that should be considered in a critical evaluation of the study's worth. In this section, we review the substantive/theoretical, methodological, interpretive, ethical, and presentational/stylistic dimensions.

Substantive and Theoretical Dimensions

The reviewer needs to determine whether the study was an important one in terms of the significance of the problem studied, the soundness of the conceptualizations, and the creativity and appropriateness of the theoretical framework. The research problem is one that should have obvious relevance to some aspect of the nursing profession. It is not enough that a problem be "interesting" if it offers no possibility of contributing to nursing knowledge or improving nursing practice. Even before the reader learns *how* a study was conducted, there should be an evaluation of whether the study should have been conducted in the first place.

The reader's own disciplinary orientation should not intrude in an objective evaluation of the study's significance. A clinical nurse might not be intrigued by a study focusing on the determinants of nursing turnover, but a nursing administrator trying to improve staffing decisions might find such a study highly useful. Similarly, a psychiatric nurse might find little value in a study of the sleep–wake patterns of low birthweight infants, but nurses in neonatal intensive care units might not agree. It is important, then, not to adopt a myopic view of the study's importance and relevance to nursing.

Many problems that are relevant to nursing are still not necessarily substantively worthwhile. The reviewer must ask a question such as, "Given what we know about this topic, is this research the right next step?" Knowledge tends to be incremental. Researchers must consider how to advance knowledge on a topic in the most beneficial way. They should avoid unnecessary replications of a study once a body of research clearly points to an answer, but they should also not leap several steps ahead when there is an insecure foundation. Sometimes replication is exactly what is needed to enhance the believability or generalizability of earlier findings.

A final issue to consider is whether the researcher has appropriately placed the research problem into some larger theoretical context. As we stressed in Chapter 7, a researcher does little to enhance the value of the study if the connection between the research problem and a conceptual framework is artificial and contrived. However, a specific research problem that is genuinely framed as a part of some larger intellectual problem can generally go much farther in advancing knowledge than a problem that ignores its theoretical underpinnings.

The substantive and theoretical dimensions of a study are normally communicated to readers in the introduction to a report. The manner in which the introductory materials are presented is vital to the proper understanding and appreciation of what the researcher has accomplished. Specific guidelines for critiquing the introduction of a research report are presented in Boxes 28-2 to 28-5.* Box 28-2 provides guidelines for critiquing the researcher's statement of the problem. Boxes 28-3 and 28-4 suggest considerations relevant to a critique of the literature review and conceptual framework, respectively. Box 28-5 includes questions for the evaluation of the study's hypotheses.

Methodological Dimensions

Once a research problem has been identified, the researcher must make a number of important decisions regarding how to go about answering the research questions or testing the research hypotheses. It is the consumer's job to critically evaluate the consequences of those decisions. In fact, the heart of the research critique lies in the analysis of the methodological decisions adopted in addressing the research ques-

---

* The questions included in the boxes in this chapter are not exhaustive. Many additional questions will need to be raised in dealing with a particular piece of research. Moreover, the boxes include many questions that do not apply to every piece of research. The questions are intended to represent a useful point of departure in undertaking a critique.

BOX 28-2   GUIDELINES FOR CRITIQUING PROBLEM STATEMENTS

1. Does the problem have significance to the nursing profession and does the researcher describe what that significance is?
2. Has the researcher explained his or her purpose in conducting the research? What does the researcher hope to accomplish?
3. Does the problem flow from prior scientific information, experience in the topic area, or a theory?
4. Has the researcher appropriately delimited the scope of the problem, or is the problem too big or complex for a single investigation?
5. Does the problem statement clearly identify the research variables and the nature of the population being studied?
6. Are the research variables adequately defined and are they measurable?
7. Is the problem statement clearly and concisely articulated? If it is worded in the declarative form, does it clearly suggest the question to be answered?
8. Was the problem statement introduced promptly?

---

tion. Although the researcher makes hundreds of methodologically relevant decisions in conducting a study, the four major decisions on which the consumer should focus critical attention are as follows:

Decision 1. What design should be used that will yield the most unambiguous and meaningful results about the study questions?

Decision 2. Who should the subjects of the study be? To what population should the research findings be generalized? How large should the sample of subjects be, where should they be recruited from, and what sampling approach should be used to select the sample?

Decision 3. How should the research variables

be operationalized? How can the variables be reliably and validly measured for each participant in the study? How should the data be collected?

Decision 4. What analyses will provide the most appropriate and meaningful tests of the research hypotheses or answers to the research questions?

Because of practical constraints, research studies almost always involve making some compromises between what is ideal and what is feasible. For example, the researcher might ideally

---

BOX 28-3 GUIDELINES FOR CRITIQUING RESEARCH LITERATURE REVIEWS

1. Does the review seem thorough? Does it appear that the review includes all or most of the major studies that have been conducted on the topic of interest? Does the review include recent literature?
2. Is there an overdependence on secondary sources when primary sources could have been obtained?
3. Is there an overreliance on opinion articles and an underemphasis on research studies?
4. Does the content of the review relate directly to the research problem, or is it only peripherally related?
5. Is the review merely a summary of past work, or does it critically appraise and compare the contributions of key studies? Does it discuss weaknesses in existing studies and identify important gaps in the literature?
6. Is the review paraphrased adequately, or is it a string of quotations from the original sources?
7. Does the review use appropriate language, suggesting the tentativeness of prior findings?
8. Is the material organized in such a way that the review builds a case for conducting a new study?
9. Does the review conclude with a brief synopsis of the state-of-the-art of the literature on the topic?

BOX 28-4 GUIDELINES FOR CRITIQUING THEORETICAL/ CONCEPTUAL FRAMEWORKS

1. Does the research report describe a theoretical or conceptual framework for the study? If not, does the absence of a theoretical framework detract from the usefulness or significance of the research?
2. Is the theory appropriate to the research problem? Would a different theoretical framework have been more appropriate?
3. Is the theoretical framework based on a conceptual model of nursing, or is it borrowed from another discipline? Is there adequate justification for the researcher's decision about the type of framework used?
4. Do the research problem and hypothesis flow naturally from the theoretical framework, or does the link between the problem and the theory seem contrived?
5. Are the deductions from the theory or conceptual framework logical?
6. Are all of the concepts adequately defined in a way that is consistent with the theory?

---

like to work with a sample of 1000 subjects but because of limited resources might have to be content with a sample of 200 subjects. The person doing a research critique cannot realistically demand that researchers attain these methodological ideals, but must be prepared to evaluate how much damage has been done by failure to achieve them.

After the reader evaluates the types of decisions that the researcher made, a further step is necessary. The reviewer must assess how well the research plan was actually executed. A well-conceived research plan may go awry because of time pressures, financial constraints, personnel changes, researcher inexperience, administrative problems, and so on. Therefore, the methodological aspects of a study must be critiqued not only as they were conceived but also as they were put into operation.

Various boxes are presented to guide the reader in performing a critical analysis of the

BOX 28-5 GUIDELINES FOR CRITIQUING RESEARCH HYPOTHESES

1. Does the research report contain formally stated hypotheses? If not, is their absence justifiable?
2. Are the hypotheses directly and logically tied to the research problem?
3. Do the hypotheses flow logically from the theoretical rationale or review of the literature? If not, what justification is offered for the researcher's predictions?
4. Does each hypothesis contain at least two variables?
5. Do the hypotheses state a predicted relationship between the variables (i.e., between the independent and dependent variables)?
6. Do the hypotheses indicate the nature of the population being studied?
7. Can the hypotheses be tested in such a way that it is clear whether the hypotheses are supported or not?
8. Are the hypotheses worded clearly, unambiguously, and objectively, and written as a stated prediction?
9. Are the hypotheses directional? If not, is there a rationale for the nondirectional hypotheses?
10. Are the hypotheses stated as research hypotheses rather than null hypotheses?

BOX 28-6 GUIDELINES FOR CRITIQUING RESEARCH DESIGNS

1. Given the nature of the research question, what type of design is most appropriate? How much flexibility does the research question call for, and how much structure is needed?
2. Does the design involve an experimental intervention? Was the full nature of any intervention described in detail?
3. If there is an intervention, was a true experimental, quasi-experimental, or pre-experimental design used? Should a more rigorous design have been used?
4. If the design is nonexperimental, what is the reason that the researcher decided not to manipulate the independent variable? Was this decision appropriate?
5. What types of comparisons are specified in the research design (e.g., before/after, the use of one or more comparison group)? Are these comparisons the most appropriate ones?
6. If the research design does not call for any comparisons, what difficulties, if any, does this pose for understanding what the results mean?
7. What procedures, if any, did the researcher use to control external (situational) factors? Were these procedures appropriate and adequate?
8. What procedures, if any, did the researcher use to control extraneous subject characteristics? Were these procedures appropriate and adequate?
9. To what extent did the design affect the internal validity of the study? What types of alternative explanations must be considered, given the design that was used?
10. To what extent did the design enhance the external validity of the study? Can the design be criticized for its artificiality, or praised for its realism?
11. Does the research design enable the researcher to draw causal inferences about the relationships among research variables?
12. How many times were data collected or observations recorded? Is this number appropriate, given the research question?
13. What are the major limitations of the design used? Are these limitations acknowledged by the researcher?

research methods, which are generally described in the methods section of a research report. Box 28-6 presents guidelines for critiquing the overall research design. The sampling strategy and the researcher's selection of a target population can be evaluated using the questions included in Box 28-7.

Four separate boxes are included here to assist with a critique of the researcher's data collection plans. Explicit guidelines are provided for evaluating self-report approaches (Box 28-8); observational methods (Box 28-9); and biophysiologic measures (Box 28-10). Criteria are not provided for evaluating infrequently used data collection techniques, such as Q sorts and records. However, in addition to questions adapted from Boxes 28-8 through 28-10, other methods

BOX 28-7 GUIDELINES FOR CRITIQUING SAMPLING PLANS

1. Is the target or accessible population identified and described? Are the eligibility criteria clearly specified?
2. Given the research problem and limitations on resources, is the target population appropriately designated?
3. Would a more limited population specification have controlled for important sources of extraneous variation not covered by the research design?
4. Are the sample selection procedures clearly described? Does the report make clear whether probability or non-probability sampling was used? Could the sampling plan be replicated?
5. Is the sampling plan one that is likely to have produced a representative sample?
6. If the sampling plan is relatively weak (such as in the case of a convenience sample) are potential sample biases identified?
7. Did some factor other than the sampling plan itself (such as a low rate of response) affect the representativeness of the sample?
8. Are the size and key characteristics of the sample described?
9. Is the sample sufficiently large? Was the sample size justified on the basis of a power analysis?
10. To whom can the study results reasonably be generalized?

can be evaluated by considering one overarching question: Did the researcher's method of measurement and data collection yield the best possible measure of the key research variables? Box 28-11 suggests some guidelines for evaluating the overall quality of the measurements.

The researcher's analytic plan is the final methodological area that requires a critical analysis. The analytic strategy is sometimes presented in the methods section of a research report, but is usually more fully explicated in the results section, where the actual findings are reported. Box 28-12 lists a number of guiding questions of relevance for evaluating quantitative analyses and Box

28-13 identifies questions for qualitative analyses. When a study has used both qualitative and quantitative analyses, questions from both boxes are likely to be applicable. In addition, the reader should ask: Were the qualitative and quantitative analyses meaningfully integrated, and did they complement each other in appropriate ways?

Interpretive Dimensions

Research reports almost always conclude with a "Discussion," "Conclusions," or "Implications" section. It is in this final section that the researcher attempts to make sense of the statistical analyses, to understand what the findings mean *vis-à-vis* the research hypotheses, to consider whether the findings support or fail to support a theoretical framework, and to discuss what the findings might mean for the nursing profession. Inevitably, the discussion section is more subjective than other sections of the report. This subjectivity is not necessarily detrimental, because great insights spring from researchers' personal experience, knowledge, and creative capacities—not from the data themselves. However, subjectivity can sometimes block insights if researchers read into the data only what they want to see.

The task of the reviewer is generally to contrast his or her own interpretation with that of the researcher and to challenge conclusions that do not appear to be warranted by the empirical results. If the reviewer's objective reading of the research methods and study findings leads to an interpretation that is notably different from that endorsed by the researcher, then the interpretive dimension of the study may well be faulty. Box 28-14 presents questions to assist readers in assessing the researcher's conclusions.

Ethical Dimensions

The person performing a research critique should consider whether there is any evidence that the rights of human subjects were violated during the course of the investigation. If there are any potential ethical problems, then the reviewer must consider the impact of those problems on the scientific merit of the study on the one hand and on subjects' well-being on the other. Guidelines for evaluating the ethical dimensions of a research report are presented in Box 28-15.

There are two main types of ethical "transgressions" in research studies. The first class consists of inadvertent actions or activities that the researcher did not interpret as creating an ethical dilemma. For example, in a study that examined married couples' experiences with sexually transmitted diseases, the researcher might inadvertently schedule the interview at a time when privacy could not be ensured.

In other cases, the researcher is aware of

having committed some violation of ethical principles, but has made a conscious decision that the violation is relatively minor in relation to the knowledge that could be gained by doing the study in a certain way. For example, the researcher may decide not to obtain informed consent from the parents of minor children attending a family planning clinic because to require such consent would probably dramatically reduce the number of minors willing to participate in the research and would lead to a biased sample of clinic users; it could also violate the minors' right to confidential treatment at the clinic. When the researcher knowingly elects not to follow the

---

BOX 28-8   GUIDELINES FOR CRITIQUING SELF-REPORTS

Interviews/Questionnaires

1. Does the research question lend itself to a self-report approach? Would an alternative method have been theoretically more appropriate?
2. Is the degree of structure of the researcher's approach consistent with the nature of the research question?
3. Do the questions included in the instrument adequately cover the complexities of the problem under investigation?
4. Did the researcher use the right mode for the collection of self-report data (i.e., personal interview, telephone interview, self-administered questionnaire), given the nature of the research question and the characteristics of the respondents? Would an alternative mode have improved the quality of data collected?
5. Was there an appropriate balance of open-ended and closed-ended questions?
6. [If an instrument is included for review] Are the questions clearly worded? Do the questions tend to bias responses in a certain direction? Do response options to closed-ended questions adequately cover the alternatives? Is the ordering of questions appropriate?
7. Was there an appropriate number of questions? Was the instrument too long? Too brief?
8. Was the instrument adequately pretested?
9. Was the response rate adequately high? Did the researcher take steps to produce a high response rate? Does the researcher discuss the nature and extent of biases (if any) resulting from non-response?

Scales

10. If a scale was used, is its relevance to the objectives of the study clearly explained? Does it, in fact, adequately capture the construct of interest?
11. If a new scale was developed, is there adequate justification for failure to use an existing one? Was the new scale pretested and refined?
12. Is the rationale for selecting one scaling procedure as opposed to another (e.g., Likert vs. semantic differential) explained? Is the rationale convincing?
13. Is the scale sufficiently long?
14. Are procedures for eliminating or minimizing response set biases described, and are they appropriate? For example, are negative and positive items counterbalanced?

BOX 28-9 GUIDELINES FOR CRITIQUING OBSERVATIONAL METHODS

1. Does the research question lend itself to an observational approach? Would an alternative method have been theoretically more appropriate?
2. Is the degree of structure of the observational method consistent with the nature of the research question?
3. Are the phenomena under observation the same as those described in the problem statement?
4. Do the categories included in the instrument (if applicable) adequately cover the relevant behaviors?
5. To what degree were the observers concealed during data collection? What effect might their presence have had on the behaviors and events they were observing?
6. What was the unit of analysis in the study? How much inference was required on the part of the observers, and to what extent did this lead to the potential for bias?
7. Where did the observations actually take place? To what extent did the setting influence the "naturalness" of the behaviors being observed?
8. How were data actually recorded (e.g., on field notes or checklists)? Did the recording procedure appear appropriate?
9. What steps were taken to minimize observer biases? For example, how were observers trained? How detailed were the explanations of the behaviors to be recorded?
10. What was the plan by which events or behaviors were sampled for observation? Did this plan appear to yield a representative sample of relevant behaviors?
11. If a category scheme was developed, was it exhaustive? Was the scheme overly demanding of observers, leading to the potential for inaccurate data? If the scheme was not exhaustive, did the omission of large realms of subject behavior lead to an inadequate context for understanding the behaviors of interest?

BOX 28-10 GUIDELINES FOR CRITIQUING BIOPHYSIOLOGIC MEASURES

1. Does the research question lend itself to a biophysiologic approach? Would an alternative method have been theoretically more appropriate?
2. Was the proper instrumentation used to obtain the biophysiologic measurements? Would an alternative instrument or method have been more appropriate? Did the researcher present a rationale for the use of the particular method, and was that rationale convincing?
3. Were the procedures for data collection adequately described? Did the procedures appear to be appropriate?
4. Does the report suggest that care was taken to obtain accurate data? For example, did the researcher's activities permit accurate recording if an instrument system with recording equipment was not used?
5. Does the researcher appear to have the skills necessary for proper interpretation of the biophysiologic measurements?

ethical principles outlined in Chapter 3, the reviewer must evaluate the decision itself *and* the researcher's rationale.

The reviewer who comments on the ethical aspects of a study based on a report of completed research is obviously "too late" to prevent an ethical transgression from occurring. Nevertheless, the critique can bring the ethical problems to the attention of those who might be replicating the research.

Presentational and Stylistic Dimensions

Although the worth of the study itself is primarily reflected in the dimensions we have reviewed thus far, the manner in which the information is communicated in the research report is also fair game in a comprehensive critical appraisal. Box 28-16 summarizes the major points

BOX 28-11 GUIDELINES FOR CRITIQUING MEASUREMENTS

1. Does there appear to be a strong congruence between the research variables as conceptualized and as operationalized? Do the measures appear to show a strong correspondence to reality?
2. At what level of measurement were the research variables measured? Could they have been measured at even higher levels than the ones used?
3. Does the report provide any evidence of the reliability of the measurements? If not, are there any indications of efforts the researcher made to minimize errors of measurement?
4. If there is evidence of reliability, what method was used? Was this method appropriate? Should an alternative or additional method of assessing reliability have been used? Was the reliability of the instrument adequate?
5. Does the report offer any evidence of the validity of the measures? If there is, what approach was used to validate the measures? Was this approach appropriate? Should there have been an alternative or additional method of validation used? Does the validity of the instrument appear to be adequate?
6. In a qualitative study, were methods of triangulation used to converge on the "truth"? What methods were used? Were these efforts sufficient, or should other forms of triangulation have been used? Did the triangulation procedures suggest that the qualitative information obtained was adequately valid and reliable?

that should be considered in evaluating the presentation of a research report.

An important consideration is whether the research report has provided sufficient information for a thoughtful critique of the other dimensions. For example, if the report does not describe how the sample was selected, then the reviewer cannot comment on the adequacy of the sampling plan, but he or she can criticize the

researcher's failure to include information on sampling. When vital pieces of information are missing, the researcher leaves the reader little choice but to assume the worst, because this would lead to the most cautious interpretation of the results.

The writing in a research report, as in any published document, should be clear, grammatically correct, concise, and well-organized. Unnecessary jargon should be kept to a minimum, although colloquialisms should also be avoided. The reader should try to observe whether the researcher's view intruded too much in the report, especially in the reporting of the results.

≡ CONCLUSION

In concluding this chapter, several points about the research critique should be made. It should be apparent to those who have glanced through the questions in the boxes in this chapter that it will not always be possible to answer the questions satisfactorily on the basis of the research report. This is especially true for journal articles in which the need for economy often translates into a severe abridgement of methodological descriptions. Furthermore, there are many questions listed that may have little or no relevance for a particular study. The inclusion of a question in the list does not necessarily imply that all reports should have all of the components mentioned. The questions are meant to suggest aspects of a study that often are deserving of consideration, and not meant to lay traps for identifying omitted and perhaps unnecessary details.

It must be admitted that the answers to many questions will call upon the reader's judgment as much as, or even more than, upon his or her knowledge. An evaluation of whether the most appropriate data collection procedure was used for the research problem necessarily involves a degree of subjectiveness. Issues concerning the appropriateness of various strategies and techniques are topics about which even experts disagree. One should strive to be as objective as possible and to indicate one's reasoning for the judgments made.

≡ SUMMARY

Evaluating research reports involves critically appraising both the merits and the limitations of the published report. A systematic assessment of the various aspects of a research report is essential in judging the utility and value of a study. This chapter offers suggestions for assessing the substantive, methodological, interpretive, ethical, and stylistic aspects of a written research report.

≡ STUDY SUGGESTIONS

1. Read the article "Effects of an experimental program on post-hospital adjustment of early discharged patients" by Wong et al. (1990) in the *International Journal of Nursing Studies,* volume 27, pages 7–20. What limitations of the research methods did the authors identify? Do these limitations alter your acceptance of the findings?

2. Read an article from any issue of *Nursing Research* or any other nursing research journal and systematically assess the article according to the questions contained in this

---

BOX 28-12   GUIDELINES FOR CRITIQUING QUANTITATIVE ANALYSES

1. Does the research question lend itself to quantitative data collection and analysis? Would a more qualitative approach to data analysis have been more appropriate?
2. Does the report include any descriptive statistics? Do these statistics sufficiently describe the major characteristics of the researcher's data set?
3. Were indices of both central tendency and variability provided in the report? If not, how does the absence of this information affect the reader's understanding of the research variables?
4. Were the correct descriptive statistics used (e.g., was a median reported when a mean would have been more appropriate)?
5. Does the report include any inferential statistics? Was a statistical test performed for each of the hypotheses or research questions? If inferential statistics were not used, should they have been?
6. What level of statistical significance was established by the researcher as acceptable? Was this level insufficiently stringent or too conservative?
7. Was the selected statistical test appropriate, given the level of measurement of the variables?
8. Was a parametric test used? Does it appear that the assumptions for the use of parametric tests were met? If a nonparametric test was used, should a more powerful parametric procedure have been used instead?
9. Were any multivariate procedures used? If so, does it appear that the researcher chose the appropriate test?
10. If multivariate procedures were not used, should they have been? Would the use of a multivariate procedure have improved the researcher's ability to draw conclusions about the relationship between the dependent and independent variables?
11. In general, does the research report provide a rationale for the researcher's decision to use certain statistical tests but not others? Does the report contain sufficient information for the reader to judge whether appropriate statistics were used?
12. Were the results of any statistical tests significant? What do the tests tell the reader about the plausibility of the research hypotheses?
13. Was there an appropriate amount of statistical information reported?
14. Were tables used judiciously to summarize large masses of statistical information? Are the tables clearly presented, with good titles and carefully labeled column headings? Is the information presented in the text consistent with the information presented in the tables? Is the information totally redundant?

BOX 28-13   GUIDELINES FOR CRITIQUING QUALITATIVE ANALYSES

1. Does the research question lend itself to qualitative analysis or would a more quantitative approach have been more appropriate?
2. Is the categorization system and thematic analysis consistent with the goals of the research?
3. Were any of the qualitative materials converted to quantitative data? Was the level of quantification appropriate? Why or why not?
4. What sources of data were used to yield the qualitative materials (e.g., unstructured interview, observation)? Are these sources sufficient to provide a broad array of information and to capture the full range of likely variation within categories?
5. What were the major themes that emerged from the qualitative analysis? If excerpts from the narrative materials are provided, do these themes appear to capture the meaning of the narratives (i.e., did the researcher adequately interpret and conceptualize the themes)?
6. Is the analysis parsimonious? That is, could two or more themes have been collapsed into some broader and perhaps more useful conceptualization of the issues?
7. What efforts did the researcher make to validate the findings? Were quasi-statistical procedures use? Did two or more researchers independently code and analyze the data? Did the researcher specifically mention a search for contrary occurrences? What evidence does the report provide that the researcher's analysis is accurate, objective, and replicable?
8. Was either a grounded theory or analytic induction approach used? If so, does it appear to have been used appropriately?

BOX 28-14   GUIDELINES FOR CRITIQUING THE INTERPRETIVE DIMENSIONS OF A RESEARCH REPORT

Interpretation of the Findings

1. Are all of the important results discussed? Are the interpretations consistent with the results?
2. Is each result interpreted in terms of the original hypothesis to which it relates and to the conceptual framework? Is each result interpreted in light of findings from similar research studies?
3. Are alternative explanations for the findings mentioned, and is the rationale for their rejection discussed?
4. Do the interpretations give due consideration to the limitations of the research methods?
5. Are any unwarranted interpretations of causality made?
6. Is there evidence of bias in the interpretations?
7. Does the interpretation distinguish between practical and statistical significance?

Implications

8. Are implications of the study ignored, although a basis for them is apparent?
9. Are the implications of the study discussed in terms of the retention, modification, or rejection of a theory/conceptual framework?
10. Are the implications of the findings for nursing practice described?
11. Are the discussed implications appropriate, given the study's limitations?
12. Are generalizations made that are not warranted on the basis of the sample used?

Recommendations

13. Are recommendations made concerning how the study's methods could be improved? Are recommendations for future research investigations made?
14. Are recommendations for specific nursing actions made on the basis of the implications?
15. Are the recommendations thorough, consistent with the findings, and consistent with related research results?

BOX 28-15 GUIDELINES FOR CRITIQUING THE ETHICAL ASPECTS OF A STUDY

1. Were the subjects unnecessarily subjected to any physical harm or psychologic distress or discomfort?
2. Did the researchers take appropriate steps to remove or prevent harm?
3. Did the benefits that accrued from the research outweigh any potential risks or actual discomfort to the subjects?
4. Was information gathered from study participants by personnel with appropriate qualifications?
5. Were the subjects told about any real or potential risks that might result from participation in the study? Were the purposes and procedures of the study fully described in advance?
6. Was any type of coercion or undue influence used in recruiting subjects for the study? Were vulnerable subjects used?
7. Did all the subjects know they were subjects in a study? Did they have an opportunity to decline participation? Were subjects deceived in any way?
8. Was informed consent obtained from all subjects or their representatives? If not, was there a valid and justifiable reason for not doing so?
9. Were appropriate steps taken to safeguard the privacy of the research subjects?
10. Was the research study approved and monitored by an Institutional Review Board or other similar committee on ethics?

BOX 28-16 GUIDELINES FOR CRITIQUING THE PRESENTATION OF A RESEARCH REPORT

1. Does the report include a sufficient amount of detail to permit a thorough critique of the study's purpose, conceptual framework, design and methods, handling of critical ethical issues, and interpretation?
2. Is the report well written? Are pretentious words or jargon used when simpler wording would have been possible? Are the grammar and spelling correct?
3. Is the report well-organized, or is the presentation confusing? Is there an orderly, logical presentation of ideas? Are transitions smooth and is the report characterized by continuity of thought and expression?
4. Is the report sufficiently concise, or does the author include a lot of irrelevant details?
5. Is the report written in an objective style, or are the author's biases and viewpoints overly intrusive? Are attributions made for any opinions presented in the report?
6. Is the report written using tentative language as befits the nature of scientific inquiry, or does the author talk about what the study did or did not "prove"?
7. Is sexist language avoided?
8. Does the title of the report adequately capture the variables and population under investigation?
9. Does the report have a summary or abstract? Does the abstract adequately summarize the research problem, the study methods, and important findings?
10. Does the author include a reference for every citation made in the text, so that readers can refer to earlier work on the topic?

chapter. What are the merits and limitations of the report?

3. Review the research critique presented in Polit and Hungler (1989) in Chapter 13.

≡ SUGGESTED READINGS

Aamodt, A.M. (1983). Problems in doing nursing research: Developing criteria for evaluating qualitative research. *Western Journal of Nursing Research, 5,* 398–402.

Burns, N. (1989). Standards for qualitative research. *Nursing Science Quarterly, 2,* 44–52.

Downs, F.S. (1977). Elements of a research critique. In F.S. Downs & M.A. Newman (Eds.), *A source book of nursing research* (2nd ed., pp. 1–12). Philadelphia: F.A. Davis.

Field, W.E. (1983). Clinical nursing research: A proposal of standards. *Nursing Leadership, 6,* 117–120.

Fleming, J.W., & Hayter, J. (1974). Reading research reports critically. *Nursing Outlook, 22,* 172–175.

Gehlbach, S.H. (1982). *Interpreting the medical literature.* Lexington, MA: The Collamore Press.

Horsley, J., & Crane, J. (1982). *Using research to improve nursing practice: A guide.* New York: Grune & Stratton.

Norbeck, J.S. (1979). The research critique. *Western Journal of Nursing Research, 1,* 296–306.

Parse, R., Coyne, A., & Smith, M. (1985). *Nursing research: Qualitative methods.* Bowie, MD: Brady Communications. (Chapter 11).

Polit, D.F., & Hungler, B.P. (1989). *Essentials of nursing research: Methods and applications* (2nd ed.). Philadelphia: J.B. Lippincott.

Sherman, K.M., & Kirsch, A.K. (1978). Can nursing educators deal effectively with nursing students' difficulty in critiquing nursing research articles? How can critical thinking be fostered? *Nursing Research, 27,* 69–70.

Topham, D.L., & DeSilva, P. (1988). Evaluating congruency between steps in the research process: A critique guide for use in clinical nursing practice. *Clinical Nurse Specialist, 2,* 97–102.

Ward, M.J., & Felter, M.E. (1978). What guidelines should be followed in critically evaluating research reports? *Nursing Research, 27,* 120–126.

29
Utilization
of Nursing
Research

Nurse researchers are usually not interested in pursuing knowledge simply for the sake of knowledge itself. In a practicing profession such as nursing, researchers generally want to have their findings incorporated into nursing protocols and into diagnostic decision making. In fact, it might be argued that the ultimate worth of a nursing research study is demonstrated by the extent to which its findings are eventually used to improve the delivery of nursing services.

Over the past two decades, a number of changes have been made in nursing education and in nursing research that were prompted by the desire to develop a better knowledge base for the practice of nursing. In education, most schools of nursing changed their curricula to include courses on nursing research. Now, almost all baccalaureate nursing programs offer courses to instill some degree of research competence in their students. In the research arena, as indicated in Chapter 1, there has been a dramatic shift toward research on clinical nursing problems. These two changes alone, however, have not in and of themselves been enough to effect widespread modifications to the delivery of nursing care on the basis of scientific research. There appears to have been an unwarranted assumption that the production of clinically relevant studies would lead automatically to improved nursing practice—if only there were an audience of practicing nurses who were competent in critically evaluating these studies. Research utilization, as the nursing community has increasingly begun to recognize, is a complex and nonlinear phenomenon. In this chapter, we discuss various aspects of the utilization of nursing research.

≡ WHAT IS RESEARCH UTILIZATION?

Broadly speaking, *research utilization* refers to the use of some aspect of a scientific investigation in an application unrelated to the original research. Current conceptions of research utilization recognize a continuum in terms of the specificity or diffuseness of the use to which knowledge is put. At one end of the continuum are discrete, clearly identifiable attempts to base some specific action on the results of research findings. For example, a series of studies in the 1960s and 1970s demonstrated that the optimum placement time for accurate oral temperature determination is nine minutes (e.g., Nichols & Verhonick, 1968). When nurses specifically alter their behavior from shorter placement times to the empirically based recommendation for nine minutes, this constitutes an instance of research utilization at this end of the continuum. Research utilization is sometimes defined in terms of such direct, specific impacts. For example, Horsley and her colleagues (1983), who were involved in a major project on the utilization of research in nursing, defined research utilization as a "process directed toward transfer of specific research-based knowledge into practice through the systematic use of a series of activities" (pp. 100–101). This type of utilization has been referred to as *instrumental utilization* (Caplan & Rich, 1975).

However, there is growing recognition that research can be utilized in a more diffuse manner—in a way that promotes cumulative awareness, understanding, or "enlightenment." Caplan and Rich (1975) refer to this end of the utilization continuum as *conceptual utilization.* Thus, a practicing nurse may read a research report in which the investigators report that nonnutritive sucking among preterm infants in a neonatal intensive care unit had a beneficial effect on the number of days to the infant's first bottle feeding and on number of days hospitalized. The nurse may be reluctant to alter his or her own behavior or suggest an intervention based on the results of

a single study. However, the nurse's reading of the research report may make the nurse more observant in his or her own work with preterm infants and may lead the nurse to collect informal "data" regarding the benefits of nonnutritive sucking in the nurse's own setting. Conceptual utilization, then, refers to situations in which users are influenced in their thinking about an issue based on their knowledge of one or more studies but do not put this knowledge to any specific, documentable use.

The middle ground of this continuum involves the partial impact of research findings on nursing activities. Here, nursing actions or decisions are based to some extent on research findings, but other factors such as first-hand experience, tradition, and situational constraints are also considered. This middle ground is frequently the result of a slow evolutionary process that does not reflect a conscious decision to use an innovative procedure, but rather reflects what Weiss (1980) termed "knowledge creep" and "decision accretion." *Knowledge creep* refers to an evolving "percolation" of research ideas and findings. *Decision accretion* refers to the manner in which momentum for a decision builds over time based on accumulated information gained through readings, informal discussions, meetings, and so on.

Research utilization at all points along this continuum appears to be an appropriate goal for nurses.

≡ RESEARCH UTILIZATION IN NURSING

Numerous commentators have noted that progress in utilizing the results of nursing research studies has proceeded slowly—too slowly for many who are anxious to establish a scientific base for nursing actions. In this section, we consider the possibilities for research utilization and evidence on the extent to which utilization has occurred.

Incorporating Research Into Practice: The Potential

The nursing process is complex and requires nurses to engage in many decision-making activities. In the course of delivering patient care, nurses collect relevant information, make assessments and diagnoses, develop plans for appropriate nursing actions, initiate interventions, and evaluate the effects of these interventions. These activities, it may be recalled from Chapter 1, correspond to the five phases of nursing outlined in the Standards of Nursing Practice established by the American Nurses' Association (1973). Within each of these phases, the findings from research can assist nurses in making more informed decisions and in taking actions that have a solid, scientifically based rationale. Thus, research conducted by nurses can potentially play a pivotal role in improving the quality of nursing care, the efficiency with which it is delivered, and the process by which the care is delivered.

Incorporating Research Into Practice: The Record

As suggested previously, considerable potential exists for utilizing research throughout the various phases of the nursing process. However, there is currently concern that nurses have thus far failed to realize this potential for using research findings as a basis for making decisions and for developing nursing interventions. This concern is based on some evidence suggesting that nurses are not always aware of research results and do not effectively incorporate these results into their practice.

One of the first pieces of evidence about the "gap" between research and practice was a study by Ketefian (1975), who reported on the oral temperature determination practices of 87 registered nurses (RNs). Ketefian's study was designed to learn what "happens to research findings relative to nursing practice after five or ten years of dissemination in the nursing literature" (p. 90). The results of a series of investigations in the late 1960s had clearly demonstrated that the optimal placement time for oral temperature determination was nine minutes. In Ketefian's study, only one out of 87 nurses reported the correct placement time, suggesting that these practicing nurses were unaware of or ignored the research findings about optimal placement time.

In another study investigating research utilization, Kirchhoff (1982) investigated the discontinuance of coronary precautions in a nationwide sample of 524 intensive care nurses. Several published studies had failed to demonstrate that the practices of restricting ice water and rectal temperature measurement were necessary, yet Kirchhoff's results indicated that these coronary precautions were still widely practiced. Only 24% of the nurses had discontinued ice water restrictions and only 35% had discontinued rectal temperature restrictions.

More recently, Brett (1987) investigated practicing nurses' adoption of 14 nursing innovations that had been reported in the nursing literature. Brett used the utilization criteria suggested by Haller and colleagues (1979) in selecting 14 studies. These criteria included scientific merit, significance and usefulness of the research findings to the practice setting, and the suitability of the finding for application to practice. A sample of 216 nurses practicing in ten hospitals of varying sizes completed questionnaires that measured the nurses' awareness and use of the study findings. The results indicated much variation across the 14 studies. For example, from 34% to 95% of the nurses reported awareness of the various innovations. Brett used an interesting scheme to categorize each study according to its stage of adoption: awareness (indicating knowledge of the innovation); persuasion (indicating the nurses' belief that nurses should use the innovation in practice); occasional use in practice; and regular use in practice. Only one of the 14 studies was at the "regular use" stage of adoption. Half of the studies were in the "persuasion" stage, indicating that the nurses knew of the innovation and thought it *ought* to be incorporated into nursing practice, but were not basing their own nursing decisions on it. Table 29-1 describes four of the 14 nursing innovations, one for each of the four stages of adoption, according to Brett's results. The results of Brett's study (and the results of a similar study undertaken by Coyle and Sokop, 1990) are more encouraging than the studies by Ketefian and Kirchhoff in that they suggest that, on average, the practicing nurses were aware of many innovations based on research results, were persuaded that the innovations ought to be used, and were beginning to use them on occasion. Of course, it is possible that the respondents overstated their awareness and use of nursing innovations in an attempt to "look good."

It is clear that a gap exists between knowledge production and knowledge utilization in

Table 29-1. *Extent of Adoption of Four Nursing Practice Innovations**

STAGE	NURSING INNOVATION	% AWARE	% PERSUADED	% USE SOMETIMES	% USE ALWAYS
Awareness	Internal rotation of the femur during injection into the dorsogluteal site, in either the prone or side-lying position, results in reduced discomfort from the injection (Kruszewski et al., 1979)	44	34	29	10
Persuasion	Accurate monitoring of oral temperatures can be achieved on patients receiving oxygen therapy by using an electronic thermometer placed in the sublingual pocket (Lim-Levy, 1982)	63	47	32	28
Occasional use	A formally planned and structured preoperative education program preceding elective surgery results in improved patient outcomes (King & Tarsitano, 1982)	87	83	36	33
Regular use	A closed sterile system of urinary drainage is effective in maintaining the sterility of urine in patients who are catheterized for fewer than 2 weeks; continuity of the closed drainage system should be maintained during irrigations, sampling procedures, and patient transport (Horsley et al., 1981)	95	92	14	79

* Based on findings reported in Brett, J.L.L. Use of nursing practice research findings. *Nursing Research, 36,* 344–349 (1987). The sample consisted of 216 practicing nurses.

nursing and in other disciplines. Some gap is inevitable and, given the imperfection of scientific research as a means of knowing, even desirable. Moreover, it seems likely that the gap as identified in studies such as those described previously is somewhat overstated for three reasons. First, utilization studies do not always consider technological changes that might make the knowledge irrelevant. Thus, as Downs (1979) has pointed out, electronic thermometers that rapidly replaced glass thermometers in the mid-1970s made the placement-time findings obsolete, and could account for Ketefian's results. Second, an important factor in research utilization is a risk/benefit analysis, as we describe later in this chapter. The subjects in Kirchhoff's study may have continued using coronary care precautions because the risk of problems that might arise by eliminating them (e.g., if the study results were incorrect) outweighed the benefits (e.g., more efficient use of staff time) that could accrue. Third, utilization studies have focused primarily on utilization at one end of the utilization continuum—the end we have referred to as instrumental utilization. That is, utilization studies have been interested primarily in the extent to which specific types of information are used in specific nursing situations. Brett's study, which found that half of the innovations were in the "persuasion" stage, supported the notion of a great "middle ground" when it comes to research utilization. No study has investigated "conceptual utilization" but we suspect that, with the growing emphasis on nursing research in nursing curriculums, there is a much higher level of conceptual utilization throughout the nursing community today than there was ten years ago. Nurses are becoming "enlightened" with regard to the value of research and enlightened by a growing body of research that is challenging traditional ways of practicing nursing.

Efforts to Improve Utilization

The need to reduce the gap between nursing research and nursing practice has been the topic of much discussion, but there have been relatively few formal efforts to achieve that goal. In this section, we briefly describe the most prominent of these efforts.

THE WICHE PROJECT

One of the earliest research utilization projects was the Western Interstate Commission for Higher Education (WICHE) Regional Program for Nursing Research Development. The project, a 6-year effort funded by the Division of Nursing of the U.S. Department of Health, Education, and Welfare, had as its original goal investigating the feasibility of increasing nursing research activities through regional collaborative activities. According to the final report (Krueger et al., 1978), the three major project activities were (1) collaborative, nontargeted research (bringing together nurses from educational and practice settings to design studies based on mutually identified nursing problems); (2) collaborative, targeted research (multiple studies in different settings all designed to investigate the concept of quality of care); and (3) research utilization. The project team visualized research utilization as part of a five-phase resource linkage model. In this model, nurses were conceived as organizational change agents who could provide a link between research and practice. Through a support system (e.g., through workshops, conferences, and consultations), participant nurses were to utilize research results to solve problems identified as occurring in practice.

Nurses who participated in the WICHE project were given the opportunity to identify problems that needed research-based solutions, and were then provided with opportunities to develop skills in reading and evaluating research for use in practice. They also developed detailed plans for introducing research innovations into their clinical practice settings. The final report indicated that the project was successful in increasing research utilization, but also identified a stumbling block. The problem that posed the greatest difficulty was finding scientifically sound, reliable nursing studies with clearly identified implications for nursing care.

THE NCAST PROJECT

The Nursing Child Assessment Satellite Training (NCAST) Project was a 2-year research dissemination project, also funded by the Division of Nursing. The primary objectives of the project were to determine whether satellite communication technology is an efficient means of disseminating nursing research and whether an interactive communication facility would promote effective application of new health-care assessment techniques (Barnard & Hoehn, 1978). The results of the study supported the use of satellite communication for research dissemination. In terms of research utilization, the project directors proposed a model with four components: (1) recruitment (i.e., the identification and recruitment of an appropriate practitioner audience); (2) translation (i.e., the transformation of research results into a format and idiom that can easily be understood by nurse practitioners); (3) dissemination (i.e., the communication of research findings in an effective and efficient manner); and (4) evaluation (i.e., the determination of the impact of the other three processes).

THE CURN PROJECT

The best-known nursing research utilization project is the Conduct and Utilization of Research in Nursing (CURN) Project, a 5-year development project awarded to the Michigan Nurses' Association by the Division of Nursing. The major objective of the CURN project was to increase the use of research findings in the daily practice of RNs by disseminating current research findings, facilitating organizational changes needed for the implementation of innovations, and encouraging the conduct of collaborative research that has relevance to nursing practice.

One of the activities of the CURN project was to stimulate the conduct of research in clinical settings. The project resulted in a set of nine volumes on various clinical problems. The titles of these volumes (e.g., *Pain, Preventing Decubitus Ulcers, Structured Preoperative Teaching,* and *Reducing Diarrhea in Tube-Fed Patients*) indicate that a wide range of clinical issues were studied.

The CURN project also focused on helping nurses to utilize research findings in their practice. The CURN project staff saw research utilization as primarily an organizational process (Horsley et al., 1978). According to their view, the commitment of organizations that employ practicing nurses to the research utilization process is essential for research to have any impact on nursing practice. They conceptualized the six phases of the research utilization process as follows (Horsley et al., 1983):

1. Identification of practice problems that need solving, and assessment of valid research bases to use in nursing practice
2. Evaluation of the relevance of the research-based knowledge as it applies to the identified clinical problem, the organization's values, current policies, and potential costs/benefits
3. Design of a nursing practice innovation that addresses the clinical problem but does not exceed the scientific limitations of the research base
4. Clinical trial and evaluation of the innovation in the practice setting
5. Decision making to adopt, revise, or reject the innovation
6. Development of strategies to extend the innovation to other appropriate settings

The CURN project team concluded that research utilization by practicing nurses is feasible, but only if the research is relevant to practice and if the results are broadly disseminated.

≡ BARRIERS TO UTILIZING NURSING RESEARCH

Typically, several years elapse between the time a researcher conceptualizes and designs a study and the time the results are reported in the research literature. Many more years may elapse between the time the results are reported and the time practicing nurses learn about the results and attempt to incorporate them into practice. Thus, it is not unusual for there to be an interim of a decade or so between the posing of a research problem and the implementation of a solution— if, in fact, there is *ever* an effort to implement. In the next section of this chapter, we discuss some strategies for bridging the gap between nursing research and nursing practice. First, however, we review some of the barriers to research utilization in nursing. These barriers can be broadly grouped into four categories relating to characteristics of the source of the barrier: (1) the research itself, (2) practicing nurses, (3) organizational settings, and (4) the nursing profession.

Research Characteristics

Because nursing research is a relatively new area of inquiry, the state-of-the-art of research knowledge on any given problem is often at a relatively rudimentary level. Studies reported in the literature often do not warrant the incorporation of their findings into practice. Flaws in research design, sample selection, data collection instruments, or data analysis often raise questions about the soundness or generalizability of the study findings. Thus, a major impediment to research utilization by practicing nurses is that there has not yet been the development of an extensive base of valid, reliable, and generalizable study results.

As we have repeatedly stressed throughout this book, most scientific studies have flaws of one type or another. The study may be flawed conceptually or methodologically; the flaws may be minor or major; but the fact remains that there are few, if any "perfect" studies. If one were to wait for the perfect study before basing clinical decisions and interventions on research findings, however, one would have a very long wait indeed. It is precisely because of the limits of the scientific approach that replication becomes essential. When repeated testings of a hypothesis in different settings and with different types of subjects yield similar results, then there can be greater confidence that the "truth" has been verified. Isolated studies can almost never provide an ade-

quate basis for making changes in nursing practice. Therefore, another constraint to research utilization is the dearth of reported replications of studies.

Nurses' Characteristics

Practicing nurses as individuals have characteristics that impede the incorporation of research findings into nursing care. Perhaps the most obvious is the educational preparation of nurses. The majority of practicing nurses—graduates of diploma or associate degree programs— have not received any formal instruction in research. They may therefore lack the skills to judge the merits of scientific projects. Furthermore, because research played a limited role in their training, these nurses may not have developed positive attitudes toward research and may not be aware of the beneficial role it can play in the delivery of nursing care. Champion and Leach (1989) found that nurses' attitudes toward research were strong predictors of the utilization of research findings. Courses on research methodology are now typically offered in baccalaureate nursing programs, but there is generally insufficient attention paid to research utilization. The ability to critique a research report is a necessary, but not sufficient, condition for effectively incorporating research results into daily decision making.

Another characteristic is one that is common to most humans. People are generally resistant to change. Change requires effort, retraining, and restructuring one's work habits. Change may also be perceived as threatening—for example, proposed changes may be perceived as potentially affecting one's job security. Thus, there is likely to be some opposition to introducing innovations in the practice setting.

Organizational Characteristics

Some of the impediments to research utilization, as the CURN project staff so astutely noted, stem from the organizations that train and employ practicing nurses. Organizations, perhaps to an even greater degree than individuals, resist change, unless there is a strong organizational perception that there is something fundamentally wrong with the *status quo*. In many settings, the organizational climate is simply not conducive to research utilization. To challenge tradition and accepted practices, a spirit of intellectual curiosity and openness must prevail.

In many practice settings, administrators have established protocols and procedures to reward expertise and competence in nursing practice. However, few practice settings have established a system to reward nurses for critiquing nursing studies, for utilizing research in practice, or for discussing research findings appropriate to clients. Thus, organizations have failed to motivate or reward nurses to seek ways to implement appropriate findings into their practice. Research review and utilization are often considered appropriate activities only when time is available. Especially today, with the nursing shortage, available time is generally quite limited.

Finally, organizations may be reluctant to expend the necessary resources for attempting utilization projects or for implementing changes to organizational policy. Resources may be required for the use of outside consultants, for staff release time, for administrative review, for evaluating the effects of an innovation, and so on. With the push toward cost containment in health-care settings, resource constraints may therefore pose a barrier to research utilization.

Characteristics of the Nursing Profession

Some of the impediments that contribute to the gap between research and practice are more global than those discussed previously and can be described as reflecting the state of the nursing profession or, even more broadly, the state of American society.

One of the difficulties is that it has sometimes been difficult to encourage clinicians and researchers to interact and collaborate. They are generally in different settings, have many differ-

ent professional concerns, interact with different networks of nurses, and operate according to different philosophical systems. Relatively few systematic attempts have been made to form collaborative arrangements, and to date even fewer of these arrangements have been institutionalized as formal, permanent entities. Moreover, attempts to develop such collaboration will not necessarily be welcomed by either group. As Phillips (1986) has observed, there is often a deep-seated lack of trust between nurse researchers and nurse clinicians.

A related issue is that communication between practitioners and researchers is problematic. The majority of practicing nurses do not read nursing research journals nor do they usually attend professional conferences where research results are reported. Many nurses involved in the direct delivery of care are too overwhelmed by the jargon, the statistical symbols, and the wealth of quantitative information contained in research reports to fully understand such reports even when they do read them. Furthermore, nurse researchers may too infrequently attend to the needs of clinical nurses as identified in specialty journals. For research utilization to happen, there must be two-way communication between the practicing nurse and the nurse researcher.

Phillips (1986) has also noted two other noteworthy barriers to bridging the research–practice gap. One is the shortage of appropriate role models. Phillips commented that "even if a nurse wants to assume the role of nursing research consumer, there are few colleagues available to give support for the endeavor and fewer still available to emulate" (p. 8). The other barrier is the historical "baggage" that has defined nursing in such a way that practicing nurses may not typically perceive themselves as independent professionals capable of recommending changes based on nursing research results. If practicing nurses believe that their role is to await direction from the medical community and if they believe they have no power to be self-directed, then they will have difficulty in initiating innovations based on nursing research results.

≡ *SCOPE OF RESPONSIBILITY FOR RESEARCH UTILIZATION*

Where does the responsibility for bridging the gap between research and practice lie? Should individual practicing nurses pursue appropriate nursing innovations? Should organizations and their administrative staff take the lead? Or should the direction come from researchers themselves? In our view, the entire nursing community must be involved in the process of putting research into practice. In this section, we discuss some research utilization strategies that various segments of the nursing community can adopt.

Strategies for Researchers

A great deal of the responsibility for research utilization rests in the hands of researchers. Indeed, there is little point in pursuing scientific investigations if the results do not get used, so it behooves researchers to take steps to ensure that utilization can occur. Some suggestions for strategies that researchers could implement to foster better adoption of their research results are as follows:

- *Do high-quality research.* A major impediment to utilizing nursing research results, as indicated in the previous section, is that there is often an inadequate scientific basis for introducing innovations or for making changes. The quality of nursing studies has improved dramatically in the past two decades, but much progress remains to be made. The inadequacy of sampling plans remains one of the greatest weaknesses of nursing studies. If a study is based on an unrepresentative sample of 50 subjects, then utilization efforts based on the study findings are simply inappropriate.
- *Replicate.* As noted earlier, utilization of research results can almost never be justified on the basis of a single isolated study, so researchers must make a real commitment to replicating studies. It is also important to publish the results of replications even if—in fact, especially if—the results are exactly the same as those obtained in an earlier investigation.

- *Collaborate with practitioners.* Academic researchers will never succeed in having much of an impact on nursing practice unless they become better attuned to the needs of practicing nurses and the clients they serve, the problems that practicing nurses face in delivering nursing care, and the constraints that operate in practice settings. Practicing nurses will be more willing to change their behaviors and modes of delivering care if they perceive that researchers are addressing issues of concern and importance to them. Researchers should seek opportunities to exchange ideas for research problems with nurse clinicians. They also need to involve clinicians in the actual conduct of research, and in the interpretation of study results.
- *Disseminate aggressively.* If a researcher fails to communicate the results of a completed study to other nurses, it is obvious that the results will never be utilized by practicing nurses. Even studies with a variety of methodological shortcomings can make a contribution, if only to illuminate the researcher's conceptualization of a practice problem, or to suggest how the research question might be better addressed in some subsequent study. It is the researcher's *responsibility* to find some means of communicating research results. Researchers should submit their manuscripts to at least two or three journals before abandoning hope of getting their reports published.
- *Disseminate broadly.* A researcher's responsibility for dissemination does not end at the point at which an article has been accepted for publication. Most nurses read only one or two professional journals, so a researcher who is truly committed to having his or her results known by the nursing community often publishes study results in several journals. It is unethical to submit *exactly* the same

manuscript to two different journals, but a study generally yields more information than can be concisely reported in a single journal anyway. It is especially important from a utilization standpoint for researchers to report their results in specialty journals, which are more likely to be read by practicing nurses than the nursing research journals. Another important communication outlet from a utilization standpoint is the journal *Applied Nursing Research,* which was specifically created "as a forum for all professional nurses, to serve as a medium in which we can advance our research and our practice" (Fitzpatrick, 1988, p.1). Researchers should also take steps to disseminate study findings at conferences, colloquia, and workshops that are known to be attended by nurse clinicians. Collaboration with practicing nurses should prove useful in developing effective dissemination plans.

- *Communicate clearly.* It is not always possible to present the results of a research project in a way that is readily comprehensible to all nonresearchers. However, researchers need to be encouraged to avoid unnecessary jargon whenever possible, to construct tables carefully so that a nonresearcher can get a sense of the findings, and to compose the abstract of the report so that virtually any intelligent reader can understand the research problem, the general approach, and the most salient findings.

- *Suggest clinical implications.* In the discussion section of research reports, researchers should suggest how the results of their research can be utilized by practicing nurses. The researcher should be careful to discuss study limitations and to make some assessment of the generalizability of the study findings. If an "implications" section with suggestions for clinical practice became a standard feature of research reports, then the burden of utilization would be much lighter for the nurse clinician.

Strategies for Scholars and Educators

There is some overlap between the categories of nurse researcher and nurse academician, but the overlap is imperfect because not all educators are researchers and not all researchers are in academia. Several of the following suggested strategies could, however, be undertaken by nonacademic researchers, as well as by educators.

- *Incorporate research findings into the curriculum.* Research findings should be integrated throughout the curriculum. Whenever possible, faculty should document the efficacy of a specific procedure or technique by referring to a relevant study. When there is no relevant research, the instructor can note the absence of empirical evidence supporting the technique—this could help to stimulate the students' interest in a research-based verification.

- *Encourage research and research utilization.* Either by acting as role models to students (e.g., by discussing their own research) or by clearly demonstrating positive attitudes toward research and its use in nursing, instructors can help to foster a spirit of inquiry and openness that are preconditions to effective utilization of research. Instructors of research methods can also encourage students to become better consumers of nursing research, to do their own research, or to develop a plan for a utilization project.

- *Prepare integrative reviews.* There is a desperate need for high-quality critical reviews of research on specific research topics. If a research question has been studied by several different researchers—in other words, if there have been several replications of a study—then the question may be ripe for a review that will summarize the state of knowledge. Such reviews can play an invaluable role for practicing nurses, who generally do not have the time to do extensive literature reviews and who may have some difficulty in critically evaluating individual studies. Integrative reviews should ideally conclude with some very strong statements about the implications of the body of research for nursing practice.

- *Place demands on researchers.* Faculty (especially if they have done research themselves) are often asked to be anonymous reviewers of research proposals and reports. Funding sources that offer financial support for the conduct of nursing research generally rely on a panel of experts to help them review research proposals before awarding any grants. Peer reviewers of such proposals should demand that researchers demonstrate the proposed study's potential for practical utility. Moreover, peer reviewers can demand that the researchers include a specific plan for dissemination or utilization. Reviewers of journal articles of completed research should also criticize reports that have failed to include a discussion of the study's implications for practice.

Strategies for Practicing Nurses and Nursing Students

Practicing nurses cannot by themselves launch institutional-wide utilization projects, but their behaviors and attitudes are nevertheless critical to the success of any efforts to base nursing interventions and nursing diagnoses on research findings. Furthermore, individual nurses can clearly engage in and benefit from "conceptual utilization." Therefore, every nurse has an important role to play in utilizing nursing research.

- *Read widely and critically.* Professionally accountable nurses continue their nursing education on an ongoing basis by keeping abreast of important developments in their field. All nurses should regularly read journals relating to their specialty and should not avoid reading research reports.

    Research reports should be critically appraised, according to guidelines such as those suggested in Chapter 28. It is especially important for nurse clinicians to read critical reviews of research that integrate numerous studies on a problem. Brett's (1987) study confirms the importance of reading. Her findings revealed that nurses who spent more time each week reading professional journals were more likely to adopt a research-based innovation than nurses who read infrequently.

- *Attend professional conferences.* Many nursing conferences include presentations of studies that have clinical relevance. It is often more rewarding to attend research presentations at a conference than to read a research report because the lag time between the conduct of a study and a conference presentation is generally less than the lag time for publication. Thus, conference attendees usually hear of an innovation much sooner than those who wait to read about it in a journal. Furthermore, those attending a conference get an opportunity to meet the researcher and to ask questions about practice implications. Brett's (1987) utilization study revealed a positive relationship between nurses' conference attendance and their degree of adopting a research-based innovation. Nurses should ask their supervisors about the possibility of obtaining stipends to defray the cost of attending such conferences.

- *Learn to expect "evidence" that a procedure is effective.* Every time nurses or nursing students are told about a standard nursing procedure, they have a right to ask: Why? Nurses need to develop expectations that the decisions they make in their clinical practice are based on sound rationales. It is not inappropriate for the nursing student or practitioner to challenge the principles and procedures that are currently in use, although tact is clearly advisable so that defensiveness is not engendered by such challenges.

- *Seek environments that support research utilization.* Organizations differ in their openness to research utilization, so nurses interested in basing their practice on research have some control through their employment decisions. Given the current shortage of nurses, if organizations perceive that nurses are basing their employment decisions on such factors as the organizational climate *vis-à-vis* research, there will be some pressure to support research utilization.

- *Become involved in a journal club.* Many organizations that employ nurses sponsor "journal clubs" that meet regularly to review research articles that have potential relevance to practice. Generally, members take turns reviewing and critically appraising a study and presenting the critique to the club's members. If there is no such club in existence, it might be possible to work with the organization to initiate one. Although the bulk of the responsibility for disseminating research results lies with the researcher, this is a responsibility that can be shared by practitioners.

- *Collaborate with a nurse researcher.* Collaboration, which we previously mentioned as a strategy for nurse researchers, is a two-way street. Practicing nurses who have identified a clinical problem in need of a solution and who lack methodological skills for the conduct of a study should consider initiating a collaborative relationship with a local nurse researcher. Collaboration with a nurse researcher could also be a useful approach for formal, institutional utilization projects.

- *Pursue and participate in institutional utilization projects.* Sometimes ideas for utilization projects come from staff nurses. Although large-scale utilization projects require organizational and administrative support, individual nurses or groups of nurses can propose such a project to the nursing department. For example, an idea for such a project may emerge in the context of a journal club. If the idea for a research utilization effort originates from within the administration, then individual nurses are still likely to play an important

role in carrying out the project. Indeed, a utilization project can easily be undermined by reluctant or uncooperative staff. Although change is not always easy, it is in the interest of the profession to have practicing nurses who are open-minded about the possibility that a new technique or procedure can improve the quality of care that nurses provide.

- *Pursue appropriate "personal utilization" projects.* Not all findings from research studies are ones that require organizational commitment or policy directives. For example, a study might reveal that the health beliefs of an immigrant group are different from those of the predominant cultural group, and this may lead a nurse to informally ask several additional questions of clients of that immigrant group during assessment. If the nurse discovers that important and relevant information is gleaned from these additional questions, it may then be appropriate to recommend to the administration a more formal utilization project, which might involve changes to the standard assessment protocols. Of course, not all research findings are amenable to such informal "personal utilization" projects. If the results of a study or series of studies suggest an action or decision that is contrary to organizational policy or that has *any* potential risk for the clients, then nurses should not pursue such projects without supervisory approval. Some criteria for research utilization are discussed in the next section of this chapter.

Strategies for Administrators

According to several models of research utilization, the organizations that employ nurses play a fundamental role in supporting or undermining the nursing profession's efforts to develop a scientific base of practice. Although it is unlikely that the readers of this book include a large audience of nursing or hospital administrators, the following suggested strategies are included primarily to alert practicing nurses to the kinds of issues facing these groups:

- *Foster a climate of intellectual curiosity.* If there is a great deal of administrative rigidity and opposition to change, then the staff's interest in research utilization is unlikely to become ignited. The administrator can take steps to encourage reading and critical thinking about the challenges facing practicing nurses. Open communication is an important ingredient in persuading staff nurses that their experiences and problems are important and that the administration is willing to consider innovative solutions.
- *Offer emotional or "moral" support.* If nurse administrators are unsupportive of research utilization, then there is little chance that any utilization efforts will get off the ground. Administrators need to make their support visible, by informing staff and prospective staff on an individual basis, by establishing research utilization committees, by helping to develop research journal clubs, and so on. Administrators can perhaps offer the greatest degree of personal support by being a role model for the staff nurses. They can accomplish this by, for example, engaging in their own program of research, by actively participating themselves in the research journal clubs, and by playing a role in any utilization projects.
- *Offer financial or resource support for utilization.* Utilization projects often require some resources, although resource demands may not be great. Resources may be required for release time for nurses engaged in utilization projects, for outside consultation, for supplies and computer time, for registration at conferences, and so on. If the administration expects nurses to engage in research utilization activities on their own time and at their own expense, then the not-so-subtle message is that research utilization is unimportant to those running the organization.
- *Reward efforts for utilization.* When administrators evaluate nursing performance, they use a number of different criteria. Although research utilization should not be a primary criterion for evaluating a nurse's performance, its inclusion as one of several important criteria is likely to have a large impact on nurses' behaviors.

☰ THE UTILIZATION PROCESS AND CRITERIA FOR UTILIZATION

In this section, we discuss how a research utilization project could be planned and executed. Although the processes described here are ones that most likely will apply to an organization or a group of nurses working together, many of the steps in the processes are important ones for individual nurses to consider as they attempt to base their clinical decisions on scientific findings.

Approaches to Research Utilization

Nurses interested in utilizing research findings in their nursing practice generally set about the task in one of two ways. One approach to utilization, shown schematically in Figure 29-1, begins with the identification of a clinical problem that needs solution. This problem identification approach, which corresponds to the first step in the six-phase process described by the CURN project team, is likely to have considerable internal staff support if the selected problem is one that numerous nurses in the practice setting have encountered. This approach to utilization is likely to be high on clinical relevance, because a specific clinical situation generated the interest in resolving the problem in the first place.

The next step is a search for relevant literature to determine whether nurse researchers have addressed the problem through scientific research. If there is no research base related to the identified problem, then there are two choices: (1) to abandon the original problem and

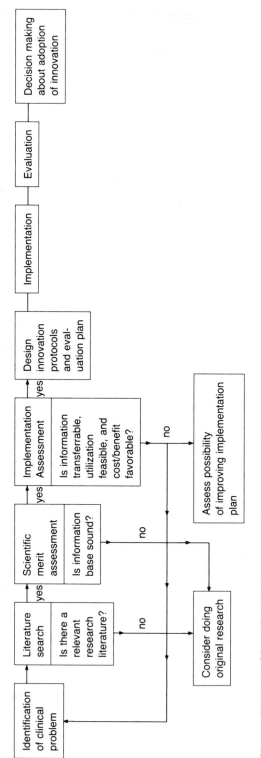

Figure 29-1. *Problem identification approach to research utilization.*

select an alternative one or (2) to consider initiating an original research project on the topic (i.e., to initiate steps to *create* a knowledge base). This decision is likely to depend on the research skills of the staff and on the availability of research consultants.

Next, the knowledge base must be assessed. If the knowledge base is sound (according to criteria to be described later), then the subsequent step is to conduct an implementation assessment. If, however, the existing knowledge base inspires little confidence that the research could effectively be utilized by nurses, then there remain the two previously suggested alternatives: (1) to "go back to the drawing board" and select a new problem or (2) to investigate the possibility of doing original research to improve the knowledge base.

The implementation assessment involves three primary aspects: (1) an assessment of the transferability of the research findings, (2) an analysis of the cost/benefit ratio, and (3) an evaluation of the feasibility of implementing the innovation. These criteria will be elaborated in the next section. If all of the implementation criteria are met, the team can then proceed to design the protocols for the innovation and its clinical evaluation, test the innovation in the practice setting, evaluate its effectiveness and costs, and then decide whether the new practice should be institutionalized. A final optional step, but one that is highly advisable, is the dissemination of the results of the utilization project so that other practicing nurses can benefit. If the implementation analysis suggests that there might be problems in testing the innovation within that particular practice setting, then the team can either identify a new problem and begin the process anew or consider adopting a plan to improve the implementation potential (e.g., seeking external resources if cost considerations were the inhibiting factor).

The second major approach to conducting a utilization project, shown schematically in Figure 29-2, has many of the same components as the first approach. The major difference, however, is the starting point. Here, the process starts with the research literature. This could occur if, for example, a utilization project emerged as a result of discussions within a journal club. In this approach, the team would proceed through most of the same steps as outlined previously, except that a preliminary assessment would need to be made of the clinical relevance of the research findings. If it is determined that the research base is not clinically relevant, then the next step involves further reading and reviewing of the research literature.

Both of these approaches involve several types of assessments, the results of which affect the appropriateness of proceeding with the utilization project. Criteria for making these assessments are presented below.

Utilization Criteria

As the two models shown in Figures 29-1 and 29-2 suggest, there are three broad classes of criteria that are important in undertaking a utilization project:

1. Clinical relevance
2. Scientific merit
3. Implementation potential

Box 29-1 presents some assessment questions for these categories, each of which is elaborated on here.

CLINICAL RELEVANCE

Of critical importance is whether the problem and its solution have a high degree of clinical relevance. The central issue here is whether a problem of significance to nurses will be solved by making some change or introducing a new intervention. There is little point in undertaking a utilization project if the nursing profession or the clients it serves cannot benefit from the effort. If, under the best of circumstances, there is little potential for solving a nursing problem or helping nurses to make important clinical decisions, then the project should probably be discontinued.

(*text continues on page 614*)

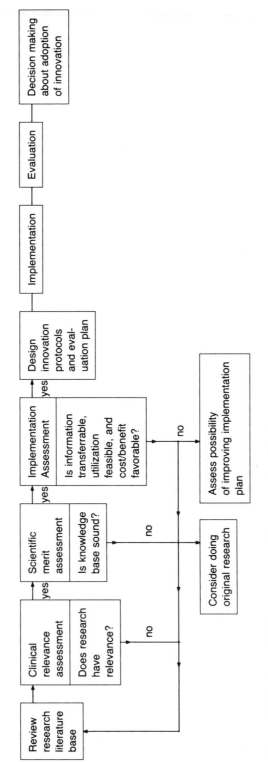

Figure 29-2. *Research literature approach to research utilization.*

BOX 29-1 CRITERIA FOR EVALUATING THE UTILIZATION POTENTIAL OF A STUDIED INNOVATION

Clinical Relevance

1. Does the research have the potential to help solve a problem that is currently being faced by practitioners today?
2. Does the research have the potential to help with clinical decision making with respect to appropriate observations to make, identifying client risks or complications, or selecting an appropriate intervention?
3. Are clinically relevant theoretical propositions tested by the research?
4. If the research involves an intervention, does the intervention have potential for implementation in clinical practice? Do nurses have control over the implementation of such interventions?
5. Can the measures used in the study be used in clinical practice?

Scientific Merit

1. Does the knowledge base include studies that are conceptually and methodologically rigorous? Do the findings appear to be accurate, internally valid, and generalizable to the target population?
2. Has the research been replicated? Has it been replicated with clinical clients? Have the replications yielded similar results, such that there is confidence that the innovation is effective?

Implementation Potential

Transferability of the Findings

1. Will the innovation "fit" in the proposed setting?
2. How similar was the target population in the research and the target population in the new setting?
3. Is the philosophy of care underlying the innovation fundamentally different from the philosophy prevailing in the practice setting? How entrenched is the prevailing philosophy?
4. Is there a sufficiently large number of clients in the practice setting who could benefit from the innovation?
5. Will the innovation take too long to implement and evaluate?

Feasibilty

1. Will nurses have the freedom to carry out the innovation? Will they have the freedom to terminate the innovation if it is considered undesirable?
2. Will the implementation of the innovation interfere inordinately with current staff functions?
3. Does the administration support the innovation? Is the organizational climate conducive to research utilization?
4. Is there a fair degree of consensus among the staff and among the administrators that the innovation could be beneficial and should be tested? Are there major pockets of resistance or uncooperativeness that could undermine efforts to implement and evaluate the innovation?
5. To what extent will the implementation of the innovation cause friction within the organization? Does the utilization project have the support and cooperation of departments outside the nursing department?
6. Are the skills needed to carry out the utilization project (both the implementation and the clinical evaluation) available on the nursing staff? If not, how difficult will it be to collaborate with or to secure the assistance of others with the necessary skills?
7. Does the organization have the equipment and facilities necessary for the innovation? If not, is there a way to obtain the needed resources?
8. If nursing staff need to be released from other practice activities to learn about and implement the innovation, then what is the likelihood that this will happen?
9. Are appropriate measuring tools available for a clinical evaluation of the innovation?

(continued)

BOX 29-1 CRITERIA FOR EVALUATING THE UTILIZATION POTENTIAL OF A STUDIED INNOVATION (*CONTINUED*)

Cost/Benefit of the Innovation

1. What are the risks to which clients would be exposed during the implementation of the innovation?
2. What are the potential benefits that could result from the implementation of the innovation?
3. What are the risks of maintaining current practices (i.e., the risks of *not* trying the innovation)?
4. What are the material costs of implementing the innovation? What are the costs in the short-term during utilization, and what are the costs in the long run, if the change is to be institutionalized?
5. What are the material costs of *not* implementing the innovation (i.e., could the new procedure result in some efficiencies that could lower the cost of providing service)?
6. What are the potential nonmaterial costs of implementing the innovation to the organization (e.g., lower staff morale, staff turnover, or absenteeism)?
7. What are the potential nonmaterial benefits of implementing the innovation (e.g., improved staff morale, improved staff recruitment, and so on)?

The five questions relating to clinical relevance, shown in Box 29-1, can be applied to a research report or set of related reports, and can generally be answered based on a reading of the introductions to the reports. According to Tanner (1987), from whom these questions were adapted, if the answer is "yes" to any one of the five questions, then the next step in the process can be pursued because the innovation has the potential for being useful in practice. If, however, the answers to all of the questions are negative, then the prospect of clinical relevance is small, and there is probably little point in pursuing the problem area any further.

SCIENTIFIC MERIT

We have discussed the criteria for scientific merit throughout this book, and in Chapter 28 we presented guidelines for assessing whether the findings and conclusions of a study are accurate, believable, and generalizable. When it comes to utilization, however, some additional concerns must be considered. First and foremost is the issue of replication, the repeating of a study in a new setting, with a new sample of subjects. It is unwise to base an entire utilization project on a single study that has not been replicated, even if the study is extremely rigorous. Ideally, there would be several replications—each providing

similar evidence of the effectiveness of the innovation being considered. At least one and ideally more of the studies should have been conducted in a clinical setting, with "real" clients.

Replications are seldom exact duplications of an earlier study; usually a replication involves making some changes to some aspects of the research methods, such as the data collection instruments, the sampling plan, and so on. It is not essential that the replications be identical to provide a useful basis for pursuing a utilization project. Rather, it is more important that the *problem* being addressed is the same, and that the innovations being tested are conceptually similar to each other. For example, several nurse researchers have investigated the use of therapeutic touch as a means of reducing stress and enhancing the psychologic well-being of patients. Although these studies have all operationalized "therapeutic touch" in somewhat different ways and have examined somewhat different outcomes, it would be reasonable for a utilization project to consider the whole body of research on therapeutic touch.

IMPLEMENTATION POTENTIAL

Even when it has been determined that a problem has clinical significance and when there is a sound knowledge base relating to that clinical problem, it is not necessarily true that a utilization project can be planned and implemented. A number of other issues must be considered, which we have grouped under three headings: (1) the transferability of the knowledge, (2) the feasibility of implementation, and (3) the cost/benefit ratio of the innovation.

The main issue in the transferability question is whether it makes good sense to attempt the selected innovation in the new practice setting. If there is some aspect of the practice setting that is fundamentally incongruent with the innovation—in terms of its philosophy, the type of clients it serves, its personnel, or its financial or administrative structure—then it clearly makes little sense to try to transfer the innovation, even if a clinically significant innovation has been shown to be effective in various research contexts.

The feasibility questions address a number of practical concerns about the availability of resources, the availability of staff, the organizational climate, the need for and availability of external assistance, and the potential for clinical evaluation. An important issue here is whether nurses will have control over the innovation (usually this means having the ability to manipulate the independent variable). When nurses do not have full control over the new procedure being introduced, it is important to recognize the interdependent nature of the utilization project and to proceed as early as possible to establish the necessary cooperative arrangements.

A critical part of any decision to proceed with a utilization project is a careful assessment of the costs and benefits of the innovation. The assessment should encompass costs and benefits to various groups, including clients, staff, the organization as a whole, and even the nursing profession as a whole. Clearly, the most important factor is the client. If the degree of risk in introducing a new procedure is high, then the potential benefits must be very great. Moreover, if there are risks to client well-being, it is essential that the knowledge base be very sound. That is, an innovation that involves client risks should only be implemented when there is a solid body of evidence

from several methodologically rigorous studies that the new practice is effective. A cost/benefit assessment should consider the reverse side of the coin as well: the costs and benefits of *not* implementing the innovation. It is sometimes easy to forget that the *status quo* bears its own risks, and that failure to change—especially when such change is based on a firm knowledge base—is costly to clients, to organizations, and to the entire nursing community.

≡ *SUMMARY*

In nursing, *research utilization* refers to the use of some aspect of a scientific investigation in a clinical application unrelated to the original research. Research utilization can best be characterized as lying on a continuum with direct utilization of some specific innovation at (*"instrumental utilization"*) one end and more diffuse situations in which users are influenced in their thinking about an issue based on some research (*"conceptual utilization"*) at the other end.

There is tremendous potential for research utilization at all points along this continuum throughout the nursing process. To date, however, there is little evidence that utilization has occurred—at least not with respect to instrumental utilization. It seems likely, though, that more diffuse forms of utilization have occurred as nurses have increased their research productivity and their awareness of the need for research. Several major utilization projects have been implemented, the most noteworthy being the WICHE, NCAST, and CURN projects. These utilization projects demonstrated that it is possible to increase research utilization, but they also shed light on some of the barriers to utilization. These barriers include such factors as an inadequate scientific base, nursing staff with little training in research and utilization, resistance to change among nurses and institutions that employ them, unfavorable organizational climates, resource constraints, limited collaboration among practitioners and researchers, poorly developed communication channels among these two groups, and the shortage of appropriate role models.

Responsibility for research utilization should be borne by the entire nursing community. Researchers, educators, members of peer review panels, practicing nurses, nursing students, and nurse administrators could adopt a number of strategies to improve the extent to which research findings form the basis for nursing practice.

In planning a major utilization project, practicing nurses can begin with the identification of an important clinical problem and then proceed to identify and critique the knowledge base and perform an assessment of the implementation potential of the innovation. Under favorable conditions, the nurses could then plan the innovation protocols, implement and evaluate the innovation, and make a rational decision regarding the adoption of the innovation based on the evaluation. Alternatively, nurses can begin with the knowledge base and then perform an evaluation of the clinical relevance of a research area before proceeding through the other steps of the utilization process. In either case, there are three major categories of criteria that must be considered before proceeding with a utilization plan: (1) clinical relevance, (2) scientific merit, and (3) implementation potential. The implementation potential category includes the dimensions of transferability of knowledge, feasibility of utilization in the particular setting, and the cost/benefit ratio of the innovation.

≡ *STUDY SUGGESTIONS*

1. Find an article in a recent issue of a nursing research journal that does not discuss the implications of the study for nursing practice. Evaluate the study's relevance to nursing practice and, if appropriate, write one to two paragraphs summarizing the implications.
2. Consider your personal situation. What are the barriers that might inhibit your use of research findings? What steps might be taken to address those barriers?

≡ *SUGGESTED READINGS*

METHODOLOGICAL REFERENCES

American Nurses' Association Congress for Practice. (1973). *Standards for practice.* Kansas City, MO: Author.

Barnard, K.E., & Hoehn, R.E. (1978). *Nursing child assessment satellite training: Final report.* Hyattsville, MD: Department of Health, Education, and Welfare, Division of Nursing.

Brodish, M.S., Tranbarger, R.E., & Chamings, P.A. (1987). Clinical nursing research: A model for collaboration. *Journal of Nursing Administration, 17,* 6, 32.

Caplan, N., & Rich, R.F. (1975). *The use of social science knowledge in policy decisions at the national level.* Ann Arbor, MI: Institute for Social Research, University of Michigan.

Downs, F.S. (1979). Clinical and theoretical research. In F.S. Downs & J.W. Fleming (Eds.), *Issues in nursing research.* New York: Appleton-Century-Crofts.

Fitzpatrick, J.J. (1988). Harmonic convergence. *Applied Nursing Research, 1,* 1.

Funk, S.G., Tornquist, E.M., & Champagne, M.T. (1989a). A model for improving the dissemination of nursing research. *Western Journal of Nursing Research, 11,* 361–367.

Funk, S.G., Tornquist, E.M., & Champagne, M.T. (1989b). Application and evaluation of the dissemination model. *Western Journal of Nursing Research, 11,* 485–491.

Haller, D., Reynolds, M., & Horsley, J. (1979). Developing research-based innovation protocols: Process, criteria, and issues. *Research in Nursing and Health, 2,* 45–51.

Horsley, J.A., Crane, J., & Bingle, J.D. (1978). Research utilization as an organizational process. *Journal of Nursing Administration, 8,* 4–6.

Horsley, J., Crane, J., Crabtree, M., & Wood, D. (1983). *Using research to improve nursing practice: A guide.* New York: Grune & Stratton.

Jackel, M. (1989). Presenting research to nurses in clinical practice. *Applied Nursing Research, 2,* 191–193.

Keefe, M.R., Pepper, G., & Stoner, M. (1988). Toward research-based nursing practice: The Denver collaborative research network. *Applied Nursing Research, 1,* 109–115.

Krueger, J.C., Nelson, A.H., & Wolanin, M.O. (1978).

Nursing research: Development, collaboration, and utilization. Germantown, MD: Aspen Systems.

Lambert, C.E., & Lambert, V.A. (1988). Clinical nursing research: Its meaning to the practicing nurse. *Applied Nursing Research, 1,* 54–57.

Larson, E. (1989). Using the CURN project to teach research utilization in a baccalaureate program. *Western Journal of Nursing Research, 11,* 593–599.

Maurin, J.T. (1990). Research utilization in the social-political arena. *Applied Nursing Research, 3,* 48–51.

Phillips, L.R.F. (1986). *A clinician's guide to the critique and utilization of nursing research.* Norwalk, CT: Appleton-Century-Crofts.

Reynolds, M.A., & Haller, K.B. (1986). Using research in practice: A case for replication in nursing. *Western Journal of Nursing Research, 8,* 113–116.

Stetler, C.B. (1985). Research utilization: Defining the concept. *Image, 17,* 40–44.

Tanner, C.A. (1987). Evaluating research for use in practice: Guidelines for the clinician. *Heart and Lung, 16,* 424–430.

Weiss, C. (1980). Knowledge creep and decision accretion. *Knowledge: Creation, Diffusion, Utilization, 1,* 381–404.

SUBSTANTIVE REFERENCES

Brett, J.L.L. (1987). Use of nursing practice research findings. *Nursing Research, 36,* 344–349.

Brett, J.L.L. (1989). Organizational integrative mechanisms and adoption of innovations by nurses. *Nursing Research, 38,* 105–110.

Champion, V.L., & Leach, A. (1989). Variables related to research utilization in nursing. *Journal of Advanced Nursing, 14,* 705–710.

Coyle, L.A., & Sokop, A.G. (1990). Innovation adoption behavior among nurses. *Nursing Research, 39,* 176–180.

Horsley, K., Crane, J., Haller, J., & Bingle, J. (1981). *Closed urinary drainage system (CURN Project).* New York: Grune & Stratton.

Ketefian, S. (1975). Application of selected nursing research findings into nursing practice. *Nursing Research, 24,* 89–92.

King, I., & Tarsitano, E. (1982). The effect of structured and unstructured preoperative teaching: A replication. *Nursing Research, 31,* 324–329.

Kirchhoff, K.T. (1982). A diffusion survey of coronary precautions. *Nursing Research, 31,* 196–201.

Kruszewski, A., Lang, S., & Johnson, J. (1979). Effect of positioning on discomfort from intramuscular injections in the dorsogluteal site. *Nursing Research, 28,* 103–105.

Lim-Levy, F. (1982). The effect of oxygen inhalation on oral temperature. *Nursing Research, 31,* 150–152.

Longman, A.J., Verran, J.A., Ayoub, J., Neff, J., & Noyes, A. (1990). Research utilization: An evaluation and critique of research related to oral temperature measurement. *Applied Nursing Research, 3,* 14–19.

Nichols, G.A., & Verhonick, P.J. (1968). Placement times for oral temperatures: A nursing study replication. *Nursing Research, 17,* 159–161.

30
Writing a Research Proposal

This chapter brings us, in a sense, full circle: back to the beginning of a research project. A *research proposal* is a written document specifying what the investigator proposes to study and is, therefore, written before the project has commenced. Proposals serve to communicate the research problem, its significance, and planned procedures for solving the problem to some interested party.

Proposals are written for various reasons. A student enrolled in a research class is often expected to submit a brief plan to the professor before data collection actually begins. Most universities require a formal proposal and a proposal hearing for students about to engage in research for a thesis or dissertation. Funding agencies that sponsor research almost always award funds competitively and use proposals as a basis for their funding decisions.

Proposals prepared for different reasons vary in the amount of detail expected but, like research reports, often have similar content. In the next section, we provide some general information regarding the content and preparation of research proposals. In a subsequent section, we offer more specific guidelines for the preparation of a proposal for the National Institutes of Health (NIH), the federal agency that sponsors a great number of nursing studies.

≡ OVERVIEW OF PROPOSAL PREPARATION

Reviewers of research proposals, whether they are faculty, funding sponsors, or peer reviewers, want a clear idea of what the researcher plans to do, how and when various tasks are to be accomplished, and whether the researcher is capable of successfully following the proposed plan of action. Proposals are generally evaluated on a number of criteria, including the importance of the research question, its theoretical relevance, the adequacy of the research methods, the availability of appropriate personnel and facilities, and, if money is being requested, the reasonableness of the budget. General guidelines for preparing research proposals follow.

Proposal Content

A researcher preparing a proposal will almost always be given a set of instructions that indicate the format to be followed. Funding agencies often supply an application kit that includes forms to be completed and a specified format for organizing the contents of the proposal. Despite the fact that formats and the amount of detail required may vary widely, there is considerable similarity in the type of information that is expected in research proposals. The major "ingredients" normally included in research proposals are described in the following sections.

ABSTRACT

Proposals often begin with a brief synopsis of the proposed research. The abstract helps to establish a frame of reference for the reviewers as they begin to read the proposal. The abstract should be brief (about 200 to 300 words in length) and should concisely state the study objectives and methods to be used.

STATEMENT OF THE PROBLEM

The problem that the intended research will address is ordinarily identified early in the proposal. The problem should be stated in such a way that its importance is apparent to the reviewer. On the other hand, the researcher should not promise more than can be produced. A broad and complex problem is unlikely to be solvable or manageable.

SIGNIFICANCE OF THE PROBLEM

The proposal needs to clearly describe how the proposed research will make a contribution to knowledge. The proposal should indicate the expected generalizability of the research, its contribution to theory, its potential for improving nursing practice and patient care, and possible applications or consequences of the knowledge to be gained.

BACKGROUND OF THE PROBLEM

A section of the proposal is often devoted to an exposition of how the intended research builds on what has already been done in an area. The background material should strengthen the author's arguments concerning the significance of the study, orient the reader to what is already known about the problem, and indicate how the proposed research will augment that knowledge; it should also serve as a demonstration of the researcher's command of current knowledge in a field.

OBJECTIVES

Specific, achievable objectives provide the reader with clear criteria against which the proposed research methods can be assessed. Objectives stated as research hypotheses or specific models to be tested are often preferred. Whenever the theoretical background of the study, existing knowledge, or the researcher's experience permit an explicit prediction of outcomes, these predictions should be included in the proposal. Avoid the use of null hypotheses, which create an amateurish impression. In exploratory or descriptive research, the formulation of hypotheses might not be feasible. Objectives may, in such cases, be most conveniently phrased as questions.

METHODS

The explanation of the research methods should be thorough enough that a reader will have no question about how the research objectives will be addressed. A thorough methods section includes a description of the sampling plan, research design, instrumentation, specific procedures, and analytic strategies, together with a discussion of the rationale for the methods, potential methodological problems, and intended strategies for handling such problems.

THE WORK PLAN

It is customary for the proposal to describe the plan according to which the various tasks and subtasks will be accomplished. In other words, the researcher indicates the sequence of tasks to be performed, the anticipated length of time required for their completion, and the personnel required for their accomplishment. The work plan indicates to the reader how realistic and thorough the researcher has been in designing the study.

PERSONNEL

In proposals addressed to funding agencies, the qualifications of key project personnel should be described. The research competencies of the project director and other team members are typically given major consideration in evaluating a proposal.

FACILITIES

The proposal should document the extent to which special facilities required by the project will be available. Access to physiologic instrumentation, libraries, data processing equipment, computers, special documents or records, and so forth should be described to reassure sponsors or advisers that the project will be able to proceed as planned. The willingness of the institution with which the researcher is affiliated to allocate space, equipment, services, or data should also be indicated.

BUDGET

The budget translates the project activities into monetary terms. It is a statement of how much money will be required to accomplish the various tasks. A well-conceived work plan greatly facilitates the preparation of the budget. If there are inordinate difficulties in detailing financial needs, there may be reason to suspect that the work plan is insufficiently developed.

General Tips on Proposal Preparation

Although it would be impossible to tell readers exactly what steps to follow to produce a successful proposal, we can offer some advice that might help to minimize the anxiety and frustration that often accompany the preparation of a proposal. Many of the tips we provide are especially relevant for researchers who are preparing a proposal for the purpose of securing funding for a research project.

1. REVIEW A SUCCESSFUL PROPOSAL

Although there is no substitute for actually doing one's own proposal as a learning experience, beginning proposal writers can often profit considerably by actually seeing the "real thing." The information in this chapter is useful in providing some guidelines, but reviewing an actual successful proposal can do more to acquaint the novice with how all the pieces fit together than all the textbooks in the world.

Chances are some of your colleagues have written a proposal that has been accepted (either by a funding sponsor or by a dissertation committee), and many people are glad to share their successful efforts with others. Also, proposals funded by the federal government are generally in the public domain. That means that you can ask to see a copy of proposals that have obtained federal funding by writing to the sponsoring agency.

In recognition of the need of beginning

researchers to become familiar with successful proposals, *The Western Journal of Nursing Research* has published proposals in their entirety (with the exception of administrative information such as budgets), together with the critique of the proposal prepared by a panel of expert reviewers. For example, the first such published proposal was a grant application funded by the Division of Nursing entitled, "Couvade: Patterns, Predictors, and Nursing Management" (Clinton, 1985). Another journal, *Grants Magazine,* also publishes successful proposals.

2. PAY ATTENTION TO REVIEWERS' CRITERIA

In most instances in which research funding is at stake, the funding agency will provide the researcher with information about the criteria that reviewers use in making funding decisions. In some cases, the criteria will simply be a listing of questions that the reviewers must address in making a global assessment of the proposal's quality. In other cases, however, the agency will be able to specify exactly how many points will be assigned to different aspects of the proposal on the basis of specified criteria. As an example, the National Institute of Child Health and Human Development funded some research projects relating to fertility regulation using the following evaluation criteria:

Conceptualization of the problem. Ability of the researcher to conceptualize the problem, including the operationalizing and quantifying of measures, and the development of a theoretical/conceptual framework.
(0 to 30 points)
Project staff qualifications and availability.
Adequacy of the relevant training and experience of the proposed staff.
(0 to 15 points)
Appropriateness of allocation of personnel and time to accomplish objectives of the project.
(0 to 10 points)
Data sources and analysis. Demonstration of capability for identifying and obtaining access to pertinent and relevant sources of data and ade-

quacy of plans for data analysis.
(0 to 20 points)
Review and analysis of literature. Adequacy of the review and analysis of the literature in terms of scope and depth and extent to which research needs in theoretical, methodological, and analytical areas are delineated.
(0 to 15 points)
Facilities and equipment. Adequacy of computer facilities and other equipment that would be needed in the performance of the research.
(0 to 10 points)

Different agencies establish different criteria for different types of research projects. The wise researcher will learn what those criteria are and pay careful attention to them in the development of the proposal. In the example of reviewers' criteria, a maximum of 100 points was awarded for each competing proposal. The proposals with the highest scores would ordinarily be most likely to obtain funding. Therefore, the researcher should pay particular attention to those aspects of the proposal that contribute most to an overall high score. In the example, it would have made little sense to put 85% of the proposal development effort into the literature review section, when a maximum of 15 points could be given for this part of the proposal.

3. BE JUDICIOUS IN DEVELOPING A RESEARCH TEAM

For projects that are funded, reviewers often give considerable weight to the qualifications of the people who will conduct the research. In the example of reviewers' criteria, a full 25 of the 100 points were based on the expertise of the research personnel and their time allocations.

The person who is in the lead role in the project—often referred to as the *Principal Investigator* or PI—should carefully scrutinize the qualifications of the research team. It is not enough to have a team of competent people. It is necessary to have the right mix of competence. A project team of three brilliant theorists without statistical skills in a project that proposes sophisticated multivariate techniques may have difficulty convincing reviewers that the project would be successful. Gaps and weaknesses can often be compensated for by the judicious use of consultants.

Another shortcoming of many project teams is that they often look as though there are too many managers. It is generally unwise to load up a project staff with five or more top-level professionals who are only able to contribute 5% to 10% of their time to the project. Such projects often run into management difficulties because no one person is ever really in control of the flow of work. Although collaborative efforts are to be commended, you should be able to *justify* the inclusion of every staff person and to identify the unique contribution that each will make to the successful completion of the project.

4. JUSTIFY AND DOCUMENT YOUR DECISIONS

Unsuccessful proposals often fail because they do not provide the reviewer with confidence that adequate thought and consideration have been given to a rationale for decisions. Almost every aspect of the proposal involves a decision— the problem selected, the population studied, the size of the sample, the data collection procedures to be used, the comparison group to be used, the extraneous variables to be controlled, the analytic procedures to be used, the personnel who will work on the project, and so on. These decisions should be carefully made, keeping in mind the costs and benefits of an alternative decision. When you are satisfied that you have made the right decision, you should be ready to defend your decision by sharing the rationale with the reviewers. In general, insufficient detail is more detrimental to the proposal than an overabundance of detail, although page constraints may make full detail impossible.

5. ARRANGE FOR A CRITIQUE OF THE PROPOSAL

Before formal submission of a proposal, a draft should be reviewed by at least one other person, preferably someone with relevant methodological and substantive strengths in the proposed area of research. (Ideally, if the proposal is being submitted for funding, then the reviewer will be someone who is knowledgeable about the funding source.) If a consultant has been proposed because of specialized expertise that you believe will strengthen the study, then it would be very advantageous to have that consultant participate in the proposal development by reviewing the draft and making recommendations for its improvement.

≡ GRANT APPLICATIONS TO NIH

The National Institutes of Health funds a considerable number of nursing research studies through the National Center for Nursing Research (NCNR) and through other institutes and agencies within NIH. Applications for grant funding through NIH are made by completing Public Health Service Grant Application Form PHS 398, which is available through the research offices of most universities and hospitals. Copies of the application kit can also be obtained by writing

Division of Research Grants
National Institutes of Health
Westwood Building
5333 Westbard Avenue
Bethesda, MD 20205

New grant applications are processed in three cycles annually. The schedule for submission and review of new grant applications is shown in Table 30-1. Proposals (grant applications) may be submitted on the proper forms at any time during the year. However, proposals received after one receipt date will be held for another cycle. For example, if a proposal is received by NIH on February 2, it will be considered with the proposals received by June 1, not February 1.

The Review Process

Grant applications submitted to NIH are received by the Division of Research Grants, where they are reviewed for relevance *vis-à-vis* the overall mission of NIH. Acceptable applications are assigned to an appropriate Institute or Center. Figure 30-1 presents the NIH Institutes and Centers, as of June 1989. Most applications by nurse researchers are assigned to NCNR, unless the content of the proposal is better suited to another Institute.

As the schedule in Table 30-1 indicates, NIH uses a dual review system for making decisions about its grant applications. The first level involves a panel of peer reviewers, who evaluate the grant application for its scientific merit. This panel (usually referred to as an Initial Review Group or *Study Section*) consists of approximately 10 to 15 scientists with backgrounds appropriate to the specific Study Section for which they have been selected. Appointments to the review panels are generally for 4-year terms, and are staggered so that approximately one fourth of each panel is new each year. The second level of review is by a National Advisory Council, which includes both scientific and lay representatives. The National Advisory Council considers not only the scientific merit of an application but the relevance of the proposed study to the programs and priorities of the Center or Institute to which the application has been submitted.

The peer review panel members, after discussing the strengths and weaknesses of a given application, normally make one of three decisions: (1) to approve an application, (2) to disapprove an application, or (3) to defer an application. Deferrals are relatively rare and usually involve an application that the review panel considers meritorious but missing some crucial information that would permit the panel to make a final determination. Most proposals are either approved or disapproved immediately. Review panels vary considerably from one Study Section to another in the proportion of applications that are approved. In part, this reflects the quality of the proposals themselves, but it also reflects the "philosophy" of different panels. Because only a relatively small percentage of proposals that are approved are actually funded, some panels decide to disapprove only a small minority of applications, reserving their disapprovals for projects that are judged to potentially "set back science." In the Nursing Research Study Section, approximately 95% of all grant applications typically are approved at each meeting.

All applications that are *approved* are assigned a priority rating by each member of the review panel. The ratings range from 1.0 (the best possible score) to 5.0 (the least favorable score), in increments of 0.1. NIH has established the following guidelines for assigning priority scores:

Outstanding: 1.0–1.5
Excellent: 1.5–2.0
Good: 2.0–2.5
Satisfactory: 2.5–3.0
Adequate: 3.0–3.5
Fair: 3.5–4.0
Acceptable: 4.0–5.0

The individual ratings from different panel members are then combined, averaged, and multiplied by 100 to yield scores that range from 100 to 500, with 100 being the best possible score.

Table 30-1. *Schedule for Processing Grant Applications*

RECEIPT DATES	INITIAL (PEER) REVIEW DATES	NATIONAL ADVISORY COUNCIL REVIEW DATES	EARLIEST POSSIBLE START DATES
February 1	June/July	September/October	December 1
June 1	October/November	January/February	April 1
October 1	February/March	May/June	July 1

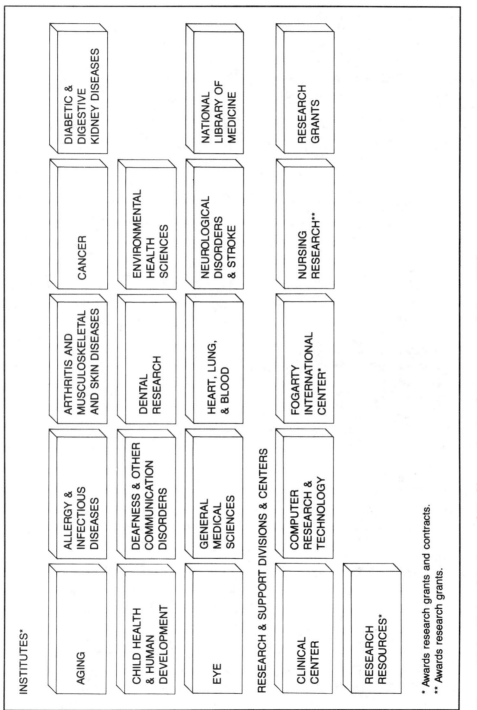

Figure 30-1. *National Institutes of Health organizational structure as of June 1989.*

INSTITUTES*

AGING	ALLERGY & INFECTIOUS DISEASES	ARTHRITIS AND MUSCULOSKELETAL AND SKIN DISEASES	CANCER	DIABETIC & DIGESTIVE KIDNEY DISEASES
CHILD HEALTH & HUMAN DEVELOPMENT	DEAFNESS & OTHER COMMUNICATION DISORDERS	DENTAL RESEARCH	ENVIRONMENTAL HEALTH SCIENCES	
EYE	GENERAL MEDICAL SCIENCES	HEART, LUNG, & BLOOD	NEUROLOGICAL DISORDERS & STROKE	NATIONAL LIBRARY OF MEDICINE

RESEARCH & SUPPORT DIVISIONS & CENTERS

| CLINICAL CENTER | COMPUTER RESEARCH & TECHNOLOGY | FOGARTY INTERNATIONAL CENTER* | NURSING RESEARCH** | RESEARCH GRANTS |
| RESEARCH RESOURCES* | | | | |

* Awards research grants and contracts.
** Awards research grants.

Among all approved applications, only those with the best priority scores actually obtain funding. Cutoff scores for funding vary from agency to agency and year to year. It is generally necessary to obtain a rating of 200 or better to become funded. Within NIH overall, fewer than 20% of all grant applications are actually funded.*

Each applicant, regardless of the decision of the Study Section, is sent a summary of the peer review panel's evaluation. These "pink sheets" (so called because they are printed on pink paper) summarize the reviewers' comments in six areas: (1) an overall description of the project; (2) a critique of the strengths and weaknesses of the methodological and conceptual aspects of the proposal; (3) an evaluation of the project team; (4) an evaluation of the facilities and resources; (5) an assessment of the reasonableness of the budget; and (6) a discussion of other considerations, with emphasis on the protection of the rights of human subjects or the welfare of animal subjects. The applicant is also advised of the panel's decision (approval, disapproval, or deferral), and, if the proposal was approved, the priority score and percentile rank.

Unless an unfunded proposal is criticized in some very fundamental way (e.g., the problem area was not judged to be significant or the basic design was considered inappropriate), it is often worthwhile to resubmit an application, making revisions that reflect the concerns of the peer review panel. Proposals that receive encouraging but unfundable priority scores (in the 200 range) are especially likely to fare well in a resubmission. When a proposal is resubmitted, the next review panel is usually given a copy of the original application and the "pink sheet" so that they can evaluate the degree to which the original criticisms have been addressed.

Types of NIH Grants

NIH awards different types of grants, and each has its own objectives and review criteria.

Three types of grants that represent the bulk of awards are discussed below, but other types are also available.

The basic grant program is the *Research Project Grant* (R01). The objective of the R01 grant is to support discrete, specific research projects in areas reflecting the interests and competencies of a Principal Investigator. The review criteria include (1) the significance and originality of the proposed research, (2) the appropriateness and adequacy of the proposed research methods, (3) the qualifications and experience of the PI and other staff, (4) the availability of needed resources, (5) the reasonableness of the proposed budget, and (6) the adequacy of proposed means for protecting human subjects or research animals.

A special program (R15) has been established for researchers working in educational institutions that have not been major participants in NIH programs. These are the *Academic Research Enhancement Awards* (AREA), the objective of which is to stimulate research in institutions that provide baccalaureate training for many individuals who go on to do health-related research. AREA grants enable qualified researchers to obtain support for small-scale research projects. The review criteria for AREA grants are basically the same as for the Research Project Grants.

Another special program has been established for new investigators. The *First Independent Research Support and Transition* or FIRST (R29) program is designed to provide an initial period of support for newly independent researcher scientists. These grants are intended to provide an opportunity for new scientists to demonstrate creativity and productivity and to assist them in making the transition to other NIH grants. FIRST awards are made for a period of 5 years and the total direct costs must not exceed $350,000 in total. The review criteria are similar to those for R01 grants, but less emphasis is placed on the investigator's experience than on his or her potential for productive research. Letters of reference must accompany the proposal and are carefully evaluated.

* Within the Nursing Research Study Section, the median priority score is typically in the 250 to 270 range.

Preparing a Grant Application for NIH

As indicated earlier, proposals to NIH must be submitted according to procedures described in the Public Health Service application kit. Each kit specifies exactly how the grant application should be prepared and what forms are to be used for supplying critical pieces of information. It is important to follow these instructions precisely. In the following sections, we describe the various components of an application and provide some tips that should be helpful in completing certain sections.*

SECTION 1

The "frontmatter" of the grant application consists primarily of forms that help in the processing of the application or that provide administrative information about the conduct of the research. Proposal writers often fail to give this section the attention it merits, because all of the intellectual work is presented in Section 2. However, we urge researchers to pay as much attention to detail in this first section as in the second. Each component of Section 1 is briefly described to acquaint the reader with its contents.

- *Title page.* Here the researcher provides the title of the application (not to exceed 56 spaces), the name of the PI, the name of the PI's institutional affiliation, the amount of money requested, the length of the proposed project, and other administrative information.
- *Abstract of research plan.* Page 2 asks for a listing of the key professional personnel who would work on the study and a half-page abstract of the investigator's aims and methods. The abstract *must* fit into the space allocated.

*The application kit for NIH grants changes periodically. Therefore, the instructions in a current version of Form PHS 398 should be carefully reviewed and followed in preparing a grant application, rather than relying exclusively on information in this chapter.

- *Table of contents.* Page 3 indicates on what pages various sections and subsections of the proposal are to be found.
- *Budget.* Pages 4 and 5 consist of budgetary forms. Page 4 asks for an itemization of all costs that would be incurred by the project during the first 12 months. Page 5 asks for a summary of the budget for the entire project period. For R01 grants, support can be requested for up to five years, but the majority of projects are completed in three years or fewer. Beginning at the bottom of page 5, the researcher must provide a narrative justification of all budgeted items. New researchers often make the mistake of submitting a budget justification that is insufficiently detailed. Remember that the reviewers need to be able to tell whether the budget is reasonable, and part of your job is to convince them that you would use funding judiciously. Normally two or three single-spaced pages are needed to justify budgetary items.

Figure 30-2 presents a hypothetical "Page 4" (detail of first-year expenditures), and Figure 30-3 presents a hypothetical "Page 5" for a study that would require two years of support. The bottom of Figure 30-2 presents the first half-page of a budget justification, showing the level of detail that is ordinarily considered appropriate. For most projects, personnel costs (wages and fringe benefits) represent the bulk of the requested funds, and personnel costs are generally represented as a percentage of a person's time (e.g., 20 hours per week would be designated as a 50% level of effort on the proposed project). Other costs include the cost for consultants, project-specific equipment, supplies, travel costs, patient care costs, costs associated with a subcontract or consortium arrangements, and other expenses. The final category might include such items as laboratory fees, subject stipends, transcriptions, computer time, and data entry expenses. Note that the NIH budget forms should indicate direct project costs only. Indirect institu- (*text continues on page 630*)

DETAILED BUDGET FOR FIRST 12-MONTH BUDGET PERIOD
DIRECT COSTS ONLY

FROM 12/1/90	THROUGH 11/30/91

PERSONNEL (Applicant organization only)		1	2	3	DOLLAR AMOUNT REQUESTED (Omit cents)		
NAME	ROLE IN PROJECT	TYPE APPT.	% OF APPT.	EFFORT ON PROJ.	SALARY	FRINGE BENEFITS	TOTALS
Cozette White	Principal Investigator	1.0	.25	.25	10,000	2,500	12,500
Alison Lupping	Co-Investigator	1.0	.10	.10	3,000	750	3,750
To Be Hired	Interviewer	1.0	.75	.75	13,500	3,375	16,875
To Be Hired	Research Asst.	.50	.50	.25	3,750	938	4,688
To Be Hired	Secretary	1.0	.40	.40	5,200	1,300	6,500
	SUBTOTALS ⟶				35,450	8,863	44,313

CONSULTANT COSTS
Wan Choi	5 days @ $250	(Statistical Consultant)	1,250
Anne Trainor	20 days @ $125	(Programming Consultant)	2,500

EQUIPMENT (Itemize)

Computer Modem	500

SUPPLIES (Itemize by category)
Office Supplies	$75./Mo. X 12	900
Xerox	$50./Mo. X 12	600
Postage	$40./Mo. X 12	480
Printing Instruments		750
Telephone (Long Distance)		500

TRAVEL	DOMESTIC 1 Conference and Interviewer Travel	1,750
	FOREIGN	
PATIENT CARE COSTS	INPATIENT	
	OUTPATIENT	

ALTERATIONS AND RENOVATIONS (Itemize by category)

CONSORTIUM/CONTRACTUAL COSTS
Subcontract to Woodlawn Hospital	9,375

OTHER EXPENSES (Itemize by category)
Subject Stipends - 200 @ $15	3,000
Data Entry - 200 X $3	600
Word Processing - 100 Hrs. @ $5/Hr.	500
Computer Time (Preliminary Analyses)	500

TOTAL DIRECT COSTS FOR FIRST 12-MONTH BUDGET PERIOD (Item 7a) ⟶	$	67,518

Figure 30-2. Example of first-year budget.

BUDGET FOR ENTIRE PROPOSED PROJECT PERIOD
DIRECT COSTS ONLY

BUDGET CATEGORY TOTALS		1st BUDGET PERIOD (from page 4)	ADDITIONAL YEARS SUPPORT REQUESTED			
			2nd	3rd	4th	5th
PERSONNEL (Salary and fringe benefits.) (Applicant organization only)		44,313	60,309			
CONSULTANT COSTS		3,750	5,000			
EQUIPMENT		500	---			
SUPPLIES		3,230	2,480			
TRAVEL	DOMESTIC	1,750	1,500			
	FOREIGN					
PATIENT CARE COSTS	INPATIENT					
	OUTPATIENT					
ALTERATIONS AND RENOVATIONS						
CONSORTIUM/ CONTRACTUAL COSTS		9,375	4,250			
OTHER EXPENSES		4,600	5,800			
TOTAL DIRECT COSTS		67,518	79,339			

TOTAL FOR ENTIRE PROPOSED PROJECT PERIOD (Also enter on page 1, item 8) ⟶ | $ 146,857

JUSTIFICATION (Use continuation pages if necessary): Describe the specific functions of the personnel and consultants. If a recurring annual increas in personnel costs is anticipated, give the percentage. For all years, justify any costs for which the need may not be obvious, such as equipment, foreig travel, alterations and renovations, and consortium/contractual costs. For any additional years of support requested, justify any significant increases i any category over the first 12 month budget period. In addition, for COMPETING CONTINUATION applications, justify any significant increases ov the current level of support.

Personnel

White, the Principal Investigator, will be responsible for overall project management, instrument development, data quality control, data analysis, and report preparation. She is budgeted for 25% effort in the first 18 months of the project. In the final 6 months, White will devote 50% of her time to the proposed project to perform the data analyses and prepare a final report.

Lupping, the Co-Investigator, will devote 10% of her time to the project throughout the 2-year period. She will participate in the instrumentation, training of the interviewer, development of a coding scheme, and analysis of the data.

The Interviewer will be hired in the fourth project month. She will work for 15 months at 100% effort and will be responsible for all data collection. A research assistant will be hired to assist with such tasks as library research, instrument pretests, and data coding. Her level of effort will be 25% throughout the project. A secretary will be hired at 40% effort to perform secretarial and clerical functions.

A 5% salary increase has been budgeted for all personnel in Year 2.

Consultants

Dr. Paul Speckman, a professor of statistics, will provide 5 days of consulting in Year 1 and 10 days of consulting in Year 2 relating to the analysis of research data.

Mr. Henry Mitchell, a doctoral student in computer sciences, will provide 20 days of consulting in both project years to assist with the establishment of data files and the processing of research data.

Equipment

A DC Hayes modem (300/1200 baud) will be purchased to permit communication between the project's mini-computer and the university mainframe. The modem will permit a more efficient analysis of the data.

Figure 30-3. Example of overall summary budget.

REMOVE AND USE FOR DRAFT COPY

tional costs (overhead) are not included in the budget. Beginning researchers are likely to need the assistance of a research administrator or an experienced, funded researcher in developing their first budget.

- *Biographical sketches.* Forms are provided to summarize salient aspects of the education and experience of key project personnel. The PI and any other proposed staff who are considered important contributors to the project's success must have their biographical sketches included. A maximum of two pages is permitted for each person.

- *Other support.* Key personnel must identify any sources of support they are now receiving or sources of support that they have pending in the form of other planned or submitted proposals. This page is designed to help reviewers determine whether important staff may be overcommitted and therefore be potentially unable to devote a sufficient amount of time to the proposed project.

- *Resources and environment.* On this form, the author must designate the availability of needed facilities and equipment, such as office space, computers, laboratories, medical apparatus, and so on.

SECTION 2

Section 2 of the NIH grant application is reserved for the investigator's research plan. This section consists of nine subsections (though not all nine are relevant to every application). Parts A through D of the research plan, combined, must not exceed 20 single-spaced pages. If the proposal does not adhere to this page restriction, then the application may be returned without review. Within the overall 20-page limitation, the text can be distributed among Parts A–D in any manner the researcher considers appropriate, although guidelines are suggested.

A. *Specific aims.* The researcher must provide a very succinct summary of the research problem and the specific objectives to be undertaken during the course of the project, in-

cluding any hypotheses to be tested. The guidelines suggest that Part A be restricted to a single page.

B. *Significance.* In Part B, the researcher must convince the review panel that the proposed study idea is sound and has important practical or theoretical relevance. In this section of the research plan, the researcher provides the context for the conduct of the study, usually through a brief analysis of existing knowledge on the topic and through a discussion of a conceptual framework. Within this context, the investigator must demonstrate the significance of, and need for, the proposed new project. Beginning researchers often have an especially difficult time with this section because only two to three pages are recommended. This is often a challenging task, especially if you have a firm grasp on the broad range of literature relating to your topic. However, we again urge researchers not to be tempted to exceed the three-page guideline. Space should be conserved for a full elaboration of the proposed research methods.

C. *Preliminary studies.* This section is reserved for a description of the project team's previous studies that are relevant to the new proposed investigation. Many novice researchers mistakenly believe that this section is designed for a literature review. If you make this mistake, it will only serve to indicate that you are a novice and unable to follow instructions. This section (although it is optional for new applications and is only required for continuation proposals) provides an opportunity to convince the reviewers that you have the skills and background needed to do the research. Because the biographical sketch is limited to only two pages, the "Preliminary Studies" section provides a forum for the description of any relevant work you and other key staff have either completed or are in the process of doing. If the only relevant research you have completed is your dissertation, here is an opportunity to describe that research in full. If you have completed relevant research that has led to publications, you should reference them in this section, and include copies of them as appendixes. Other items that might be described in this section include previous uses of an instrument or an experimental procedure that will be used in the new study, relevant clinical or teaching experience, membership on task forces or in organizations that have provided you with a perspective on the research problem, or the results of a pilot study that involved the same research problem. The point is that this section allows you to demonstrate that the proposed work grew out of some ongoing commitment to, interest in, or experience with the topic. For new applications, no more than 5 to 6 pages should be devoted to Part C, and fewer pages are often sufficient.

D. *Experimental design and methods.* It is in Part D that you must describe the methods you will use to conduct the study. This section should be succinct, but with sufficient detail to persuade reviewers that you have a good rationale for your methodological decisions. Although there are no specific page limitations associated with this section of the application, keep in mind that you have up to 20 pages in total for Parts A through D combined.

The number of subsections in the methods section varies from one application to another. Each subsection should be labeled clearly to facilitate the review process. As is true in organizing any written material, it is often useful to begin with an outline. Here is an outline of the sections used in a successful grant application for a nonexperimental study of parenting behavior and family environments among low-income teenage mothers:

- Overview of the Research Design
- Sampling Considerations
- Research Variables and Measuring Instruments
- Data Collection Procedures
- Data Analysis

- Research Products
- Project Schedule

If there is an experimental intervention, then that intervention should be described in full. Protocols for the implementation of the intervention also need to be discussed. If there is to be a control group, clearly identify how the control group will be selected. If the control group is an intact group, then you will need to discuss your rationale for the selection of the specified group, any shortcomings in using this group, and why this group is preferable to some alternative. For example, if you were to study the psychologic consequences of an abortion in an effort to determine the need for follow-up interventions, there are at least four alternative control groups: (1) same-aged, never-pregnant women; (2) same-aged women who had had a miscarriage; (3) same-aged women who were still pregnant and had not decided how to resolve the pregnancy; or (4) same-aged women who had delivered a baby. Each group might be expected to introduce different types of selection biases, so your rationale for selecting one over the other would be a critical reflection of your conceptualization of the problem and your methodological sophistication.

The design section should also indicate how (if at all) the research situation will be structured to control for extraneous variables. The proposal should specify what variables might represent contaminating sources of influence; which variables will be controlled (and how); why other variables will not be controlled; and what the probable impact of the uncontrolled variables on the study outcome will be. Krathwohl (1988) observed that "probably nobody knows better than the researcher the multiple sources of contamination which might affect the study. Convincingly indicate the nature and basis of the particular compromise which is being proposed and the reasons for accepting it" (p. 31).

A number of things should be included

in a section on sampling. The reviewer normally expects to find a description of the population, the proposed sampling design, and the number of subjects to be included in the study. This information has an important bearing on the generalizability of the results. The section should include both a description of the sampling plan and a justification for its use. If you cannot use random sampling, explain the constraints (e.g., the costs of implementing such a design) and discuss steps you would take to make the sample as representative as possible and to document any biases. Increasingly, review panels expect to see a power analysis that justifies the adequacy of the specified sample size. It is also advisable to document your access to the specified subject pool. For instance, if the proposal indicates that patients and personnel from Park Memorial Hospital will participate in the study, then you should include a letter of cooperation from an administrator of the hospital with the application. The reviewer needs to have confidence that the proposed study, if funded, would actually be done as planned.

Normally, a subsection is devoted to instrumentation. The use of particular measuring instruments should be justified as appropriate for the purposes of the study. It is inadequate to select a well-known measure without explicitly demonstrating its relevance and valued qualities. For established measures, the proposal should describe reported evidence of the measure's reliability and validity. If a new instrument is to be developed, then the anticipated procedures for its development *and* evaluation should be described. If possible, sample items or the entire instrument should be included in an appendix.

A subsection should be devoted to the specific procedures that will be used to collect the research data. This subsection should include such information as where and when the data will be collected, how subjects will be recruited, how research personnel such as interviewers or observers will be trained, whether subjects will be paid a stipend for their time, what quality control procedures will be implemented to ensure the integrity of the data, and how the security of the data will be maintained. If the study is longitudinal, then it is also important to describe the schedule for waves of data collection (and a rationale for the schedule), as well as information on how the problem of attrition will be managed.

The grant application should include, in as much detail as possible, the plan for the analysis of data. This is typically one of the weakest sections of proposals. Some applications say little more than, "Trust me—I'll figure out what to do with the data once I have collected them." You may not be able to tell in advance every analytic strategy you will try, but you should be able to work through the general procedures you will use in testing the hypotheses. Earlier in this section, we presented an outline of a grant application relating to parenting among low-income teenage mothers. The Data Analysis subsection of this grant application described the proposed plan with respect to the following analytic tasks:

a. Data Cleaning and Descriptive Analyses
b. Exploratory Analyses
c. Analysis of Bias
d. Testing Individual Hypotheses
e. Path Analysis

Although the grant application kit does not specifically request a project schedule or work plan, it is often useful to include one (unless the page limitation makes it impossible to do so). A work plan helps reviewers assess how realistic you have been in planning the project, and it should help you to develop an estimate of needed resources (i.e., your budget). Flowcharts and other diagrams are often useful for highlighting the sequencing and interrelationships of project activities. One of the simplest and most effective types of charts is called a *Gantt chart,* named after its inventor Henry Gantt. Figure

30-4 presents a Gantt chart for the 30-month study on teenage parents. Other more sophisticated charting techniques, such as the *Program Evaluation Review Technique (PERT)* and the *Critical Path Method,* are sometimes used for complex projects. These are briefly described by Krathwohl (1988).

E. *Human subjects.* If the research involves data collected from human subjects, then this section must describe the procedures that will be used to protect their rights and to minimize the risks that they will take. The application kit specifies six questions that need to be addressed (an example is presented in Appendix A). This section of the proposal often serves as the cornerstone of the document submitted to the Institutional Review Board (IRB) of your institution before funding (check with your office of research administration for IRB requirements).

F. *Vertebrate animals.* If your proposed re-search involves the use of vertebrate animals, then this section must contain a justification of their use and a description of the procedures used to safeguard their welfare.

G. *Consultants/collaborators.* If you plan to include consultants to help with specific tasks on the proposed project, you must include a letter from each consultant, confirming his or her willingness to serve on the project. Letters are also needed from collaborators on the project, if they are affiliated with an institution different from your own.

H. *Consortium/contractual arrangements.* If the proposed project will involve the collaboration of two or more different institutions (e.g., if a separate organization will be used to perform laboratory analyses, under a subcontract agreement), then details about the nature of the arrangements must be described in this section.

I. *Literature cited.* The final subsection of the

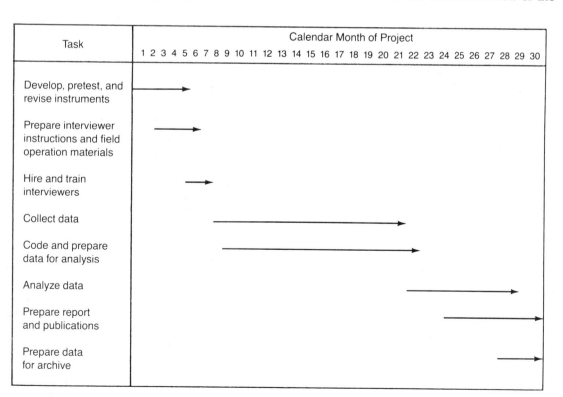

Figure 30-4. *Example of a Gantt chart.*

Research Plan consists of a list of references used in the text of the grant application. Any reference style is acceptable. This section is restricted to four pages.

SECTION 3

The concluding section of the grant application is reserved for appended materials. These materials might include actual instruments to be used in the project, detailed calculations on sample size estimates, scoring or coding instructions for instruments, proposed letters of consent, letters of cooperation from institutions that will provide access to subjects, complex statistical models, and other supplementary material in support of the application. The researcher can also submit copies of published papers or papers accepted for publication (but *not* papers submitted for publication but not yet accepted). The appended materials are not made available to the entire review panel, so essential information should not be relegated to the appendix.

☰ FUNDING FOR RESEARCH PROPOSALS

Funding for research projects is becoming more and more difficult to obtain. The problem lies not only in research cutbacks and inflation but also in the extremely keen and growing competition among researchers. As increasing numbers of nurses become prepared to carry out significant research, so, too, will applications for research funds increase. Successful proposal writers need to have good research and proposal-writing skills, and they must also know how and from whom funding is available. The combined set of skills and knowledge is sometimes referred to as *"grantsmanship."*

Federal Funding

The federal government is the largest contributor to the support of research activities. The two major types of federal disbursements are grants and contracts. *Grants* are awarded for pro-

posals in which the research idea is developed by the investigator. The researcher who identifies an important research problem can seek federal funds through a grant program of one or more agencies of the government.

There are two basic mechanisms for the funding of federal grants. One mechanism is for agencies and institutes to issue broad objectives and priorities and to invite grant applications that address these objectives. Researchers apply for funding from this grants program through the process described in the preceding section.

There are several ways to find out about such grant programs. *The Catalogue of Federal Domestic Assistance* publishes information about all federal programs that provide any kind of aid. The programs of such agencies as NIH, National Institute of Mental Health (NIMH), National Institute on Drug Abuse (NIDA), and so on are described in terms of objectives, types of assistance, award processes, and so on. There are also commercially available guides to programs, such as the annual *Federal Funding Guide*. (This guide, if purchased through Government Information Services in Arlington, Virginia, includes 12 monthly grant updates.) Programs identified as particularly promising through such sources can then be contacted for further information.

The second grant-funding mechanism offers federal agencies a mechanism for identifying a topic area in which they are especially interested in receiving applications. An agency may announce, for instance, that it is soliciting grant applications for studies relating to infertility. Such an announcement is referred to as a *Request for Applications* (RFA). Unlike the more general grants programs, the RFA usually specifies a deadline for the receipt of proposals. General guidelines and goals for the competition are also specified, but the researcher has considerable liberty to develop the specific research problem. Notices of such grant competitions are published in *The Federal Register*.

The second type of government funding (and this may occur at both the federal and state level) is in the form of *contracts*. An agency that identifies the need for a specific study issues a

Request for Proposals (RFP), which details the exact work that the government wants done. Proposals in response to RFPs describe the methods the researcher would use in addressing the research problem, the project staff and facilities, and the cost of doing the study in the proposed way. Contracts are usually awarded to only one of the competitors. Clearly, the contract method of securing research support severely constrains the kinds of work in which investigators can engage. For this reason, most nurse researchers probably will want to compete for grants rather than contracts. Nevertheless, many interesting RFPs have been issued by NIH and other agencies. For example, one recent NIH RFP called for proposals for a study of "Ethnic Differences in Life Style, Psychological Factors, and Medical Care During Pregnancy."

A summary of each federal RFP is printed in the *Commerce Business Daily,* which is published every government workday. Also, NIH publishes a weekly bulletin called the *NIH Guide for Grants and Contracts.* This bulletin announces new NIH initiatives, including the announcement of RFAs and RFPs issued by NIH.*

Private Funds

Health-care research is supported by a number of philanthropic foundations, professional organizations, and corporations. Many investigators prefer private funding to government support because there is often less red tape. Private organizations typically are less rigid in their proposal regulations, their reporting requirements, clearance of instruments, and their monitoring of progress. Not surprisingly, private organizations are besieged with proposed research projects.

Information about philanthropic foundations that support research is available in *The Foundation Directory,* published by the Foundation Center. This volume, which is updated periodically, lists more than 2500 foundations whose annual grants are at least $500,000. The directory lists the purposes and activities of the foundations and the addresses for contacting them. Also available through the Foundation Center is a directory entitled *National Guide to Foundation Funding in Health.* Information on foundations (as well as federal programs) is also available through the Sponsored Programs Information Network (SPIN), which is a computerized data base to which most universities and research institutions have access.

Professional associations such as the American Nurses' Foundation, Sigma Theta Tau, the American Association of University Women, and the Social Science Research Council offer funds for conducting research. Health organizations such as the American Heart Association and the American Cancer Society also support research activities. Finally, funds for research are sometimes donated by private corporations, particularly those dealing with health-care products. Additional information concerning the requirements and interests of such groups should be obtained either from the organization directly or from personnel in research administration offices of universities, hospitals, or other agencies with which you are affiliated.

Information regarding funding opportunities is also available in a publication offered by the American Association of Colleges of Nursing entitled *The Complete Grants Sourcebook for Nursing and Health.* Finally, announcements relating to grants competitions and funding sources are published in the "Research Reporter" section of the journal *Nursing Research.*

≡ *CONCLUSION*

Proposals represent the means for opening communication between researchers and parties interested in the conduct of research. Those "parties" may be funding agencies, faculty advisers, or institutional officers, depending on the circumstances. An accepted proposal is a two-way contract: those accepting the proposal are effectively

*The *NIH Guide* is usually available through institutional research offices, or may be obtained by writing to Printing and Reproduction Branch, National Institutes of Health, Room B4BN08, Building 31, Bethesda, MD 20892.

saying, "We are willing to offer our [emotional or financial] support, as long as the investigation proceeds as proposed," and those writing the proposal are saying, "If you will offer support, then I will conduct the project as proposed." Therefore, the proposal offers some assurance that neither party will be disappointed.

Beginning proposal writers sometimes forget that, in essence, they are selling a product: themselves and their ideas. It is not inappropriate, therefore, to do a little "marketing." If the researcher does not sound convinced that the proposed study is important and will be executed with skill, then the reviewers will not be convinced either. The proposal should be written in a positive, confident tone. Instead of saying, "The study will *try* to . . . ," it is better to indicate more positively that the study *will* achieve some goals. Similarly, it is more optimistic to specify what the investigator *will* do, rather than what it *would* do, if approved. There is no need to brag or promise what cannot be accomplished. Rather, it is a question of putting the actual project accomplishments and significance in a positive light.

As another aspect of marketing, the proposal should be as physically attractive as possible. A neat and pleasing appearance invites the reviewer to read a proposal and suggests that care has been devoted to its preparation. Flashy and expensive binders, figures, and so forth are unnecessary, but the physical presentation should not leave a bad impression on readers either.

Grantsmanship, like research skills, is both a skill and an art. The skill can be acquired through further reading, by attending a course on grantsmanship, or by working with a mentor. We also hope that we have been helpful in communicating some of what goes into the "skill" part and offer all readers our best wishes in cultivating the art of doing and writing about research and acquiring support to pursue it.

≡ SUMMARY

A *research proposal* is a written document specifying what a researcher intends to study, and is written with the intent of obtaining approval and support—often financial support. The major components of a research proposal include the following: an abstract, statement of the problem, significance of the problem, background, objectives, methods, work plan, personnel, facilities, and a budget.

A major source of funding for nurse researchers is the National Institutes of Health (NIH), within which is housed the National Center for Nursing Research (NCNR). Nurses can apply for a variety of grants from NIH, the most common being the Research Project Grant (*R01* grant), *FIRST* grant, or *AREA* grant. Grant applications to NIH, which are submitted on special forms and that must follow strict formatting guidelines, are reviewed three times a year in a dual review process. The first phase involves a review by a peer *Study Section* that evaluates each proposal's scientific merit, and the second phase is a review by a National Advisory Council. The Study Section assigns *priority scores* to all approved proposals; a score of 100 represents the most meritorious ranking, and a score of 500 is the lowest possible score. A detailed critique of the proposal, together with information on the priority score and percentile ranking, are sent back to the researcher in the form of a *pink sheet*.

The federal government is the largest source of research funds for health researchers. In addition to regular grants programs, agencies of the federal government announce special funding programs in the form of *Requests for Applications (RFAs)* (for *grants*) and *Requests for Proposals (RFPs)* (for *contracts*). Other sources of funding include foundations, professional associations, and private corporations. The set of skills associated with learning about funding opportunities and developing fundable proposals is sometimes referred to as *"grantsmanship."*

≡ STUDY SUGGESTIONS

1. Suppose that you were planning to study the problem of role conflict among nursing administrators.

a. Outline the methods you would recommend adopting.
b. Develop a work plan.
c. Prepare a hypothetical budget.
2. Suppose that you were interested in studying separation anxiety in hospitalized children. Using the references cited in this chapter, identify potential funding sources for your project.

≡ *SUGGESTED READINGS*

Bauer, D.G., & the American Association of Colleges of Nursing (1988). *The complete grants source book for nursing and health.* New York: Macmillan.

Bloch, D. (1990). Strategies for setting and implementing the National Center for Nursing Research priorities. *Applied Nursing Research, 3,* 2–6.

Brodsky, J. (1976). *The proposal writer's swipe file II.* Washington, DC: Taft Products.

Brooten, D., Munro, B.H., Roncoli, M., Arnold, L., Brown, L., York, R., Hollingsworth, A., Cohen, S., & Rubin, M. (1989). Developing a program grant for use in model testing. *Nursing and Health Care, 10,* 315–318.

Clinton, J. (1985). Couvade: Patterns, predictors and nursing management: A research proposal submitted to the Division of Nursing. *Western Journal of Nursing Research, 7,* 221–248.

Foundation Center Staff. (1989a). *The Foundation directory* (12th ed.). New York: The Foundation Center.

Foundation Center Staff. (1989b). *National guide to foundation funding in health.* New York: The Foundation Center.

Fuller, E.O. (1982). The pink sheet syndrome. *Nursing Research, 31,* 185–186.

Gortner, S. (1980). Researchmanship: The judges and their judgments. *Western Journal of Nursing Research, 2,* 434–437.

Gortner, S. (1982). Research funding sources. *Western Journal of Nursing Research, 4,* 248–250.

Hinshaw, A.S. (1988a). The National Center for Nursing Research: Challenges and initiatives. *Nursing Outlook, 36,* 54, 56.

Hinshaw, A.S. (1988b). The new National Center for Nursing Research: Patient care research programs. *Applied Nursing Research, 1,* 2–4.

Jackson, N.E. (1982). Choosing and using a statistical consultant. *Nursing Research, 31,* 248–250.

Krathwohl, D.R. (1988). *How to prepare a research proposal* (3rd ed.). Syracuse, NY: Syracuse University Bookstore.

Sandelowski, M., Davis, D., & Harris, B. (1989). Artful design: Writing the proposal for research in the naturalist paradigm. *Research in Nursing and Health, 12,* 77–84.

Stewart, R., & Stewart, A.L. (1984). *Proposal preparation.* New York: John Wiley and Sons.

Tornquist, E.M., & Funk, S.G. (1990). How to write a research grant proposal. *Image, 22,* 44–51.

White, V.P. (1975). *Grants: How to find out about them and what to do next.* New York: Plenum Press.

Glossary

abstract A brief description of a completed or proposed research investigation; in research journals, usually located at the beginning of an article.

accessible population The population of subjects available for a particular study; often a nonrandom subset of the target population.

accidental sampling Selection of the most readily available persons (or units) as subjects in a study; also known as *convenience sampling*.

acquiescence response set A bias in self-report instruments, especially in social psychologic scales, created when subjects characteristically agree with statements ("yea-say") independent of their content.

active variables Variables that the researcher creates or manipulates.

adjusted means The mean value of the dependent variable for different groups, after removing the effects of covariates.

after-only design An experimental design in which data are collected from subjects only after the experimental intervention has been introduced.

alpha (α) (1) In tests of statistical significance, the level designating the probability of committing a Type I error, also known as the p value; (2) in estimates of internal consistency, a reliability coefficient, as in Cronbach's alpha.

analysis Methods of organizing data in such a way that research questions can be answered.

analysis of covariance (ANCOVA) A statistical procedure used to test the effect of one or more treatments on different groups while controlling for one or more extraneous variables (covariates).

analysis of variance (ANOVA) A statistical procedure for testing the effect of one or more treatments on different groups by comparing the variability between groups to the variability within groups.

analytic induction A method of analyzing qualitative data that involves an iterative approach to testing research hypotheses.

anonymity Protection of the participant in a study such that even the researcher cannot link him or her with the information provided.

applied research Research that concentrates on finding a solution to an immediate practical problem.

assumptions Basic principles that are accepted as being true on the basis of logic or reason, without proof or verification.

asymmetrical distribution A distribution of values that is skewed, i.e., has two halves that are not mirror images of the each other.

attribute variables Preexisting characteristics of the entity under investigation, which the researcher simply observes and measures.

attrition The loss of participants during the course of a study; can introduce an unknown amount of bias by changing the composition of the sample initially drawn—particularly if more subjects are lost from one group than another; can thereby be a threat to the internal validity of a study.

baseline measure The measurement of the dependent variable prior to the introduction of an experimental intervention.

basic research Research designed to extend the base of knowledge in a discipline for the sake of knowledge production or theory construction, rather than for solving an immediate problem.

batch processing mode A method of communicating with a mainframe computer in which a batch of programs is assembled for execution during the same computer run.

before-after design An experimental design in which data are collected from research subjects both before and after the introduction of the experimental intervention.

behavioral objective An intended outcome of a program or intervention, stated in terms of the behavior of the persons at whom the program is aimed.

beneficence A fundamental ethical principle that seeks to prevent harm and exploitation of, and maximize benefits for, human subjects.

beta (β) (1) In multiple regression, the standardized coefficients indicating the relative weights of the independent variables in the regression equation; (2) in statistical testing, the probability of a Type II error.

bias Any influence that produces a distortion in the results of a study.

bimodal distribution A distibution of values with two peaks (high frequencies).

bivariate statistics Statistics derived from the analysis of two variables simultaneously for the purpose of assessing the empirical relationship between them.

blind review The review of a manuscript or proposal such that neither the author nor the reviewer is identified to the other party.

borrowed theory A theory borrowed from another discipline or field to guide nursing practice or research.

byte A single character, such as a number, letter or specialized symbol, in a computer's memory.

canonical correlation A statistical procedure for examining the relationship between two or more independent variables *and* two or more dependent variables.

case study A research method that involves a thorough, in-depth analysis of an individual, group, institution or other social unit.

categorical variable A variable with discrete values rather than incremental placement along a continuum (e.g., a person's marital status).

category system In observational studies, the pre-specified plan for organizing and recording the behaviors and events to be observed.

causal relationship A relationship between two variables such that the presence or absence of one variable (the "cause") determines the presence or absence, or value, of the other (the "effect").

cell The intersection of a row and column in a table with two or more dimensions. In an experimental design, a cell is the representation of an experimental condition in a schematic diagram.

census A survey covering an entire population.

central processing unit (CPU) The portion of a

computer, comprising the control unit and arithmetic/logic unit, where all decisions and calculations are performed.

central tendency A statistical index of the "typicalness" of a set of scores that comes from the center of the distribution of scores. The three most common indices of central tendency are the mode, the median, and the mean.

chi-square test A nonparametric test of statistical significance used to assess whether a relationship exists between two nominal-level variables. Symbolized as χ^2.

clinical research Research designed to generate knowledge to guide nursing practice.

clinical trial An experiment involving a test of the effectiveness of a clinical treatment, generally involving a large and heterogeneous sample of subjects.

closed-ended question A question that offers respondents a set of mutually exclusive and jointly exhaustive alternative replies, from which the one that most closely approximates the "right" answer must be chosen.

cluster analysis A multivariate statistical procedure used to cluster people or things based on patterns of association.

cluster sampling A form of multistage sampling in which large groupings ("clusters") are selected first (e.g., nursing schools), with successive subsampling of smaller units (e.g., nursing students).

code of ethics The fundamental ethical principles that are established by a discipline or institution to guide researchers' conduct in research with humans.

codebook The documentation used in data processing that indicates the location and values of all the variables in a data file.

coding The process of transforming raw data into standardized form (usually numerical) for data processing and analysis.

coefficient alpha (Cronbach's alpha) A reliability index that estimates the internal consistency or homogeneity of a measure composed of several items or subparts.

coefficient of determination The proportion of variance in the dependent variable accounted for or "explained" by a group of independent variables, more commonly referred to as R^2.

cohort study A kind of trend study that focuses on a specific subpopulation (which is often an age-related subgroup) from which different samples are selected at different points in time (e.g., the cohort of nursing students graduated in 1970-1974).

comparison group A group of subjects whose scores on a dependent variable are used as a basis for evaluating the scores of the target group or group of primary interest. The term comparison group is generally used instead of control group when the investigation does not use a true experimental design.

compiler A computer program that translates programming language into machine language.

computer An electronic device that performs simple operations with extreme accuracy and speed.

computer program A set of instructions to a computer.

concept An abstraction based on observations of certain behaviors or characteristics (e.g., stress, pain).

conceptual framework (*conceptual model*) Interrelated concepts or abstractions that are assembled together in some rational scheme by virtue of their relevance to a common theme.

conceptual utilization The use of research findings in a general, conceptual way to broaden one's thinking about an issue, but the knowledge is not put to any specific, documentable use.

concurrent validity The degree to which scores on an an instrument are correlated with some external criterion, measured at the same time.

confidence interval The range of values within which a population parameter is estimated to lie.

confidence level The estimated probability that a population parameter lies within a given confidence interval.

confidentiality Protection of participants in a study such that their individual identities will not be linked to the information they provided and will never be publicly divulged

consent form A written agreement signed by a

subject and a researcher concerning the terms and conditions of a subject's voluntary participation in a study.

consistency check A procedure performed in cleaning a set of data to ensure that the data are internally consistent.

constant comparison A procedure often used in qualitative analysis wherein newly collected data are compared in an ongoing fashion with data obtained earlier, to refine theoretically relevant categories.

construct An abstraction or concept that is deliberately invented (constructed) by researchers for a scientific purpose (e.g., health locus of control).

construct validity The degree to which an instrument measures the construct under investigation.

consumer An individual who reads, reviews, and critiques research findings and who attempts to use and apply the findings in their nursing practice.

content analysis A procedure for analyzing written or verbal communications in a systematic and objective fashion, typically with the goal of quantitatively measuring variables.

content validity The degree to which the items in an instrument adequately represent the universe of content.

contingency table A two-dimensional table that permits a crosstabulation of the frequencies of two nominal-level or ordinal-level variables.

continuous variable A variable that can take on a large range of values representing a continuum (e.g., height).

control The process of holding constant possible influences on the dependent variable under investigation.

control group Subjects in an experiment who do not receive the experimental treatment and whose performance provides a baseline against which the effects of the treatment can be measured (see also *comparison group*).

convenience sampling Selection of the most readily available persons (or units) as subjects in a study; also known as *accidental sampling*.

convergent validity An approach to construct validation that involves assessing the degree to which two methods of measuring a construct are similar (i.e., converge).

correlation A tendency for variation in one variable to be related to variation in another variable.

correlation coefficient An index that summarizes the degree of relationship between two variables. Correlation coefficients typically range from +1.00 (for a perfect direct relationship) through 0.0 (for no relationship) to -1.00 (for a perfect inverse relationship).

correlation matrix A two-dimenensional display showing the correlation coefficients between all combinations of variables of interest.

correlational research Investigations that explore the interrelationships among variables of interest without any active intervention on the part of the researcher.

cost-benefit analysis An evaluation comparing the financial costs of a program or intervention with the financial gains attributable to it.

counterbalancing The process of systematically varying the order of presentation of stimuli, treatments, or items in a scale to control for ordering effects, as in counterbalancing the order of treatments in a repeated measures design.

covariate A variable that is statistically controlled (held constant) in analysis of covariance. The covariate is typically an extraneous, confounding influence on the dependent variable or a pretest measure of the dependent variable.

covert data collection The collection of information in a study without the subject's knowledge.

Cramer's V An index describing the magnitude of relationship between nominal-level data, used when the contingency table to which it is applied is larger than 2×2.

criterion variable (criterion measure) The quality or attribute used to measure the effect of an independent variable; sometimes used instead of *dependent variable*.

criterion-related validity The degree to which scores on an instrument are correlated with some external criterion.

critical incident technique A method of obtaining data from study participants by in-depth exploration of specific incidents and behaviors related to the matter under investigation.

critique An objective, critical, and balanced appraisal of a research report's various dimensions (e.g., conceptual, methodological, ethical).

Cronbach's alpha A widely-used reliability index that estimates the internal consistency or homogeneity of a measure composed of several subparts; also referred to as coefficient alpha.

cross-sectional study A study based on observations of different age or developmental groups at a single point in time for the purpose of inferring trends over time.

crosstabulation A determination of the number of cases occurring when simultaneous consideration is given to the values of two or more variables (e.g., sex—male/female—crosstabulated with smoking status—smoker/nonsmoker). The results are typically presented in a table with rows and columns divided according to the values of the variables.

data The pieces of information obtained in the course of a study (singular is *datum*).

data analysis The systematic organization and synthesis of research data, and the testing of research hypotheses using those data.

data cleaning The preparation of data for analysis by performing checks to ensure that the data are meaningful and consistent.

data collection The gathering of information needed to address a research problem.

data entry The process of entering data (usually in coded form) onto an input medium for computer analysis.

data transformation A step often undertaken prior to the analysis of research data, to put the data in a form that can be meaningfully analyzed (e.g., recoding of values).

debriefing Communication with research subjects, generally after their participation has been completed, regarding various aspects of the study.

deception The deliberate withholding of information, or the provision of false information, to research subjects, usually used to reduce potential biases.

deductive reasoning The process of develop-ing specific predictions from general principles (see also *inductive reasoning*).

degrees of freedom (*df*) A concept used in tests of statistical significance, referring to the number of sample values that cannot be calculated from knowledge of other values and a calculated statistic (e.g., by knowing a sample mean, all but one value would be free to vary); degrees of freedom is usually N - 1, but different formulas are relevant for different tests.

Delphi technique A method of obtaining judgments from a panel of experts. The experts are questioned individually, and a summary of the judgments is circulated to the entire panel. The experts are questioned again, with further iterations introduced as needed until there is some consensus.

demonstration A program or intervention that is being tested, often on a large scale, to determine its effectiveness and the desirability of changing policies or procedures.

dependent variable The outcome variable of interest; the variable that is hypothesized to depend on or be caused by another variable (called the *independent variable*); sometimes referred to as the *criterion variable*.

descriptive research Research studies that have as their main objective the accurate portrayal of the characteristics of persons, situations, or groups, and the frequency with which certain phenomena occur.

descriptive statistics Statistics used to describe and summarize the researcher's data set (e.g., mean, standard deviation).

determinism The belief that phenomena are not haphazard or random, but rather have antecedent causes.

deviation score A score computed by subtracting an individual score value from the mean of the distribution of scores.

dichotomous variable A variable having only two values or categories (e.g., sex).

directional hypothesis A hypothesis that makes a specific prediction about the direction and nature of the relationship between two variables.

discriminant function analysis A statistical procedure used to predict group membership or status on a categorical (nominal level) variable on the basis of two or more independent variables.

discriminant validity An approach to construct validation that involves assessing the degree to which a single method of measuring two constructs yields different results (i.e., discriminates the two).

disproportional sampling design A sampling strategy wherein the researcher samples differing proportions of subjects from different strata in the population to ensure adequate representation of subjects from strata that are comparatively smaller.

double-blind experiment An experiment in which neither the subjects nor those who administer the treatment know who is in the experimental or control group.

effect size A statistical expression of the magnitude of the relationship between two variables, or the magnitude of the difference between two groups, with regard to some attribute of interest.

eigenvalues In factor analysis, the value equal to the sum of the squared weights for each factor.

element The most basic unit of a population, from which a sample will be drawn; in nursing research, the element is typically humans.

eligibility criteria The criteria used by a researcher to designate the specific attributes of the target population, and by which subjects are selected for participation in a study.

empirical evidence Evidence that is rooted in objective reality and that is gathered through the collection of data using one's senses; used as the basis for generating knowledge through the scientific approach

endogenous variable In path analysis, a variable whose variation is determined by other variables in the model.

error of measurement The degree of deviation between true scores and obtained scores when measuring a characteristic.

eta squared A statistic calculated, in ANOVA, to indicate the proportion of variance in the dependent variable explained by the independent variables, analogous to R^2 in multiple regression; computed by dividing the sum of squares between groups by the total sum of squares.

ethics The quality of research procedures with respect to their adherence to professional, legal, and social obligations to the research subjects.

equivalence The degree of similarity between alternate forms of a measuring instrument.

ethnographic research Research that focuses on the lifeways of a particular culture or subculture, using in-depth procedures.

evaluation research Research that investigates how well a program, practice, or policy is working.

event sampling In observational studies, a sampling plan that involved the selection of integral behaviors or events.

ex post facto research Research conducted after the variations in the independent variable have occurred in the natural course of events; a form of nonexperimental research in which causal explanations are inferred "after the fact."

exogenous variable In path analysis, a variable whose determinants lie outside the model.

experiment A research study in which the investigator controls (manipulates) the independent variable and randomly assigns subjects to different conditions.

experimental intervention (experimental treatment) See intervention; treatment.

experimental group The subjects who receive the experimental treatment or intervention.

exploratory research A preliminary study designed to develop or refine hypotheses, or to test and refine the data collection methods.

external criticism In historical research, the systematic evaluation of the authenticity and genuineness of data.

external storage device A device associated with computers for long-term storage of data and programs (e.g., a magnetic tape).

external validity The degree to which the results of a study can be generalized to settings or samples other than the ones studied.

extraneous variable A variable that confounds the relationship between the independent and dependent variables and that needs to be controlled either in the research design or through statistical procedures (e.g., in a study of the effect of a mother's age on the rate of premature deliveries, social class and ethnicity would be extraneous variables).

extreme response set A bias in self-report instruments, especially in social psychologic scales, created when subjects characteristically express their opinions in terms of extreme response alternatives (e.g., "strongly agree") independent of the question's content.

F-ratio The statistic obtained in several statistical tests (e.g., ANOVA) in which variation attributable to different sources (e.g., between groups and within groups) is compared.

factor analysis a statistical procedure for reducing a large set of variables into a smaller set of variables with common characteristics or underlying dimensions.

factorial design An experimental design in which two or more independent variables are simultaneously manipulated; this design permits an analysis of the main effects of the independent variables separately, plus the interaction effects of these variables.

field notes The notes taken by researchers regarding the unstructured observations they have made in the field, and their interpretation of those observations.

field study A study in which the data are collected "in the field" from individuals in their normal roles, with the aim of understanding the practices, behaviors and beliefs of individuals or groups as they normally function in real life.

findings The results of the analysis of the research data; the results of the hypothesis tests.

Fisher's exact test A statistical procedure used to test the significance of the differnce in proportions, used when the sample size is small or cells in the contingency table have no observations.

fixed alternative question A question that offers respondents a set of prespecified responses, from which the respondent must choose the alternative that most closely approximates the correct response.

focus group interview An interview in which the respondents are a group of individuals assembled to answer questions on a given topic.

focused interview A loosely structured interview in which the interviewer guides the respondent through a set of questions using a topic guide.

follow-up study A study undertaken to determine the subsequent development of individuals with a specified condition or who have received a specified treatment.

formative evaluation An ongoing assessment of a product or program as it is being developed, designed to optimize the ultimate quality of that product or program.

frequency distribution A systematic array of numerical values from the lowest to the highest, together with a count of the number of times each value was obtained.

frequency polygon Graphic display of a frequency distribution, in which dots connected by a straight line indicate the number of times a score value occurs in a set of data.

Freidman test A nonparametric analog of ANOVA, used when the researcher is working with paired groups or a repeated measures situation.

full disclosure The communication of complete information to potential research subjects regarding the nature of the study, the subject's right to refuse participation, and the likely risks and benefits that would be incurred.

functional relationship A relationship or association between two variables wherein it cannot be assumed that one variable caused the other; however, it can be said that the variable X changes values as a function of changes in variable Y.

Gantt chart A chart depicting the scheduling of activities (tasks) of a research study and highlighting the sequencing and interrelationships among activities.

generalizability The degree to which the research procedures justify the inference that the findings represent something beyond the specific observations on which they are based; in particular, the inference that the findings can be generalized from the sample to the entire population.

grand theory A broad theory aimed at describing large segments of the physical, social, or behavioral world; also referred to as a macrotheory.

grant An award made to a researcher or team of

researchers, enabling the conduct of a proposed study through the provision of financial support.

grantsmanship The combined set of skills and knowledge needed to secure financial support for one's research ideas.

graphic rating scale A scale in which respondents are asked to rate something (e.g., a concept, issue, institution) along an ordered bipolar continuum (e.g., "excellent" to "very poor").

grounded theory An approach to collecting and analyzing qualitative data with the aim of developing theories and theoretical propositions "grounded" in real-world observations.

Guttman scale A method of measuring attitudes that makes use of a set of cumulative (monotone) items with which respondents are asked to agree or disagree.

hardware The physical electronic equipment that makes a computer.

Hawthorne effect The effect on the dependent variable caused by subjects' awareness that they are "special" participants under study.

heterogeneity The degree to which objects are dissimilar with respect to some attribute (i.e., characterized by high variability).

histogram A graphic presentation of frequency distribution data.

historical research Systematic studies designed to establish facts and relationships concerning past events.

history A threat to the internal validity of a study; refers to the occurrence of events external to the treatment but concurrent with it, which can affect the dependent variable of interest.

homogeneity (1) In terms of the reliability of an instrument, the degree to which the subparts are internally consistent (i.e., are measuring the same critical attribute). (2) More generally, the degree to which objects are similar (i.e., characterized by low variability).

hypothesis A statement of predicted relationships between the variables under investigation; hypotheses lead to empirical studies that seek to confirm or disconfirm those predictions.

impact analysis An evaluation of the effects of a program or intervention on some outcomes of interest, net of other factors influencing those outcomes.

implementation analysis An evaluation that describes the process by which a program or intervention was implemented in practice.

independent variable The variable that is believed to cause or influence the dependent variable; in experimental research, the independent variable is the variable that is manipulated.

inductive reasoning The process of reasoning from specific observations to more general rules (see also *deductive reasoning*).

inferential statistics Statistics that permit us to infer whether relationships observed in a sample are likely to occur in a larger population of concern.

informed consent An ethical principle that requires researchers to obtain the voluntary participation of subjects, after informing them of possible risks and benefits.

input devices Those parts of a computer system that allow data and commands to be entered into the computer.

Institutional Review Board (IRB) A group of individuals who convene to review proposed and ongoing studies with respect to ethical considerations.

instrument The device or technique that a researcher uses to collect data (e.g., questionnaires, tests, observation schedules, etc.).

instrumental utilization Clearly identifiable attempts to base some specific action or intervention on the results of research findings.

instrumentation system The entire set of devices and apparatus used to collect in vivo physiological measurements; includes the subject, stimulus, sensing equipment, signal-conditioning equipment, display equipment, and recording equipment.

interaction effect The effect on a dependent variable of two or more independent variables acting in combination (interactively) rather than as unconnected factors.

interactive mode A mode of communicating with a computer wherein the user interacts directly with the computer and obtains feedback almost immediately.

intercoder reliability The degree to which two coders, operating independently, assign the same codes to variables.

internal consistency A form of reliability, referring to the degree to which the subparts of an instrument are all measuring the same attribute or dimension.

internal criticism In historical research, an evaluation of the worth of the historical evidence.

internal validity The degree to which it can be inferred that the experimental treatment (independent variable), rather than uncontrolled, extraneous factors, is responsible for observed effects.

interrater (interobserver) reliability The degree to which two raters or obervers, operating independently, assign the same ratings or values for an attribute being measured; such ratings normally occur in the context of observational research.

interval estimation An estimation approach in which the researcher establishes a range of values that are likely, within a given level of confidence, to contain the true population parameter.

interval measure A level of measurement in which an attribute of a variable is rank ordered on a scale that has equal distances between points on that scale (e.g., Fahrenheit degrees).

intervention (1) In experimental research, the experimental treatment or manipulation. (2) More generally, the structure the investigator imposes on the research setting prior to making observations.

interview A method of data collection in which one person (an interviewer) asks questions of another person (a respondent); interviews are conducted either face-to-face or by telephone.

interview schedule The formal instrument, used in structured self-report studies, that specifies the wording of all questions to be asked of respondents.

inverse relationship A negative correlation between two variables; i.e., a relationship characterized by the tendency of high values on one variable to be associated with low values on a second variable.

isomorphism In measurement, the correpondence between the measures an instrument yields and reality.

item A term used to refer to a single question on a test or questionnaire, or a single statement on an attitude or other scale (e.g., a final examination might consist of 100 items).

judgmental sampling A type of nonprobability sampling method in which the researcher selects subjects for the study on the basis of personal judgment about which ones will be most representative or productive; also referred to as *purposive sampling.*

Kendall's tau A correlation coefficient used to indicate the magnitude of a relationship between ordinal-level data.

key informant A person well-versed in the phenomenon of research interest and who is willing to share the information and insight with the researcher; key informants are often used in needs assessments.

known-groups technique A technique for estimating the construct validity of an instrument through an analysis of the degree to which the instrument separates groups that are predicted to differ on the basis of some theory or known characteristic.

Kruskal-Wallis test A nonparametric test used to test the difference between three or more independent groups, based on ranked scores.

Kuder-Richardson (KR-20) formula A reliability coefficient indicating the degree of internal consistency of a scaled set of items, used when the items are dichotomous.

law A theory that has accrued such persuasive empirical support that it is accepted as truth (e.g., Boyle's law of gases).

least squares estimation A commonly-used method of statistical estimation in which the solution minimizes the sums of squares of error terms; sometimes referred to as "OLS" (ordinary least squares).

level of significance The risk of making a Type I error, established by the researcher before the statistical analysis (e.g., the .05 level).

life history A narrative self-report about a person's life experiences vis-à-vis some theme of interest to the researcher.

life table analysis A statistical procedure used when the dependent variable represents a time interval between an initial event (e.g., onset of a disease) and an end event (e.g., death).

Likert scale A type of composite measure of

attitudes that involves summation of scores on a set of items (statements) to which respondents are asked to indicate their degree of agreement or disagreement.

LISREL The widely-used acronym for linear structural relation analysis, typically used for testing causal models using procedures based on maximum likelihood estimation.

literature review A critical summary of research on a topic of interest, generally prepared to put a research problem in context or to identify gaps and weaknesses in prior studies so as to justify a new investigation.

log In participant observation studies, the observer's daily record of events and conversations that took place.

logical positivism The philosophy underlying the traditional scientific approach.

logistic regression A multivariate regression procedure that uses maximum likelihood estimation for analyzing relationships between multiple independent variables and categorical dependent variables; also referred to as logit analysis.

longitudinal study A study designed to collect data at more than one point in time, in contrast to a cross-sectional study.

macrotheory A broad theory aimed at describing large segments of the physical, social, or behavioral world; also referred to as a grand theory.

main effects In a study with multiple independent variables, the effects of a single independent variable on the dependent variable.

mainframe A large, multi-user computer system.

manipulation An intervention or treatment introduced by the researcher in an experimental or quasi-experimental study; the researcher manipulates the independent variable to asssess its impact on the dependent variable.

Mann-Whitney U test A nonparametric test used to test the difference between two independent groups, based on ranked scores.

matching The pairing of subjects in one group with those in another group based on their similarity in one or more dimension, done in order to enhance the overall comparability of groups;

when matching is performed in the context of an experiment, the procedure results in a randomized block design.

maturation A threat to the internal validity of a study that results when factors influence the outcome measure (dependent variable) as a result of time passing.

maximum likelihood estimation An estimation approach (sometimes used in lieu of the least square approach) in which the estimators are ones that estimate the parameters most likely to have generated the observed measurements.

McNemar test A statistical test for comparing differences in proportions, when the values are derived from paired (nonindependent) groups.

mean A descriptive statistic that is a measure of central tendency, computed by summing all scores and dividing by the number of subjects.

measurement The assignment of numbers to objects according to specified rules to characterize quantities of some attribute.

median A descriptive statistic that is a measure of central tendency, representing the exact middle score or value in a distribution of scores; the median is the value above and below which 50 percent of the scores lie.

median test A nonparamteric statistical test that involves the comparison of median values of two independent groups, to determine if the groups derive from populations with different medians.

mediating variable A variable that mediates or acts like a "go-between" in a chain linking two other variables (e.g., coping skills may be said to mediate the relationship between stressful events and anxiety).

meta-analysis A technique for quantitatively combining and thus integrating the results of multiple studies on a given topic.

methodological notes In observational field studies, the notes kept by the researcher regarding the methods used in collecting the data.

methodological research Research designed to develop or refine procedures for obtaining, organizing, or analyzing data.

methods (research) The steps, procedures, and

strategies for gathering and analyzing the data in a research investigation.

microcomputer A small computer used by individual users; also referred to as a personal computer.

middle range theory A theory that focuses on only a piece of reality or human experience, involved a selected number of concepts (e.g., theories of stress).

minimal risk Anticipated risks that are no greater than those ordinarily encountered in daily life or during the performance of routine tests or procedures.

missing values Values missing from a data set for some subjects, due, for example, to subject noncompliance, researcher error, or skip patterns.

modality A characteristic of a frequency distribution describing the number of "peaks" or values with high frequencies.

mode A descriptive statistic that is a measure of central tendency; the score or value that occurs most frequently in a distribution of scores.

model A symbolic representation of concepts or variables, and interrelationships among them.

molar approach A way of making observations about behaviors that entails studying large units of behavior and treating them as a whole.

molecular approach A way of making observations about behavior that uses small and highly specific behaviors as the unit of observation.

mortality A threat to the internal validity of a study, referring to the differential loss of subjects (attrition) from different groups.

multimethod research Generally, research in which multiple approaches are used to address the research problem; often used to designate research in which both qualitative and quantitative data are collected and analyzed.

multimodal distribution A distribution of values with more than one peak (high frequency).

multiple classification analysis A variant of multiple regression that yields means on the dependent variable adjusted for the effects of covariates.

multiple comparison procedures Statistical tests, normally applied after ANOVA results indicate statistically significant group differences, that compare different pairs of groups.

multiple correlation coefficient An index that summarizes the degree of relationship between two or more independent variables and a dependent variable; symbolized as R.

multiple regression A statistical procedure for understanding the simultaneous effects of two or more independent (or extraneous) variables on a dependent variable; the dependent variable must be measured on an interval or ratio scale.

multi-stage sampling A sampling strategy that proceeds through a set of stages from larger to smaller sampling units (e.g., from states, to nursing schools, to faculty members).

multitrait-multimethod matrix approach A method of establishing the construct validity of an instrument that involves the use of multiple measures for a set of subjects; the target instrument is valid to the extent that there is a strong relationship between it and other measures purporting to measure the same attribute (*convergence*) and a weak relationship between it and other measures purporting to measure a different attribute (*discriminability*).

multivariate analysis of variance (MANOVA) A statistical procedure used to test the significance of difference between the means of two or more groups on two or more dependent variables, considered simultaneously.

multivariate statistics Statistical procedures designed to analyze the relationships among three or more variables; commonly used multivariate statistics include multiple regression, analysis of covariance, and factor analysis.

N Often used to designate the total number of subjects in a study (e.g., "the total *N* was 500").

n Often used to designate the number of subjects in a subgroup or in a cell of a study (e.g., "each of the four groups had an *n* of 125, for a total *N* of 500").

needs assessment A study in which a researcher collects data for estimating the needs of a group, community, or organization; usually used as a guide to resource allocation.

negative relationship A relationship between

two variables in which there is a tendency for higher values on one variable to be associated with lower values on the other (e.g., as temperature increases, people's productivity may decrease); also referred to as an *inverse relationship*.

negative results Research results that are contrary to the researcher's hypotheses.

negatively skewed distribution An asymmetrical distribution of values such that a disproportionately high number of cases have high values— i.e., fall at the upper end of the distribution; when displayed graphically, the "tail" points to the left.

network sampling The sampling of subjects based on referrals from other subjects already in the sample.

nominal measure The lowest level of measurement that involves the assignment of characteristics into categories (e.g., males, category 1; females, category 2).

nondirectional hypothesis A research hypothesis that does not stipulate in advance the direction and nature of the relationship between variables.

nonequivalent control group A comparison group that was not developed on the basis of random assignment; when randomization is not used, there is no way of ensuring the initial equivalence among different groups.

nonexperimental research Studies in which the researcher collects data without introducing any new treatments or changes.

nonparametric statistics A general class of inferential statistics that does not involve rigorous assumptions about the distribution of the critical variables; most often used when the data are measured on the nominal or ordinal scales.

nonprobability sampling The selection of subjects or sampling units from a population using nonrandom procedures; examples include convenience, judgmental, and quota sampling.

normal distribution A theoretical distribution that is bell-shaped and symmetrical; also referred to as a normal curve.

norms Test-performance standards, based on the collection of test score information from a large, representative sample.

null hypothesis The hypothesis that states there is no relationship between the variables under study; used primarily in connection with tests of statistical significance as the hypothesis to be rejected.

objectivity A desired quality of research using the scientific approach; refers to the extent to which two independent researchers would arrive at similar judgments or conclusions (i.e., judgments not biased by personal values or beliefs).

observational notes In field studies, the observer's descriptions about observed events and conversations.

observational research Studies in which the data are collected by means of observing and recording behaviors or activities of interest.

obtained (observed) score The actual score or numerical value assigned to a subject on a measure.

one-tailed test A test of statistical significance in which only values at one extreme (tail) of a distribution are considered in determining significance; used when the researcher has predicted the direction of a relationship (see *directional hypothesis*).

open-ended question A question in an interview or questionnaire that does not restrict the respondents' answers to preestablished alternatives.

operational definition The definition of a concept or variable in terms of the operations or procedures by which it is to be measured.

operationalization The process of translating research concepts into measureable phenomena.

ordinal measure A level of measurement that yields rank orders of a variable along some dimension.

outcome analysis An evaluation of what transpires with respect to outcomes of interest after implementing a program or intervention, without use of an experimental design to assess net effects. (see also *Impact analysis*)

outcome measure A term sometimes used to refer to the dependent variable in experimental research, i.e., the measure that captures the outcome of the experimental intervention.

outliers Wild codes or numerical values that are not a part of the coding scheme.

output devices Those parts of a computer system that communicate information back to the computer user (e.g., a line printer).

p value In statistical testing, the probability that the obtained results result from chance alone; the probability of committing a Type I error.

panel study A type of longitudinal study in which the same subjects are used to provide data at two or more points in time.

paradigm A way of looking at natural phenomena that encompasses a set of philosophical assumptions and that guides one's approach to inquiry.

parameter A characteristic of a population (e.g., the mean age of all U.S. citizens).

parametric statistics A class of inferential statistics that involves (a) assumptions about the distribution of the variables, (b) the estimation of a parameter, and (c) the use of interval measures.

participant observation A method of collecting data through the observation of a group or organization in which the researcher participates as a member.

path analysis A regression-based procedure for testing causal models, typically using nonexperimental data.

Pearson's r The most widely-used correlation coefficient, designating the magnitude of relationship between two variables measured on at least an interval scale; also referred to as the product-moment correlation.

peer reviewer A person who reviews and critiques a research report or research proposal, who himself/herself is a researcher (usually working on similar types of research problems as those in the research report under review), and who makes a recommendation about publishing or funding the research.

perfect correlation A correlation between two variables such that the values of one variable permit perfect prediction of the values of the other; designated as 1.00 or -1.00.

personal notes In field studies, comments about the observer's own feelings during the research process.

phenomenology An approach to human inquiry that emphasizes the complexity of human experience and the need to study that experience holistically as it is actually lived.

phi coefficient An index describing the magnitude of relationship between two dichotomous variables.

pilot study A small scale version, or trial run, done in preparation for a major study.

pink sheet For grant applications submitted to the National Institutes of Health, the evaluation form containing the comments and priority score of the peer review panel.

point estimation An estimation procedure in which the researcher uses information from a sample to estimate the single value (statistic) that would best represent the value of the population parameter.

policy research Research conducted specifically to inform persons who create or implement policies, typically ones affecting large groups of people (e.g., federal policies on health care).

population The entire set of individuals (or objects) having some common characteristic(s) (e.g., all RNs in the state of California); sometimes referred to as *universe*.

positive relationship A relationship between two variables in which there is a tendency for high values on one variable to be associated with high values on the other (e.g., as physical activity increases, pulse rate also increases).

positive results Research results that are consistent with the researcher's hypotheses.

positively skewed distribution An asymmetrical distribution of values such that a disproportionately high number of cases have low values— i.e., fall at the lower end of the distribution; when displayed graphically, the "tail" points to the right.

posttest The collection of data after the introduction of an experimental intervention.

posttest-only design An experimental design in which data are collected from subjects only after the experimental intervention has been introduced.

power The ability of a research design to detect existing relationships among variables.

power analysis A procedure for estimating either the likelihood of committing a Type II error or sample size requirements.

prediction   One of the aims of the scientific approach; the use of empirical evidence to make forecasts about how variables of interest will behave in a new setting and with different individuals.

predictive validity   The degree to which an instrument can predict some criterion observed at a future time.

pre-experimental design   A research design that does not include controls to compensate for the absence of either randomization or a control group.

pretest   (1) The collection of data prior to the experimental intervention; sometimes referred to as *baseline data.* (2) The trial administration of a newly developed instrument to identify flaws or assess time requirements.

pretest-posttest design   An experimental design in which data are collected from research subjects both before and after the introduction of the experimental intervention.

primary source   First-hand reports of facts, findings or events; in terms of research, the primary source is the original research report as prepared by the investigator who conducted the study.

Principal Investigator (PI)   In research grants, the person who is the lead researcher and who will have primary responsibility for administering the grant.

probability sampling   The selection of subjects or sampling units from a population using random procedures; examples include simple random sampling, cluster sampling, and systematic sampling.

probing   Eliciting more useful or detailed information from a respondent in an interview than was volunteered in the first reply.

problem statement   The statement that identifies the key research variables, specifies the nature of the population, and suggests the possibility of empirical testing.

process evaluation   An evaluation focusing on the process by which a program or intervention gets implemented and used in practice.

product moment correlation coefficient (r)   The most widely-used correlation coefficient, designating the magnitude of relationship between two variables measured on at least an interval scale; also referred to as Pearson's *r.*

projective techniques   Methods for measuring psychological attributes (values, attitudes, personality) by providing respondents with unstructured stimuli to which to respond.

proportional hazards model   A model applied in multivariate analyses in which independent variables are used to predict the risk (hazard) of experiencing an event at a given point in time.

proposal   A document specifying what the researcher proposes to study; it communicates the research problem, its significance, planned procedures for solving the problem, and, when funding is sought, how much the research will cost.

prospective study   A study that begins with an examination of presumed causes (e.g., cigarette smoking) and then goes forward in time to observe presumed effects (e.g., lung cancer).

psychometric assessment   An evaluation of the quality of an instrument, based primarily on evidence of its reliability and validity.

psychometrics   The theory underlying principles of measurement and the application of the theory in the development of measuring tools.

purposive sampling   A type of nonprobability sampling method in which the researcher selects subjects for the study on the basis of personal judgment about which ones will be most representative or productive; also referred to as *judgmental sampling.*

Q-sort   A method of scaling in which the subject sorts statements into a number of piles (usually nine or 11) according to some bipolar dimension (e.g., most like me/least like me; most useful/least useful).

qualitative analysis   The organization and interpretation of nonnumerical observations for the purpose of discovering important underlying dimensions and patterns of relationships.

qualitative data   Information collected in the course of a study that is in narrative (nonnumerical) form, such as the transcript of an unstructured interview.

quantitative analysis   The manipulation of numerical data through statistical procedures for the purpose of describing phenomena or assessing the magnitude and reliability of relationships among them.

quantitative data Information collected in the course of a study that is in a quantified (numerical) form.

quasi-experiment A study in which subjects cannot be randomly assigned to treatment conditions, although the researcher does manipulate the independent variable and exercises certain controls to enhance the internal validity of the results.

quasi-statistics An "accounting" system used to assess the validity of conclusions derived from qualitative analysis.

questionnaire A method of gathering self-report information from respondents through self-administration of questions in a paper-and-pencil format.

quota sampling The nonrandom selection of subjects in which the researcher pre-specifies characteristics of the sample to increase its representativeness.

r The symbol typically used to designate a bivariate correlation coefficient, summarizing the magnitude and direction of a relationship between two variables.

R The symbol used to designate the multiple correlation coefficient, indicating the magnitude (but not direction) of the relationship between the dependent variable and multiple indpendent variables, taken together.

R^2 The squared multiple correlation coefficient, indicating the proportion of variance in the dependent variable accounted for or "explained" by a group of independent variables; also referred to as the coefficient of determination.

random assignment The assignment of subjects to treatment conditions in a random manner (i.e., in a manner determined by chance alone); also known as *randomization.*

random number table A table of digits from 0 to 9 set up in such a way that each number is equally likely to follow any other; used in randomization or random sampling.

random sampling The selection of a sample such that each member of a population (or subpopulation) has an equal probability of being included.

randomization The assignment of subjects to treatment conditions in a random manner (i.e., in a manner determined by chance alone); also known as *random assignment.*

range A measure of variability, consisting of the difference between the highest and lowest values in a distribution of scores.

ratio measure A level of measurement in which there are equal distances between score units and which has a true meaningful zero point; the highest level of measurement (e.g., age).

reactivity A measurement distortion arising from the subject's awareness of being observed, or, more generally, from the effect of the measurement procedure itself.

recursive model A path model in which the causal flow is unidirectional, without any feedback loops; opposite of a nonrecursive model.

regression A statistical procedure for predicting values of a dependent variable based on the values of one or more independent variables.

relationship A bond or a connection between two or more variables.

reliability The degree of consistency or dependability with which an instrument measures the attribute it is designed to measure.

reliability coefficient A quantitative index, usually ranging in value from .00 to 1.00, that provides an estimate of how reliable an instrument is; computed through such procedures as Cronbach's alpha technique, the split-half technique, test-retest approach, and interrater approaches.

repeated-measures design An experimental design in which one group of subjects is exposed to more than one condition or treatment.

replication The duplication of research procedures in a second investigation for the purpose of determining if earlier results can be repeated.

representative sample A sample whose characteristics are highly similar to those of the population from which it is drawn.

research Systematic inquiry that uses orderly scientific methods to answer questions or solve problems.

research design The overall plan for collecting and analyzing data, including specifications for enhancing the internal and external validity of the study.

research proposal See *proposal.*

research utilization The use of some aspect of a scientific investigation in an application unrelated to the original research.

residuals In multiple regression, the error terms or unexplained variance.

respondent In a self-report study, the research subject.

response rate The rate of participation in a survey; calculated by dividing the number of persons participating by the number of persons sampled.

response set bias The measurement error introduced by the tendency of some individuals to respond to items in characteristic ways (e.g., always agreeing), independently of the item's content.

retrospective study A study that begins with the manifestation of the dependent variable in the present (e.g., lung cancer) and then links this effect to some presumed cause occurring in the past (e.g., cigarette smoking).

right justification A convention used in data entry, when a fixed format mode is used, such that values are placed as far to the right as possible within a designated field (e.g., the value 1 in a 2-column field would be entered 01).

risk-benefit ratio The relative costs and benefits, to an individual subject and to society at large, of participation in a scientific study.

rival hypothesis An alternative explanation, competing with the researcher's hypothesis, for understanding the results of a study.

sample A subset of a population selected to participate in a research study.

sampling The process of selecting a portion of the population to represent the entire population.

sampling bias Distortions that arise from the selection of a sample that is not representative of the population from which it was drawn.

sampling distribution A theoretical distribution of a statistic using an infinite number of samples as a basis and the values of the statistic computed from these samples as the data points in the distribution.

sampling error The fluctuation of the value of a statistic from one sample to another drawn from the same population.

sampling frame A list of all the elements in the population, from which the sample is drawn.

scale A composite measure of an attribute, consisting of several items that have a logical or empirical relationship to each other; involves the assignment of a score to place subjects on a continuum with respect to the attribute.

scatter plot A graphic representation of the relationship between two variables.

scientific approach A set of orderly, systematic, controlled procedures for acquiring dependable, empirical information.

scientific merit The degree to which a study is methodologically and conceptually sound and possesses theoretical relevance and internal and external validity.

secondary analysis A form of research in which the data collected by one researcher are reanalyzed by another investigator, usually to test new research hypotheses.

secondary source Second-had accounts of events or facts; in a research context, a description of a study or studies prepared by someone other than the original researcher.

selection bias (*self-selection*) A threat to the internal validity of the study resulting from pre-existing differences between the groups under study; the differences affect the dependent variable in ways extraneous to the effect of the independent variable.

self-determination A person's ability to voluntarily decide whether or not to participate as a subject in a study.

self-report Any procedure for collecting data that involves a direct report of information by the person who is being studied (e.g., by interview or questionnaire).

semantic differential A technique used to measure attitudes that asks respondents to rate a concept of interest on a series of seven-point bipolar rating scales.

sensitivity In measurement, the ability of the measuring tool to make fine discriminations between objects with differing amounts of the attribute being measured.

setting The physical location and conditions in which data collection takes place in a study.

sign system In structured observational research, a system for listing the behaviors of interest to the researchers, in situations where the observation focuses on specific behaviors that may or may not be manfiested by the subjects.

sign test A nonparametric statistical test for comparing two paired groups, based on the relative ranking of values between the pairs.

significance level The probability that an observed relationship could be caused by chance (i.e., because of sampling error); significance at the .05 level indicates the probability that a relationship of the observed magnitude would be found by chance only five times out of 100.

simple random sampling The most basic type of probability sampling, wherein a sampling frame is created by enumerating all members of a population of interest, and then selecting a sample from the sampling frame through completely random procedures.

skewness A quality of a set of scores relating to their asymmetrical distribution around a central point.

snowball sampling The selection of subjects by means of nominations or referrals from earlier subjects.

social desirability response set A bias in self-report instruments created when subjects have a tendency to misrepresent their opinions in the direction of answers consistent with prevailing social norms.

software The instructions for performing operations made to a computer, and the documentation for those instructions.

Solomon four-group design An experimental design that uses a before-after design for one pair of experimental/control groups, and an after-only design for a second pair.

Spearman-Brown prophecy formula An equation for making corrections to a reliability estimate that was calculated by the split-half method.

Spearman's rho A correlation coefficient indicating the magnitude of a relationship between variables measured on the ordinal scale.

split-half technique A method for estimating the internal consistency (reliability) of an instrument by correlating scores on half of the measure with scores on the other half.

standard deviation The most frequently used statistic for measuring the degree of variability in a set of scores.

standard error The standard deviation of a sampling distribution (usually the sampling distribution of means).

standard scores Scores expressed in terms of standard deviations from the mean; raw scores are transformed to scores with a mean of zero and a standard deviation of one; sometimes referred to as z scores.

statistic An estimate of a parameter, calculated from sample data.

statistical inference The process of inferring attributes about the population based on information from a sample.

statistical significance A term indicating that the results obtained in an analysis of sample data are unlikely to have been caused by chance, at some specified level of probability.

statistical test An analytic procedure that allows a researcher to determine the likelihood that obtained results reflect true results, according to the laws of probability.

strata Subdivisions of the population according to some characteristic (e.g., males and females); singular is *stratum*.

stratified random sampling The random selection of subjects from two or more strata of the population independently.

structured data collection An approach to collecting information from subjects, either through self-report or observations, wherein the researcher determines in advance the response categories of interest.

Study Section Within the National Institutes of Health, the Initial Review Group (consisting of peers) that evaluates grant applications.

subject An individual who participates and provides data in a study; subjects are sometimes designated as ss, as "there were 50 ss in the experiment."

subject stipend A monetary payment to individuals participating in a study to serve as an incentive for participation and/or to compensate for time and expenses.

summated rating scale See *Likert scale*.

summative evaluation Research designed to

assess the usefulness or worth of a program or practice after it is already in operation.

survey research A type of nonexperimental research that focusses on obtaining information regarding the status quo of some situation, often via direct questioning of a sample of respondents.

survival analysis A statistical procedure used when the dependent variable represents a time interval between an initial event (e.g., onset of a disease) and an end event (e.g., death).

symmetrical distribution A distribution of values that has two halves that are mirror images of the each other; a distribution that is not skewed.

systematic sampling The selection of subjects such that every *k*th (e.g., every tenth) person (or element) in a sampling frame or list is chosen.

target population The entire population in which the researcher is interested and to which he or she would like to generalize the results of a study.

test statistic A statistic used to test for the statistical significance of relationships between variables; the sampling distributions of test statistics are known for circumstances in which the null hypothesis is true; examples include chi-square, *F*-ratio, *t*, and Person's *r*.

testing A threat to the internal validity of a study that occurs when the administration of a pretest or baseline measure of a dependent variable results in changes on the variable, independent of any treatment.

test-retest reliability Assessment of the stability of an instrument by correlating the scores obtained on repeated administrations.

theoretical notes In field studies, notes about the observer's interpretations of observed activities.

theory An abstract generalization that presents a systematic explanation about the relationships among phenomena.

Thurstone scale A type of attitude scale in which a panel of judges first rates the degree of favorability of a set of statements about some attitudinal object (e.g., abortion), and then subjects identify the statements with which they agree.

time sampling In observational research, the selection of time periods during which observations will take place.

time series design A quasi-experimental design that involves the collection of information over an extended period of time, with multiple data collection points both prior to and after the introduction of a treatment.

time sharing A method of operating mainframe computers such that several different users have access to the computer in a round robin fashion, giving the impression of simultaneous use.

topic guide A list of broad question areas to be covered in a semi-structured interview or focus group interview.

treatment The experimental intervention under study; the condition being manipulated.

treatment group The group receiving the intervention being tested; the experimental group.

trend study A form of longitudinal study in which different samples from a population are studied over time with respect to some phenomenon (e.g., a series of Gallup polls of political preferences).

triangulation The use of multiple methods or perspectives to collect and interpret data about some phenomenon, in order to converge on an accurate representation of reality.

true score A hypothetical score that would be obtained if a measure were infallible; it is the portion of the observed score not due to random error or measurement bias.

t-test A parametric statistical test used for analyzing the difference between two means.

two-tailed test A test of statistical significance in which values at both extremes (tails) of a distribution are considered in determining significance; used when the researcher has not predicted the direction of a relationship (see *nondirectional hypothesis*).

Type I error A decision to reject the null hypothesis when it is true (i.e., the researcher concludes that a relationship exists when in fact it does not).

Type II error A decision to accept the null hypothesis when it is false (i.e., the researcher concludes that *no* relationship exists when in fact it does).

unimodal distribution A distibution of values with one peak (high frequency).

unit of analysis The basic unit or focus of a researcher's analysis; in nursing research, the unit of analysis is typically the individual subject.

univariate descriptive study A study that gathers information on the occurrence, frequency of occurrence, or average value of the variables of interest, one variable at a time, without focusing on interrelationships among variables.

univariate statistics Statistical procedures for analyzing a single variable for purposes of description.

unstructured interview An oral self-report in which the researcher asks respondents questions without preconceived views regarding the specific content or flow of information to be gathered.

unstructured observation The collection of descriptive information through direct observation, whereby the observer is guided by some general research questions but does not follow a pre-specified plan for observing, enumerating, or recording the information.

utilization See *research utilization.*

validity The degree to which an instrument measures what it is intended to measure.

validity coefficient A quantitative index, usually ranging in value from .00 to 1.00, that provides an estimate of how valid an instrument is; usually computed in conjunction with the criterion-related approach to validating an instrument.

variability The degree to which values on a set of scores are widely different or dispersed (e.g., one would expect higher variability of age within a hospital than within a nursing home).

variable A characteristic or attribute of a person or object that varies (i.e., takes on different values) within the population under study (e.g., body temperature, age, heart rate).

variance A measure of variability or dispersion, equal to the square of the standard deviation.

vignette A brief description of an event, person, or situation to which respondents are asked to react.

visual analogue scale A scaling procedure used to measure a variety of clinical symptoms (e.g., pain, fatigue) by having subjects indicate on a straight line the intensity of the attribute being measured.

vulnerable subjects Special groups of people whose rights in research studies need to be protected through additional procedures because of their inability to provide meaningful informed consent or because their circumstances place them at higher-than-average-risk of deleterious effects; examples include young children, the mentally retarded, and unconscious patients.

weighting A correction procedure used to arrive at population values when a disproportional sampling design has been used.

Wilcoxon signed ranks test A nonparametric statistical test for comparing two paired groups, based on the relative ranking of values between the pairs.

Wilk's lambda An index used in discriminant function analysis to indicate the proportion of variance in the dependent variable *un*accounted for by predictors; $(\lambda) = 1 - R^2$.

z score A standard score, expressed in terms of standard deviations from the mean.

Appendix A
Human
Subjects
Protocol*

(1) *Describe the characteristics of the subject population, such as their anticipated number, age ranges, sex, ethnic background, and health status. Identify the criteria for inclusion or exclusion. Explain the rationale for the use of special classes of subjects, such as fetuses, pregnant women, children, institutionalized mentally disabled, prisoners, or others who are likely to be vulnerable.*

1. Characteristics of the population. The sample for the proposed research will consist of approximately 300 women aged 18–22 who first became pregnant before their eighteenth birthday and who subsequently delivered a child. The women were interviewed initially in 1980–1981 as part of an evaluation of a special program for teenage mothers—Project Redirection. At the time of the initial interview, the women were residing in 6 communities: Phoenix, San Antonio, Fresno, Riverside (CA), Harlem and Bedford-Stuyvesant (NY).

    The initial eligibility criteria for the Project Redirection study are indicated below:

- either pregnant or a parent;
- living in a household that met certain poverty guidelines;
- 17 years old or younger; and
- without a high school diploma or GED certificate.

* Grant applications under the Public Health Service (see Chapter 30) must include a section on the protection of human subjects, which must address six specific questions. This appendix contains the actual responses to those six questions for a funded study of parenting among low-income teenage mothers. Such a protocol often serves as the focal point of an evaluation by an Institutional Review Board.

The sample size for the proposed study is based on the teens in the six sites who completed three rounds of interviews thus far:

- Phoenix, AZ   81
- San Antonio, TX   86
- Harlem, NY   38
- Bedford-Stuyvesant, NY   54
- Riverside, CA   32
- Fresno, CA   38

TOTAL   329

This sample size is substantially larger than that used in most studies of teenage parenting and, as noted earlier, has the advantage of not depending on teens in a single site. The sample will also be heterogeneous with respect to ethnicity; of the 329 teens to be followed, the approximate ethnic distribution will be as follows: Blacks—58%; Hispanics—31%; and Whites—11%.

(2) Identify the sources of research material obtained from individually identifiable living human subjects in the form of specimens, records, or data. Indicate whether the material or data will be obtained specifically for research purposes or whether use will be made of existing specimens, records, or data.

2. Sources of Data. Three rounds of interviews have already been completed with the research sample, and information from these earlier interviews will be used in the present study. Additionally, data will be gathered in a fourth round of in-home interviews, to be collected in 1986–1987 if the proposed research is funded. Data will be gathered by a combined interview/observation approach, using a specially constructed interview schedule and several standardized instruments.

(3) Describe plans for the recruitment of subjects and the consent procedures to be followed, including the circumstances under which consent will be sought and obtained,

who will seek it, the nature of the information to be provided to prospective subjects and the method of documenting consent.

3. Recruitment and Consent. Subjects have already been recruited for this study—i.e., they were participants in three earlier rounds of interviewing as part of another research project. For the present study, letters will be mailed to respondents at their most recently known address and they will be asked to verify their current address and telephone number (if available). For respondents for whom there is no return postcard, tracking procedures to ascertain the respondents' present address will be undertaken.

For those respondents who are located through these procedures, an interviewer will contact them and explain the general nature and purpose of the research, the confidential nature of the interviews, the time commitments, and the stipend ($25) that would be paid to them in compensation for their time. The respondents will also be told that their children should be present at the time of the interview, so that appropriate observations can be made. Upon consent to be included in this wave of the research, an interview will be scheduled. At the time of the interview, the interviewers, who will receive extensive training for this project, will repeat the description of the research prior to commencing. The respondent will be told that her participation is voluntary; that no information she gives will be divulged to anyone other than research staff; that her participation will have no effect on any services that she might be receiving; that she can stop the interview at any time; and that she can decline to answer individual questions if she so chooses. This information will be included in a Consent Form, which each respondent will be requested to sign prior to the interview.

(4) Describe any potential risks—physical, psychological, social, legal, or other—and as-

sess their likelihood and seriousness. Where appropriate, describe alternative treatments and procedures that might be advantageous to the subjects.

4. Risks. There is relatively minor risk, in interviewing these young women about their family life, that the interview will be stressful to them. Furthermore, our procedures are designed to minimize any discomfort on the respondents' parts. We will use female interviewers who will be trained not only with respect to the research instrument but also with regard to the stresses of parenthood in disadvantaged populations. In the event of any signs of distress during the interview, interviewers will be instructed to refrain from further questioning, proceeding only if the respondent desires. Our experience in dealing with this sample leads us to believe, however, that the women are more likely to find a conversation with an objective but sympathetic listener therapeutic rather than stressful.

(5) Describe the procedures for protecting against or minimizing any potential risks, including risks to confidentiality, and assess their likely effectiveness. Where appropriate, discuss provisions for insuring necessary medical or professional intervention in the event of adverse effects to the subjects. Also, where appropriate, describe the provisions for monitoring the data collected to insure the safety of subjects.

5. Confidentiality. Measures to protect the confidentiality of the respondents will be instituted throughout the course of this project. Data security procedures to protect the identity of individuals will be implemented during interviewer training, data collection, data analysis, and after completion of the project. Respondents will be fully informed

as to these confidentiality procedures at the outset of the interview.

The issue of confidentiality and data security will be stressed during the training of data collectors. The need for confidentiality and the specific policies and procedures related to this issue will be explained to all interviewers. Thereafter, the interviewers will be required to sign a confidentiality statement prior to conducting interviews.

All identifying information will be removed from the interview schedule upon receipt from the field staff. Names, addresses, telephone numbers and any other identifying information will be recorded *only* on a cover sheet of the interview. The interview form itself, which will be kept in a locked file, will bear only a numeric identification code. The cover sheet will be removed from completed interviews and kept in a separate locked file. Access to this file will be restricted to key project personnel.

(6) Discuss why the risks to subjects are reasonable in relation to the anticipated benefits to subjects and in relation to the importance of the knowledge that may reasonably be expected to result.

6. Anticipated Benefits. In theory, no direct benefits to the respondents are anticipated. However, as mentioned above, we have found that respondents often enjoy the interview experience. Nevertheless, the primary benefit expected from the project is indirect. The study is expected to generate knowledge that will be useful in the formulation of social policy and in the design and delivery of appropriate services for young disadvantaged mothers and their children. Since we believe that the risks to subjects are negligible, we believe that the benefits provide justification for the conduct of this research.

Appendix B
Statistical
Tables

Table B-1. *Distribution of* t *Probability*

	LEVEL OF SIGNIFICANCE FOR ONE-TAILED TEST					
	.10	.05	.025	.01	.005	.0005
			Level of Significance for Two-Tailed Test			
df	.20	.10	.05	.02	.01	.001
1	3·078	6·314	12·706	31·821	63·657	636·619
2	1·886	2·920	4·303	6·965	9·925	31·598
3	1·638	2·353	3·182	4·541	5·841	12·941
4	1·533	2·132	2·776	3·747	4·604	8·610
5	1·476	2·015	2·571	3·365	4·032	6·859
6	1·440	1·943	2·447	3·143	3·707	5·959
7	1·415	1·895	2·365	2·998	3·449	5·405
8	1·397	1·860	2·306	2·896	3·355	5·041
9	1·383	1·833	2·262	2·821	3·250	4·781
10	1·372	1·812	2·228	2·764	3·169	4·587
11	1·363	1·796	2·201	2·718	3·106	4·437
12	1·356	1·782	2·179	2·681	3·055	4·318
13	1·350	1·771	2·160	2·650	3·012	4·221
14	1·345	1·761	2·145	2·624	2·977	4·140
15	1·341	1·753	2·131	2·602	2·947	4·073
16	1·337	1·746	2·120	2·583	2·921	4·015
17	1·333	1·740	2·110	2·567	2·898	3·965
18	1·330	1·734	2·101	2·552	2·878	3·922
19	1·328	1·729	2·093	2·539	2·861	3·883
20	1·325	1·725	2·086	2·528	2·845	3·850
21	1·323	1·721	2·080	2·518	2·831	3·819
22	1·321	1·717	2·074	2·508	2·819	3·792
23	1·319	1·714	2·069	2·500	2·807	3·767
24	1·318	1·711	2·064	2·492	2·797	3·745
25	1·316	1·708	2·060	2·485	2·787	3·725
26	1·315	1·706	2·056	2·479	2·779	3·707
27	1·314	1·703	2·052	2·473	2·771	3·690
28	1·313	1·701	2·048	2·467	2·763	3·674
29	1·311	1·699	2·045	2·462	2·756	3·659
30	1·310	1·697	2·042	2·457	2·750	3·646
40	1·303	1·684	2·021	2·423	2·704	3·551
60	1·296	1·671	2·000	2·390	2·660	3·460
120	1·289	1·658	1·980	2·358	2·617	3·373
∞	1·282	1·645	1·960	2·326	2·576	3·291

Table B-2. *Significant values of* F

α = .05 *(two-tailed)*   α = .025 *(one-tailed)*

$\frac{df_B}{df_w}$	1	2	3	4	5	6	8	12	24	∞
1	161·4	199·5	215·7	224·6	230·2	234·0	238·9	243·9	249·0	254·3
2	18·51	19·00	19·16	19·25	19·30	19·33	19·37	19·41	19·45	19·50
3	10·13	9·55	9·28	9·12	9·01	8·94	8·84	8·74	8·64	8·53
4	7·71	6·94	6·59	6·39	6·26	6·16	6·04	5·91	5·77	5·63
5	6·61	5·79	5·41	5·19	5·05	4·95	4·82	4·68	4·53	4·36
6	5·99	5·14	4·76	4·53	4·39	4·28	4·15	4·00	3·84	3·67
7	5·59	4·74	4·35	4·12	3·97	3·87	3·73	3·57	3·41	3·23
8	5·32	4·46	4·07	3·84	3·69	3·58	3·44	3·28	3·12	2·93
9	5·12	4·26	3·86	3·63	3·48	3·37	3·23	3·07	2·90	2·71
10	4·96	4·10	3·71	3·48	3·33	3·22	3·07	2·91	2·74	2·54
11	4·84	3·98	3·59	3·36	3·20	3·09	2·95	2·79	2·61	2·40
12	4·75	3·88	3·49	3·26	3·11	3·00	2·85	2·69	2·50	2·30
13	4·67	3·80	3·41	3·18	3·02	2·92	2·77	2·60	2·42	2·21
14	4·60	3·74	3·34	3·11	2·96	2·85	2·70	2·53	2·35	2·13
15	4·54	3·68	3·29	3·06	2·90	2·79	2·64	2·48	2·29	2·07
16	4·49	3·63	3·24	3·01	2·85	2·74	2·59	2·42	2·24	2·01
17	4·45	3·59	3·20	2·96	2·81	2·70	2·55	2·38	2·19	1·96
18	4·41	3·55	3·16	2·93	2·77	2·66	2·51	2·34	2·15	1·92
19	4·38	3·52	3·13	2·90	2·74	2·63	2·48	2·31	2·11	1·88
20	4·35	3·49	3·10	2·87	2·71	2·60	2·45	2·28	2·08	1·84
21	4·32	3·47	3·07	2·84	2·68	2·57	2·42	2·25	2·05	1·81
22	4·30	3·44	3·05	2·82	2·66	2·55	2·40	2·23	2·03	1·78
23	4·28	3·42	3·03	2·80	2·64	2·53	2·38	2·20	2·00	1·76
24	4·26	3·40	3·01	2·78	2·62	2·51	2·36	2·18	1·98	1·73
25	4·24	3·38	2·99	2·76	2·60	2·49	2·34	2·16	1·96	1·71
26	4·22	3·37	2·98	2·74	2·59	2·47	2·32	2·15	1·95	1·69
27	4·21	3·35	2·96	2·73	2·57	2·46	2·30	2·13	1·93	1·67
28	4·20	3·34	2·95	2·71	2·56	2·44	2·29	2·12	1·91	1·65
29	4·18	3·33	2·93	2·70	2·54	2·43	2·28	2·10	1·90	1·64
30	4·17	3·32	2·92	2·69	2·53	2·42	2·27	2·09	1·89	1·62
40	4·08	3·23	2·84	2·61	2·45	2·34	2·18	2·00	1·79	1·51
60	4·00	3·15	2·76	2·52	2·37	2·25	2·10	1·92	1·70	1·39
120	3·92	3·07	2·68	2·45	2·29	2·17	2·02	1·83	1·61	1·25
∞	3·84	2·99	2·60	2·37	2·21	2·09	1·94	1·75	1·52	1·00

(continued)

Table B-2. (continued)
Significant values of F
$\alpha = .01$ *(two-tailed)*

$\alpha = .005$ *(one-tailed)*

$\dfrac{df_B}{df_w}$	1	2	3	4	5	6	8	12	24	∞
1	4052	4999	5403	5625	5764	5859	5981	6106	6234	6366
2	98·49	99·00	99·17	99·25	99·30	99·33	99·36	99·42	99·46	99·50
3	34·12	30·81	29·46	28·71	28·24	27·91	27·49	27·05	26·60	26·12
4	21·20	18·00	16·69	15·98	15·52	15·21	14·80	14·37	13·93	13·46
5	16·26	13·27	12·06	11·39	10·97	10·67	10·29	9·89	9·47	9·02
6	13·74	10·92	9·78	9·15	8·75	8·47	8·10	7·72	7·31	6·88
7	12·25	9·55	8·45	7·85	7·46	7·19	6·84	6·47	6·07	5·65
8	11·26	8·65	7·59	7·01	6·63	6·37	6·03	5·67	5·28	4·86
9	10·56	8·02	6·99	6·42	6·06	5·80	5·47	5·11	4·73	4·31
10	10·04	7·56	6·55	5·99	5·64	5·39	5·06	4·71	4·33	3·91
11	9·65	7·20	6·22	5·67	5·32	5·07	4·74	4·40	4·02	3·60
12	9·33	6·93	5·95	5·41	5·06	4·82	4·50	4·16	3·78	3·36
13	9·07	6·70	5·74	5·20	4·86	4·62	4·30	3·96	3·59	3·16
14	8·86	6·51	5·56	5·03	4·69	4·46	4·14	3·80	3·43	3·00
15	8·68	6·36	5·42	4·89	4·56	4·32	4·00	3·67	3·29	2·87
16	8·53	6·23	5·29	4·77	4·44	4·20	3·89	3·55	3·18	2·75
17	8·40	6·11	5·18	4·67	4·34	4·10	3·79	3·45	3·08	2·65
18	8·28	6·01	5·09	4·58	4·25	4·01	3·71	3·37	3·00	2·57
19	8·18	5·93	5·01	4·50	4·17	3·94	3·63	3·30	2·92	2·49
20	8·10	5·85	4·94	4·43	4·10	3·87	3·56	3·23	2·86	2·42
21	8·02	5·78	4·87	4·37	4·04	3·81	3·51	3·17	2·80	2·36
22	7·94	5·72	4·82	4·31	3·99	3·76	3·45	3·12	2·75	2·31
23	7·88	5·66	4·76	4·26	3·94	3·71	3·41	3·07	2·70	2·26
24	7·82	5·61	4·72	4·22	3·90	3·67	3·36	3·03	2·66	2·21
25	7·77	5·57	4·68	4·18	3·86	3·63	3·32	2·99	2·62	2·17
26	7·72	5·53	4·64	4·14	3·82	3·59	3·29	2·96	2·58	2·13
27	7·68	5·49	4·60	4·11	3·78	3·56	3·26	2·93	2·55	2·10
28	7·64	5·45	4·57	4·07	3·75	3·53	3·23	2·90	2·52	2·06
29	7·60	5·42	4·54	4·04	3·73	3·50	3·20	2·87	2·49	2·03
30	7·56	5·39	4·51	4·02	3·70	3·47	3·17	2·84	2·47	2·01
40	7·31	5·18	4·31	3·83	3·51	3·29	2·99	2·66	2·29	1·80
60	7·08	4·98	4·13	3·65	3·34	3·12	2·82	2·50	2·12	1·60
120	6·85	4·79	3·95	3·48	3·17	2·96	2·66	2·34	1·95	1·38
∞	6·64	4·60	3·78	3·32	3·02	2·80	2·51	2·18	1·79	1·00

Table B-2. (continued)
Significant values of F
α = .001 (two-tailed)   *α = .0005 (one-tailed)*

$\frac{df_B}{df_w}$	1	2	3	4	5	6	8	12	24	∞
1	405284	500000	540379	562500	576405	585937	598144	610667	623497	636619
2	998·5	999·0	999·2	999·2	999·3	999·3	999·4	999·4	999·5	999·5
3	167·5	148·5	141·1	137·1	134·6	132·8	130·6	128·3	125·9	123·5
4	74·14	61·25	56·18	53·44	51·71	50·53	49·00	47·41	45·77	44·05
5	47·04	36·61	33·20	31·09	29·75	28·84	27·64	26·42	25·14	23·78
6	35·51	27·00	23·70	21·90	20·81	20·03	19·03	17·99	16·89	15·75
7	29·22	21·69	18·77	17·19	16·21	15·52	14·63	13·71	12·73	11·69
8	25·42	18·49	15·83	14·39	13·49	12·86	12·04	11·19	10·30	9·34
9	22·86	16·39	13·90	12·56	11·71	11·13	10·37	9·57	8·72	7·81
10	21·04	14·91	12·55	11·28	10·48	9·92	9·20	8·45	7·64	6·76
11	19·69	13·81	11·56	10·35	9·58	9·05	8·35	7·63	6·85	6·00
12	18·64	12·97	10·80	9·63	8·89	8·38	7·71	7·00	6·25	5·42
13	17·81	12·31	10·21	9·07	8·35	7·86	7·21	6·52	5·78	4·97
14	17·14	11·78	9·73	8·62	7·92	7·43	6·80	6·13	5·41	4·60
15	16·59	11·34	9·34	8·25	7·57	7·09	6·47	5·81	5·10	4·31
16	16·12	10·97	9·00	7·94	7·27	6·81	6·19	5·55	4·85	4·06
17	15·72	10·66	8·73	7·68	7·02	6·56	5·96	5·32	4·63	3·85
18	15·38	10·39	8·49	7·46	6·81	6·35	5·76	5·13	4·45	3·67
19	15·08	10·16	8·28	7·26	6·61	6·18	5·59	4·97	4·29	3·52
20	14·82	9·95	8·10	7·10	6·46	6·02	5·44	4·82	4·15	3·38
21	14·59	9·77	7·94	6·95	6·32	5·88	5·31	4·70	4·03	3·26
22	14·38	9·61	7·80	6·81	6·19	5·76	5·19	4·58	3·92	3·15
23	14·19	9·47	7·67	6·69	6·08	5·65	5·09	4·48	3·82	3·05
24	14·03	9·34	7·55	6·59	5·98	5·55	4·99	4·39	3·74	2·97
25	13·88	9·22	7·45	6·49	5·88	5·46	4·91	4·31	3·66	2·89
26	13·74	9·12	7·36	6·41	5·80	5·38	4·83	4·24	3·59	2·82
27	13·61	9·02	7·27	6·33	5·73	5·31	4·76	4·17	3·52	2·75
28	13·50	8·93	7·19	6·25	5·66	5·24	4·69	4·11	3·46	2·70
29	13·39	8·85	7·12	6·19	5·59	5·18	4·64	4·05	3·41	2·64
30	13·29	8·77	7·05	6·12	5·53	5·12	4·58	4·00	3·36	2·59
40	12·61	8·25	6·60	5·70	5·13	4·73	4·21	3·64	3·01	2·23
60	11·97	7·76	6·17	5·31	4·76	4·37	3·87	3·31	2·69	1·90
120	11·38	7·31	5·79	4·95	4·42	4·04	3·55	3·02	2·40	1·56
∞	10·83	6·91	5·42	4·62	4·10	3·74	3·27	2·74	2·13	1·00

Table B-3. *Distribution of χ^2 probability*

df	LEVEL OF SIGNIFICANCE				
	.10	.05	.02	.01	.001
1	2·71	3·84	5·41	6·63	10·83
2	4·61	5·99	7·82	9·21	13·82
3	6·25	7·82	9·84	11·34	16·27
4	7·78	9·49	11·67	13·28	18·46
5	9·24	11·07	13·39	15·09	20·52
6	10·64	12·59	15·03	16·81	22·46
7	12·02	14·07	16·62	18·48	24·32
8	13·36	15·51	18·17	20·09	26·12
9	14·68	16·92	19·68	21·67	27·88
10	15·99	18·31	21·16	23·21	29·59
11	17·28	19·68	22·62	24·72	31·26
12	18·55	21·03	24·05	26·22	32·91
13	19·81	22·36	25·47	27·69	34·53
14	21·06	23·68	26·87	29·14	36·12
15	22·31	25·00	28·26	30·58	37·70
16	23·54	26·30	29·63	32·00	39·25
17	24·77	27·59	31·00	33·41	40·79
18	25·99	28·87	32·35	34·81	42·31
19	27·20	30·14	33·69	36·19	43·82
20	28·41	31·41	35·02	37·57	45·32
21	29·62	32·67	36·34	38·93	46·80
22	30·81	33·92	37·66	40·29	48·27
23	32·01	35·17	38·97	41·64	49·73
24	33·20	36·42	40·27	42·98	51·18
25	34·38	37·65	41·57	44·31	52·62
26	35·56	38·89	42·86	45·64	54·05
27	36·74	40·11	44·14	46·96	55·48
28	37·92	41·34	45·42	48·28	56·89
29	39·09	42·56	46·69	49·59	58·30
30	40·26	43·77	47·96	50·89	59·70

Table B-4. *Significant values of the correlation coefficient*

df	LEVEL OF SIGNIFICANCE FOR ONE-TAILED TEST				
	.05	.025	.01	.005	.0005
	Level of Significance for Two-Tailed Test				
	.1	.05	.02	.01	.001
1	·98769	·99692	·999507	·999877	·9999988
2	·90000	·95000	·98000	·990000	·99900
3	·8054	·8783	·93433	·95873	·99116
4	·7293	·8114	·8822	·91720	·97406
5	·6694	·7545	·8329	·8745	·95074
6	·6215	·7067	·7887	·8343	·92493
7	·5822	·6664	·7498	·7977	·8982
8	·5494	·6319	·7155	·7646	·8721
9	·5214	·6021	·6851	·7348	·8471
10	·4973	·5760	·6581	·7079	·8233
11	·4762	·5529	·6339	·6835	·8010
12	·4575	·5324	·6120	·6614	·7800
13	·4409	·5139	·5923	·6411	·7603
14	·4259	·4973	·5742	·6226	·7420
15	·4124	·4821	·5577	·6055	·7246
16	·4000	·4683	·5425	·5897	·7084
17	·3887	·4555	·5285	·5751	·6932
18	·3783	·4438	·5155	·5614	·6787
19	·3687	·4329	·5034	·5487	·6652
20	·3598	·4227	·4921	·5368	·6524
25	·3233	·3809	·4451	·4869	·5974
30	·2960	·3494	·4093	·4487	·5541
35	·2746	·3246	·3810	·4182	·5189
40	·2573	·3044	·3578	·3932	·4896
45	·2428	·2875	·3384	·3721	·4648
50	·2306	·2732	·3218	·3541	·4433
60	·2108	·2500	·2948	·3248	·4078
70	·1954	·2319	·2737	·3017	·3799
80	·1829	·2172	·2565	·2830	·3568
90	·1726	·2050	·2422	·2673	·3375
100	·1638	·1946	·2301	·2540	·3211

Index

Page numbers followed by t designate tabular material; numbers in italics *designate figures; numbers in* **boldface** *designate definitions of indexed topics.*

≡ NAME INDEX